GW00670001

17 - 11 - 86

ELECTRODIAGNOSIS

JENNIFER CHU-ANDREWS, M.D.

Assistant Professor and Director
Electrodiagnostic Unit
Department of Physical Medicine and Rehabilitation
University of Pennsylvania
Philadelphia, Pennsylvania

ROBERT J. JOHNSON, M.D.

Professor Emeritus
Departments of Anatomy and Surgery
School of Medicine, and
Former Chairman, Department of Anatomy
Graduate School of Medicine
University of Pennsylvania
Philadelphia, Pennsylvania

With contributions from

FRANCIS L. BRUYNINCKX, M.D.

Staff Physician
Department of Physical Medicine and Rehabilitation, and Active Staff Member
Department of Biomedical Research
Faculty of Medicine
University of Leuven
Leuven, Belgium

RAI-CHI CHAN, M.D.

Clinical Associate Professor
Department of Physical Medicine and Rehabilitation
National Yang-Ming Medical College, and
Section Chief of Neurorehabilitation
Department of Physical Medicine and Rehabilitation
Veterans General Hospital
Taipei, Taiwan, Republic of China

ELECTRODIAGNOSIS

An Anatomical and Clinical Approach

J. B. LIPPINCOTT COMPANY

Philadelphia
London Mexico City New York St. Louis
São Paulo Sydney

Sponsoring Editor: Sanford J. Robinson
Manuscript Editor: Lee Henderson
Indexer: Ann Cassar
Design Director: Tracy Baldwin
Designer: Arlene Putterman
Production Supervisor: J. Corey Gray
Production Assistant: Kathleen R. Diamond
Compositor: Ruttle, Shaw & Wetherill, Inc.
Printer/Binder: Halliday Lithograph

 Printed in the United States of America. For information write J. B. Lippincott Company, East Washington Square, Philadelphia, Pennsylvania 19105.

6 5 4 3 2 1

Library of Congress Cataloging-in-Publication Data

Chu-Andrews, Jennifer.
Electrodiagnosis: an anatomical and clinical approach.

Includes bibliographies and index.
1. Neuromuscular diseases—Diagnosis. 2. Electrodiagnosis. 3. Electromyography. I. Johnson, Robert J. (Robert Joseph), DATE. II. Title. [DNLM: 1. Anatomy. 2. Electrodiagnosis. WB 141 C5587e]
RC925.7.C48 1986 616.7'4'07547 85-19884
ISBN 0-397-50687-2

To Waverly, Justin, and Jasmine Stanford Andrews
and Dorothy E. Johnson

Whatever you can do, or dream you can, begin it;
boldness has genius, power, and magic in it.

Goethe

FOREWORDS

What does the physician in training need to know in order to start practicing electrodiagnostic medicine? There is a need to learn various electromyographic (EMG) and nerve conduction techniques. There is a need to know where the EMG needle (the "pin" or, as I call it, the "intramuscular electrode") must be placed in order to evaluate the electrical activity of muscles supplied by different nerve roots and peripheral nerves. The physician must recognize the different electrodiagnostic abnormalities seen in various clinical conditions. And, finally, he should have studied exemplary cases and the EMG approach to them, as well as being familiar with current EMG terminology.

On the other hand, the experienced electromyographer has different requirements of a text. He needs a convenient reference to demonstrate where an electrode should be placed in order to evaluate rarely studied muscles, as well as a convenient listing of the nerve roots and peripheral nerves supplying those muscles. He also needs information about new techniques that were not readily available at the time of his training. Examples of these techniques are quantitative motor unit analysis, single-fiber EMG, and macro EMG. He also needs a reference source of the most recent standardized EMG terminology.

It is rare that a text can appeal to the novice as well as the experienced clinician. However, Drs. Chu-Andrews and Johnson have succeeded marvelously in producing such a book. It contains those elements needed by the beginner, as well as information that will be valuable to the experienced electromyographer. Nowhere have I seen a better rendering of the topographical anatomy and specific photographic documentation of sites of EMG pin placement. The beginner will appreciate the photographic topographical and dissection illustrations of the frequently evaluated muscles, and the experienced electromyographer will value the photographs of less commonly studied muscles; they are all here in one book. As a bonus, the authors have gone beyond any current EMG anatomy text and tell the electromyographer the exact instructions to give the patient to produce minimal or maximal contraction of a muscle—and even how to relax the muscle!

For several years I have known of Dr. Chu-Andrews' interest in producing a book of this type and have encouraged her to do so. Initially, she was aware of the need for a more comprehensive photographic rendering of the anatomical sites required for pin placement. The book expanded from this to be the comprehensive volume it currently is.

Dr. Chu-Andrews is a fine clinical electromyographer who completed her sabbatical time with Dr. Erik Stålberg in the Department of Clinical Neurophysiology, University Hospital, Uppsala, Sweden. She is currently on the faculty at the University of Pennsylvania, where she is a stimulating and active member of the residency training program.

I have taught the course entitled "Electromyography and Clinical Neurophysiology" at the University of Washington for more than 15 years and look forward to the publication of this volume; it will be an asset to our students and residents. I recommend it to the beginner as well as to the experienced electromyographer as a very useful reference text.

George H. Kraft, M.D.
Professor
Department of Physical Medicine and Rehabilitation
University of Washington
Seattle, Washington

In recent years a number of excellent books on electrodiagnosis covering both electromyography (EMG) and nerve conduction studies have been published. Is there really a need for another? Certainly, but only if it contains new material or covers an area in which information has previously been insufficient in quality or quantity. These are the reasons making this book worthwhile; it contains aspects not discussed in most EMG books, aspects that are of importance for today's electromyographer.

The first part of the book reviews anatomy for the electromyographer. Dr. Chu-Andrews, an experienced electromyographer from the Department of Physical Medicine and Rehabilitation at the University of Pennsylvania, has written this review in consultation with Dr. Johnson, Professor Emeritus of Anatomy and Surgery at the University of Pennsylvania. In daily electrodiagnostic routine, surface or needle electrodes are placed to record activity from a particular muscle or nerve. The investigator aims for a very specific location for the electrode and makes his interpretation from the assumption that he has studied the intended structure. Herein is one of the first problems in achieving a good study. If one does not know the innervation and gross anatomy of the muscle or its exact function (*i.e.*, body positions in which it is relaxed and activated) or about nerve anatomy, then the general quality of the investigation is likely to be poor and the interpretations erroneous. There are a number of good books available on this topic, ranging from the schematic to photographic atlases, which are often consulted before an electrophysiologic study. This book specifically addresses the needs of the electromyographer and reflects Dr. Chu-Andrews' understanding of common problems when one is performing electrodiagnostic tests. It has excellent photographs of muscles, both from dissections and from patients. Dr. Johnson's superb dissections have helped to make this part of the book unique and invaluable. Dr. Chu-Andrews has given lucid instructions on how to insert the "pin," a term that she prefers to "electrode." There is also clearly organized information about innervation levels (spinal cord segment, plexus, peripheral nerve) and function. The instructions to the patient as to how to relax or to give slight or strong activation are more detailed than given in most EMG books. This is of great help, particularly during one's training in clinical neurophysiology. This part alone would probably have been sufficient for a publication, but Dr. Chu-Andrews wished to add material to make a more complete book for the electromyographer.

The second part, which Dr. Chu-Andrews has principally authored together with contributions from Dr. Johnson and additional co-authors, concerns clinical electrodiagnosis. The reader is referred to other books for basic neurophysiology. She considers an electrophysiological procedure an extension of the clinical examination and feels that it should thus be considered a consultation. It is intended not only for confirming clinical findings but also for explaining the pathophysiological mechanisms underlying the patient's symptoms, clinically evident or not, as well as for quantifying abnormality. A number of valuable introductory comments are given here in a personal style. Succeeding chapters cover the various clinical situations seen in an EMG laboratory. The spectrum of diagnostic problems occurring in an EMG laboratory is covered to such an extent that this book could be used as a standard reference for the electromyographer. The importance of quantitative data in electrophysiology is repeatedly stressed in the book. As a result of Dr. Chu-Andrews' interest and ambition, the book contains an impressive amount of original normative data on motor unit parameters recorded with monopolar needle electrodes, previously not available in such extensive form. Nerve conduction parameters are also listed in detail.

Electrophysiology is a dynamic field. The development of new data and concepts emphasize the need for quality volumes such as this one. This book fulfills its aim to help improve the quality of clinical electrodiagnosis by giving detailed guidelines in pertinent anatomy, in principles of performing EMG and nerve conduction studies, and in analysis of the signals. Dr. Chu-Andrews, together with Dr. Johnson and their co-authors, have made an important contribution. Dr. Chu-Andrews' enthusiasm for the field, her capacity to compile information from many sources, and her concern for patients have made her great undertaking in the writing of this book successful. We are grateful to her and her co-authors for investing their time and effort to collect this information and share it with us.

Erik Stålberg, M.D.
Associate Professor and Chief
Neuromuscular Unit
Department of Clinical Neurophysiology
University of Uppsala
Uppsala, Sweden

PREFACE

The decision to write *Electrodiagnosis: An Anatomical and Clinical Approach* came after several years of teaching the practical aspects of electrodiagnosis. The electrodiagnostician must be well versed in anatomy and peripheral neurology, as well as in the theory of electrodiagnosis. The emphasis in this book is thus on the clinical anatomy that is the foundation of electrodiagnosis. More than 5 years have usually elapsed between the time that most physicians studied anatomy in medical school and the time that this knowledge must be applied in a clinical setting. Moreover, the classroom knowledge gained from dissection is not easily transferred to the clinical situation. Anatomy courses are not in general geared toward teaching the surface anatomy that an electrodiagnostician must know. Many training programs focus on the electrodiagnostic information rather than on anatomy. However, a thorough knowledge of anatomy is essential to the electrodiagnostician. Consequently, an effective method to teach applied anatomy in a way that is relevant for the electrodiagnostician is needed. *Electrodiagnosis* was written to address that need.

Electrodiagnosis is divided into two parts, one part on anatomy and one part on clinical electrodiagnosis. The anatomy portion of the book, Chapters 1 and 2, will enable the clinician to locate individual muscles and isolate the action of each muscle. This is the information that is, unfortunately, missing from the education of many electrodiagnosticians. Chapter 1 includes a number of photographs of cadaver dissections, and diagrams of muscle origins and insertions, dermatomes, and peripheral nerves can be found in the appendix.

Chapter 2, on clinical anatomy, describes the muscles individually both as to location and as to action so that the examiner can locate each muscle and can effect relaxation of that muscle or initiate minimal or maximal contraction. Photographs of the surface anatomy accompany the text. At the beginning of the textual description of each muscle, the figure numbers of the relevant cadaver dissection photographs are included. Some muscles of the body have intentionally been omitted from this section either because they are not clinically useful to the electrodiagnostician at present or because the methods of recording from them entail unjustifiable hazards. To include methods whose risks outweigh the possible benefits of the data gained could lead the inexperienced electrodiagnostician astray. In certain situations, such as examination of the extraocular muscles, it is advisable that only the ophthalmologist insert the electrode.

The second part of the book is on clinical electrodiagnosis. This section is written in synopsis form, and each of the sections is accompanied by numerous references. This part of the book is not intended to supplant the basic texts on this subject. I have not included any of the basic science, such as neurophysiology, underlying electromyography (EMG). Rather, it is my hope that this part of the text will serve as a useful reference for the busy clinician.

The section of the book on clinical electrodiagnosis consists of Chapters 3 through 7. Chapter 3 deals with the principles of electrodiagnosis. It includes a section on the principles of nerve conduction studies and a section each on the principles of EMG examination at rest, on minimal contraction, and on maximal contraction. I have included in the portions on EMG examination on minimal and maximal contraction a description of quantitative EMG, one of the newer techniques of EMG, because of my own research interests.

Chapter 4 covers the electrodiagnostic features of commonly encountered clinical situations. These include diseases of the anterior horn cells, roots, plexi, peripheral nerves, neuromuscular junctions, and muscles.

Chapter 5 covers nerve conduction studies of the individual peripheral nerves. Also included in this section is the applied anatomy of the peripheral nerves. Electrodiagnostic features of peripheral nerve injuries and common entrapment syndromes are described. Chapter 6 covers the H reflex and F wave. Chapter 7 is on the newer techniques of electrodiagnosis such as single-fiber EMG and macro EMG. An appendix consisting of the "Glossary of Terms Used in Clinical Electromyography" from the American Association of Electromyography and Electrodiagnosis is included. Also included in the appendix are some suggestions for compiling the electrodiagnostic report and a number of useful anatomical diagrams.

In the course of writing *Electrodiagnosis* I have learned a tremendous amount about anatomy, as well as about electrodiagnosis itself. It is my hope that others will benefit from this book as well. I will have achieved my goal for writing this book if the reader can confidently and comfortably transfer the principles from it to the clinical situation.

Jennifer Chu-Andrews, M.D.

ACKNOWLEDGMENTS

The preparation of this book has involved many long and difficult hours of dedicated work. As a working mother, I made many personal sacrifices because there was no other way to complete the book. However, a project of this magnitude cannot be carried out alone. The number of people who contributed to it with their time, advice, skills, or support are almost too numerous to mention.

I would like to express my sincere gratitude to Robert J. Johnson, M.D., for his help in the book's development. His meticulous dissections and his contributions to the anatomical text in Chapter 5 have made this book an exceptional reference in anatomy for electrodiagnosticians. Dr. Johnson's dedication to excellence is seen in the superb attention given to detail in his dissections. Many of the dissections were done late at night because during the preparation of the book, he also carried out his full academic and administrative duties as Professor in Anatomy at the School of Medicine of the University of Pennsylvania. I am highly honored to have him as my co-author.

My heartfelt gratitude is due to George Kraft, M.D., for his expert advice on the preparation of this volume.

I owe a special debt to Erik Stålberg, M.D., who has given me motivation, inspiration, and encouragement throughout my career. I would also like to thank him for his superb editing. I attribute my knowledge in the newer techniques in electromyography (EMG), such as automatic analysis of EMG signals, single-fiber EMG, and macro EMG, entirely to Dr. Stålberg. The warmth and hospitality of his superb staff and gracious family made my stay in Uppsala, Sweden, a very rewarding, pleasant, and memorable one.

I thank the American Association of Electromyography and Electrodiagnosis for giving me permission to reproduce its "Glossary of Terms Used in Clinical Electromyography."

My eternal gratitude is owed to William J. Erdman, M.D., Chairman of the Department of Physical Medicine and Rehabilitation at the University of Pennsylvania, for his faith in me. His support has enabled me to develop and grow as a competent electrodiagnostician. I deeply appreciate his generosity in bestowing on me a sizable grant for the preparation of this book.

Eleanor Bendler, M.D., is gratefully acknowledged for her teaching in electromyography and muscle function.

I appreciate the help and understanding given to me by Emery K. Stoner, M.D., Chief, and Duncan Van Dusen, Business Administrator, of the Department of Physical Medicine and Rehabilitation.

My deep gratitude goes to Francis L. Bruyninckx, M.D., for his invaluable help in the collection and analysis of the normal data, in my laboratory, for quantitation of motor unit potentials and nerve conduction studies.

I would like to thank Rai-Chi Chan, M.D., for his willingness to participate in the project on MUP analysis. Alan Welner, M.D., Robert Harmon, M.D., Barry Stein, M.D., and Martin Kiel, M.D., provided helpful technical assistance.

Special acknowledgement is due to Celia Witten, M.D., Ph.D., for her dedicated and careful review of the entire manuscript. I was born and educated in Burma, and English is my second language. Dr. Witten's suggestions contributed immeasurably to the technical and organizational, as well as the linguistic, aspects of this book.

The Biomedical Communications Department of the University of Pennsylvania School of Medicine did superb work in photography for this book. To Art Siegel (director), Jordan Denner, especially, and Paul Barrow (chief photographers), Greg McDonald (photographer), and Karen Ott (artist) I owe special thanks both for their high-quality work and for their flexibility in coordinating their schedules with mine.

I am grateful to Randolph Meadows for his help in modeling for the book. His well-toned, well-defined muscles were so well suited to the purposes of this book that I had him model for almost the entire volume. The help given by Ernest Williams, John Lindsay, and Raquel Ferrer is also appreciated.

My dedicated secretary, Patricia Doring, received all assignments graciously and participated in the production of the book while carrying out her routine secretarial duties.

For their continued faith, trust, and confidence in my work, I acknowledge all of the physicians who have referred their patients to me.

On the family scene I am eternally indebted to my father, C. A. Chu, M.D., for instilling in me his hope and encouragement at an early age, and for making me believe that if you try hard enough, "only the sky is the limit." My long-departed mother, Jane Shek, is remembered with this volume.

My uncle, P. H. Shek of Hong Kong, the family patriarch, provided me with financial assistance when I emigrated to the United States in 1973.

My parents-in-law, Charles and Mary Andrews, showed extraordinary understanding and contributed materially to this book with their willingness to make frequent trips between their home in Pittsburgh and ours in Philadelphia so that they could help out with my toddler son and infant daughter.

I could not have completed this book without the patience (many times impatience), understanding, and support of my husband, Waverly S. Andrews, M.D. We finally made it through after all.

I would like to thank my loyal and loving babysitter, Dora, for her devoted care of Justin and Jasmine.

And last, I would like to thank J. B. Lippincott Company for the generous grant they gave me to start this project. The medical division staff has helped in every step of development of the book. I have truly enjoyed working with J. Stuart Freeman (Editor-in-Chief), Micaela Palumbo (then Editor), Sanford Robinson (Developmental Editor), Lee Henderson (Manuscript Editor), and Tracy Baldwin (Design Director). Micaela Palumbo deserves special credit for her strong belief in the viability of this project. Her conviction helped put this book into existence.

Jennifer Chu-Andrews, M.D.

CONTENTS

Part One
ANATOMY

1
Applied Anatomy

Robert J. Johnson
Jennifer Chu-Andrews

DISSECTIONS OF THE FACE

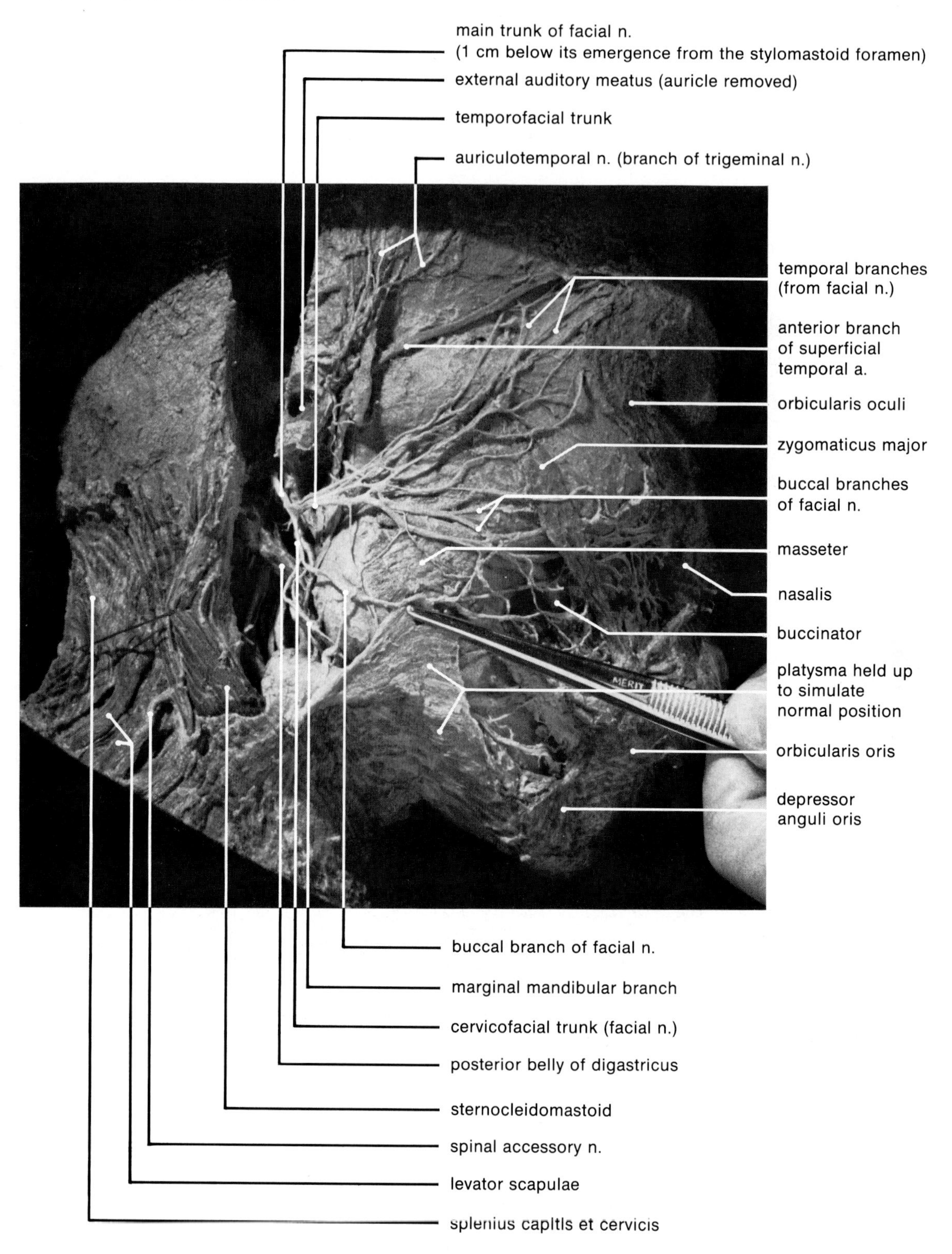

FIGURE 1-1 Face—lateral view, showing the distribution of the facial nerve.

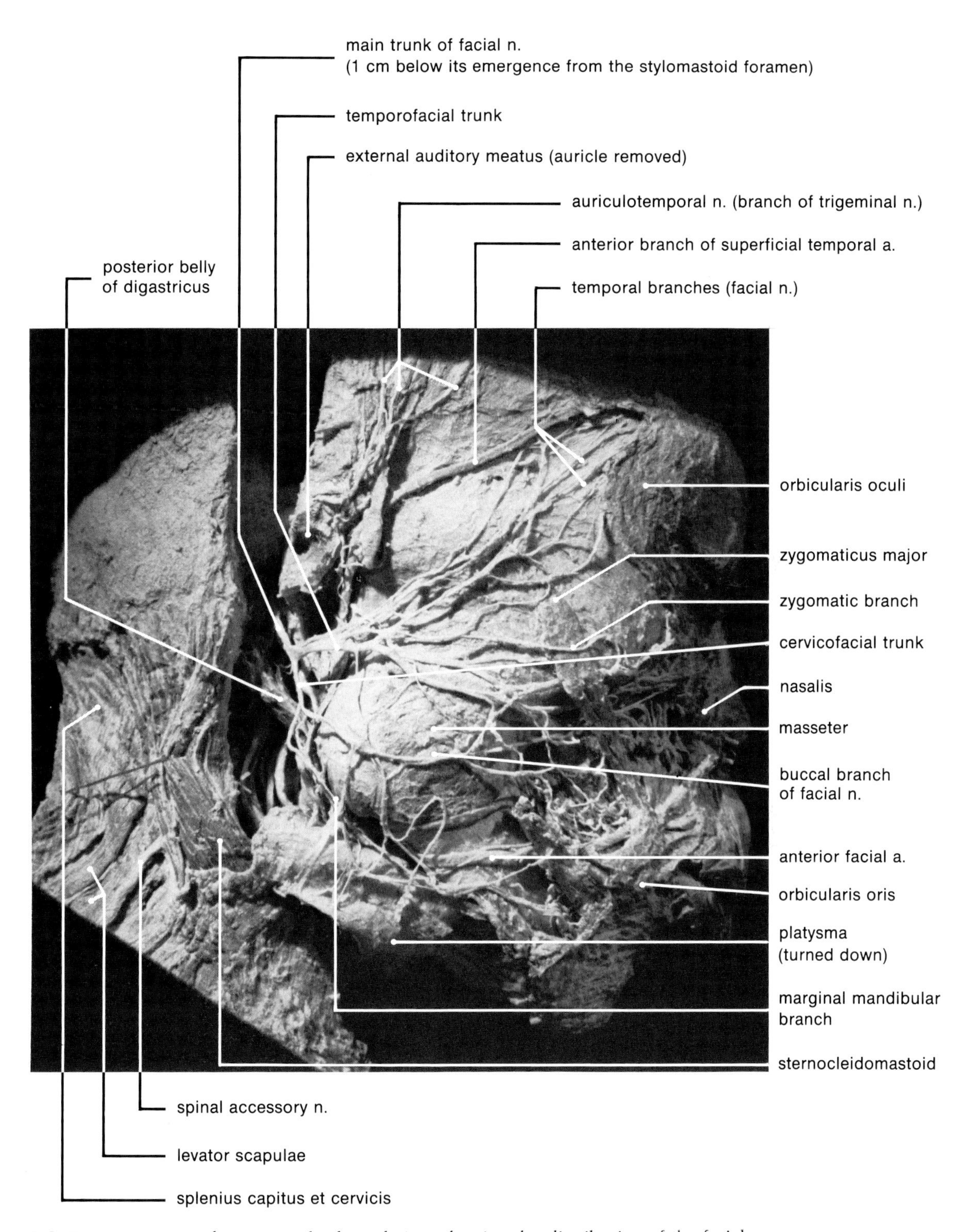

FIGURE 1-2 Face and upper neck—lateral view, showing the distribution of the facial nerve.

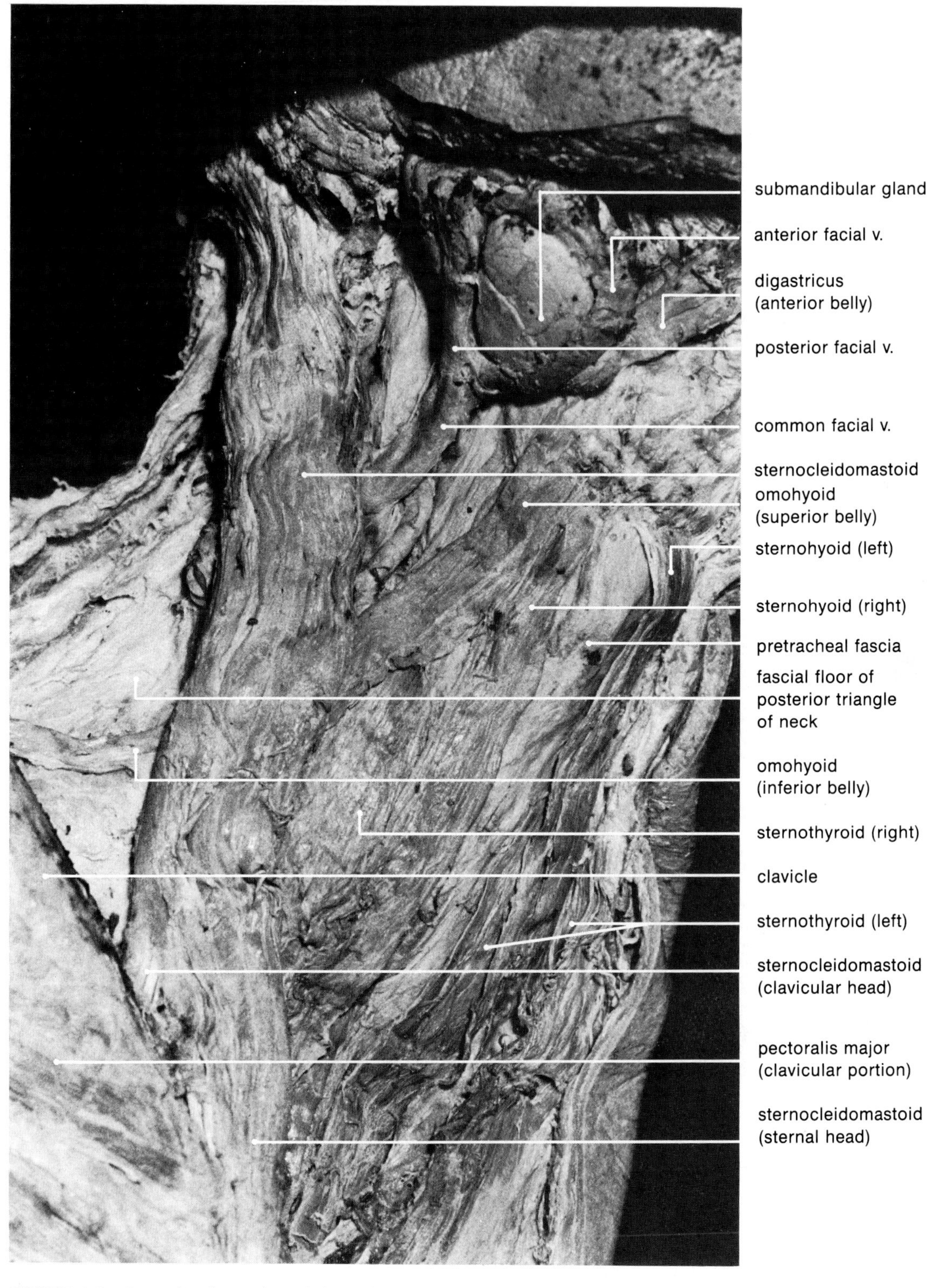

FIGURE 1-3 Superficial muscles of the right side of the neck—anterior view.

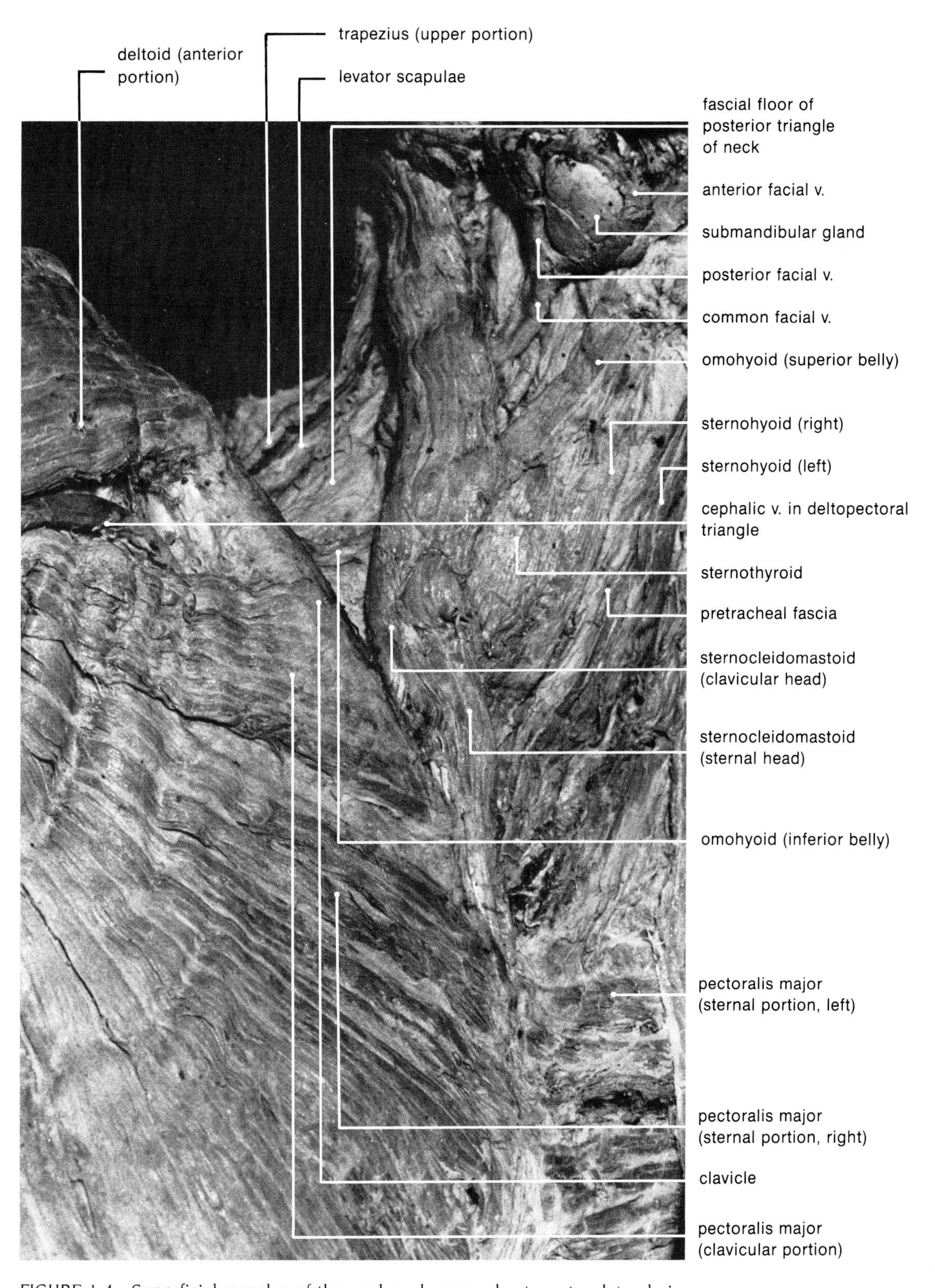

FIGURE 1-4 Superficial muscles of the neck and upper chest—anterolateral view.

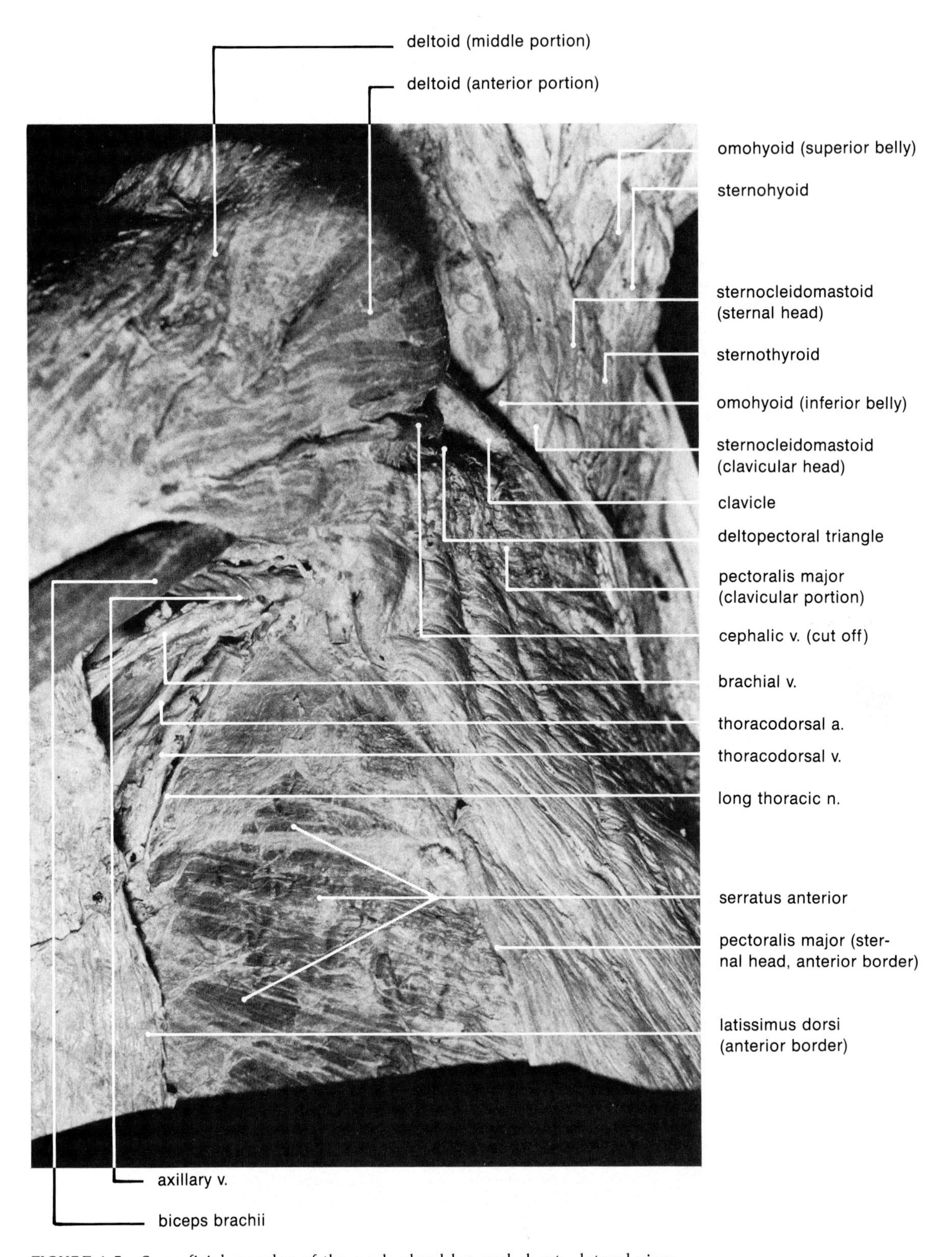

FIGURE 1-5 Superficial muscles of the neck, shoulder, and chest—lateral view.

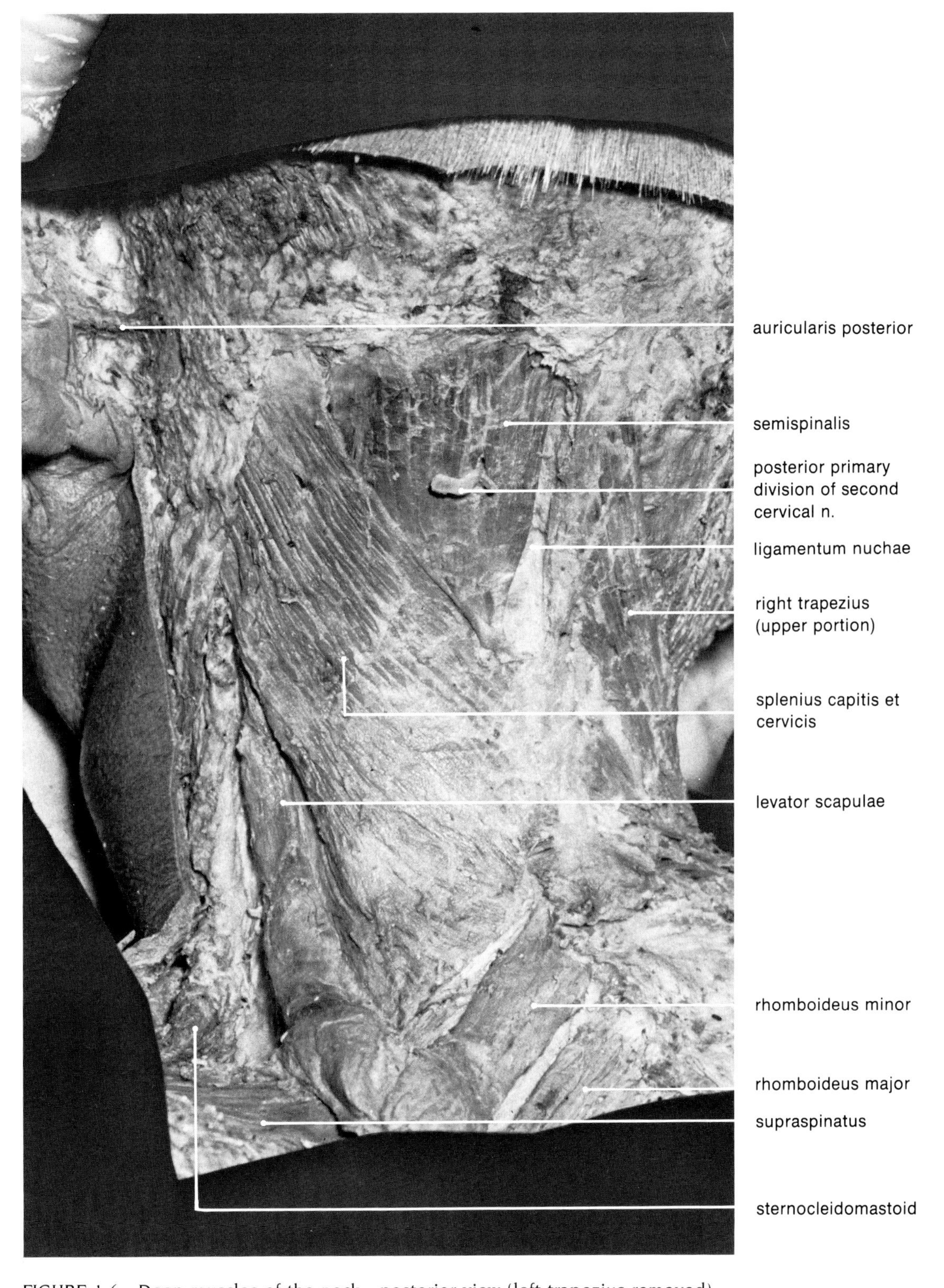

FIGURE 1-6 Deep muscles of the neck—posterior view (left trapezius removed).

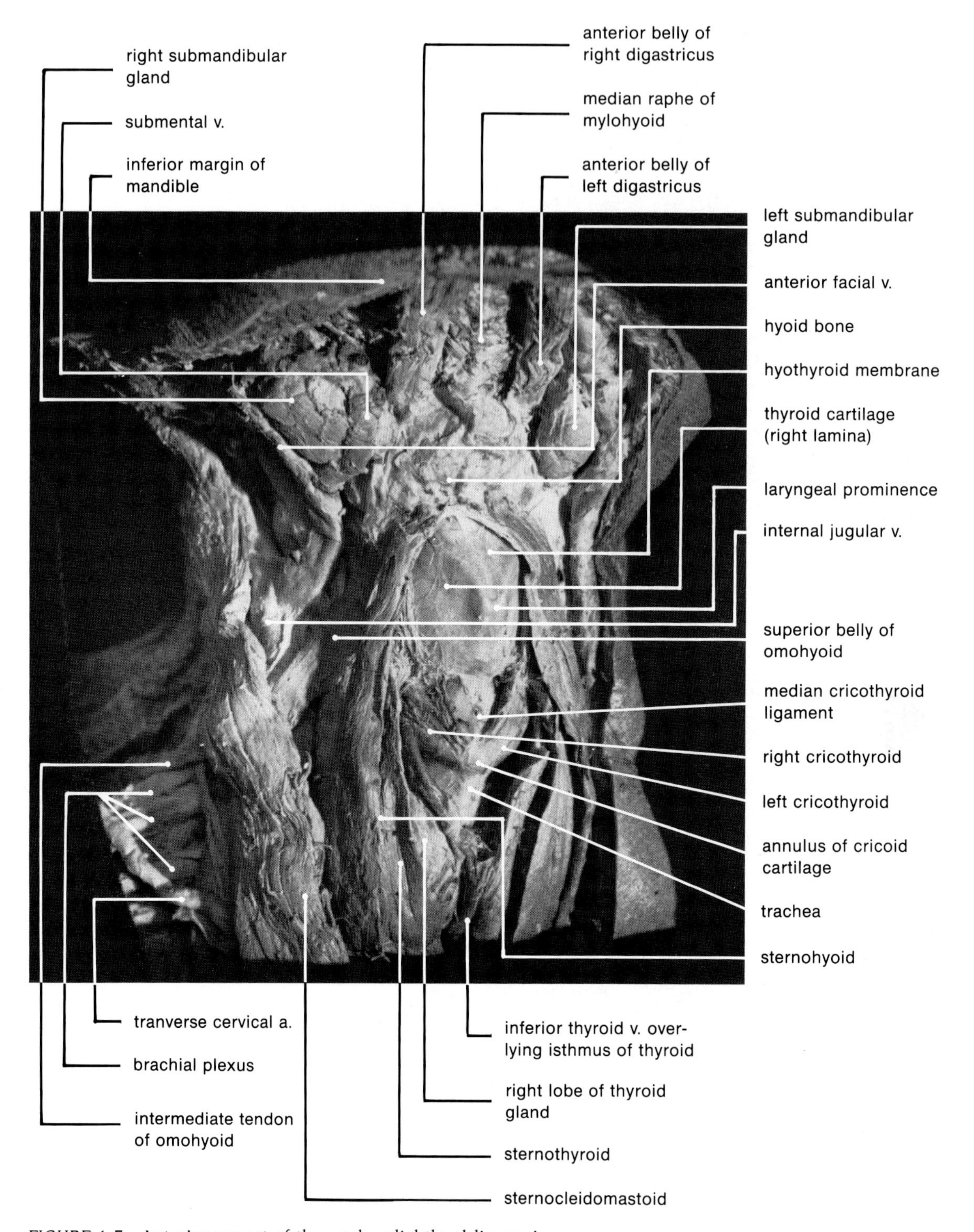

FIGURE 1-7 Anterior aspect of the neck—slightly oblique view.

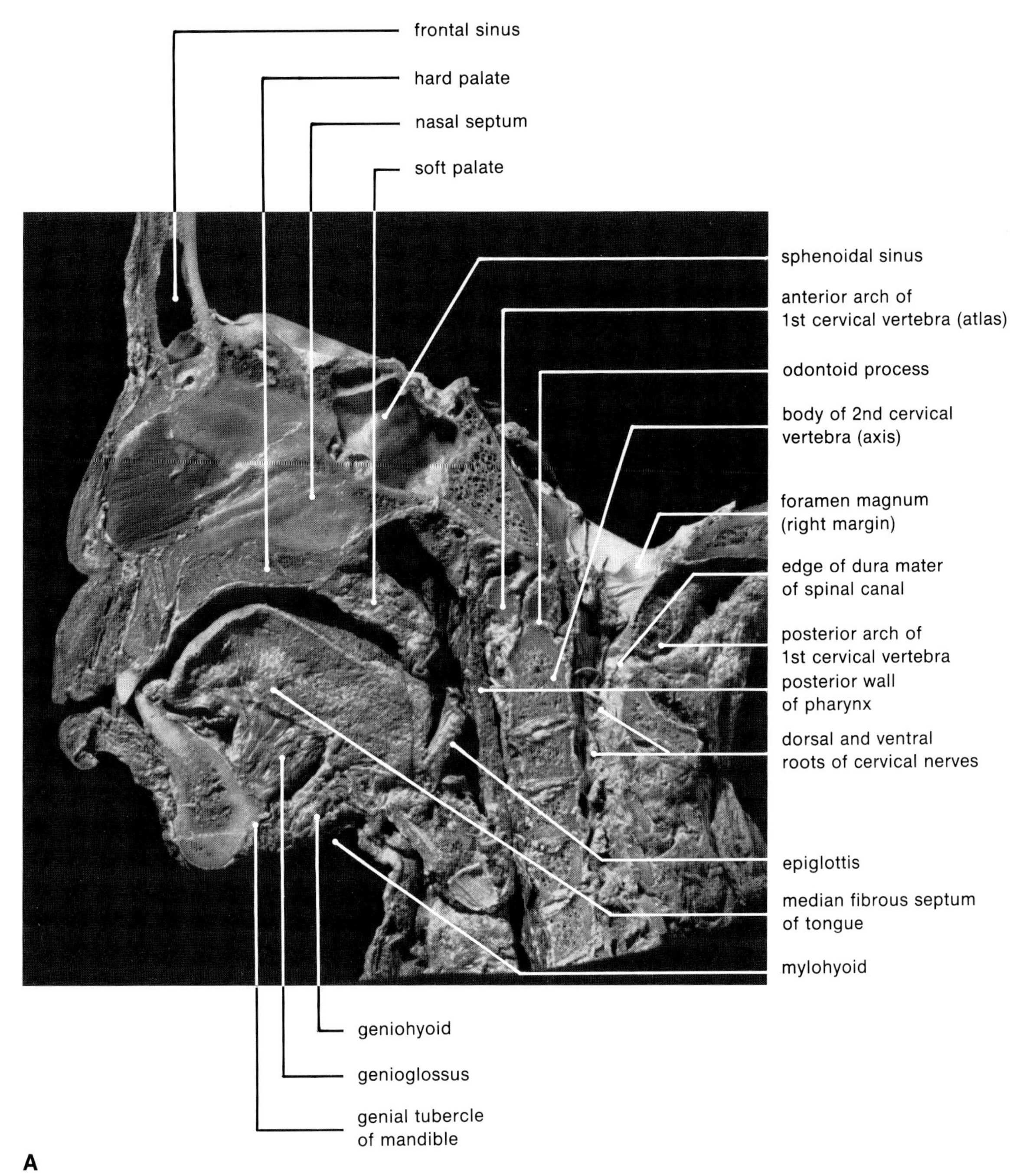

FIGURE 1-8 (A and B) Midsagittal sections of the head. (*Figure continues on next page.*)

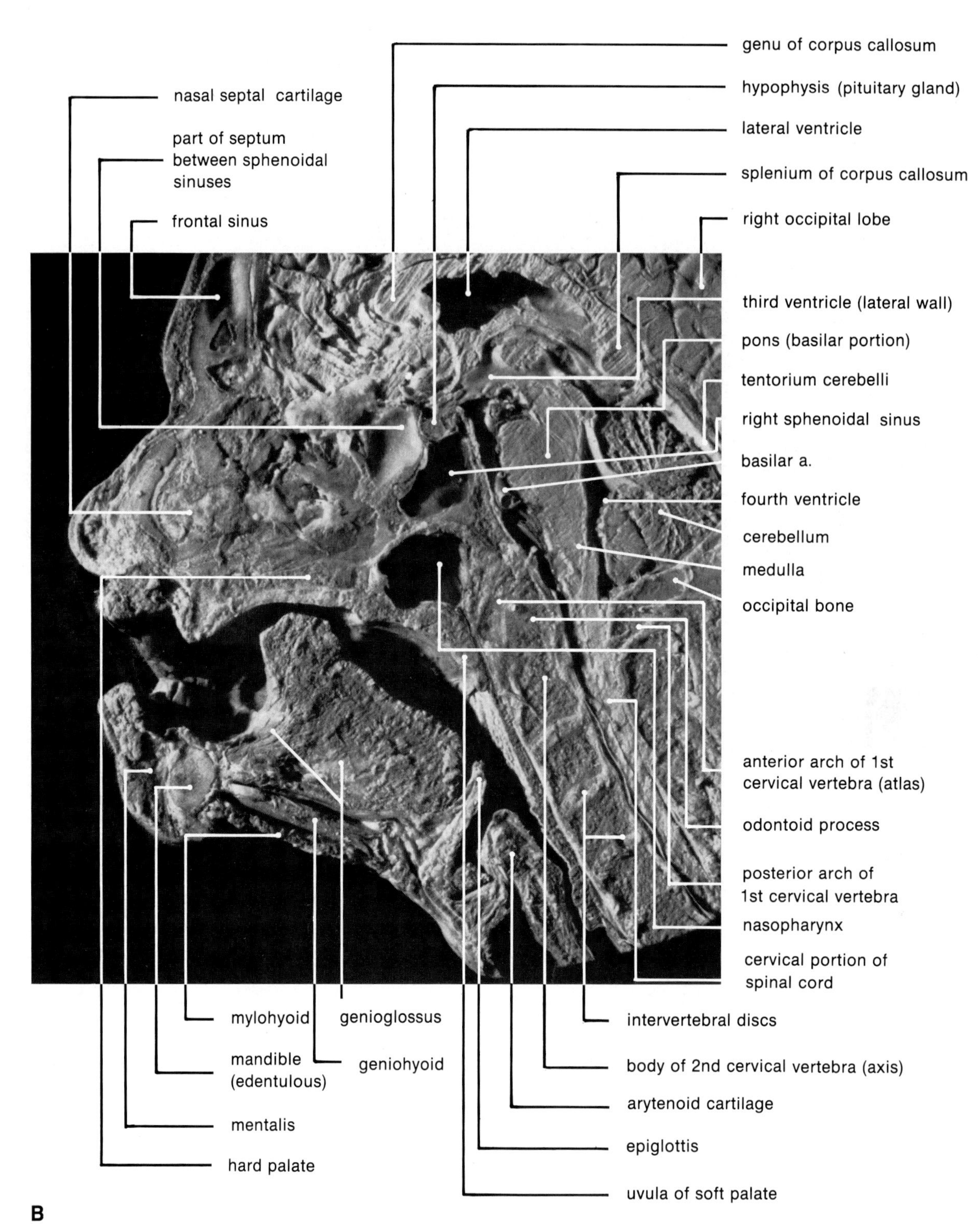

FIGURE 1-8 (B) Oral region.
Note: Tip of tongue forced backward in B (artifact of specimen).

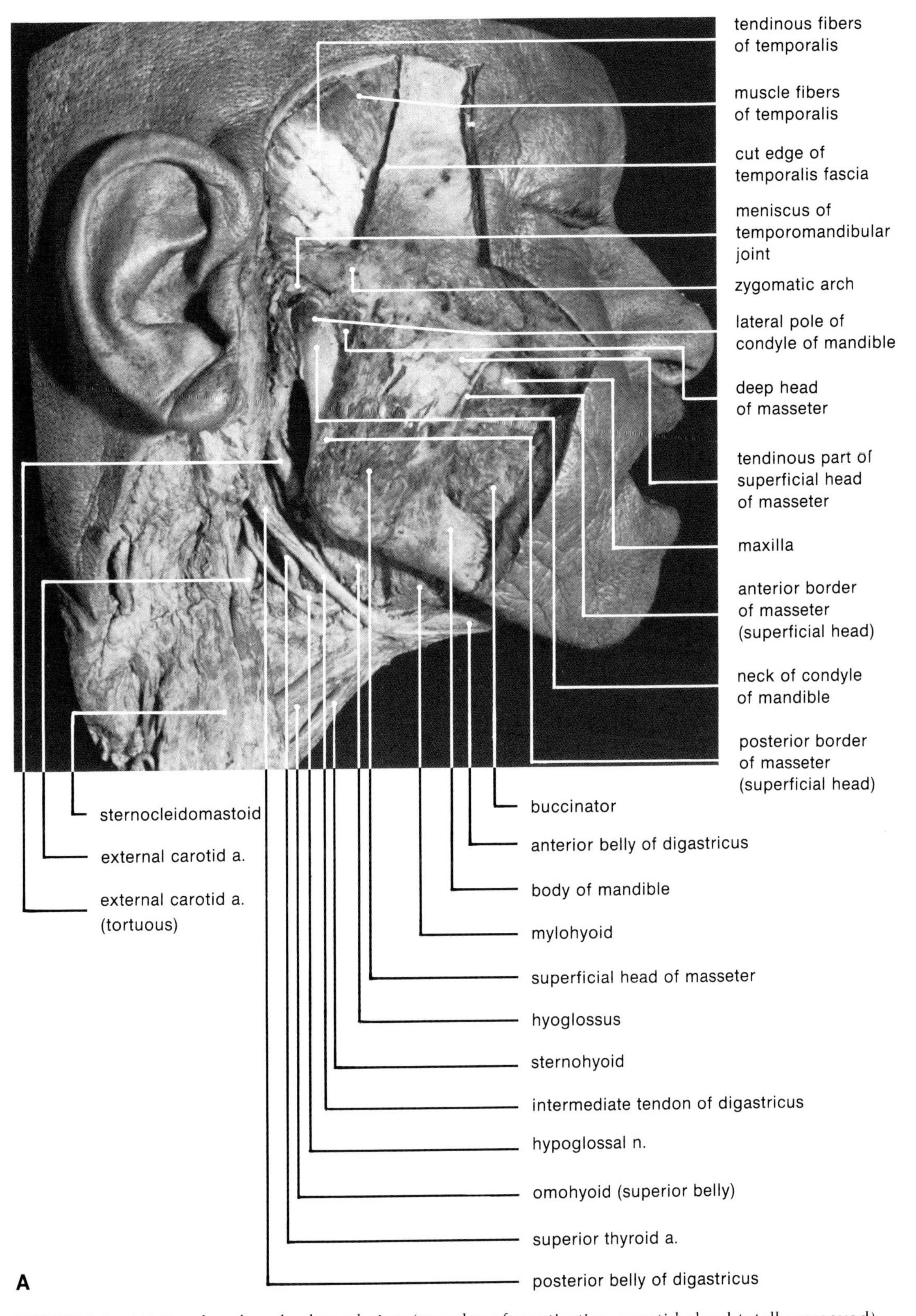

FIGURE 1-9 (A) Head and neck—lateral view (muscles of mastication, parotid gland totally removed). (*Figure continues on next page.*)

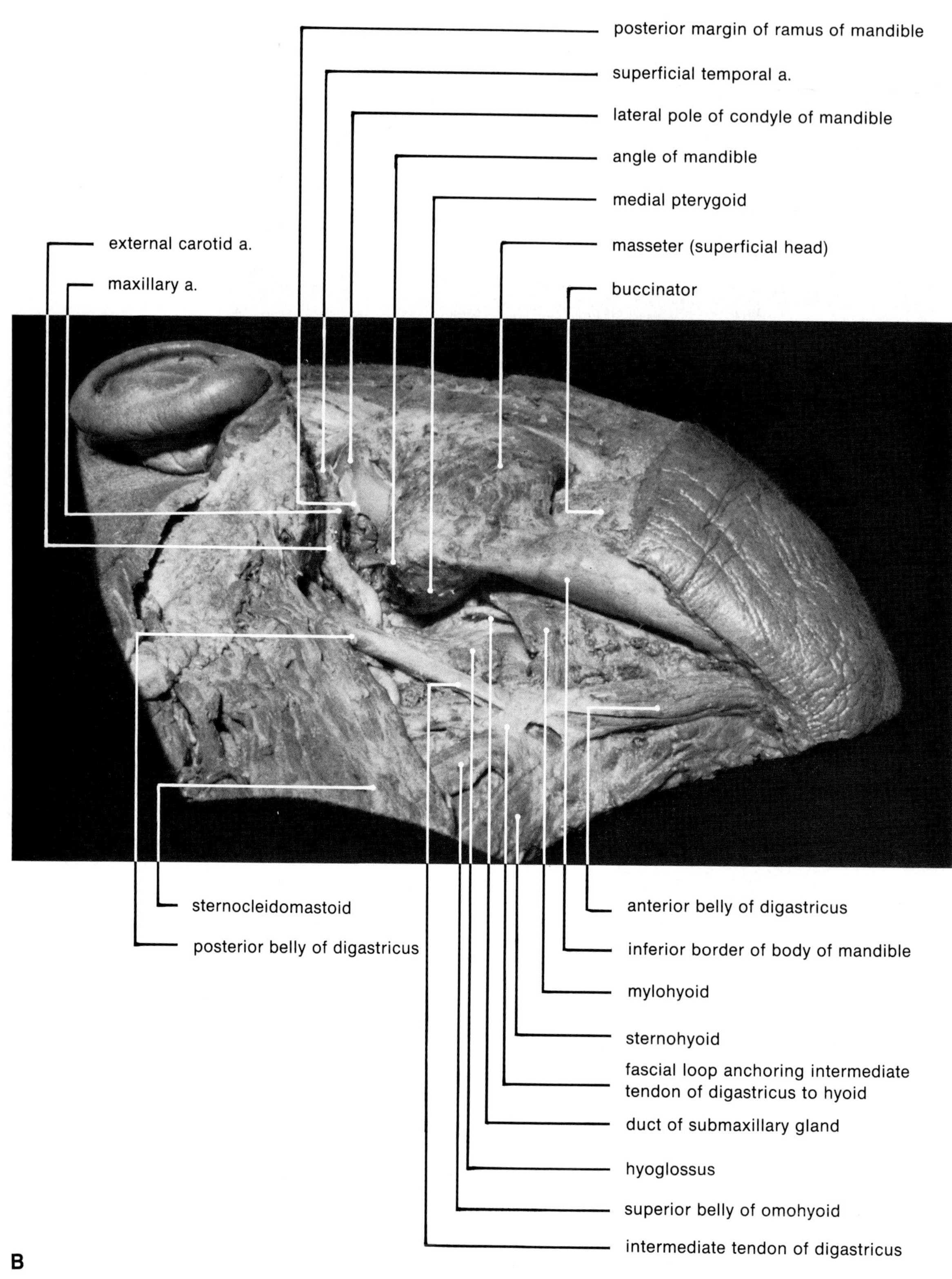

FIGURE 1-9 (B) Muscles of the head and neck—inferior view.

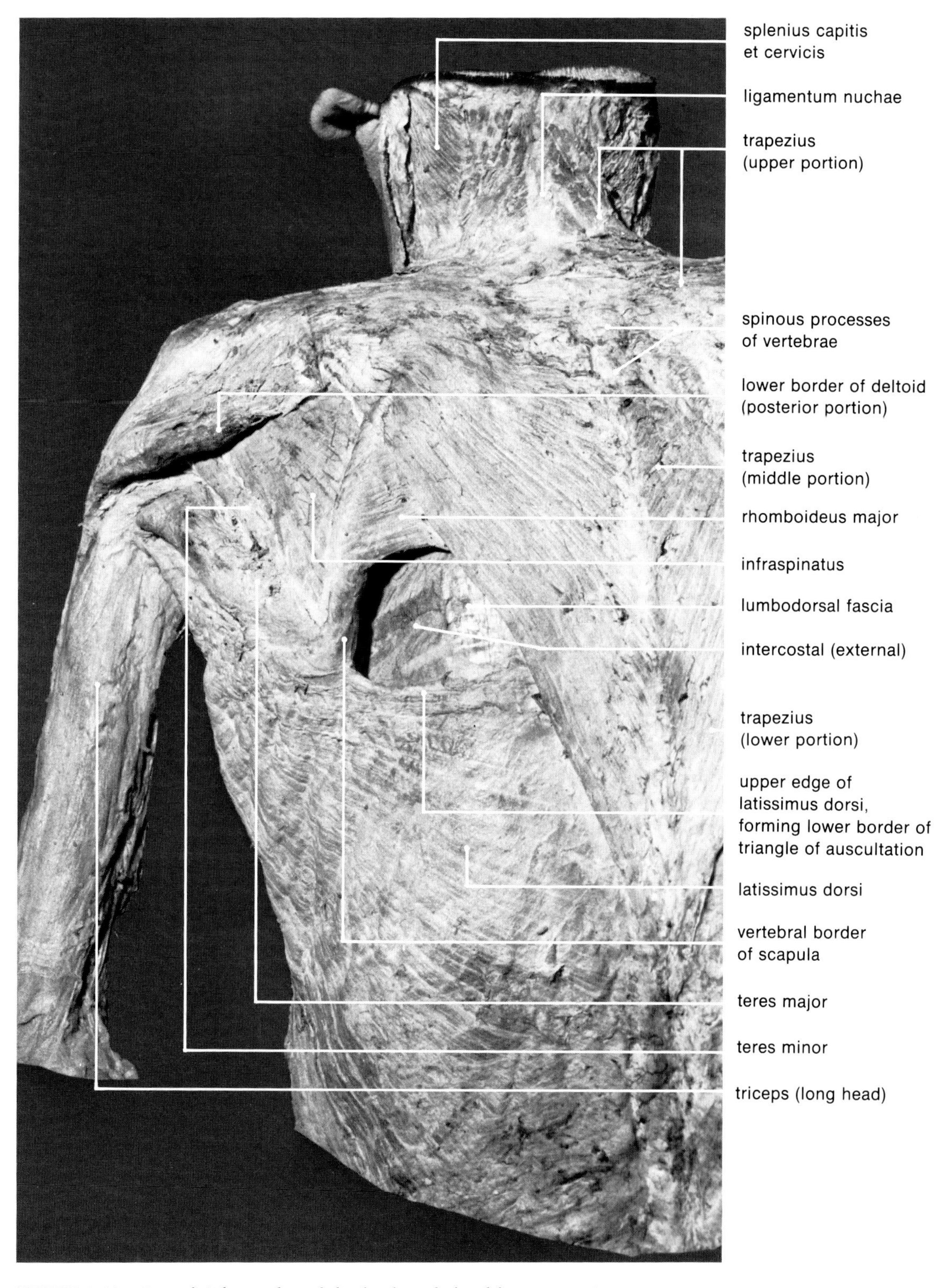

FIGURE 1-10 Superficial muscles of the back and shoulder—posterior view.

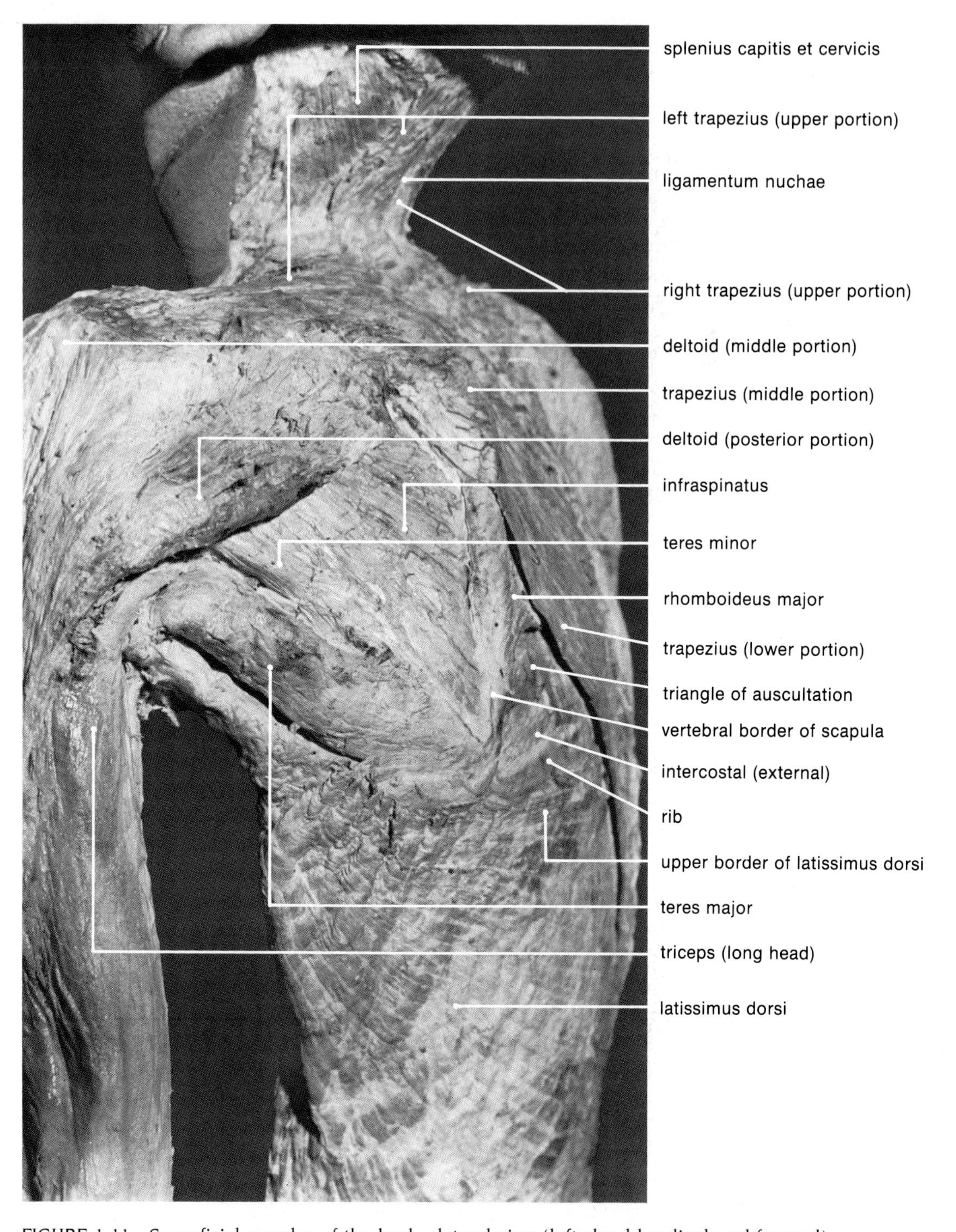

FIGURE 1-11 Superficial muscles of the back—lateral view (left shoulder displaced forward).

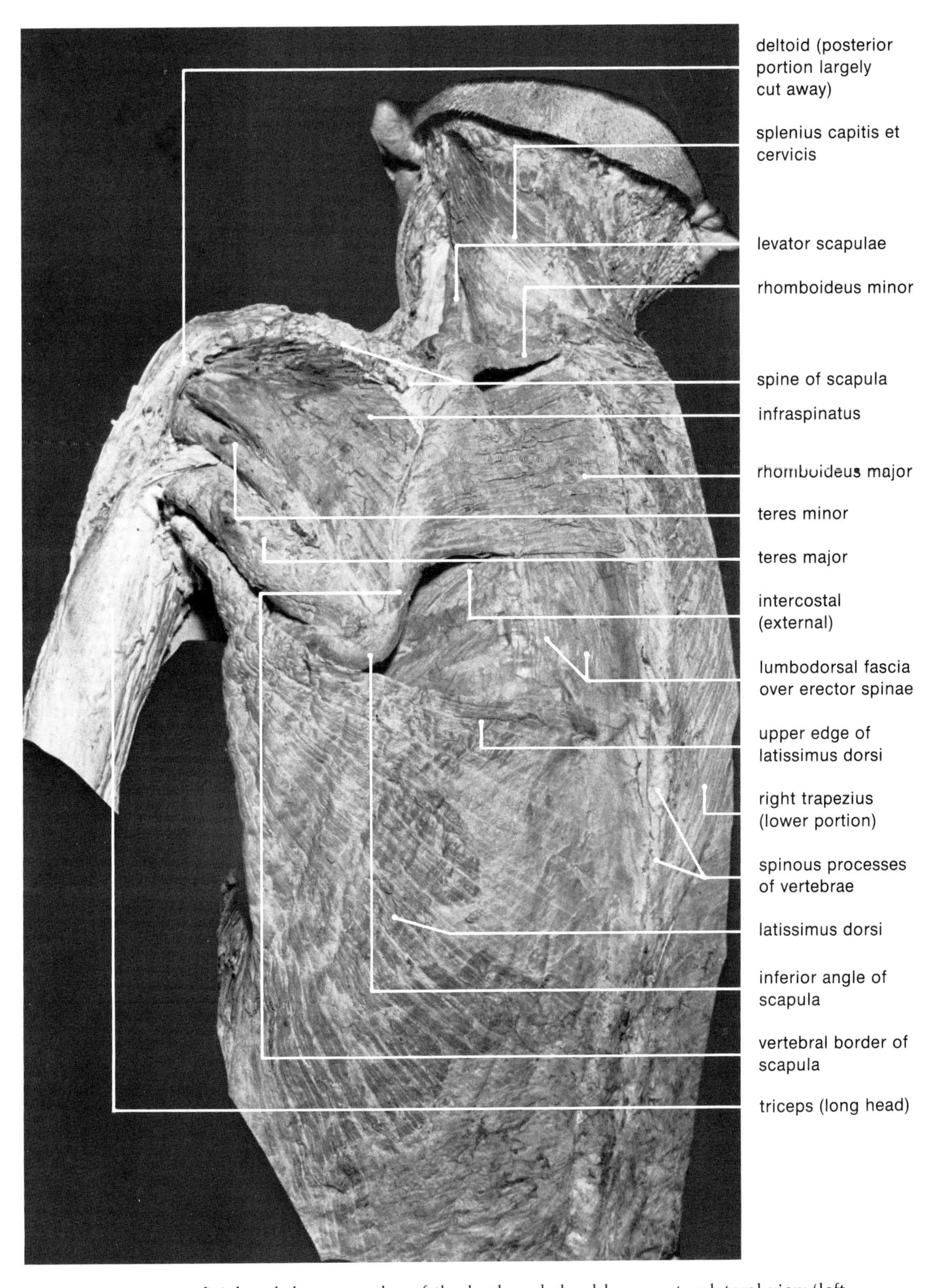

FIGURE 1-12 Superficial and deep muscles of the back and shoulder—posterolateral view (left trapezius removed).

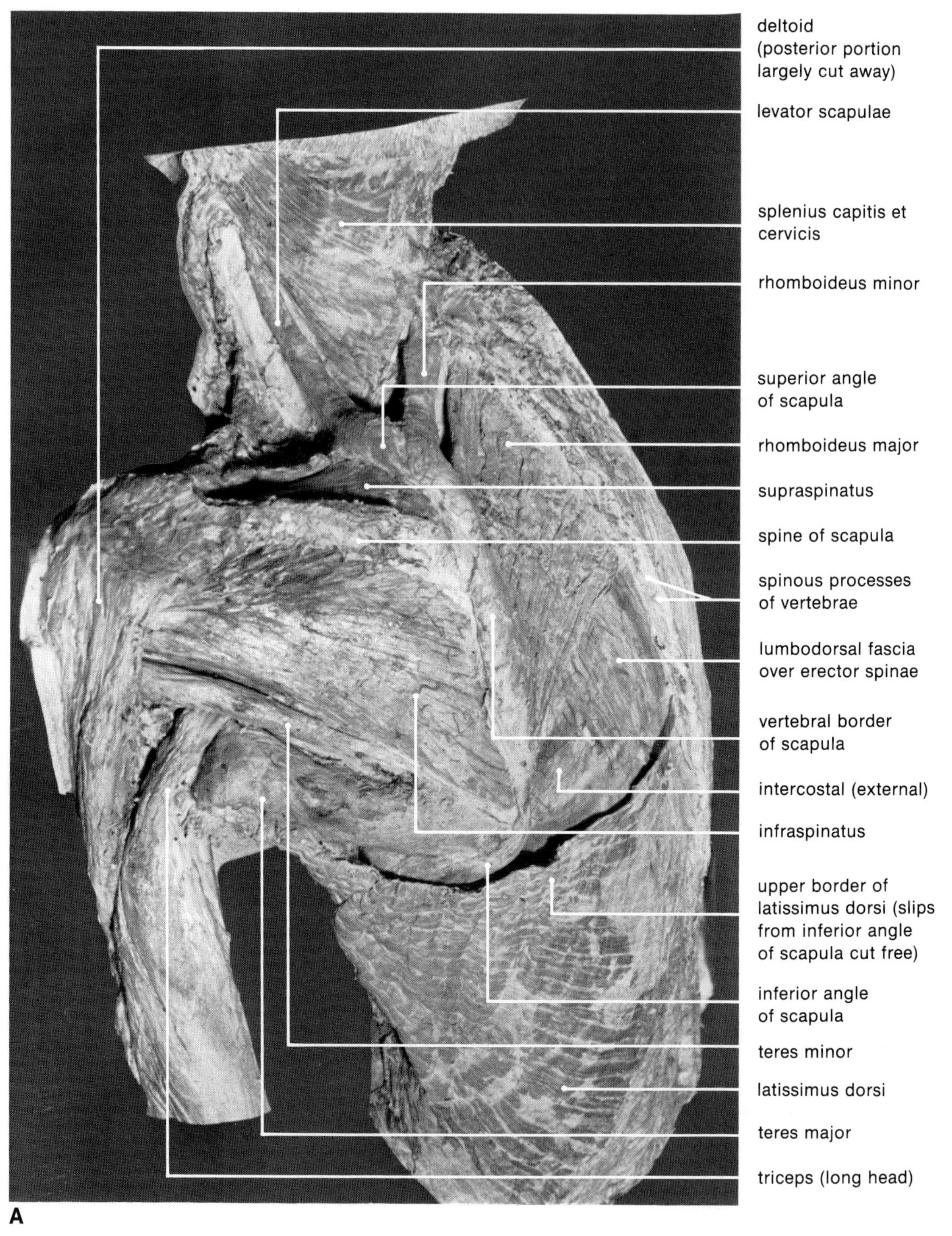

FIGURE 1-13 (A) Superficial and deep muscles of the neck, shoulder, and back—posterolateral view (left trapezius removed). (B) Shoulder—dorsal view, course and distribution of the suprascapular nerve.

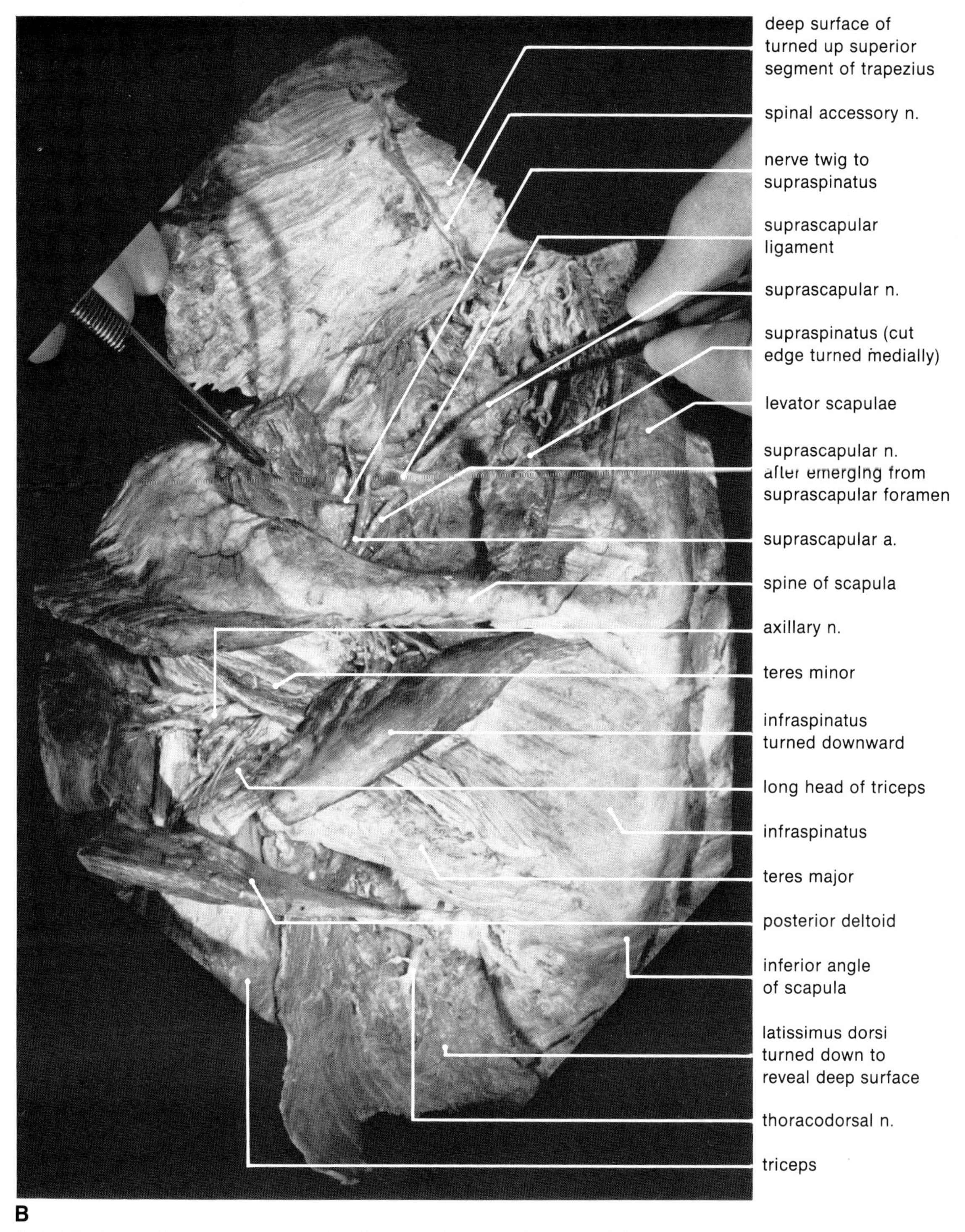

B

Note: The infraspinatus is transected and turned downward to reveal the branches of the suprascapular nerve entering its deep surface. The supraspinatus has been transected and the parts reflected to reveal the suprascapular nerve in the supraspinous fossa. The right forceps grasps the suprascapular nerve near its origin from the upper trunk of the brachial plexus. The left forceps retracts the distal segment of the supraspinatus toward the acromion. One inch below the acromion, the deltoid has been horizontally transected and the parts separated to reveal the axillary nerve. The posterior deltoid has been cut from the spinous process and displaced downward. Note the two small twigs of the axillary nerve supplying it.

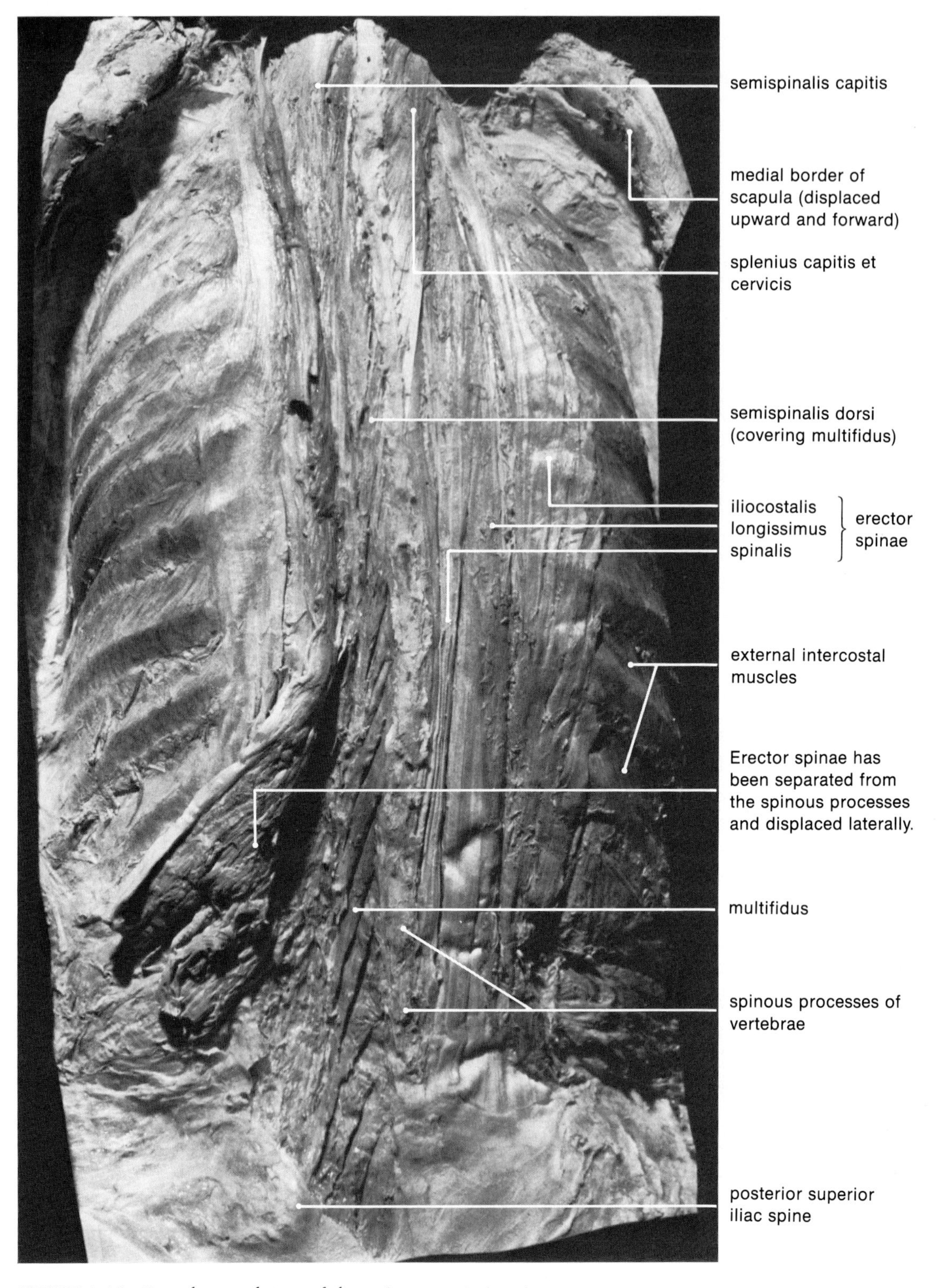

FIGURE 1-14 Dorsal musculature of the spine—posterior view.

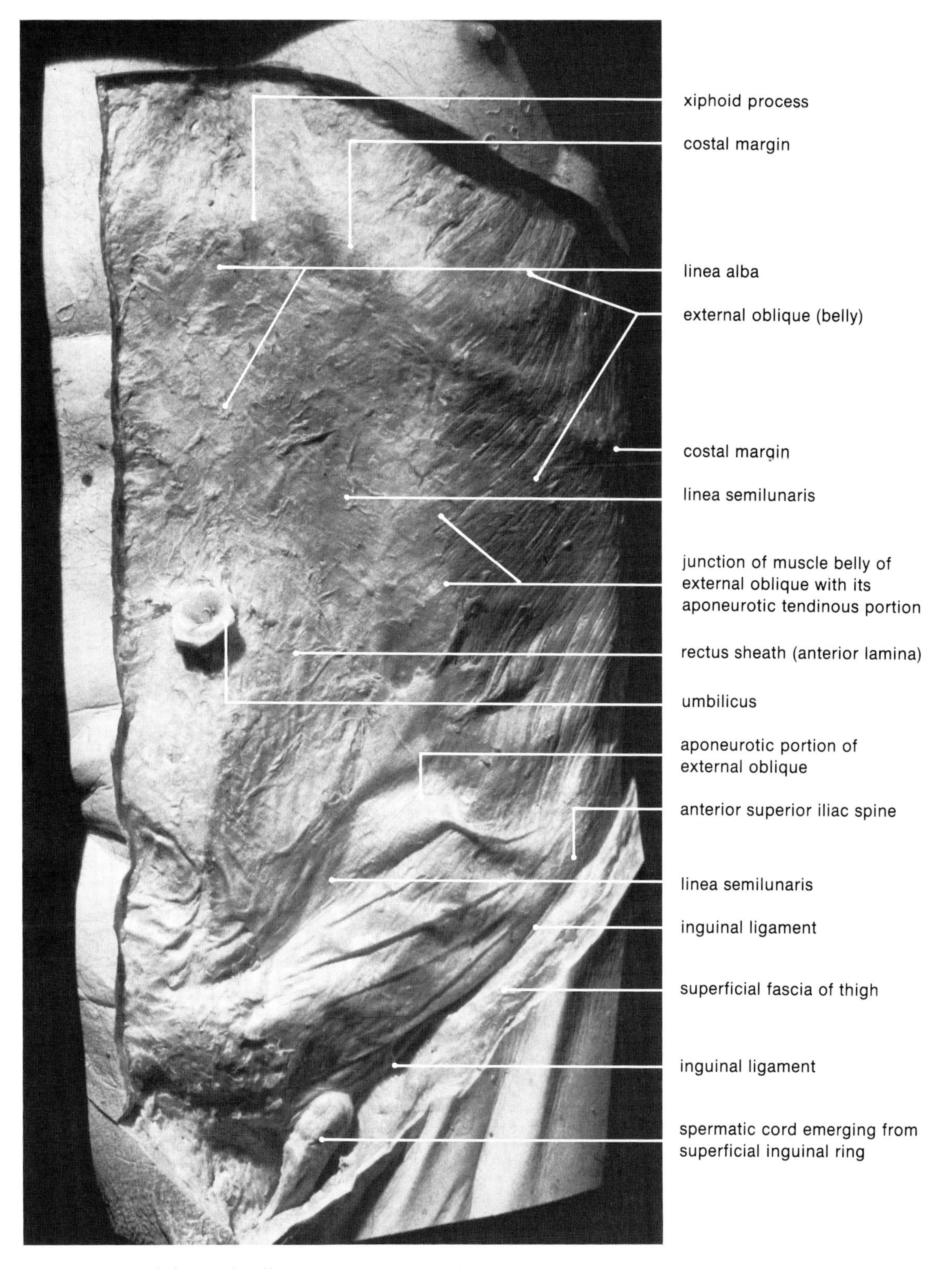

FIGURE 1-15 Abdominal wall—anterior view, with the skin and fascia removed.

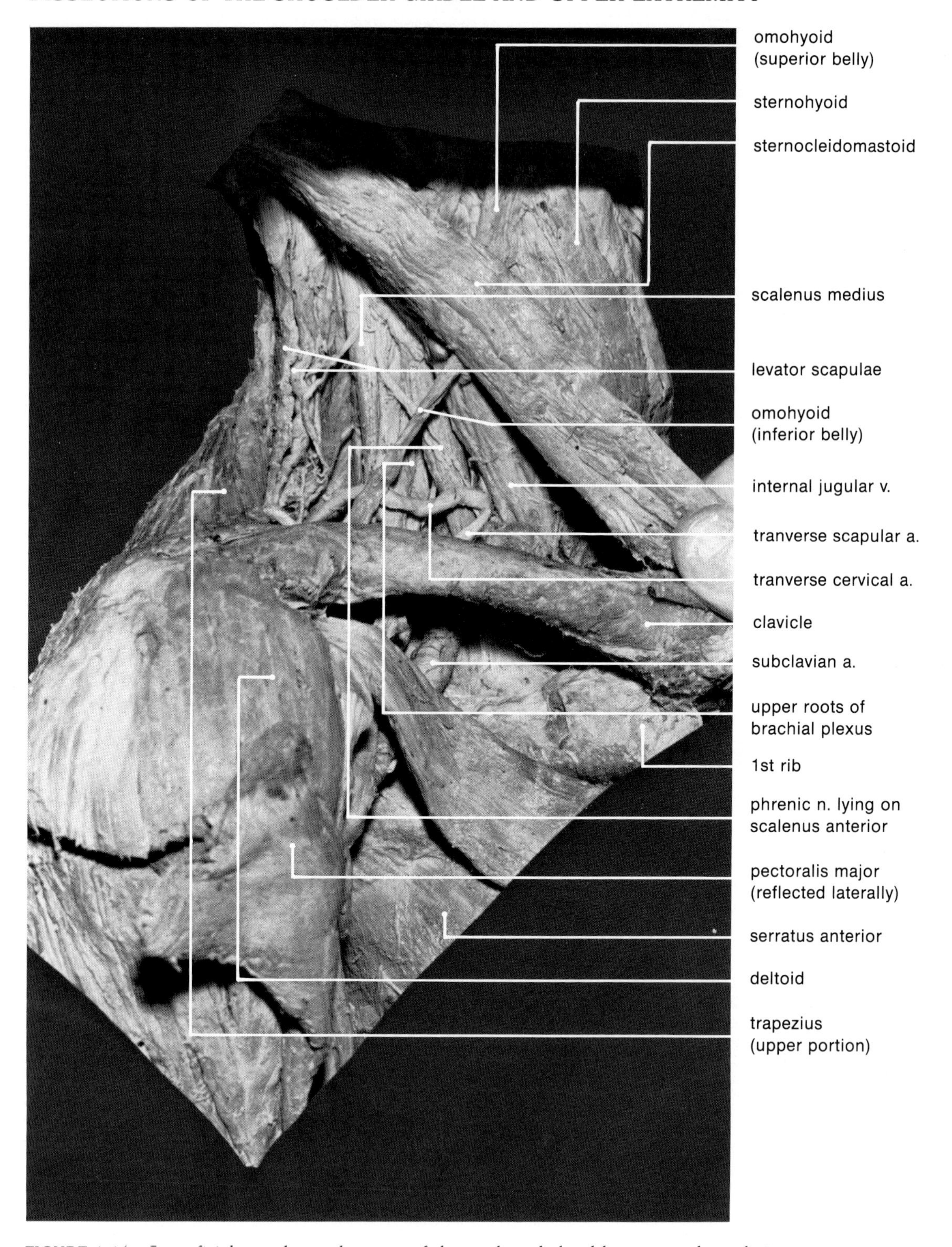

FIGURE 1-16 Superficial muscles and nerves of the neck and shoulder—anterolateral view.

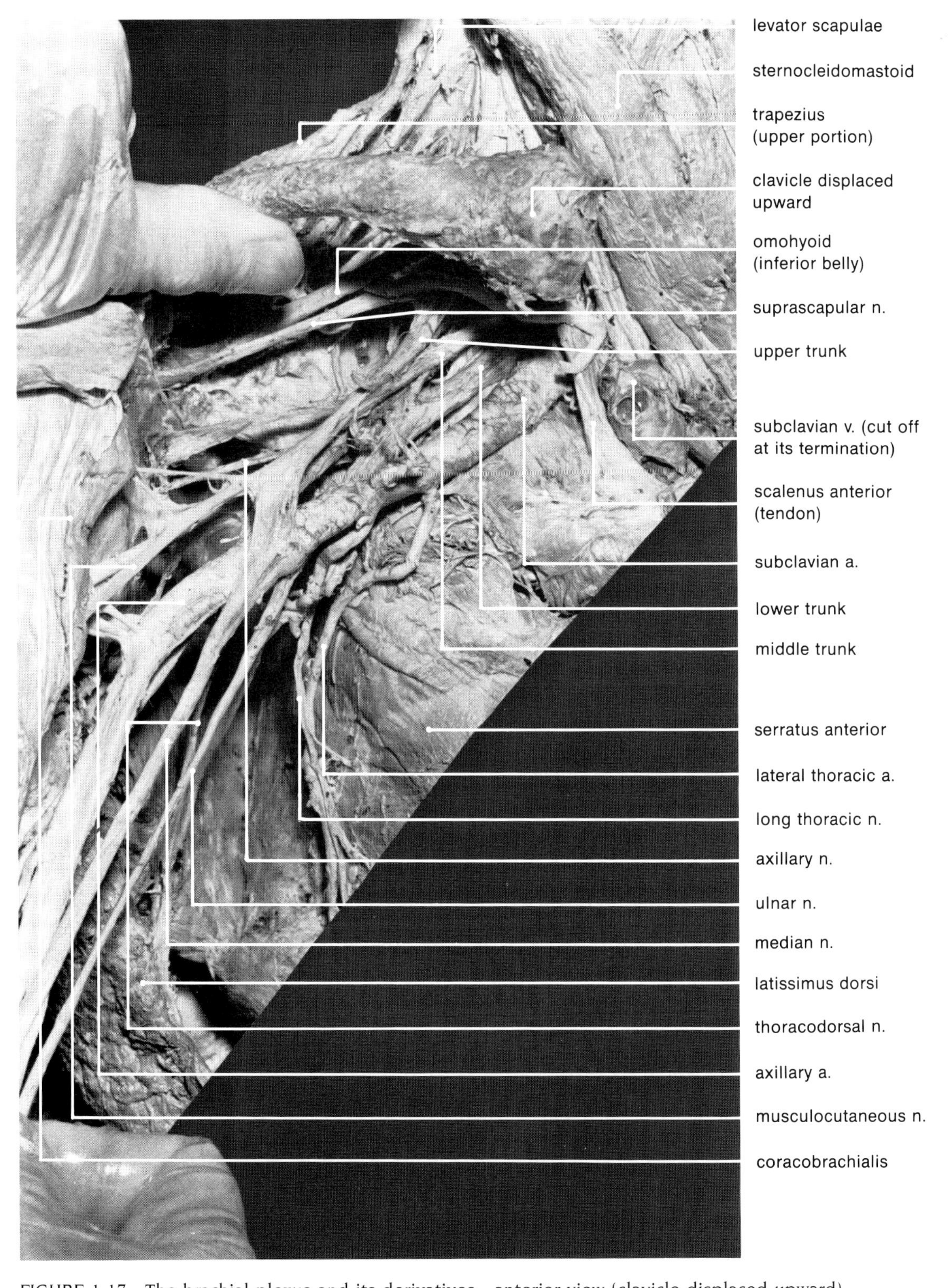

FIGURE 1-17 The brachial plexus and its derivatives—anterior view (clavicle displaced upward).

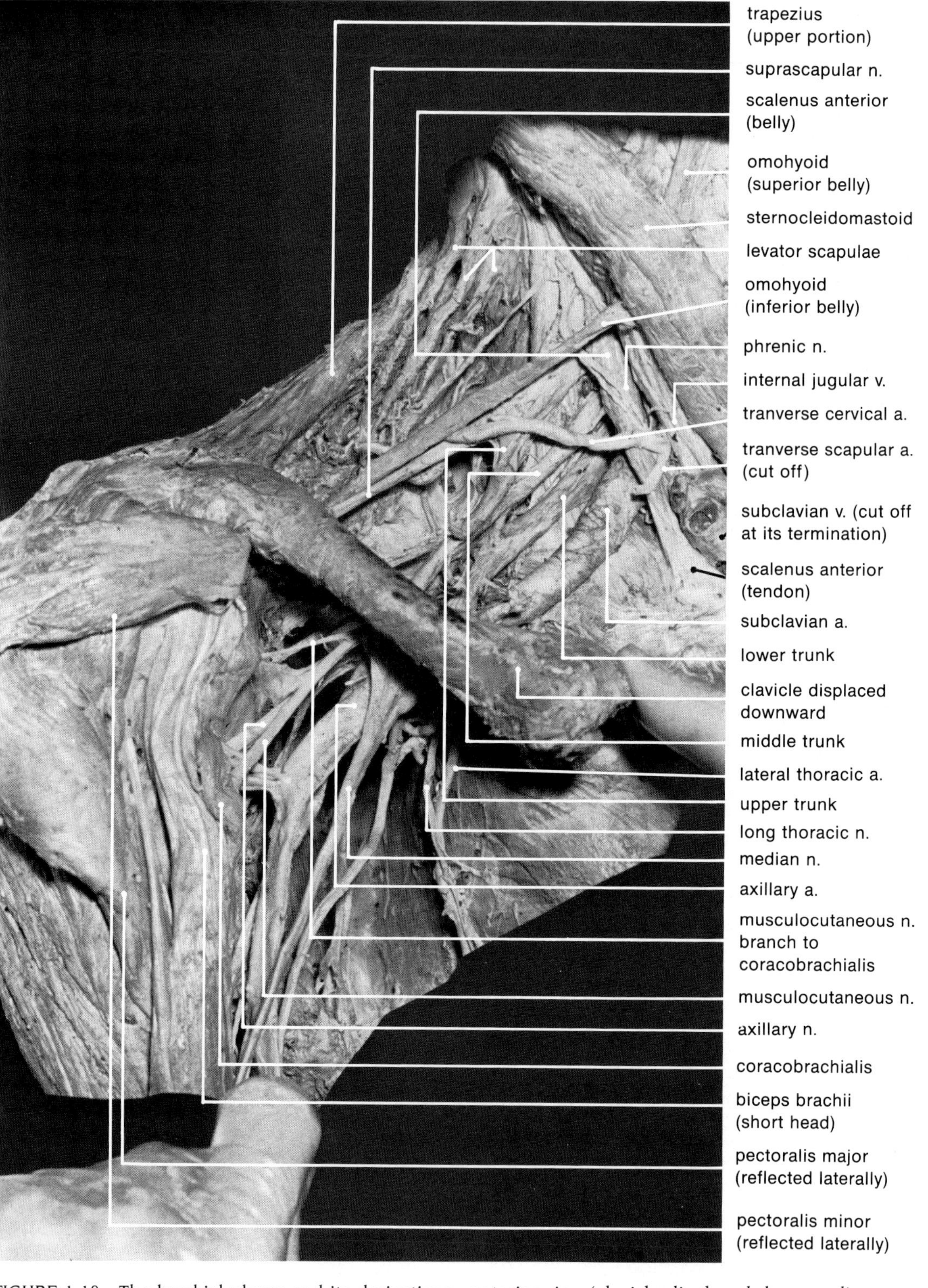

FIGURE 1-18 The brachial plexus and its derivatives—anterior view (clavicle displaced downward).

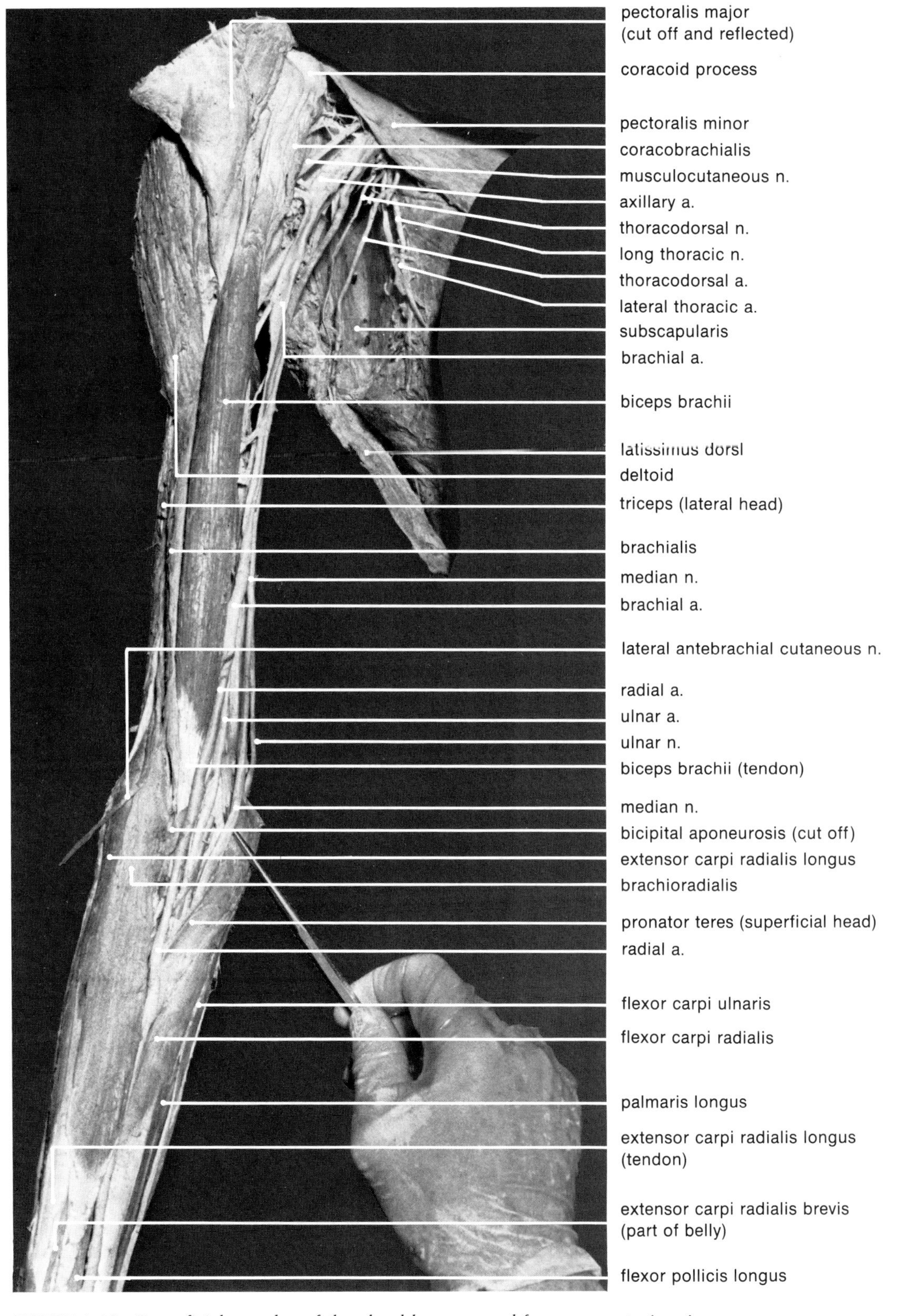

FIGURE 1-19 Superficial muscles of the shoulder, arm, and forearm—anterior view.
Note: This is a case of high division of the brachial artery, in which it divides into its radial and ulnar branches high in the arm.

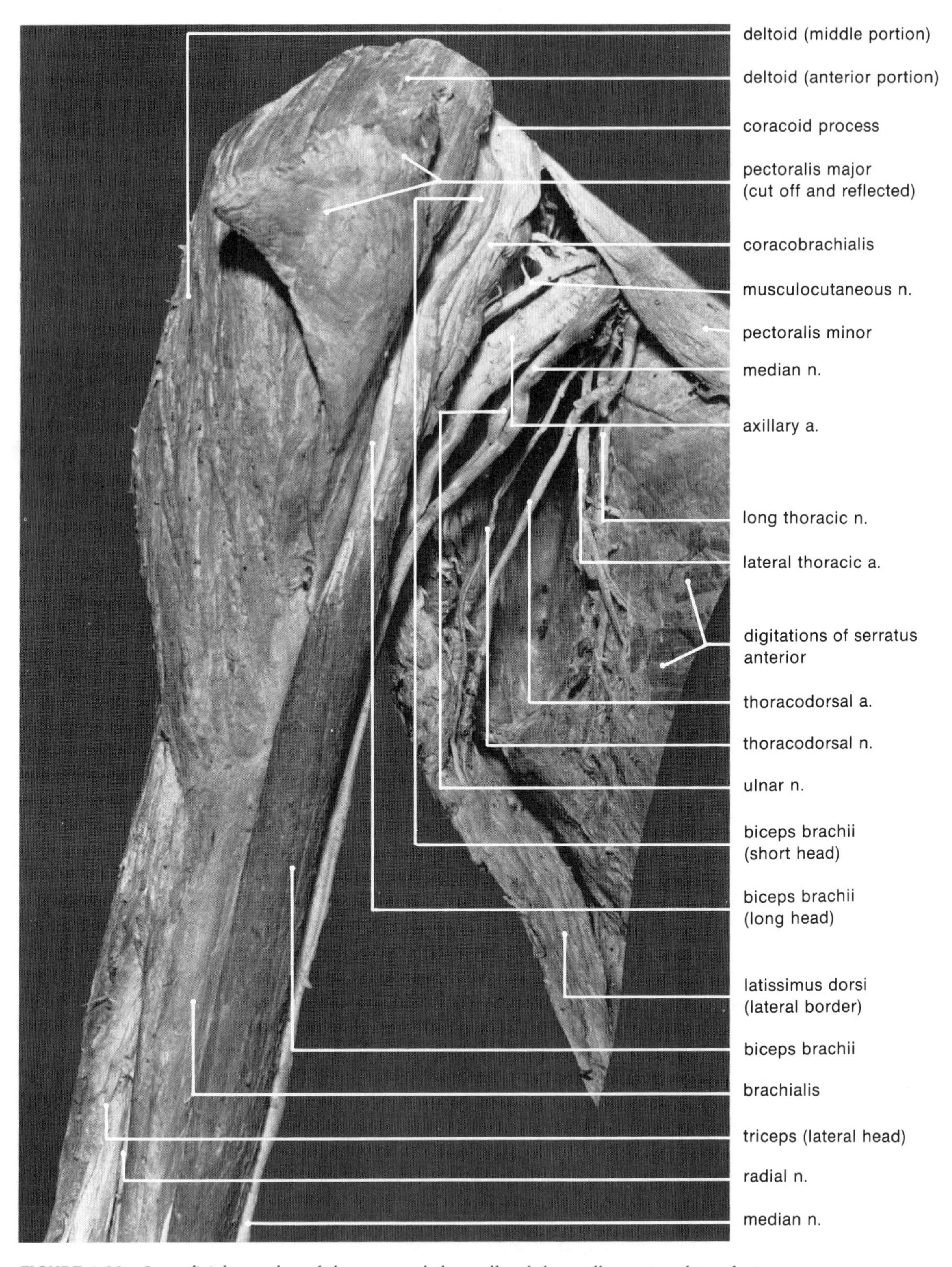

FIGURE 1-20 Superficial muscles of the arm and the walls of the axilla—anterolateral view.

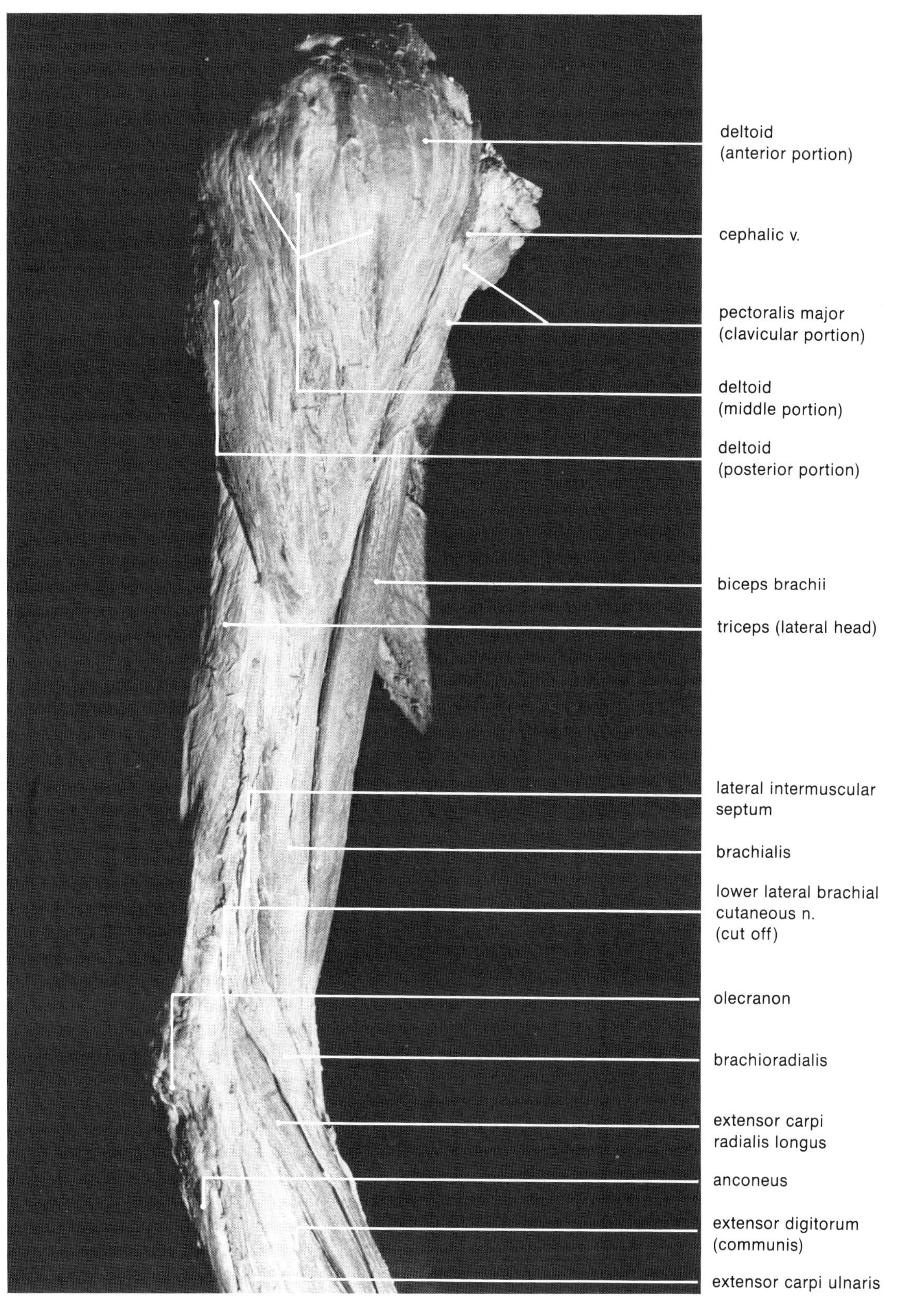

FIGURE 1-21 Superficial muscles of the arm—lateral view.

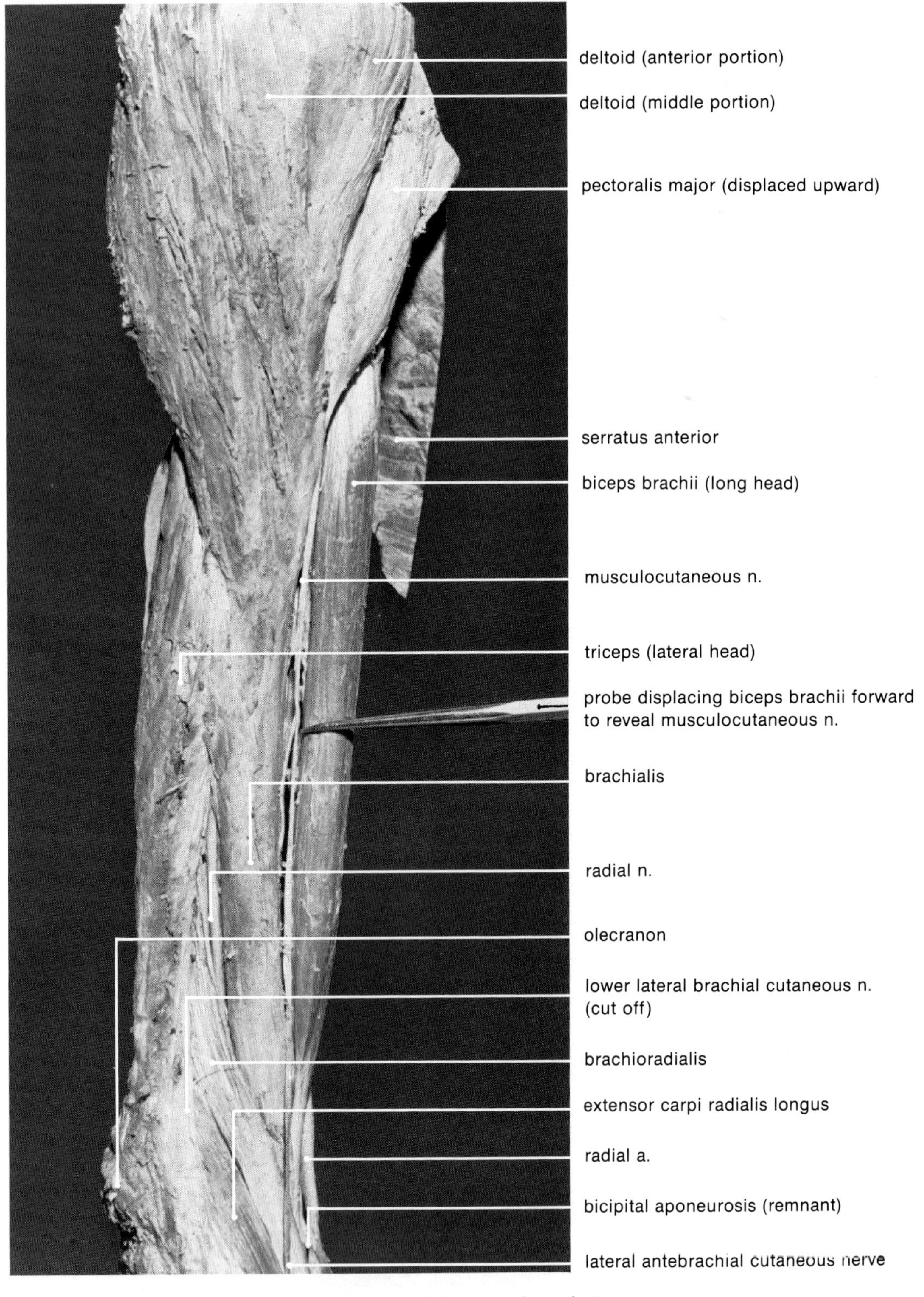

FIGURE 1-22 Superficial muscles and nerves of the arm—lateral view.
Note: In the usual specimen the position of the radial artery seen here would be the position of the brachial artery. Since this is a case of high division of the brachial artery, the vessel showing is the radial artery.

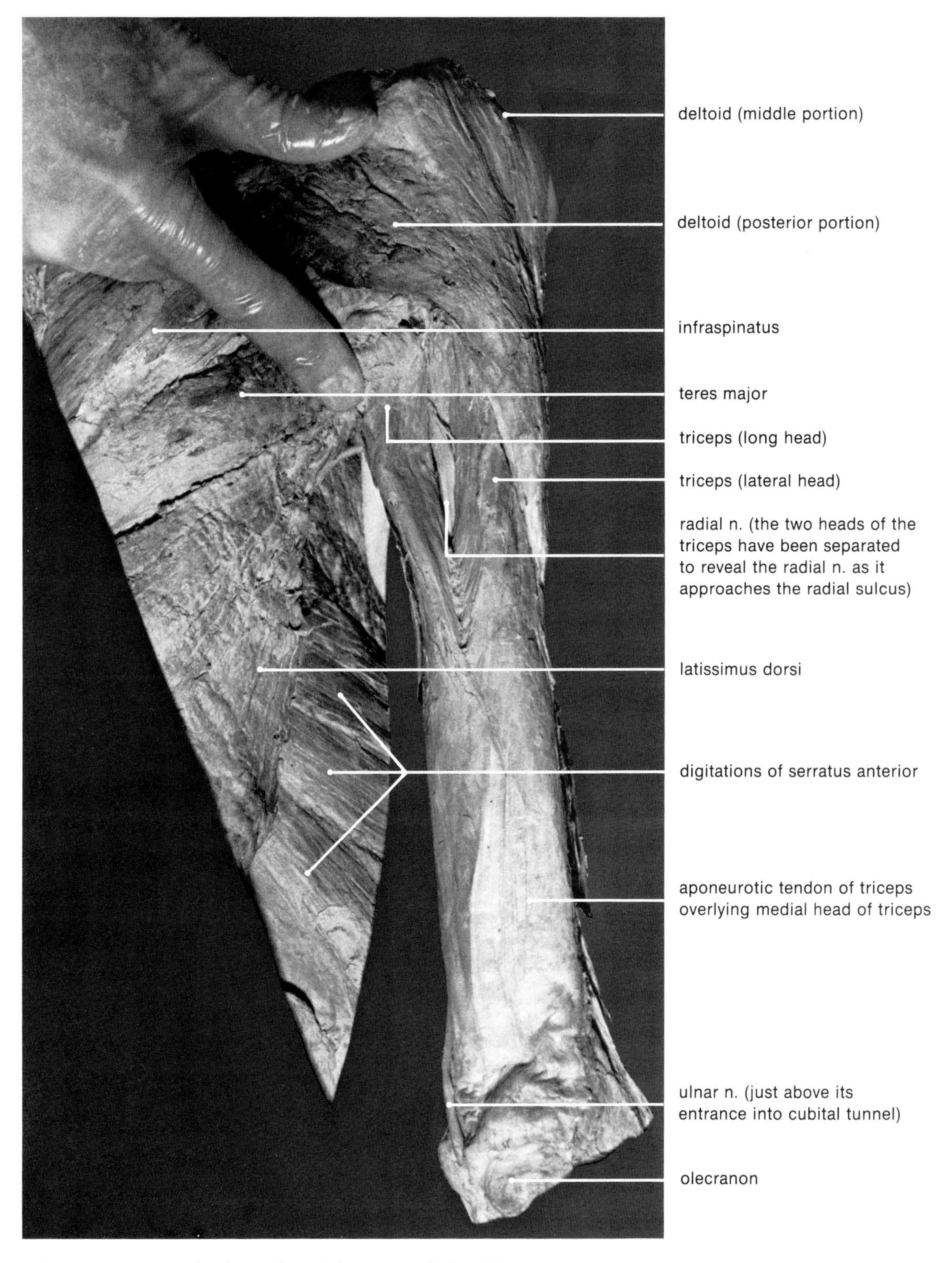

FIGURE 1-23 Superficial muscles of the arm and shoulder—posterior view.

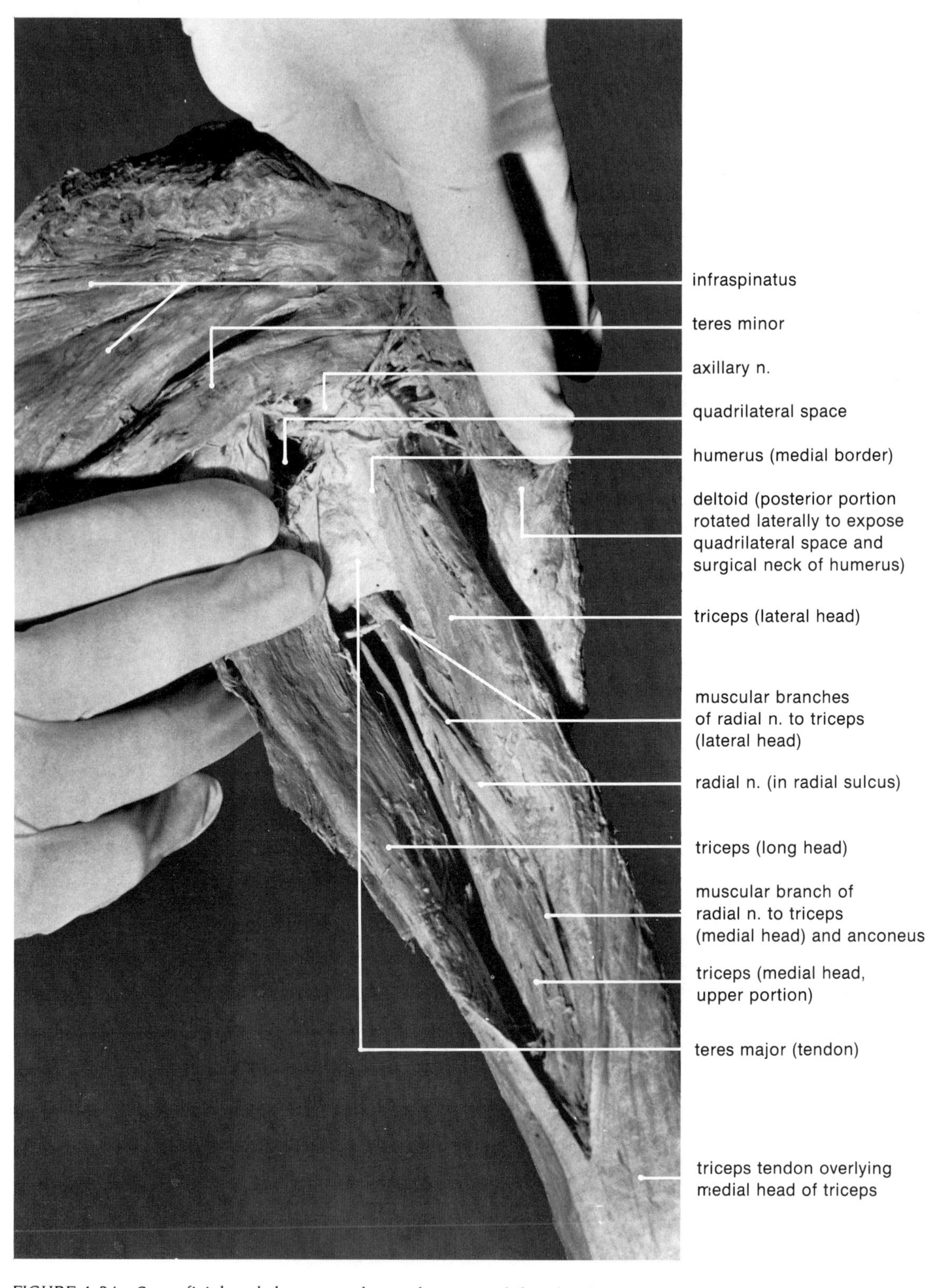

FIGURE 1-24 Superficial and deep muscles and nerves of the shoulder and arm—posterior view. *Note*: The long head and the lateral head of the triceps have been split apart along their line of fusion to reveal the radial sulcus and the upper part of the medial head of the triceps.

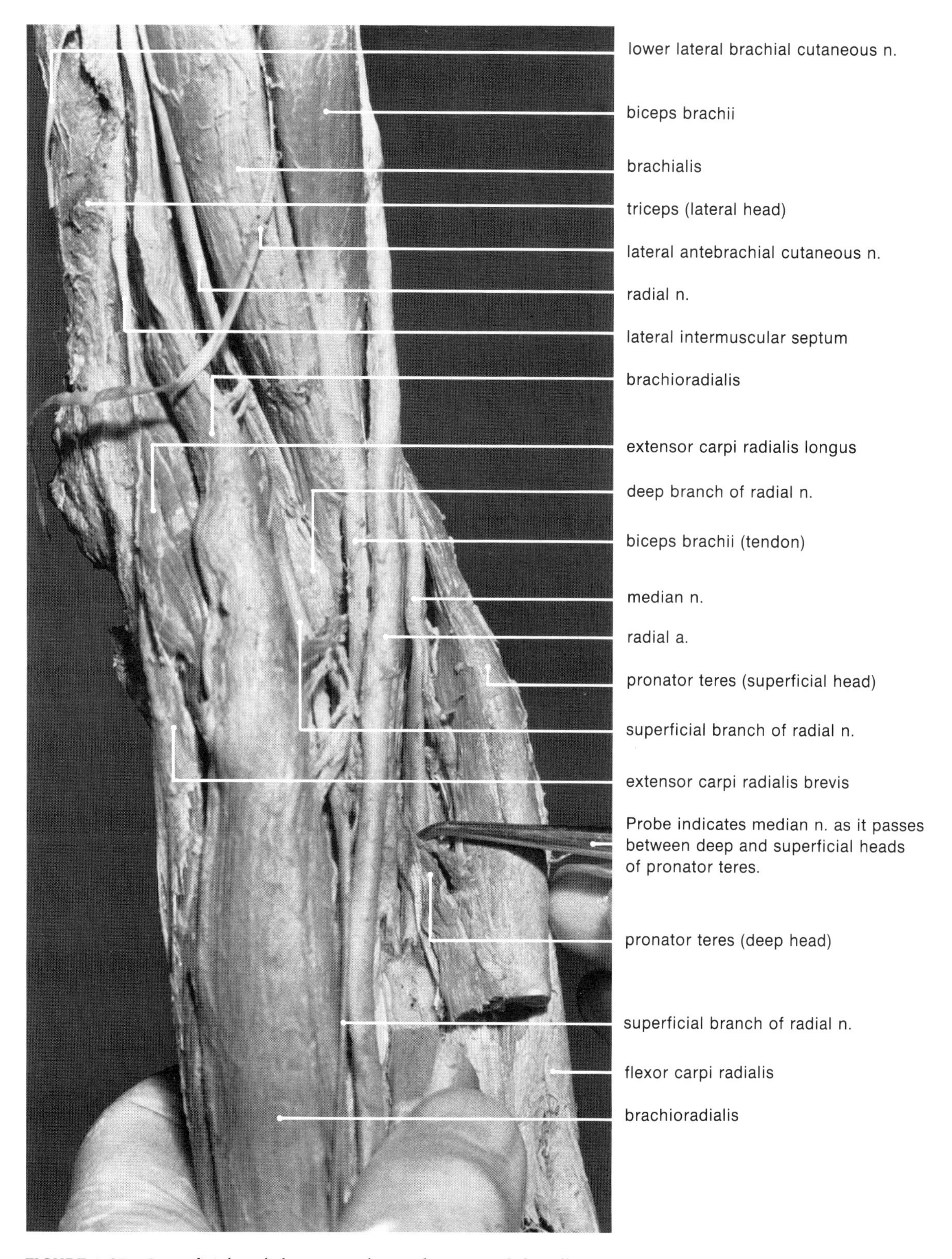

FIGURE 1-25 Superficial and deep muscles and nerves of the elbow region—anterior view.

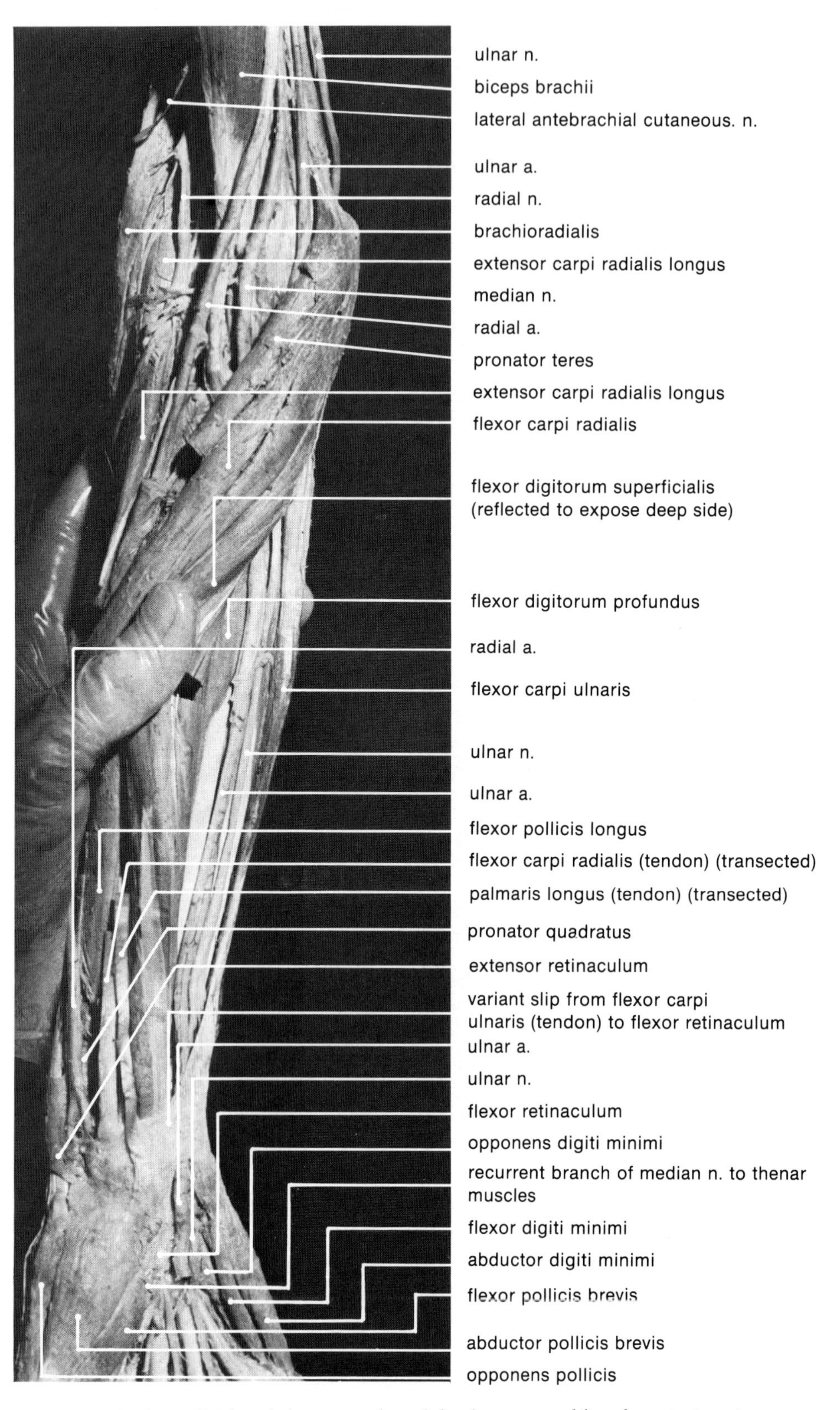

FIGURE 1-26 Superficial and deep muscles of the forearm and hand—anterior view.

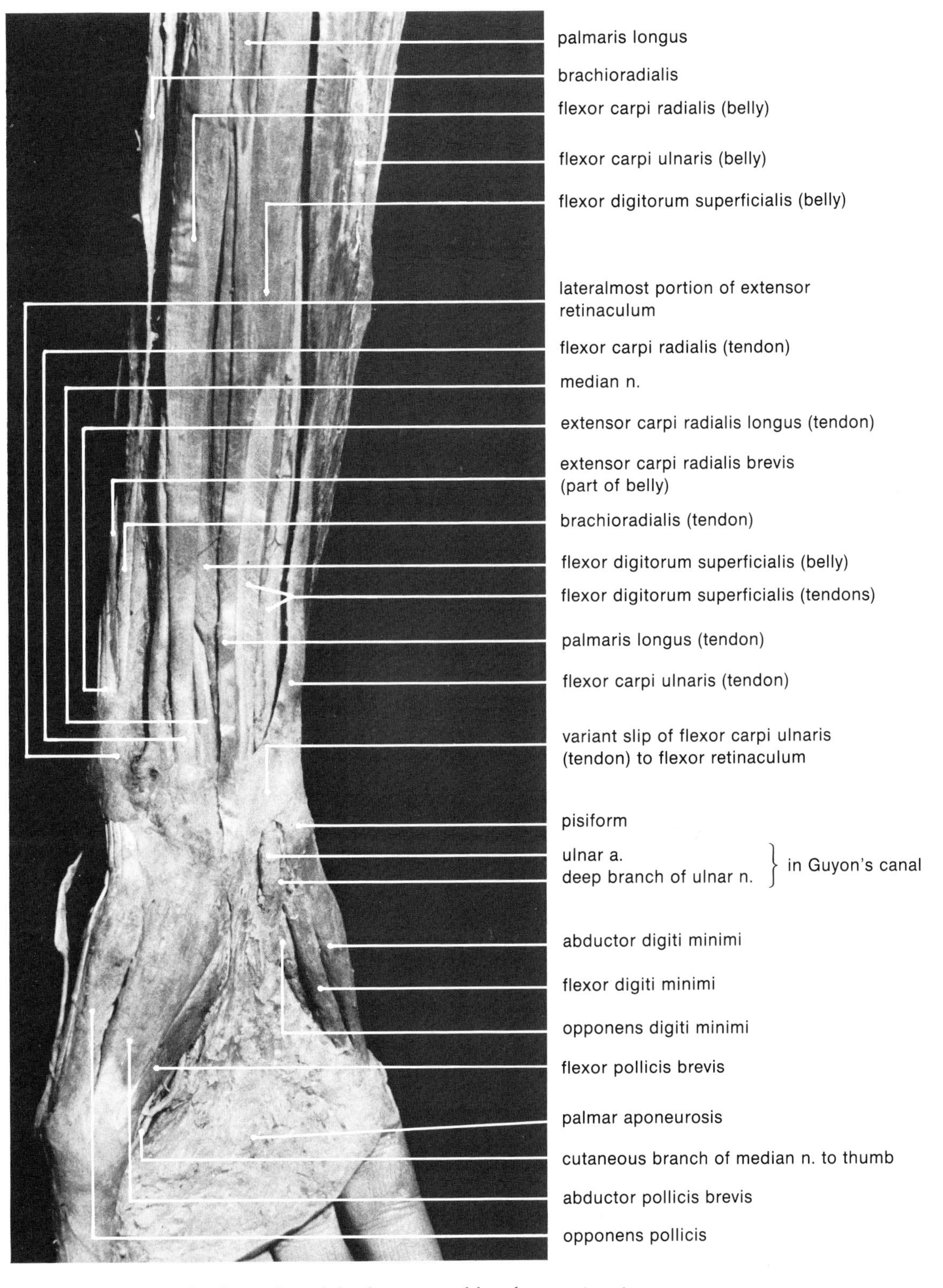

FIGURE 1-27 Superficial muscles of the forearm and hand—anterior view.

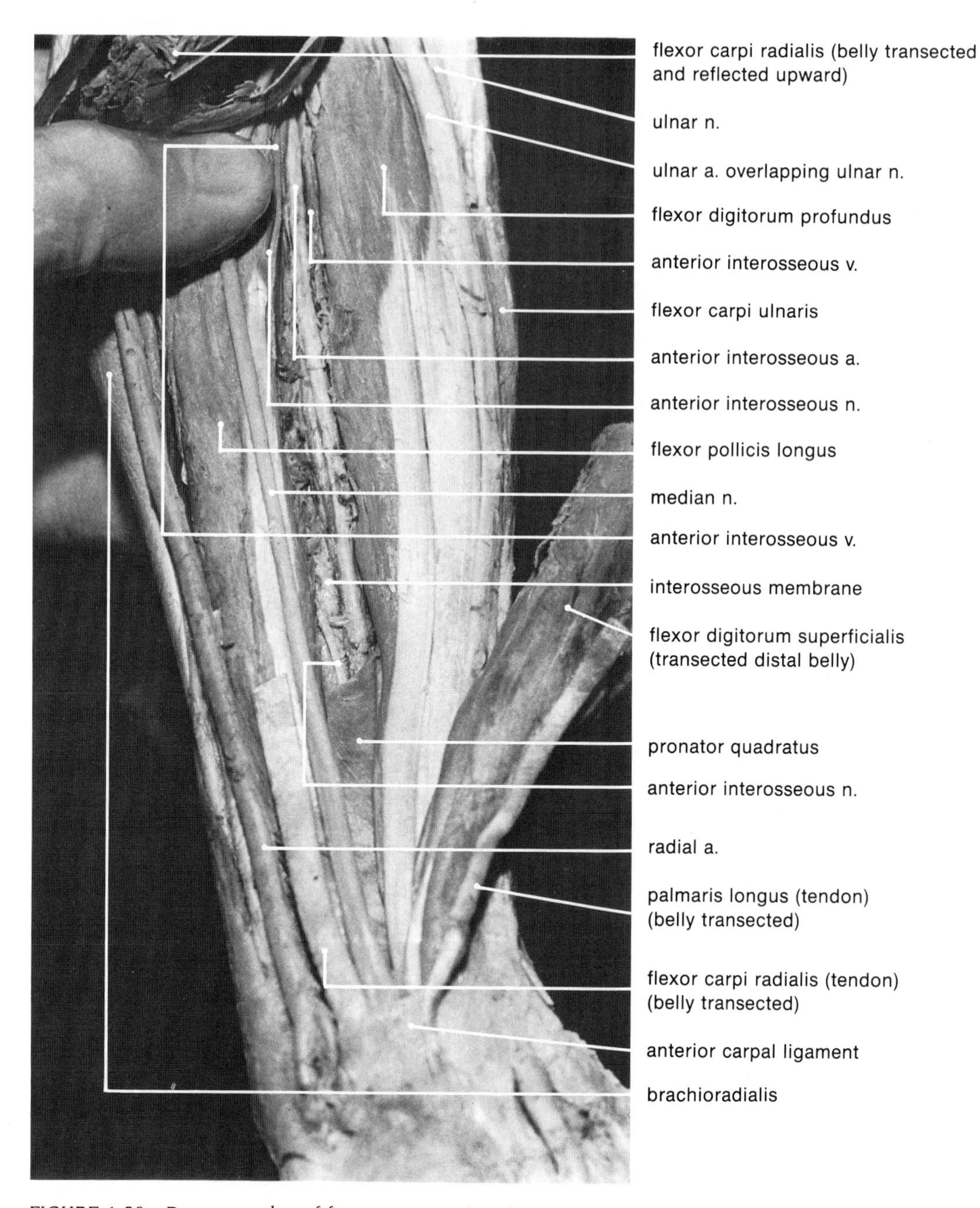

FIGURE 1-28 Deep muscles of forearm—anterior view.

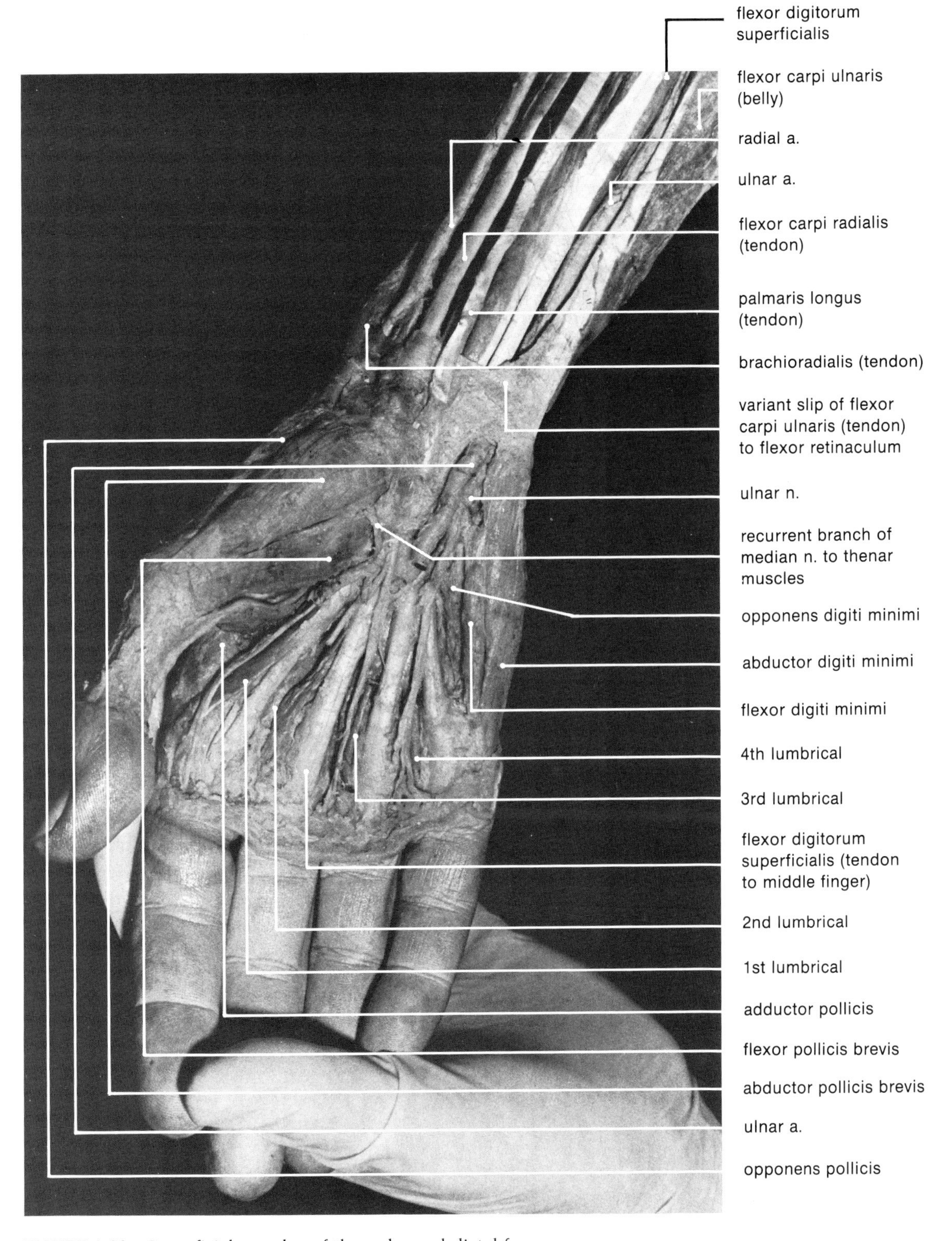

FIGURE 1-29 Superficial muscles of the palm and distal forearm.

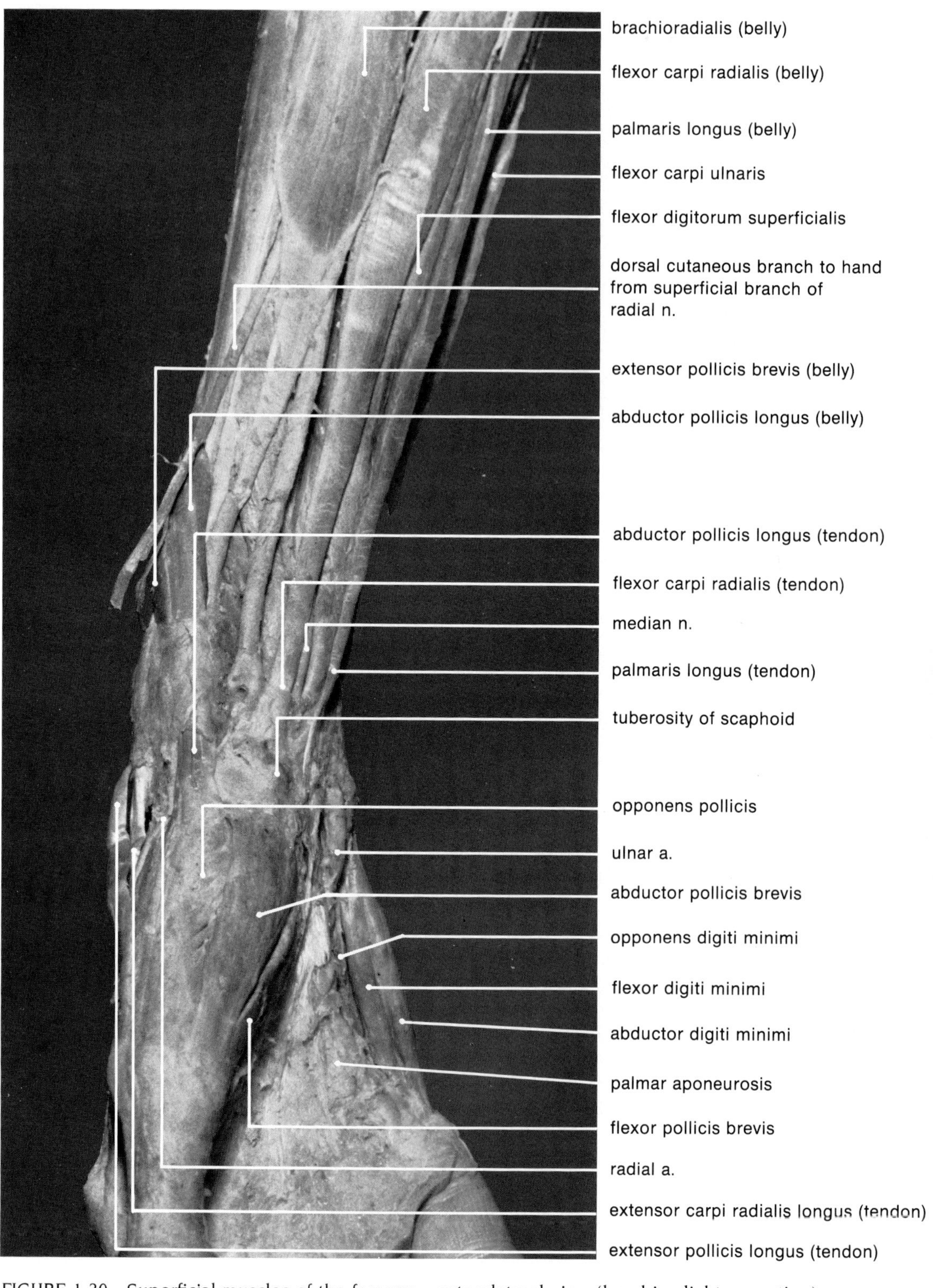

FIGURE 1-30 Superficial muscles of the forearm—anterolateral view (hand in slight pronation).

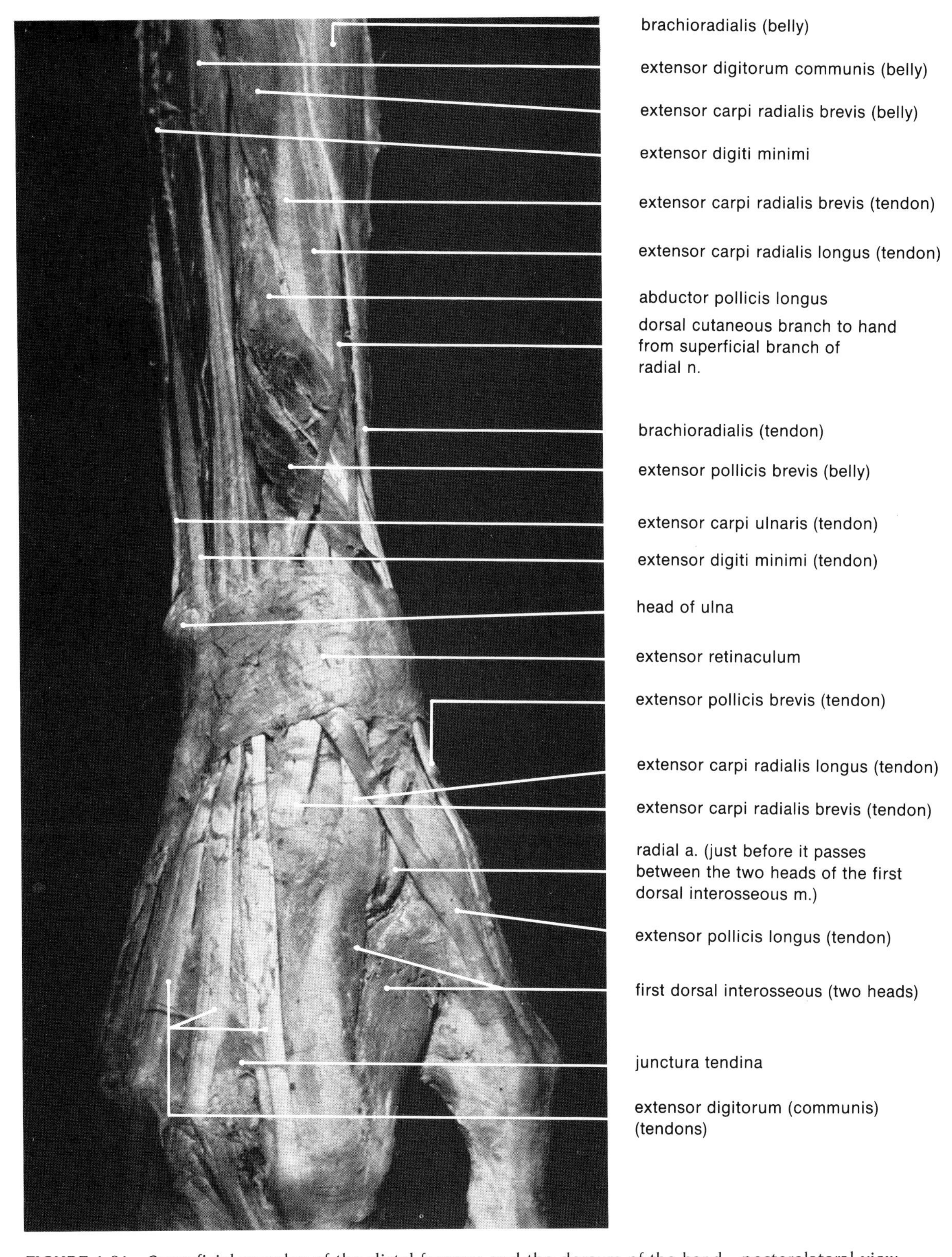

FIGURE 1-31 Superficial muscles of the distal forearm and the dorsum of the hand—posterolateral view.

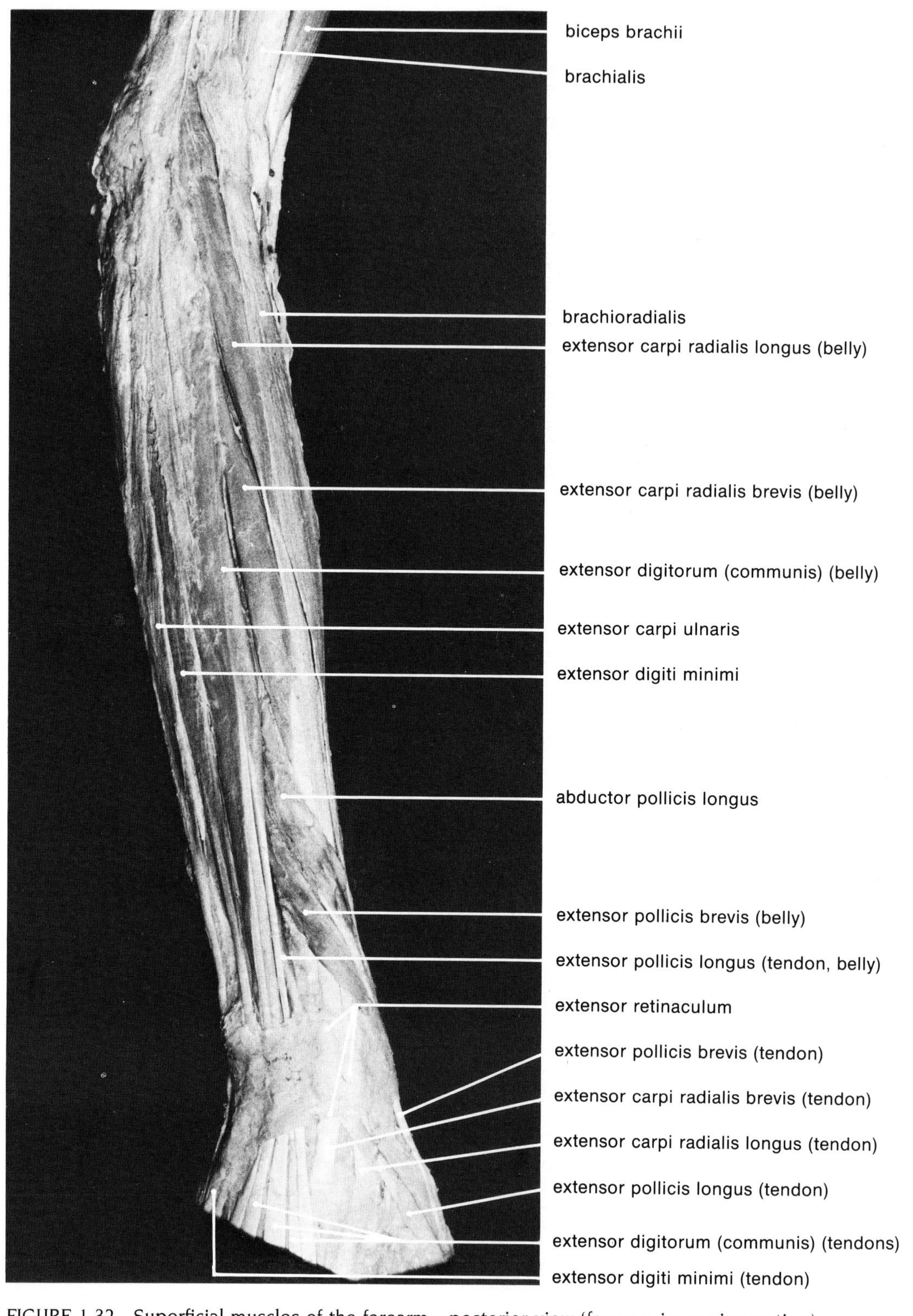

FIGURE 1-32 Superficial muscles of the forearm—posterior view (forearm in semipronation).

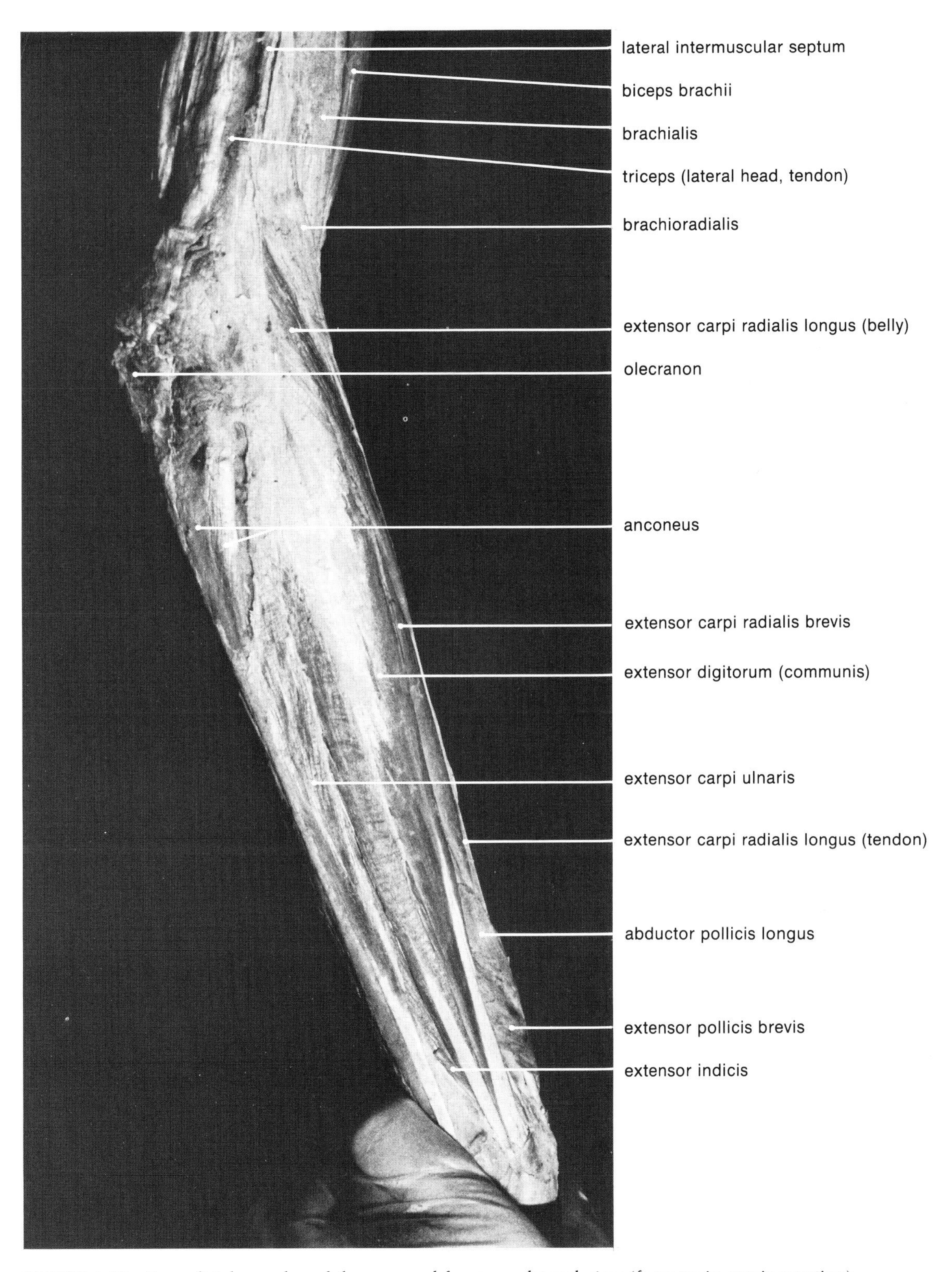

FIGURE 1-33 Superficial muscles of the arm and forearm—lateral view (forearm in semipronation).

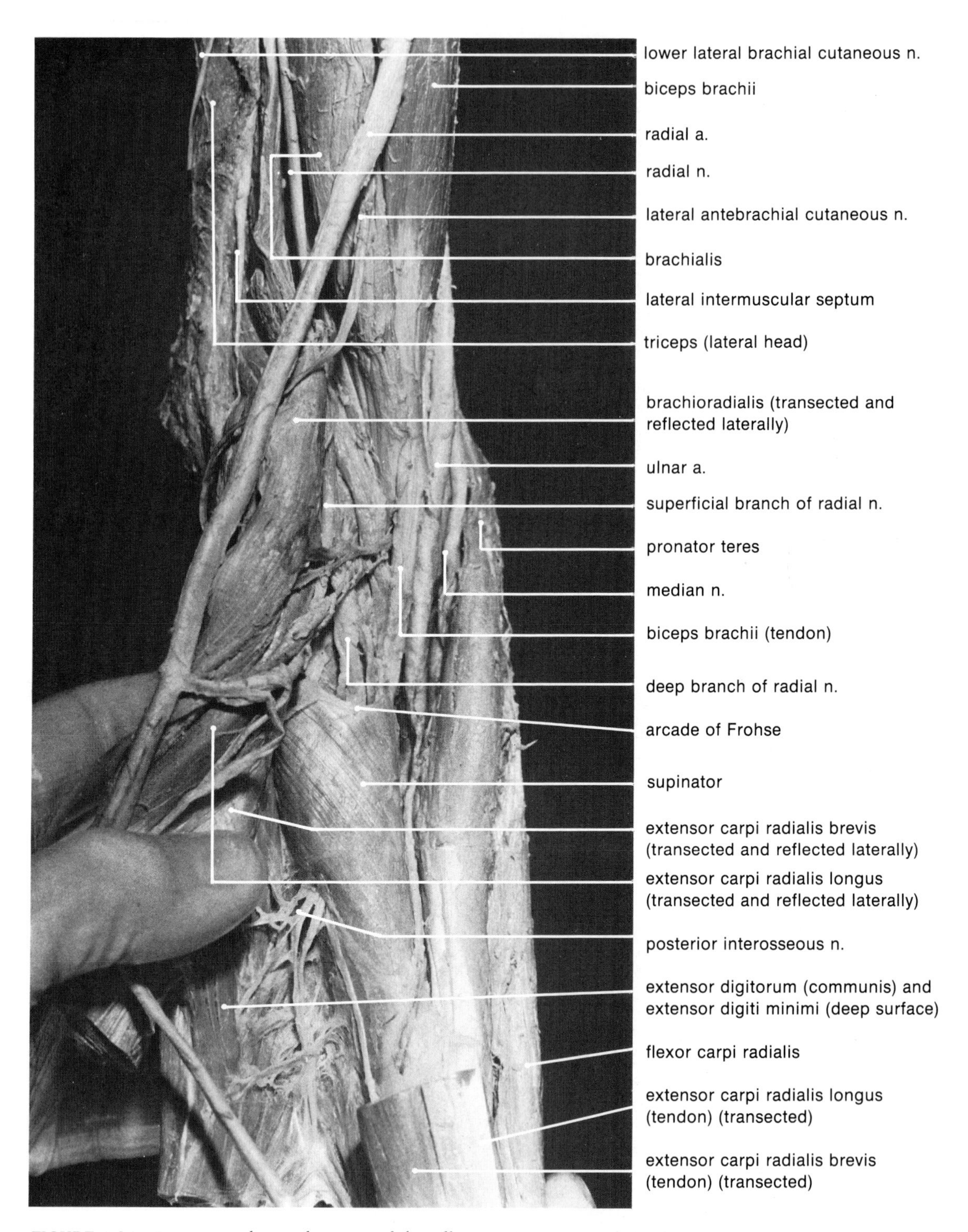

FIGURE 1-34 Deep muscles and nerves of the elbow region—anterolateral view (forearm in semipronation).
Note: The radial artery is continued from the superficial brachial artery in this case of high division of the brachial artery.

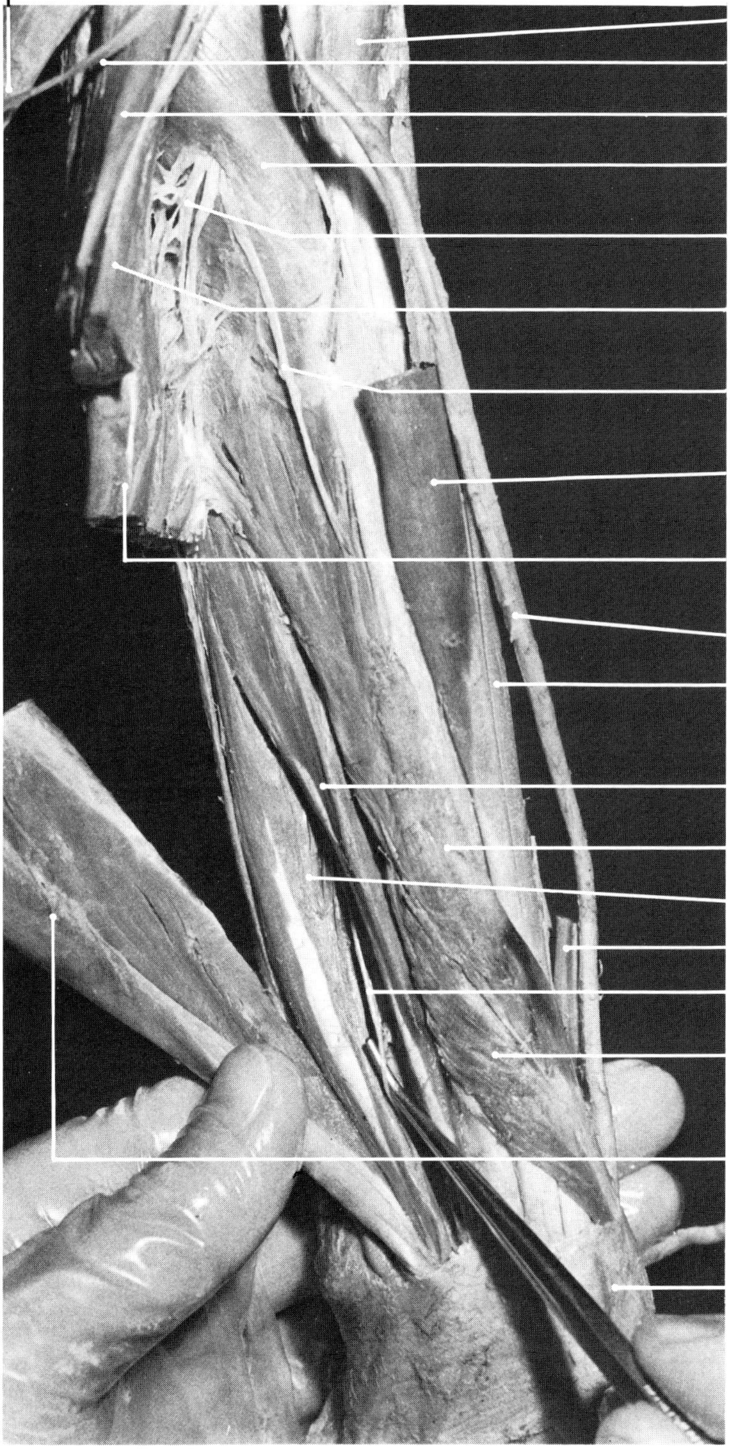

brachioradialis (transected proximal belly)

biceps brachii

lateral antebrachial cutaneous n.

extensor carpi radialis longus (transected proximal belly)

supinator

posterior interosseous n. emerging from under cover of supinator

extensor carpi radialis brevis (transected proximal belly)

branch of posterior interosseous nerve to abductor pollicis longus

extensor carpi radialis brevis (transected distal belly)

extensor digitorum (communis) and extensor digiti minimi (transected proximal bellies)

radial a.

extensor carpi radialis longus (tendon)

extensor pollicis longus

abductor pollicis longus

extensor indicis

brachioradialis (tendon) (cut end)

posterior interosseous n.

extensor pollicis brevis

extensor digitorum (communis) and extensor digiti minimi (transected distal bellies)

extensor retinaculum

FIGURE 1-35 Deep muscles of the forearm—posterior view (hand in semipronation).
Note: The probe is elevating the posterior interosseous nerve in the distal forearm.

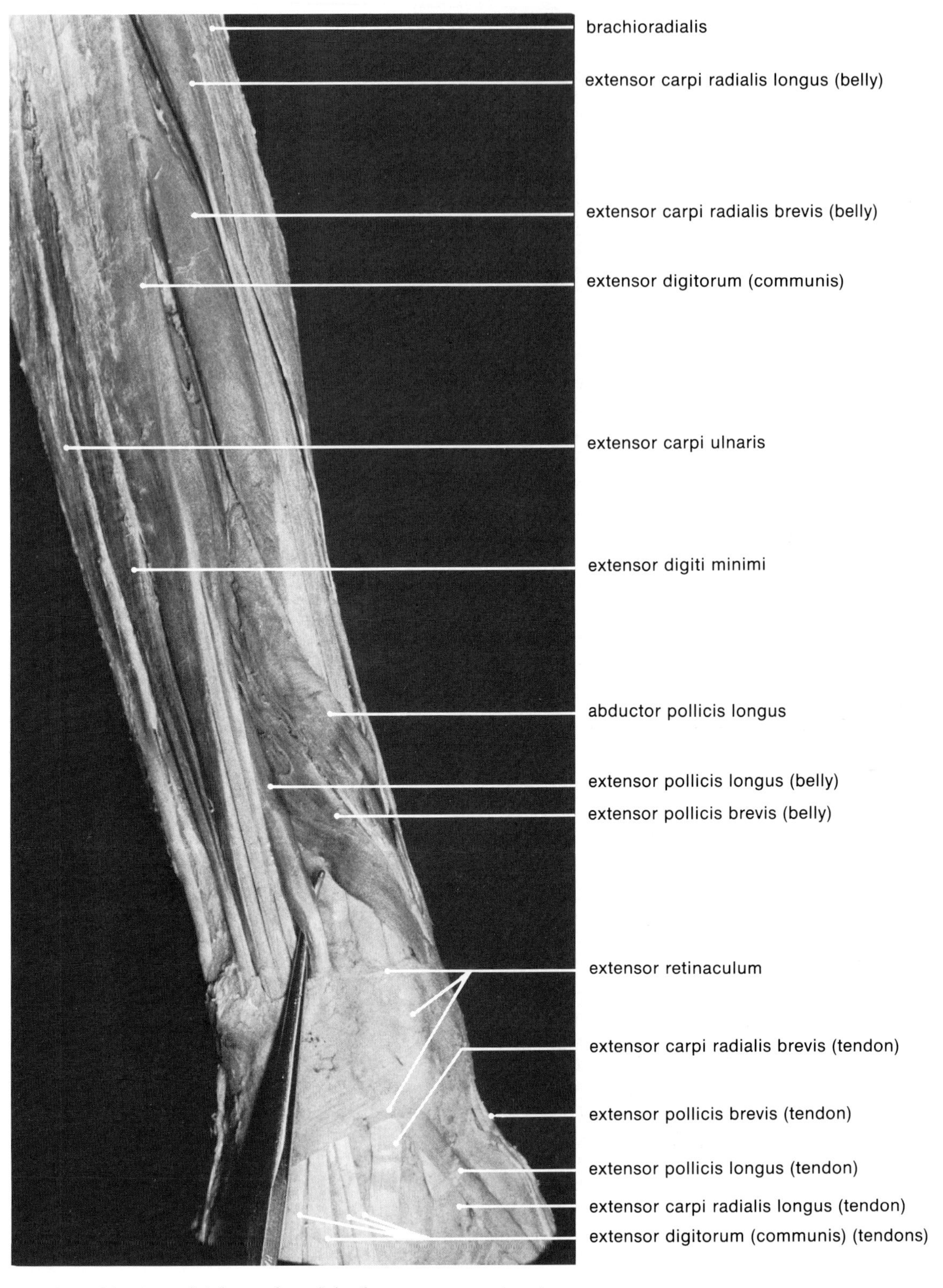

FIGURE 1-36 Superficial muscles of the forearm—posterior view.

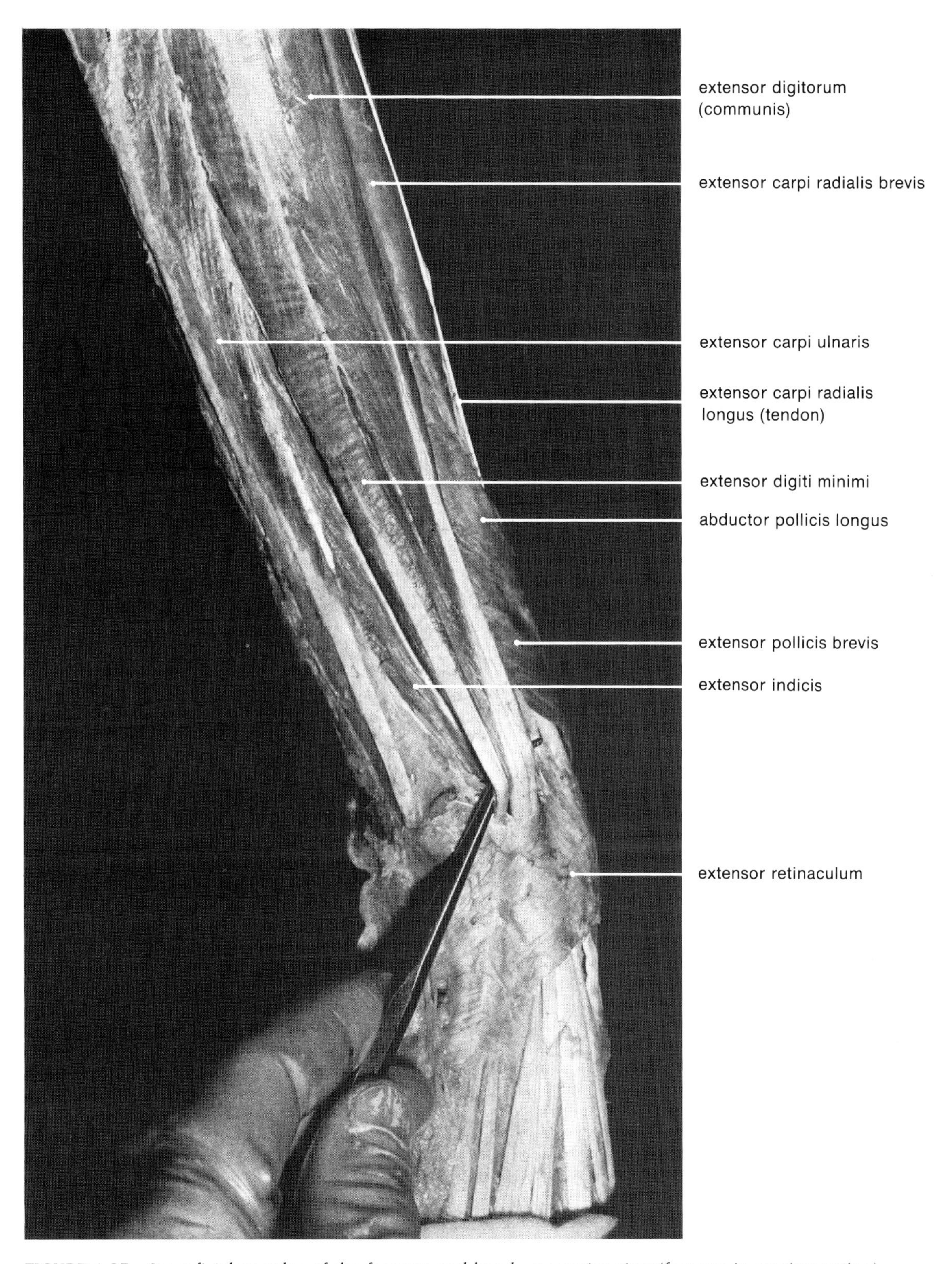

FIGURE 1-37 Superficial muscles of the forearm and hand—posterior view (forearm in semipronation).

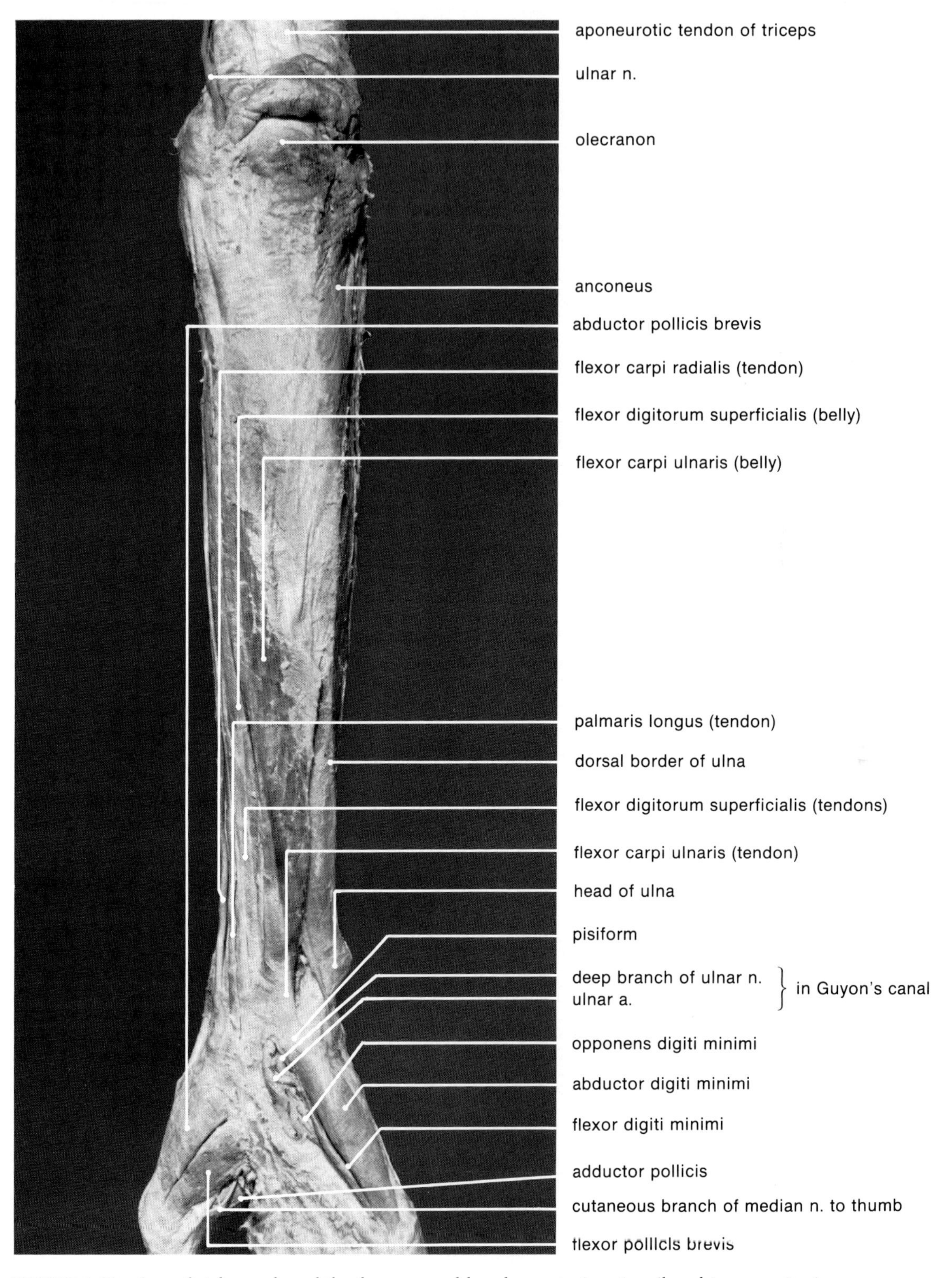

FIGURE 1-38 Superficial muscles of the forearm and hand—posterior view (hand in pronation).

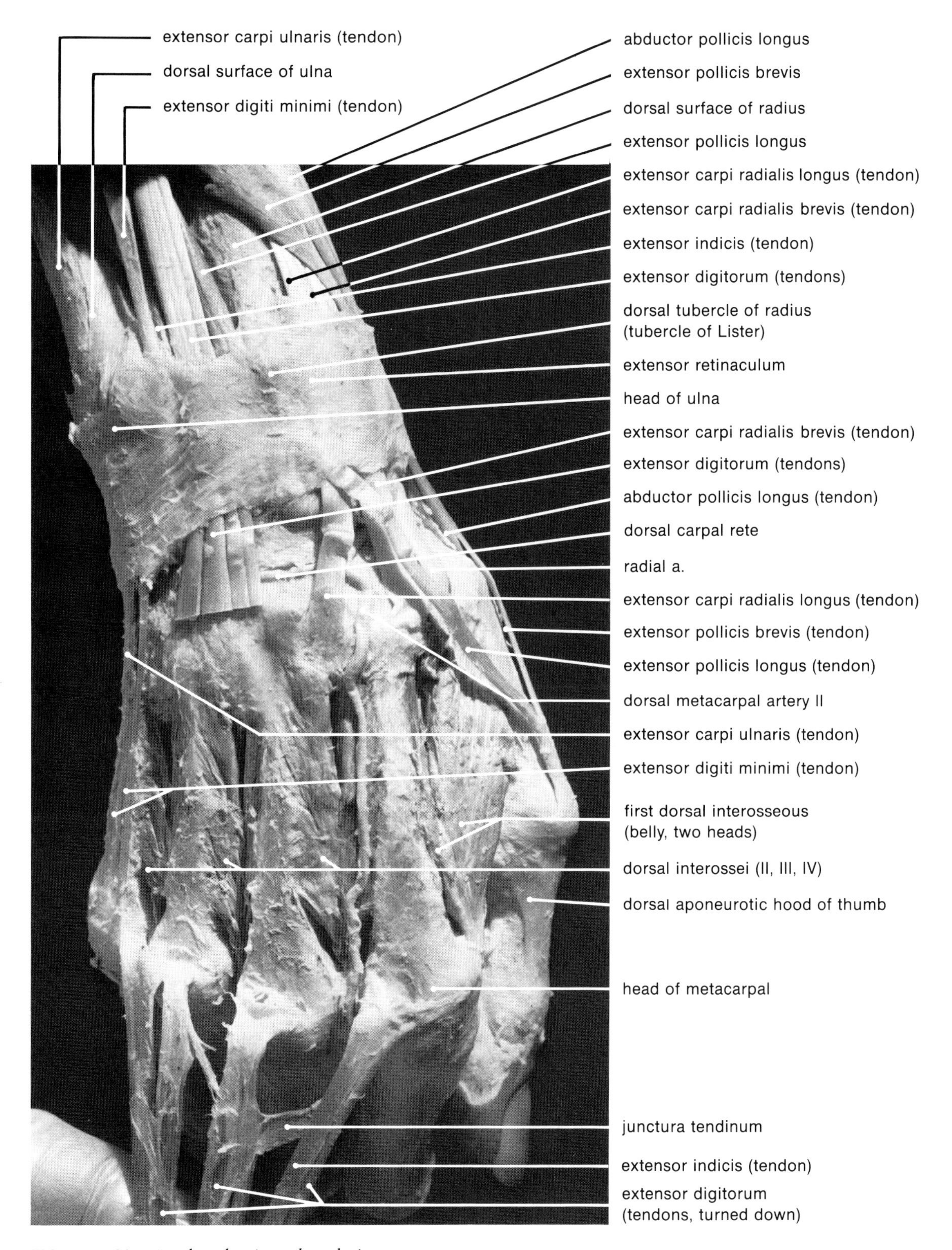

FIGURE 1-39 Hand and wrist—dorsal view.

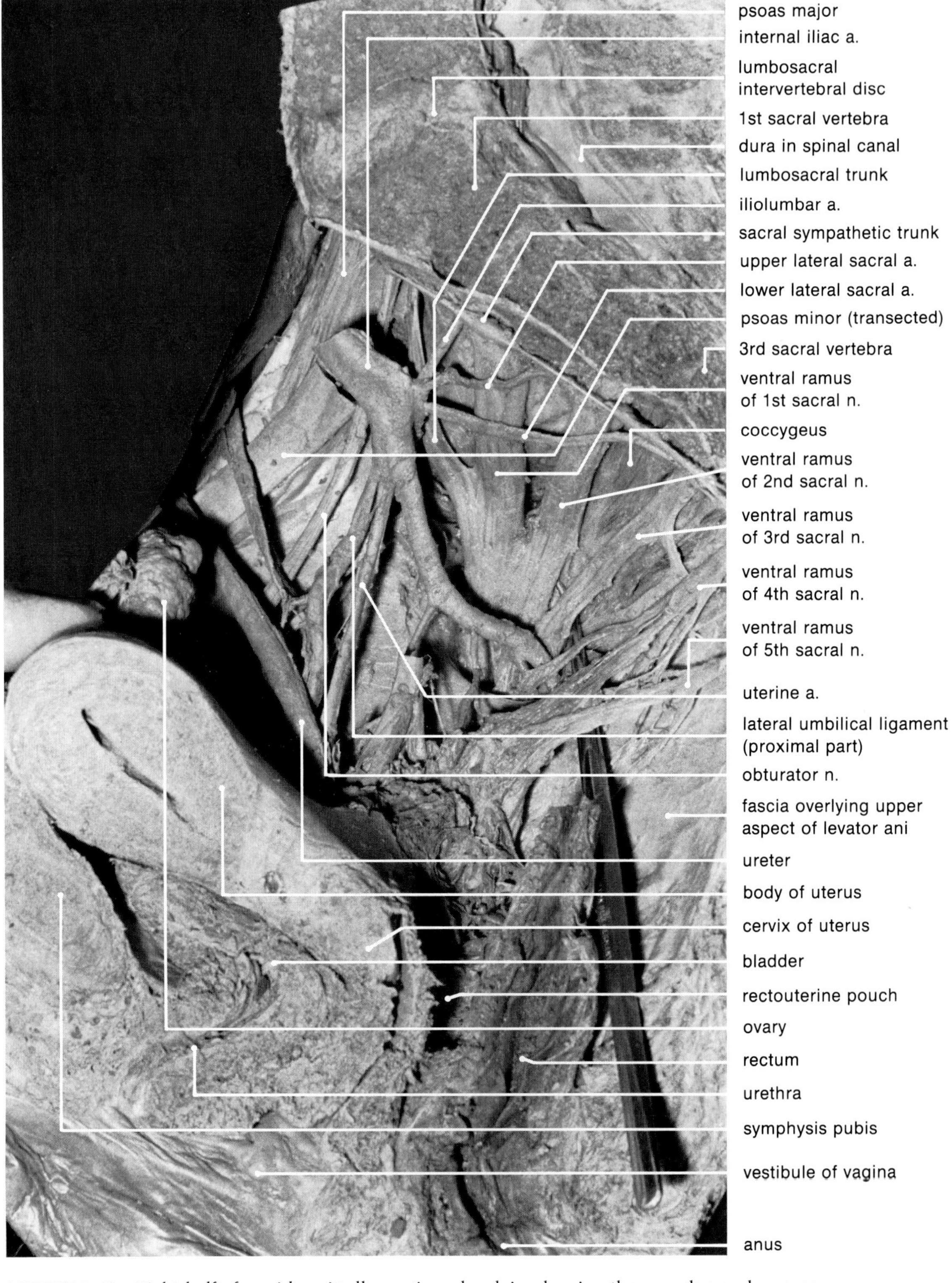

FIGURE 1-40 Right half of a mid-sagittally sectioned pelvis, showing the muscles and nerves.

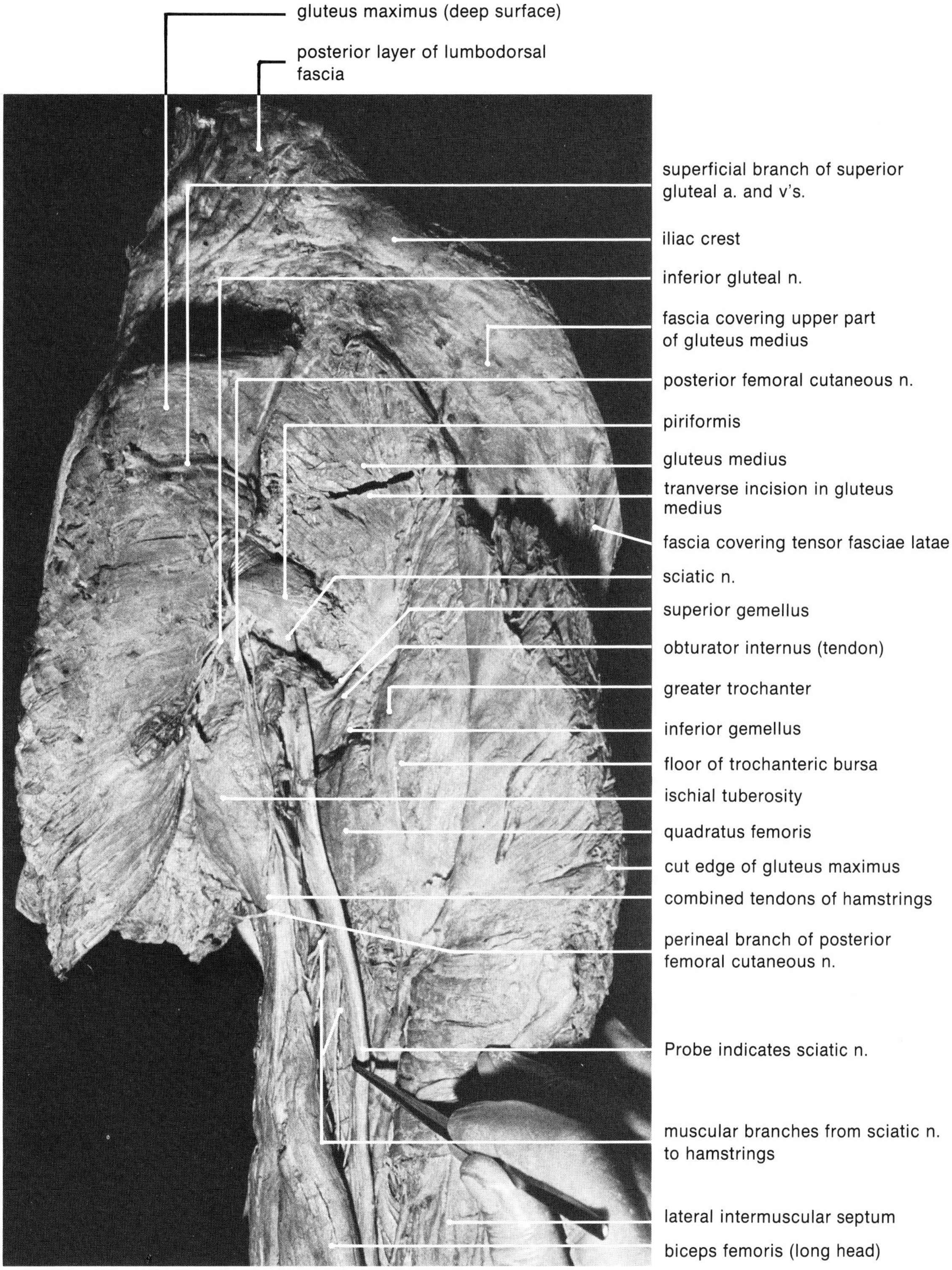

gluteus maximus (deep surface)

posterior layer of lumbodorsal fascia

superficial branch of superior gluteal a. and v's.

iliac crest

inferior gluteal n.

fascia covering upper part of gluteus medius

posterior femoral cutaneous n.

piriformis

gluteus medius

tranverse incision in gluteus medius

fascia covering tensor fasciae latae

sciatic n.

superior gemellus

obturator internus (tendon)

greater trochanter

inferior gemellus

floor of trochanteric bursa

ischial tuberosity

quadratus femoris

cut edge of gluteus maximus

combined tendons of hamstrings

perineal branch of posterior femoral cutaneous n.

Probe indicates sciatic n.

muscular branches from sciatic n. to hamstrings

lateral intermuscular septum

biceps femoris (long head)

FIGURE 1-41 Superficial dissection of the muscles and nerves of the gluteal region and upper thigh—posterior view.
Note: The gluteus maximus has been divided vertically and the medial and lateral portions reflected.

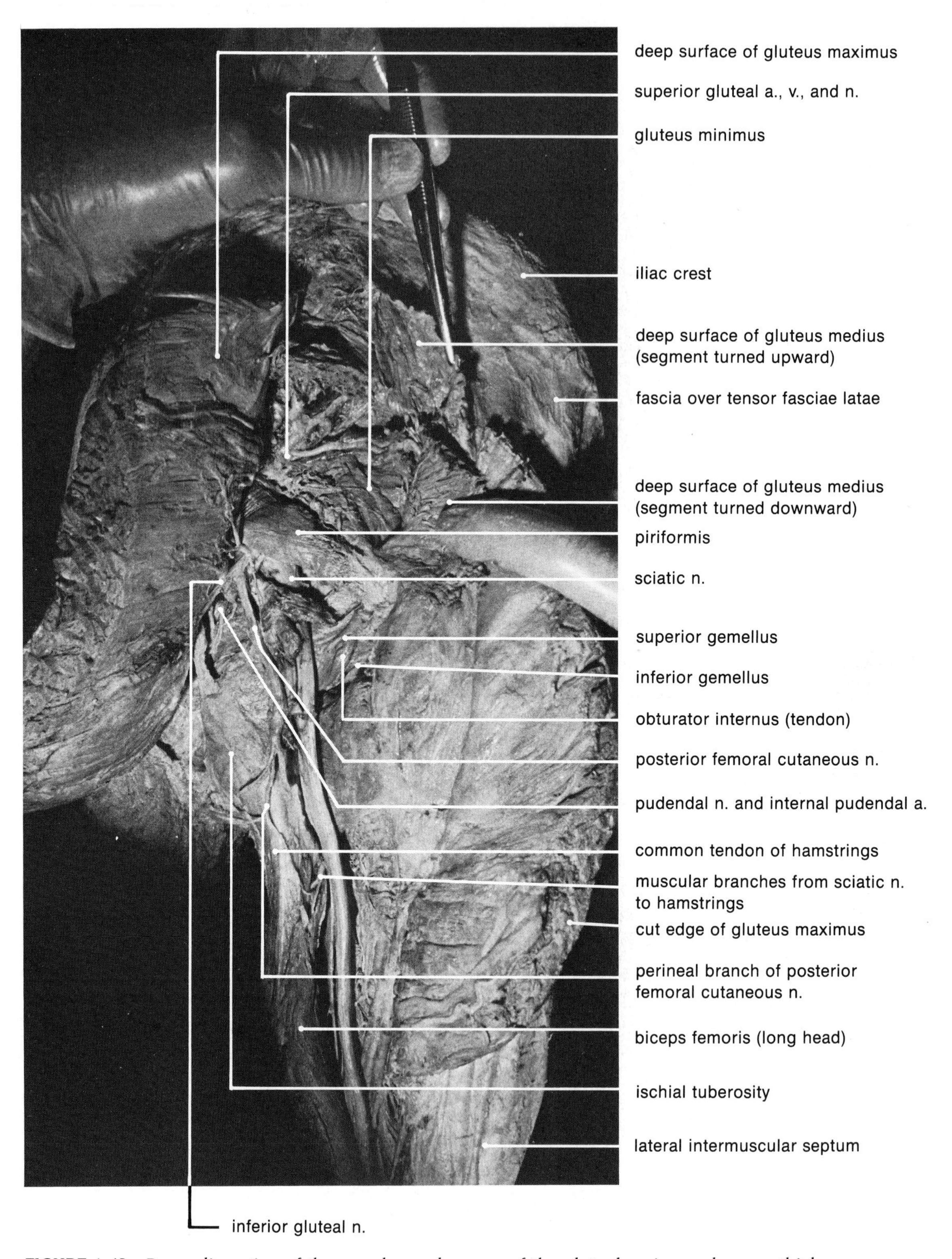

FIGURE 1-42 Deep dissection of the muscles and nerves of the gluteal region and upper thigh—posterior view.

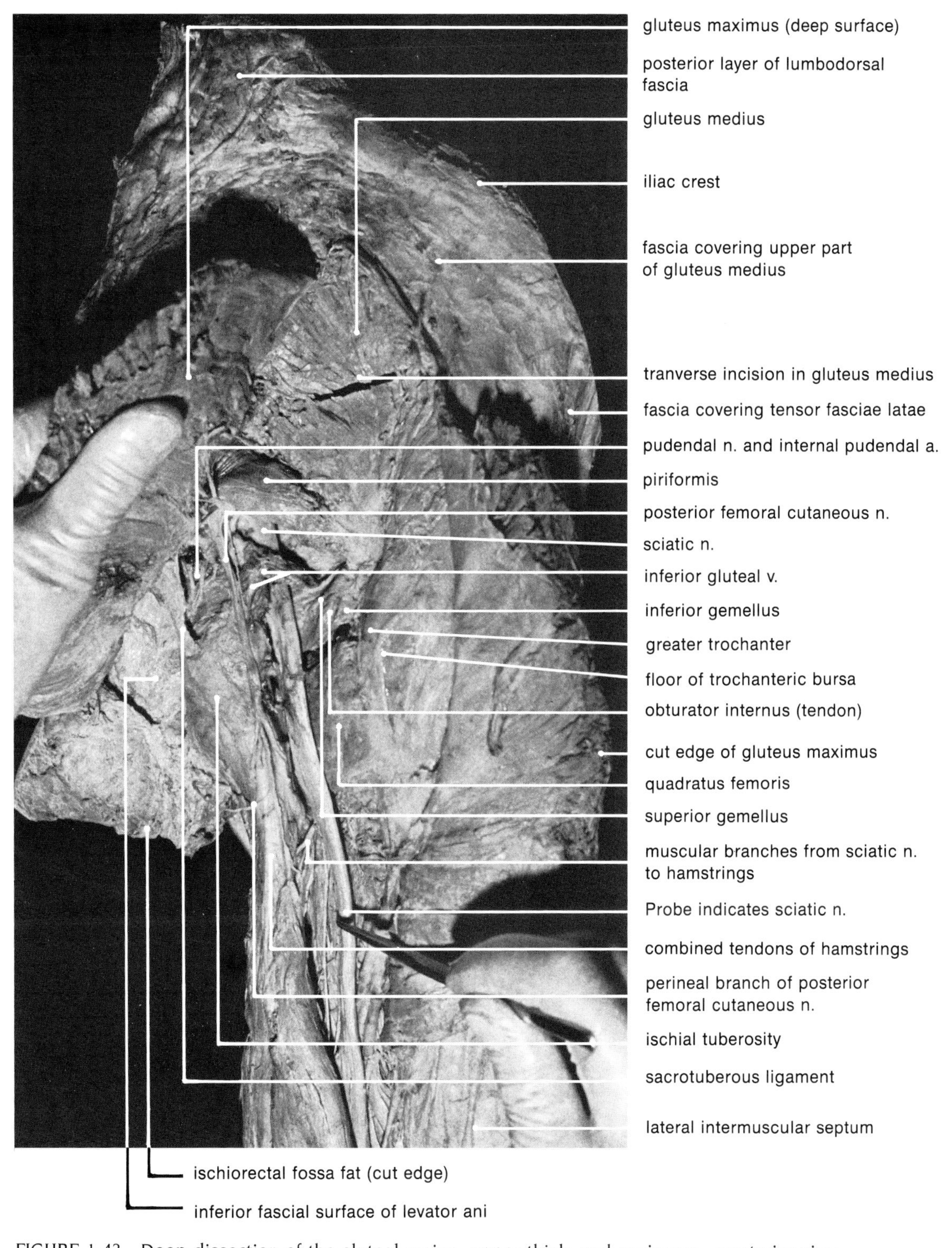

FIGURE 1-43 Deep dissection of the gluteal region, upper thigh, and perineum—posterior view.

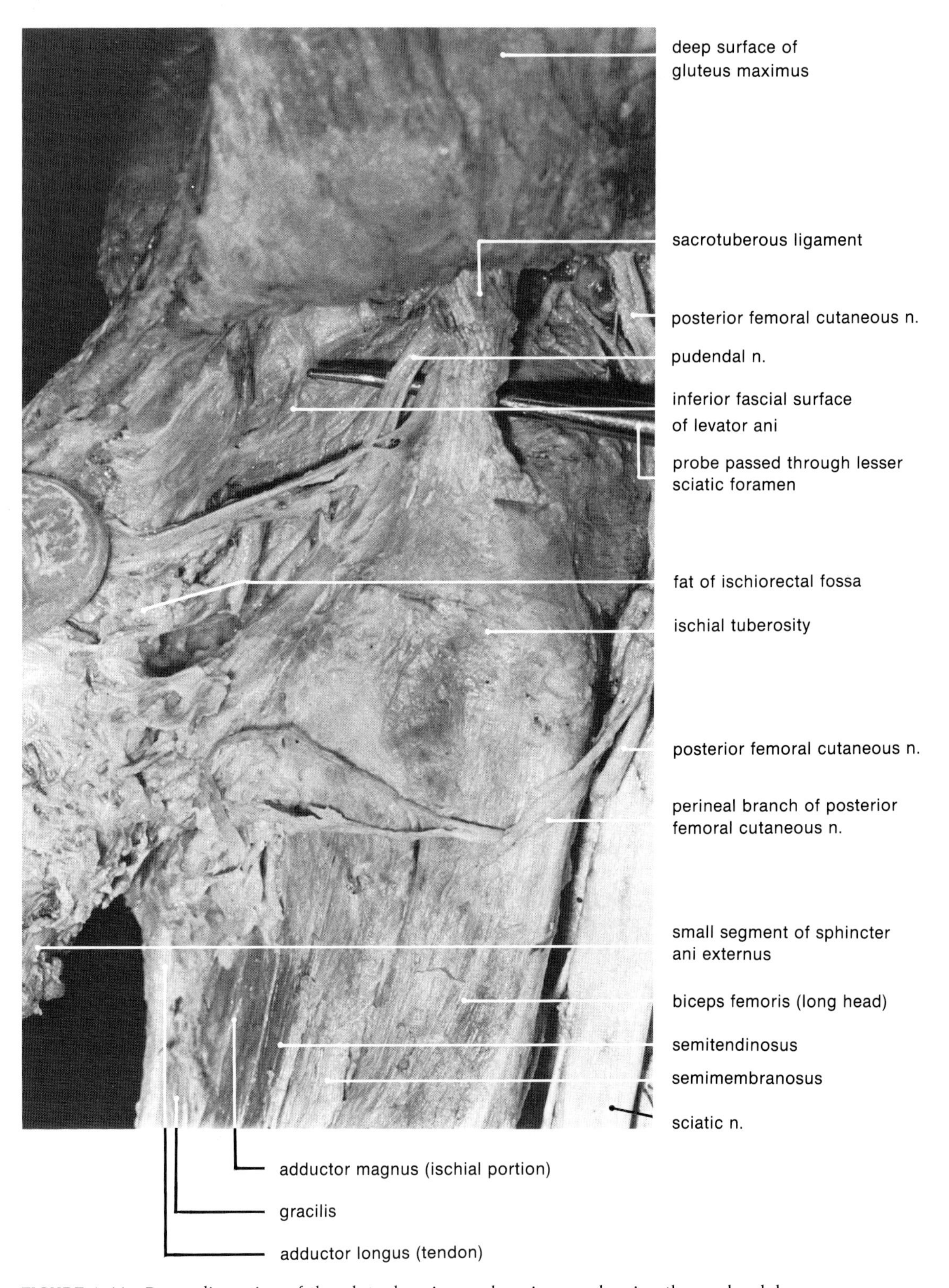

FIGURE 1-44 Deep dissection of the gluteal region and perineum showing the pudendal nerve.

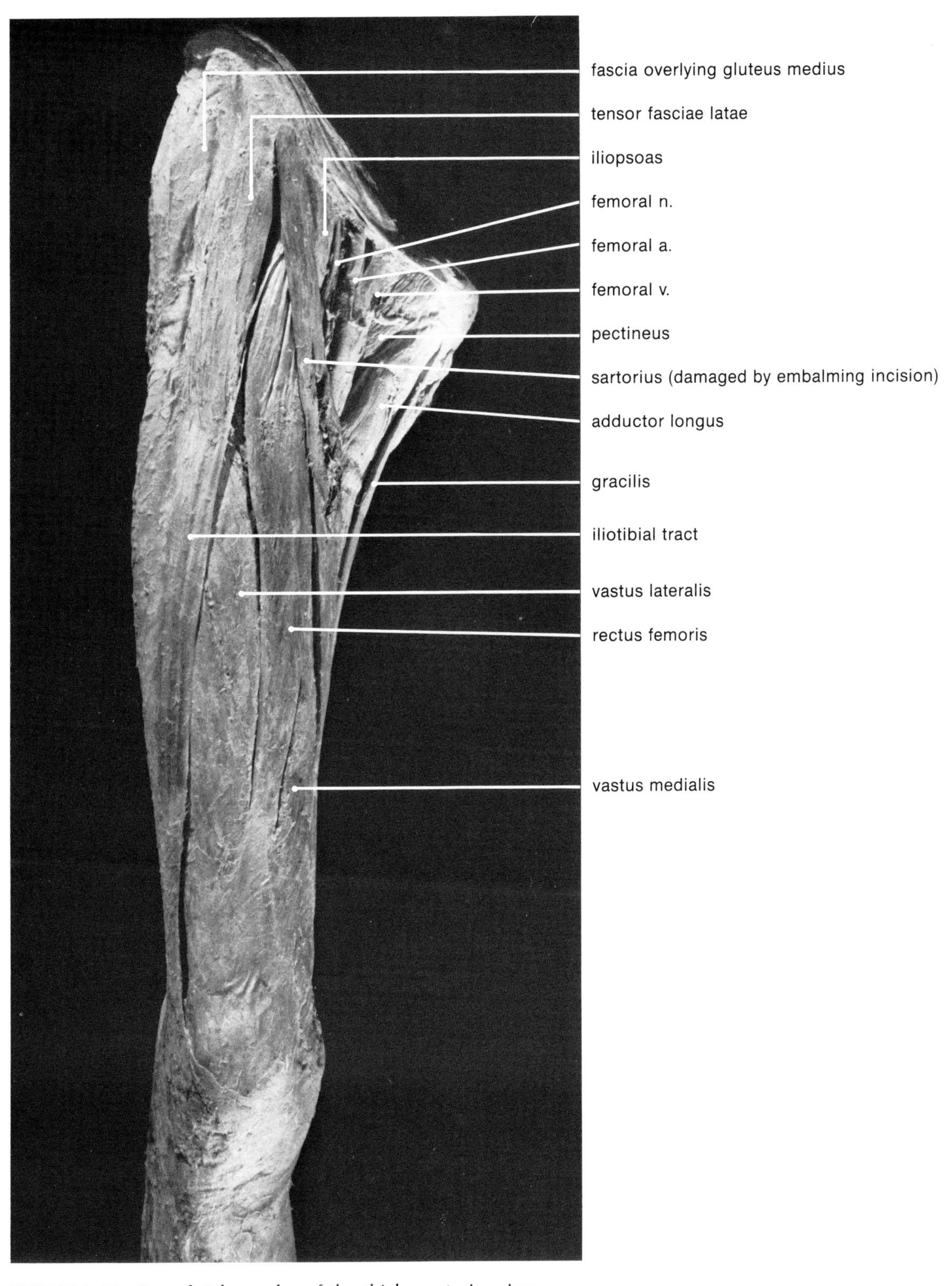

FIGURE 1-45 Superficial muscles of the thigh—anterior view.

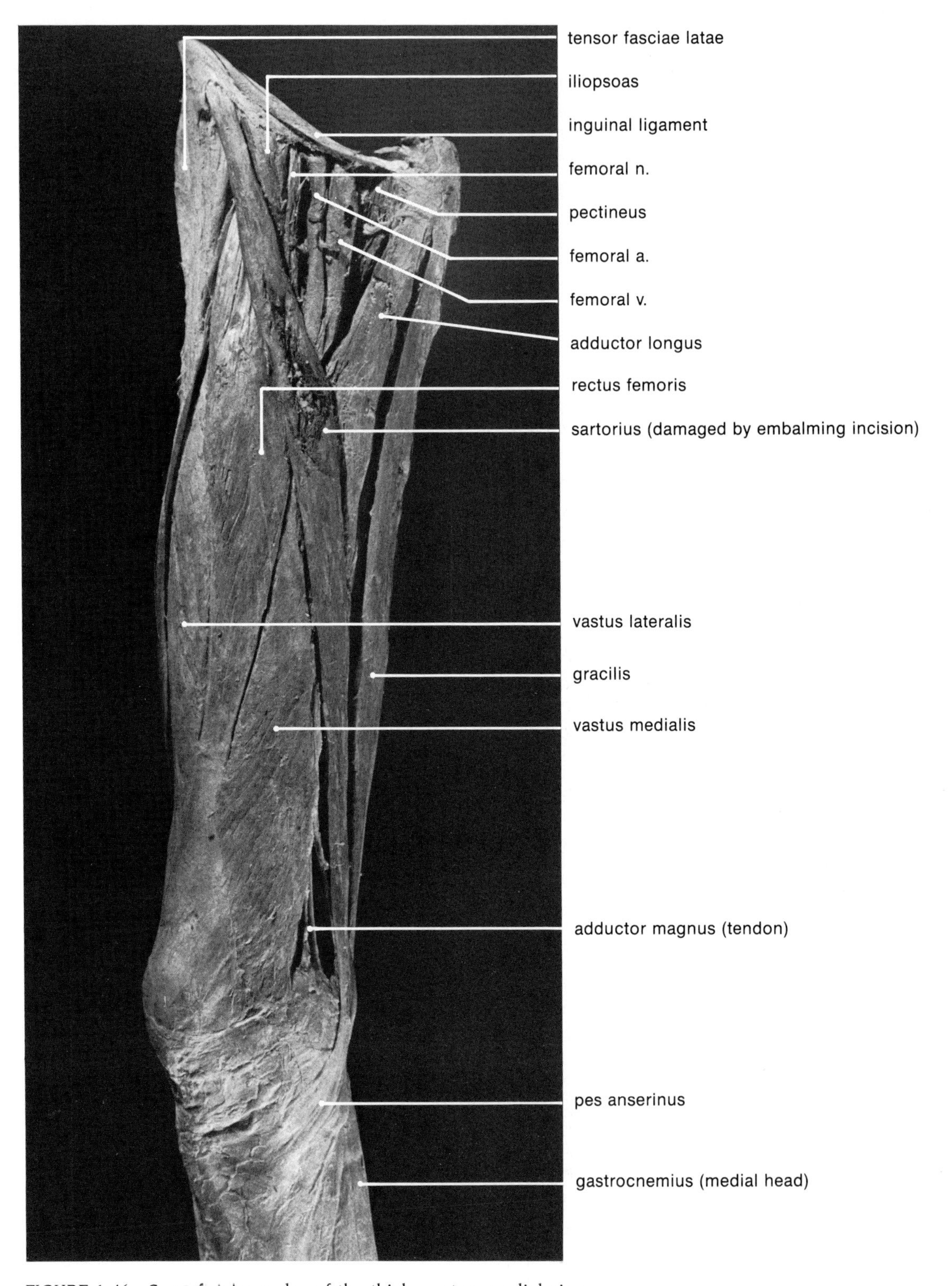

FIGURE 1-46 Superficial muscles of the thigh—anteromedial view.

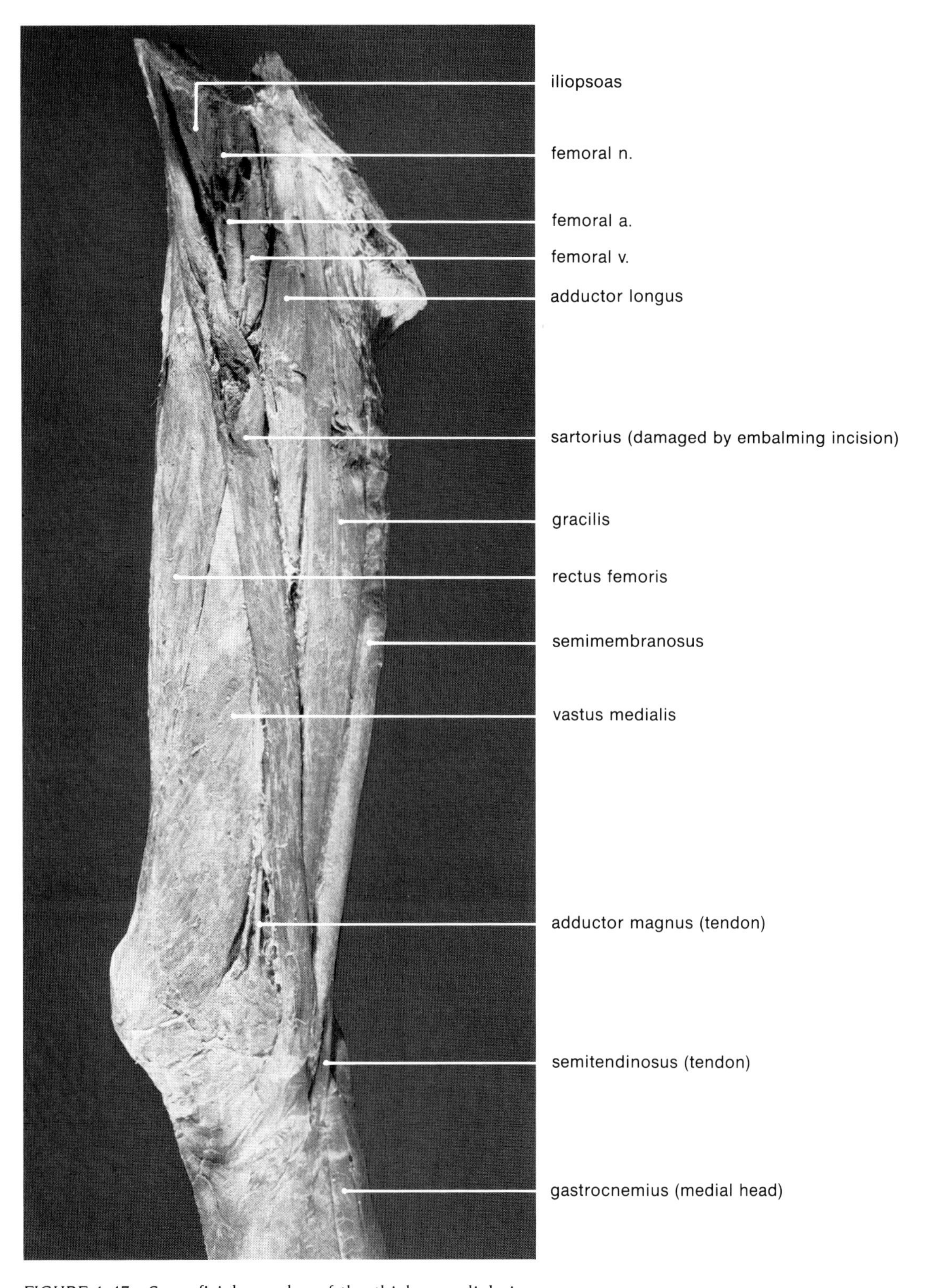

FIGURE 1-47 Superficial muscles of the thigh—medial view.

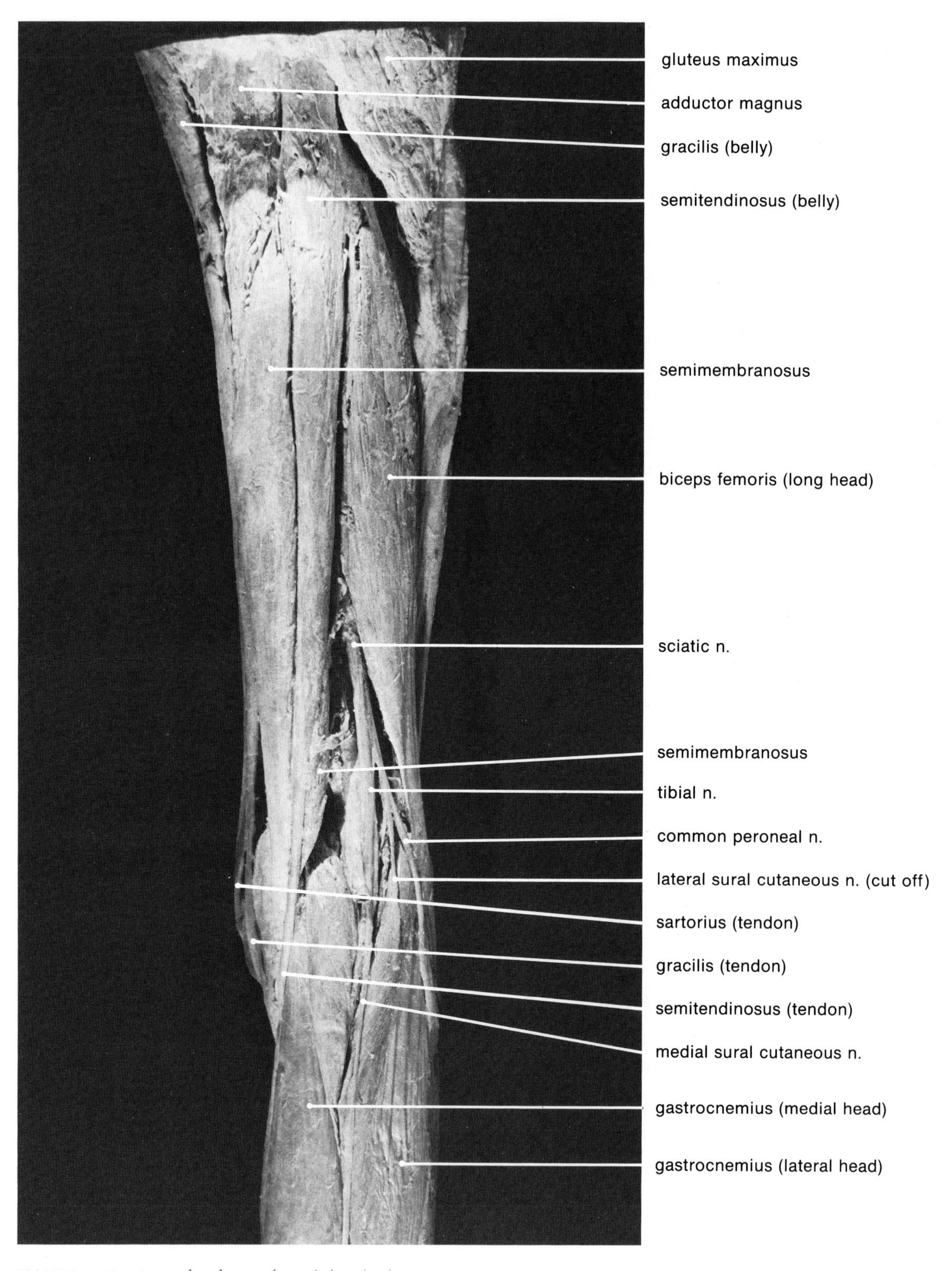

FIGURE 1-48 Superficial muscles of the thigh—posterior view.

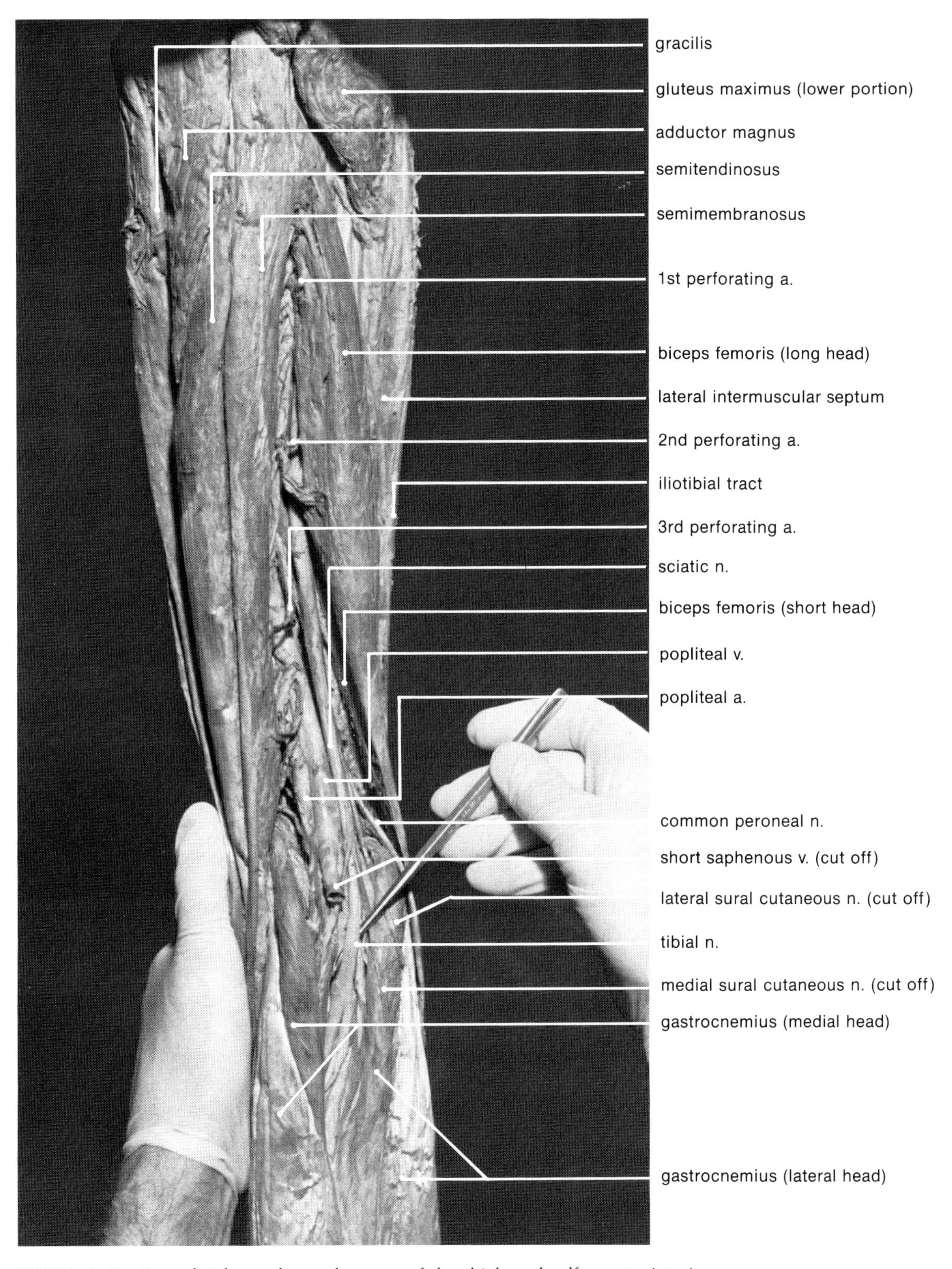

FIGURE 1-49 Superficial muscles and nerves of the thigh and calf—posterior view.
Note: The medial and lateral heads of the gastrocnemius are separated to expose the tibial nerve, which is elevated by the probe.

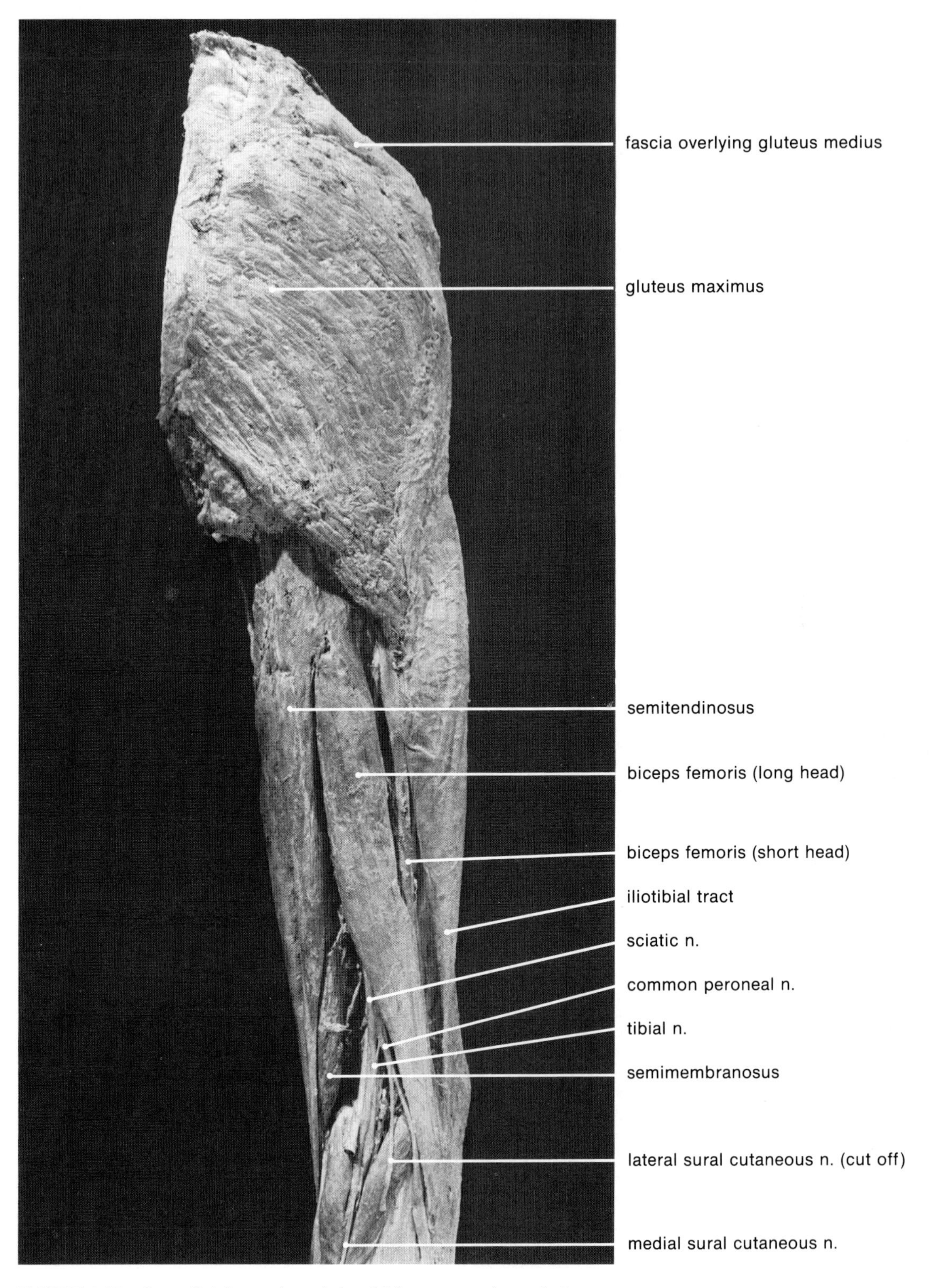

FIGURE 1-50 Superficial muscles of the thigh—posterolateral view.

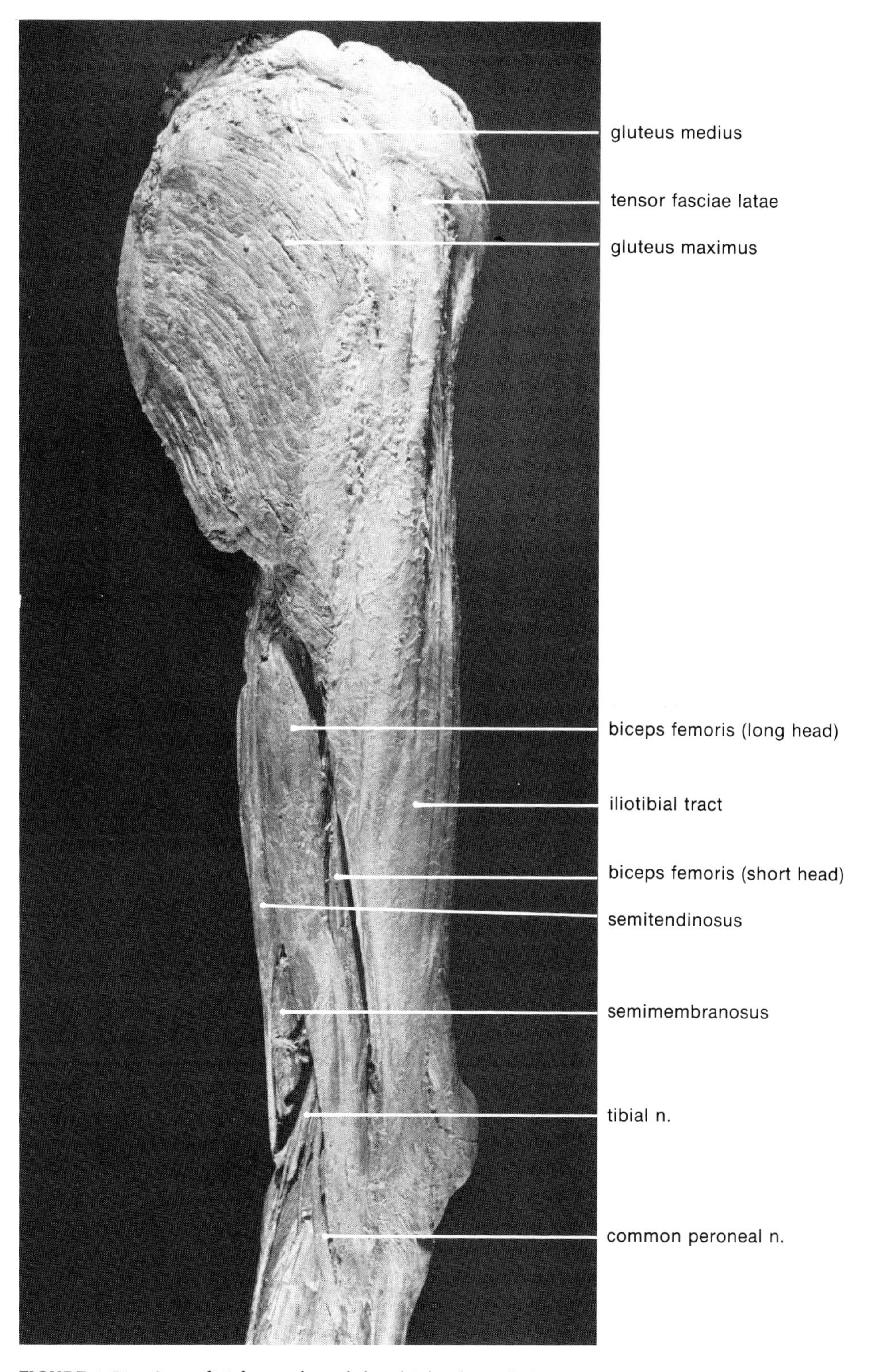

FIGURE 1-51 Superficial muscles of the thigh—lateral view.

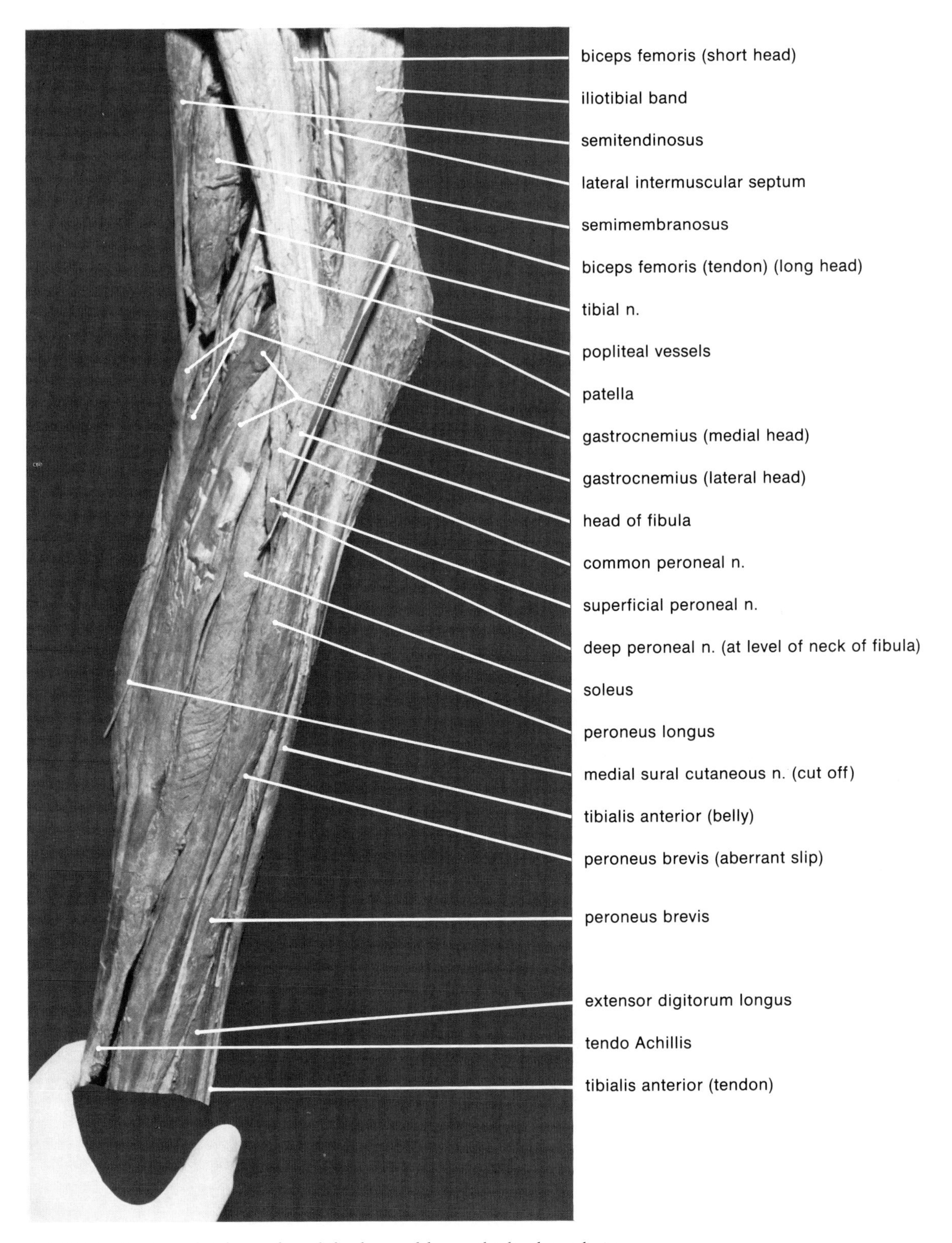

FIGURE 1-52 Superficial muscles of the leg and lower thigh—lateral view.
Note: The tip of the probe elevates the deep peroneal nerve.

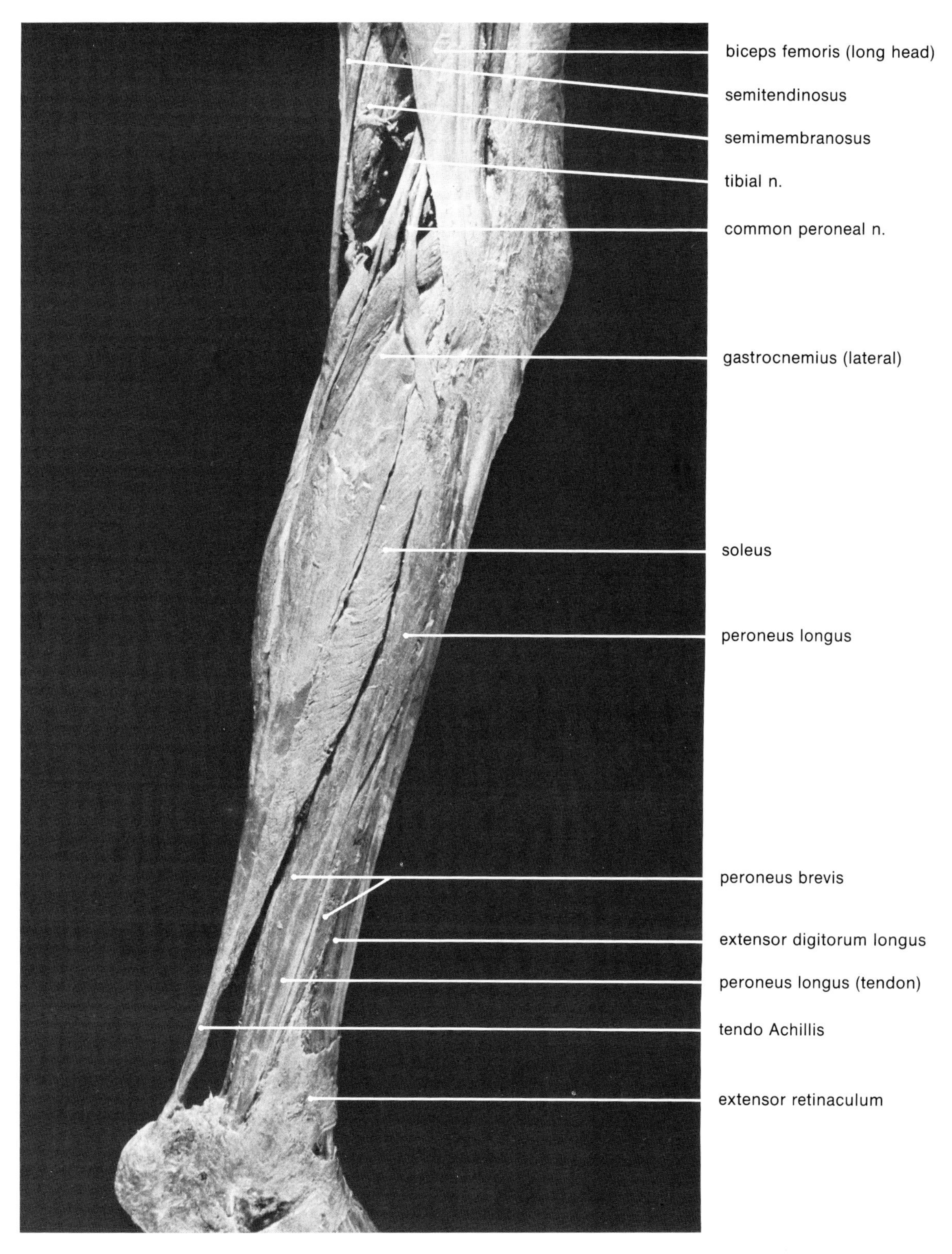

FIGURE 1-53 Superficial muscles of the leg—lateral view.

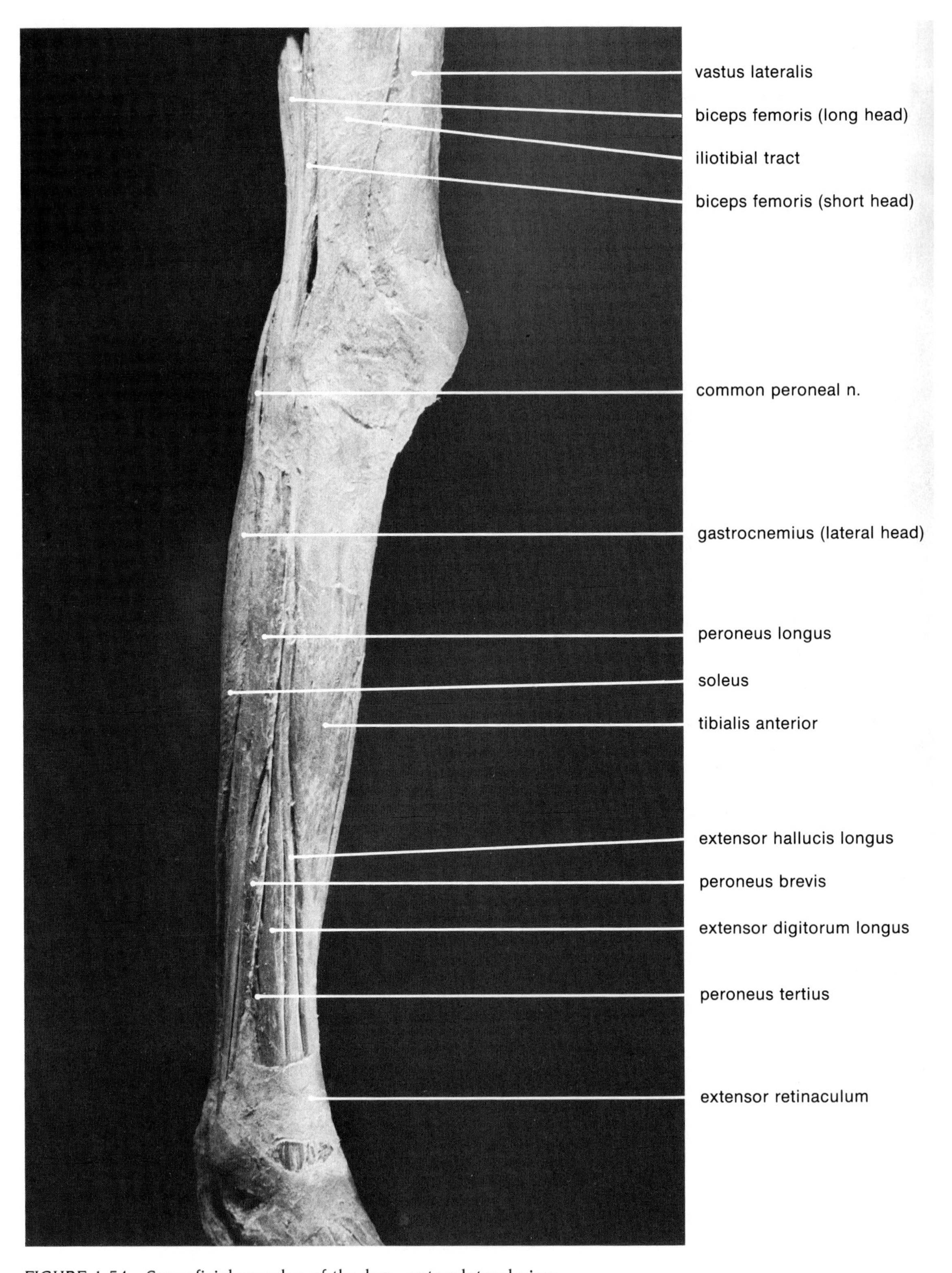

FIGURE 1-54 Superficial muscles of the leg—anterolateral view.

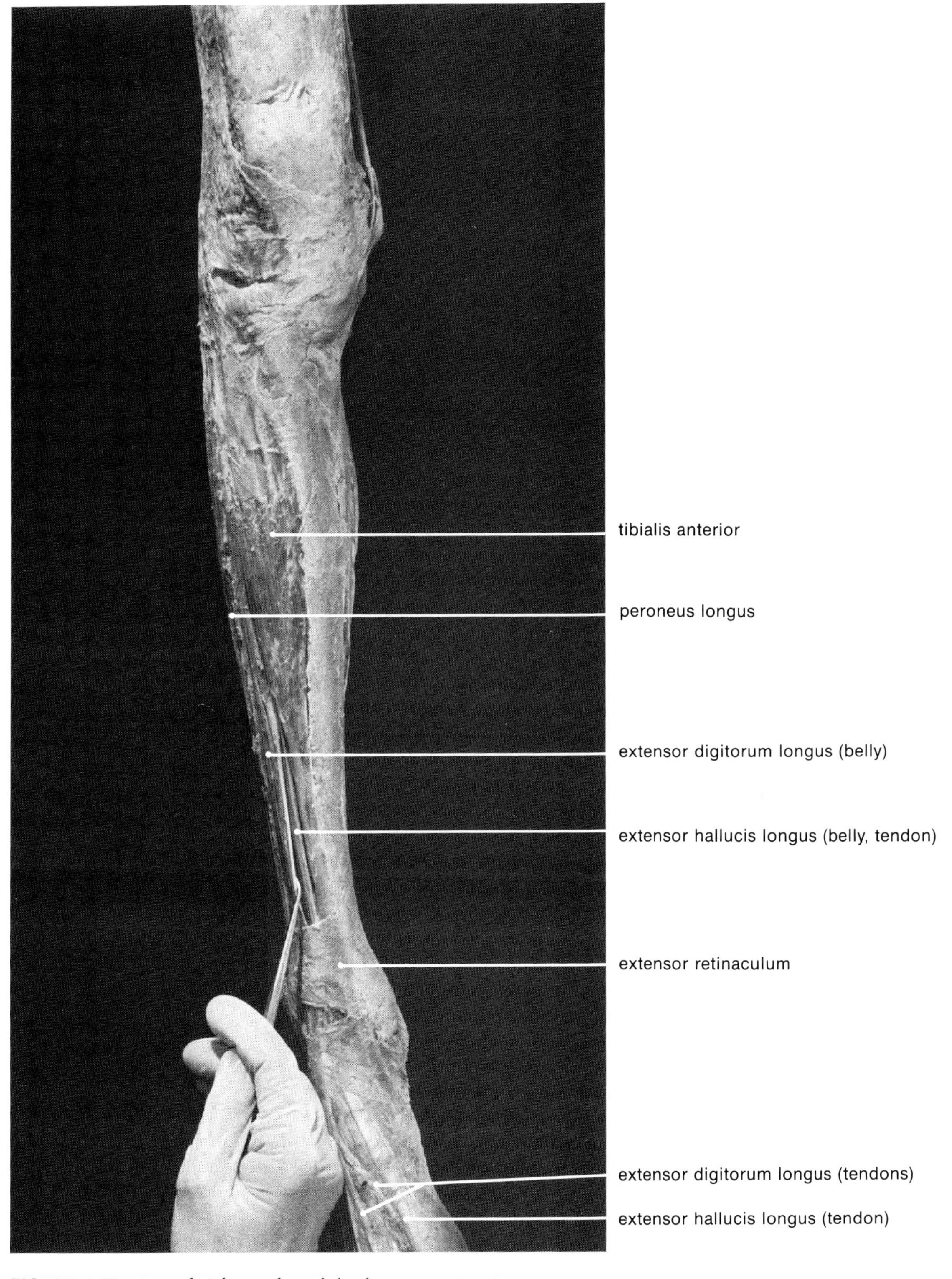

FIGURE 1-55 Superficial muscles of the leg—anterior view.

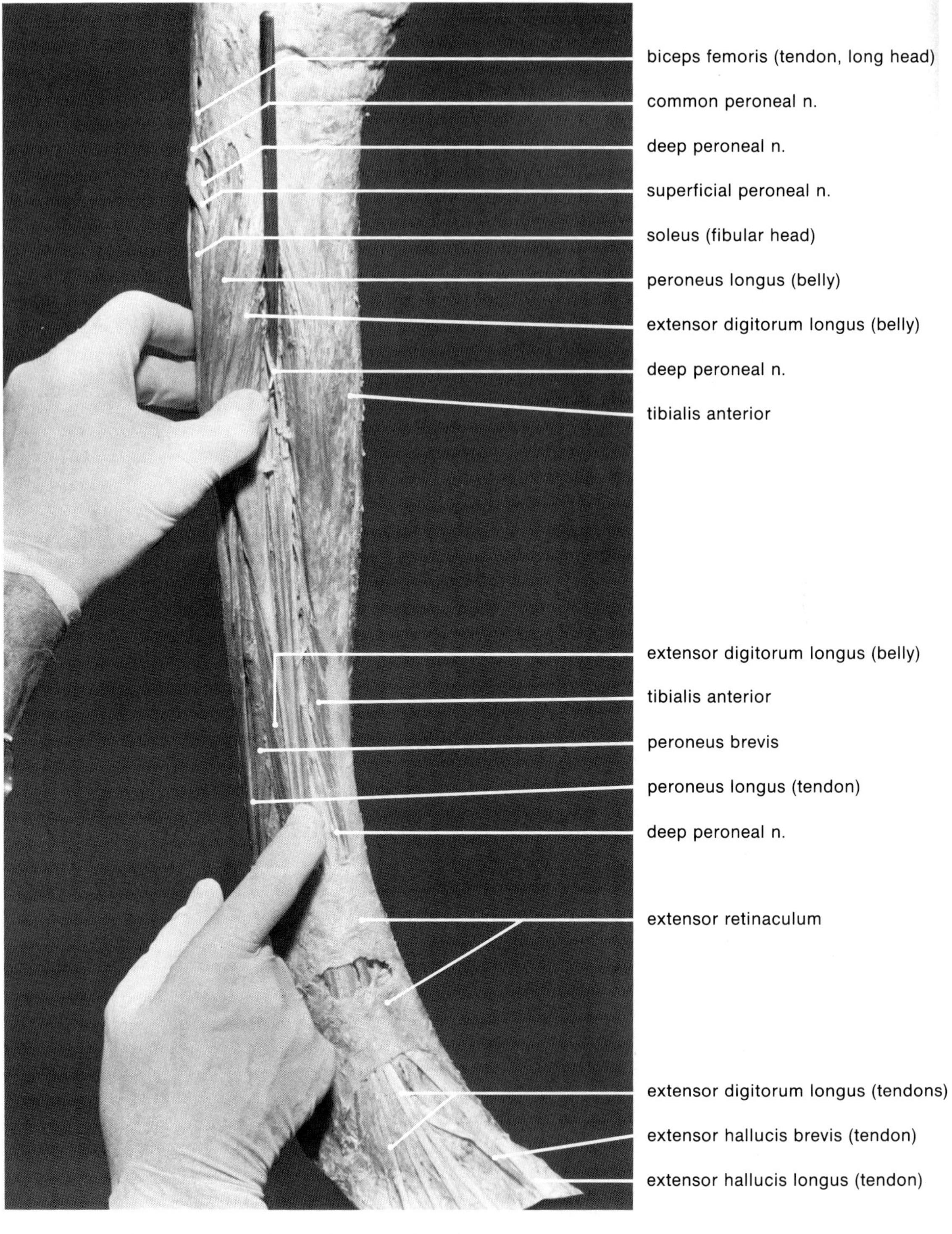

FIGURE 1-56 Superficial muscles and nerves of the leg—anterior view. *Note*: The tip of the probe is elevating the deep peroneal nerve.

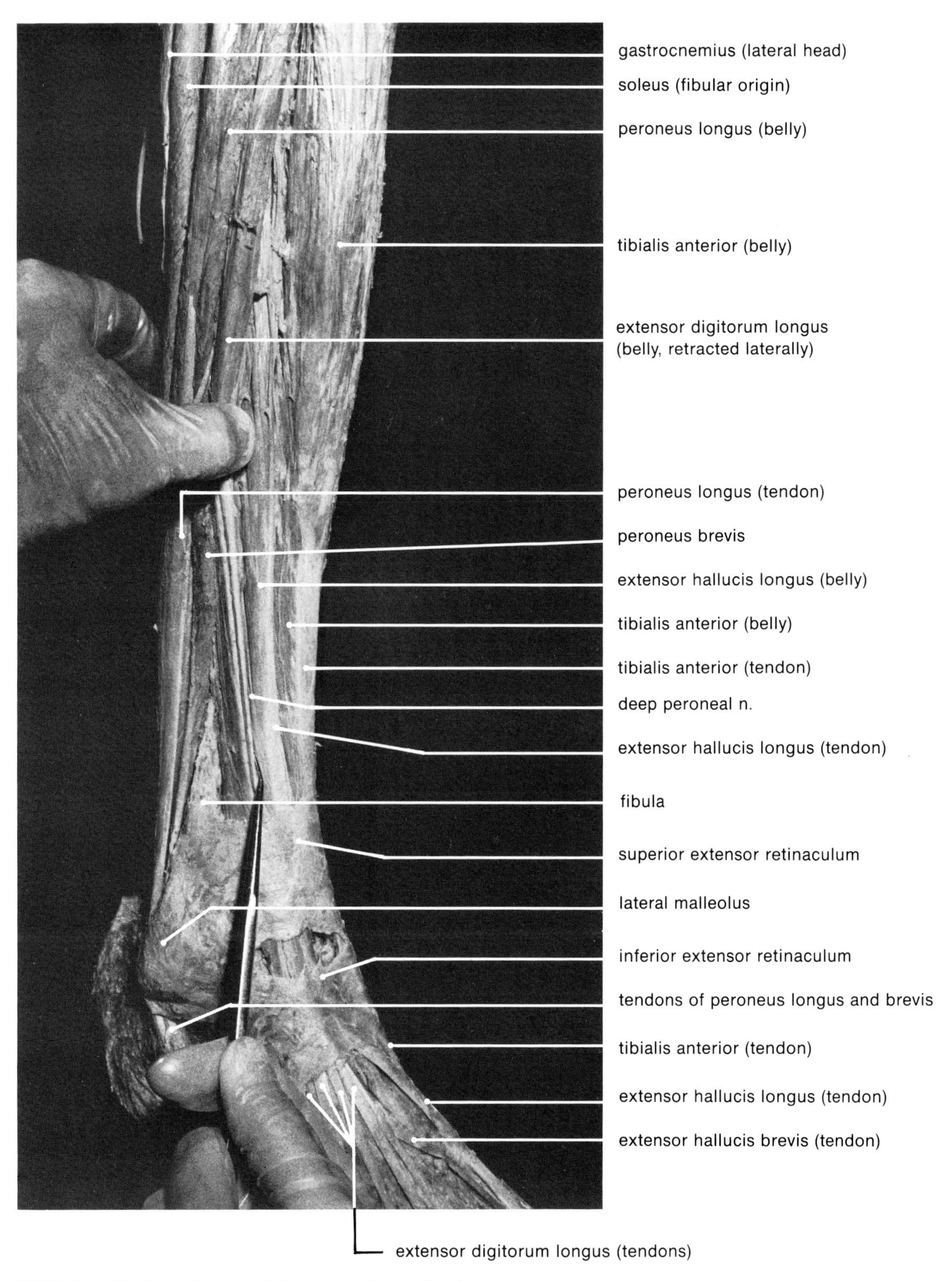

FIGURE 1-57 Superficial and deep muscles of the leg—anterolateral view.

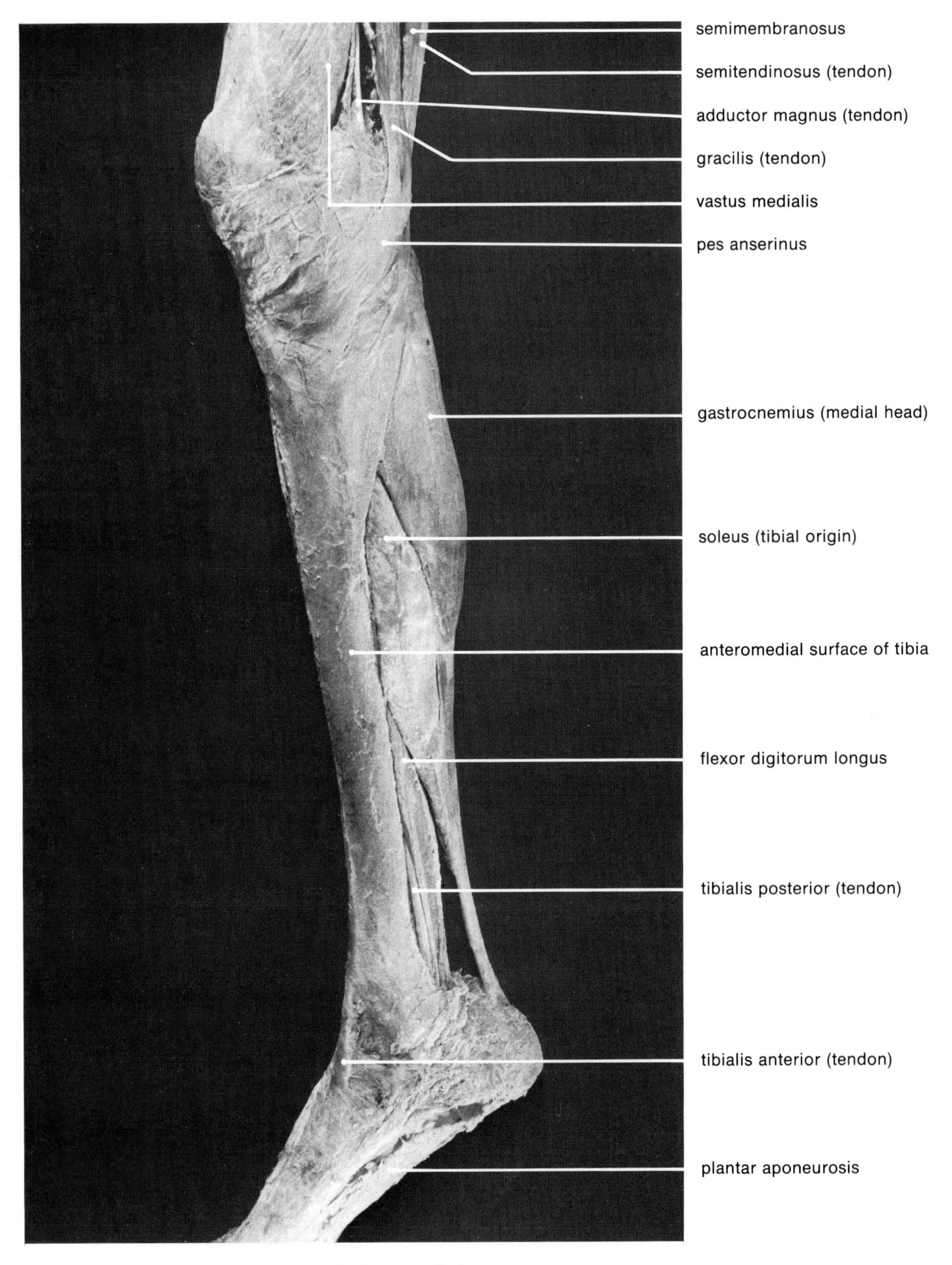

FIGURE 1-58 Superficial muscles of the leg—medial view.

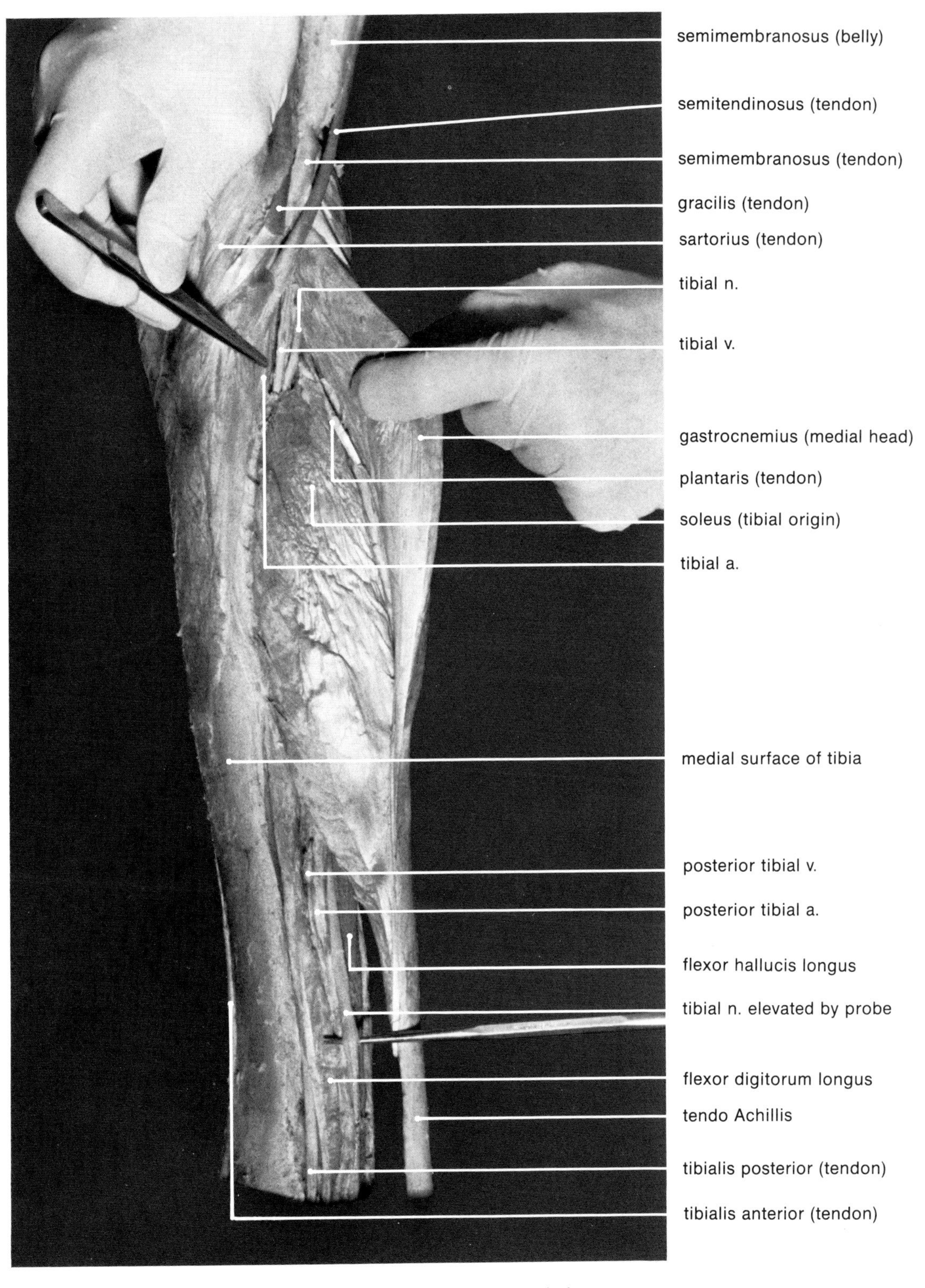

FIGURE 1-59 Superficial muscles and nerves of the leg—medial view.

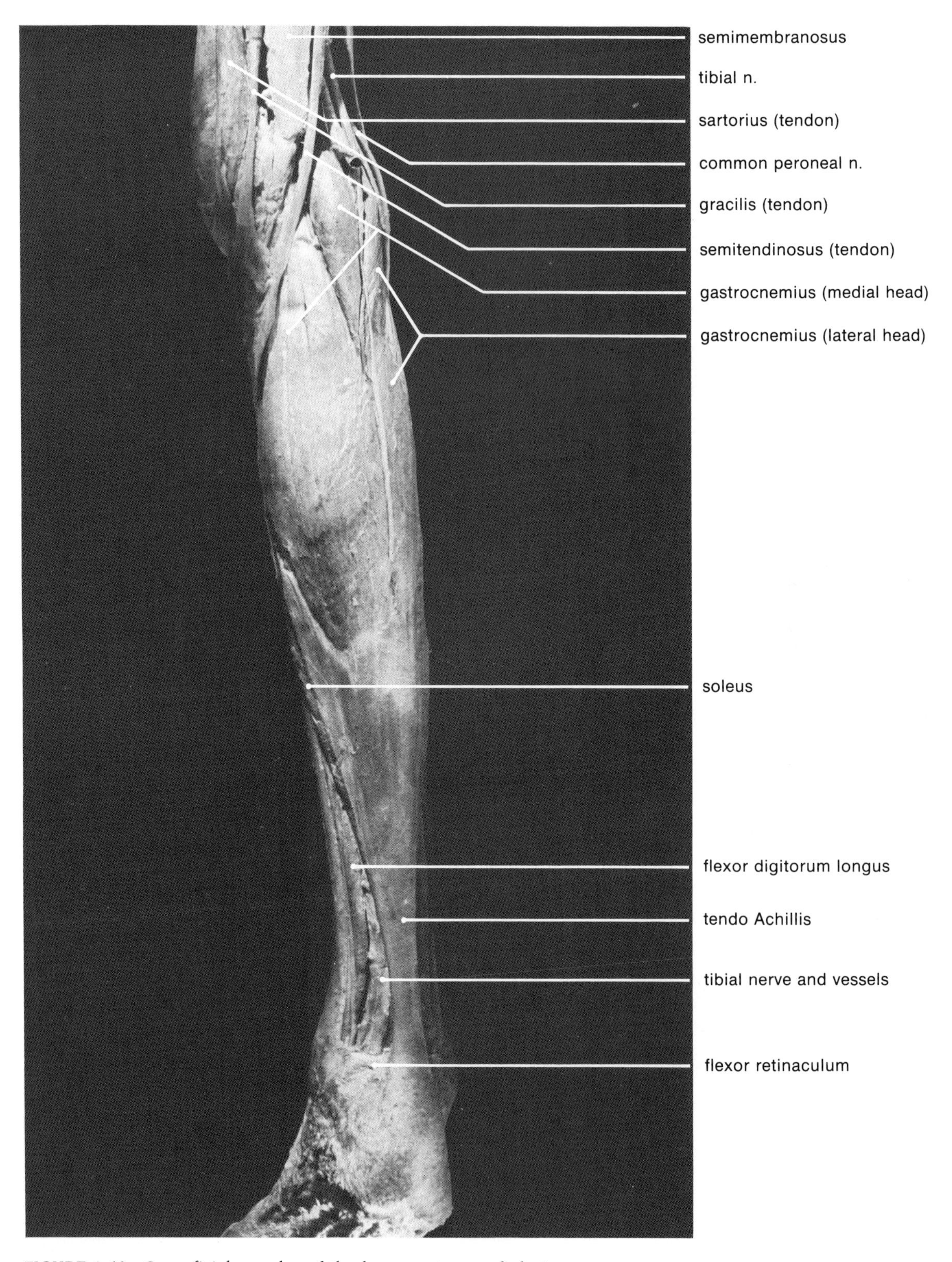

FIGURE 1-60 Superficial muscles of the leg—posteromedial view.

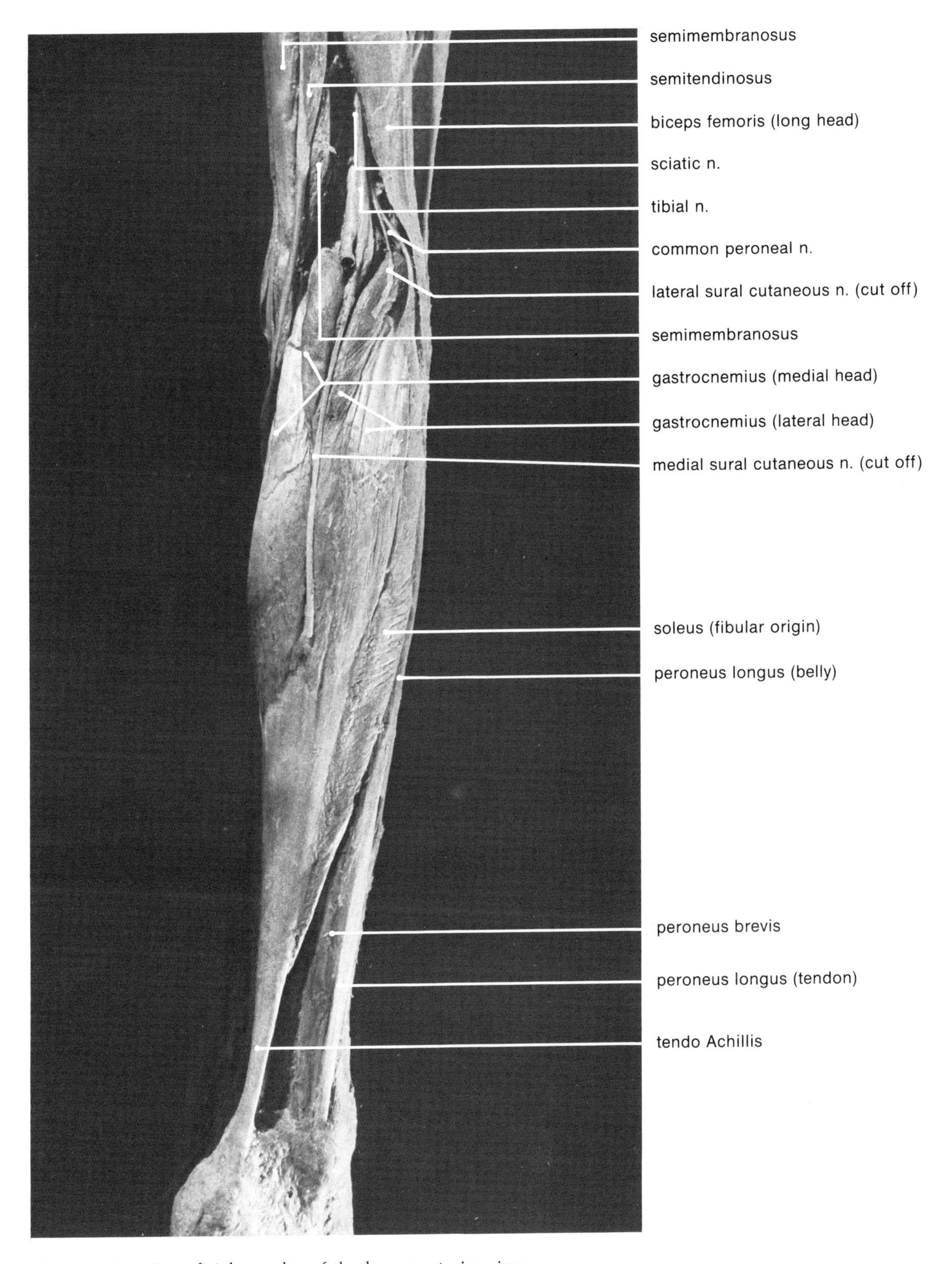

FIGURE 1-61 Superficial muscles of the leg—posterior view.

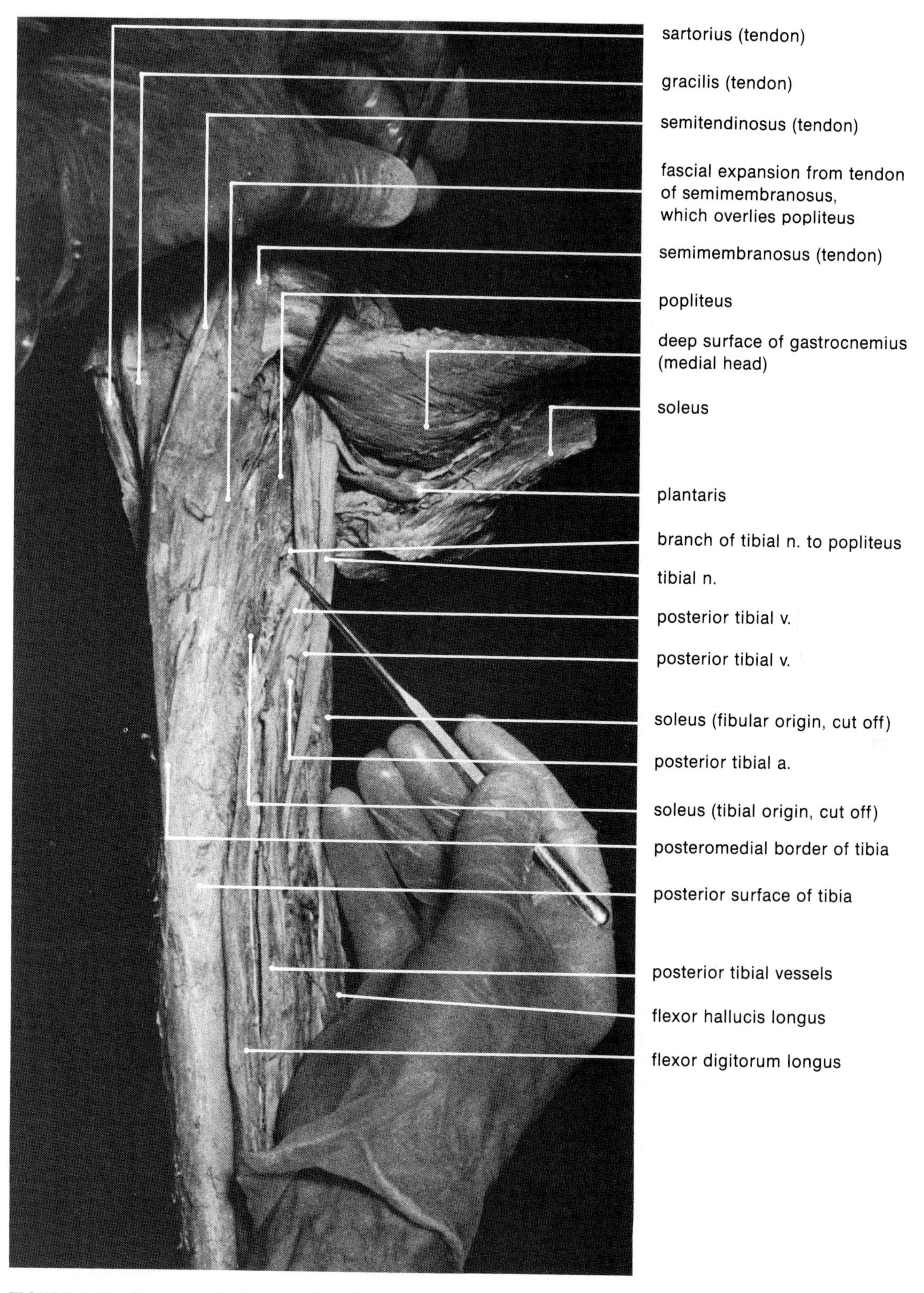

FIGURE 1-62 Deep posterior muscles of the upper part of the leg—posterior view.
Note: The two probes mark the upper and lower borders of the popliteus. The tip of the lower probe marks the site of the recurrent branch of the tibial nerve, which proceeds upward to reach and innervate the popliteus.

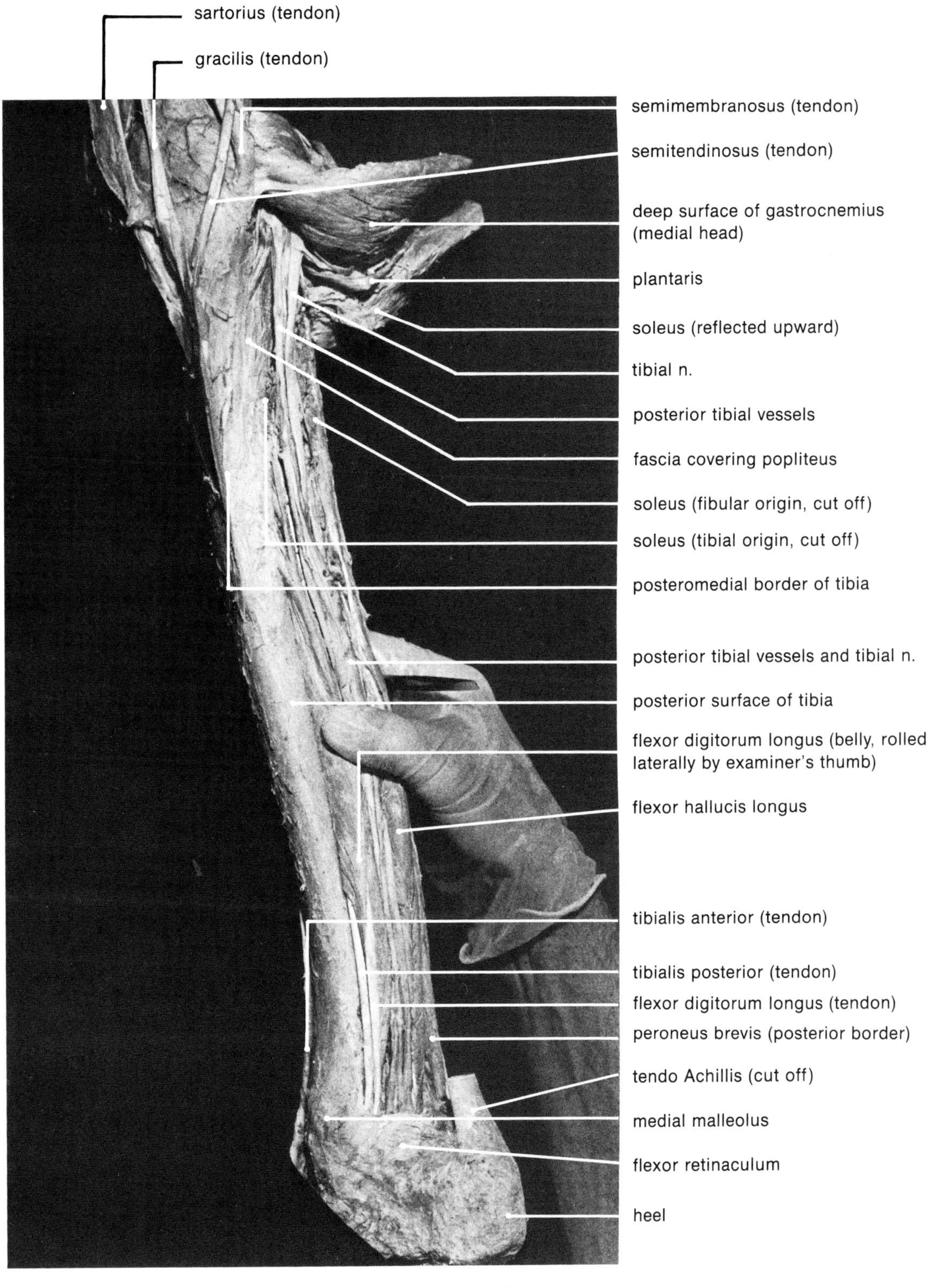

sartorius (tendon)
gracilis (tendon)
semimembranosus (tendon)
semitendinosus (tendon)
deep surface of gastrocnemius (medial head)
plantaris
soleus (reflected upward)
tibial n.
posterior tibial vessels
fascia covering popliteus
soleus (fibular origin, cut off)
soleus (tibial origin, cut off)
posteromedial border of tibia
posterior tibial vessels and tibial n.
posterior surface of tibia
flexor digitorum longus (belly, rolled laterally by examiner's thumb)
flexor hallucis longus
tibialis anterior (tendon)
tibialis posterior (tendon)
flexor digitorum longus (tendon)
peroneus brevis (posterior border)
tendo Achillis (cut off)
medial malleolus
flexor retinaculum
heel

FIGURE 1-63 Deep posterior muscles of the leg—medial view.
Note: The posterior tibial vessels and the tibial nerve have been drawn laterally by the thumb.

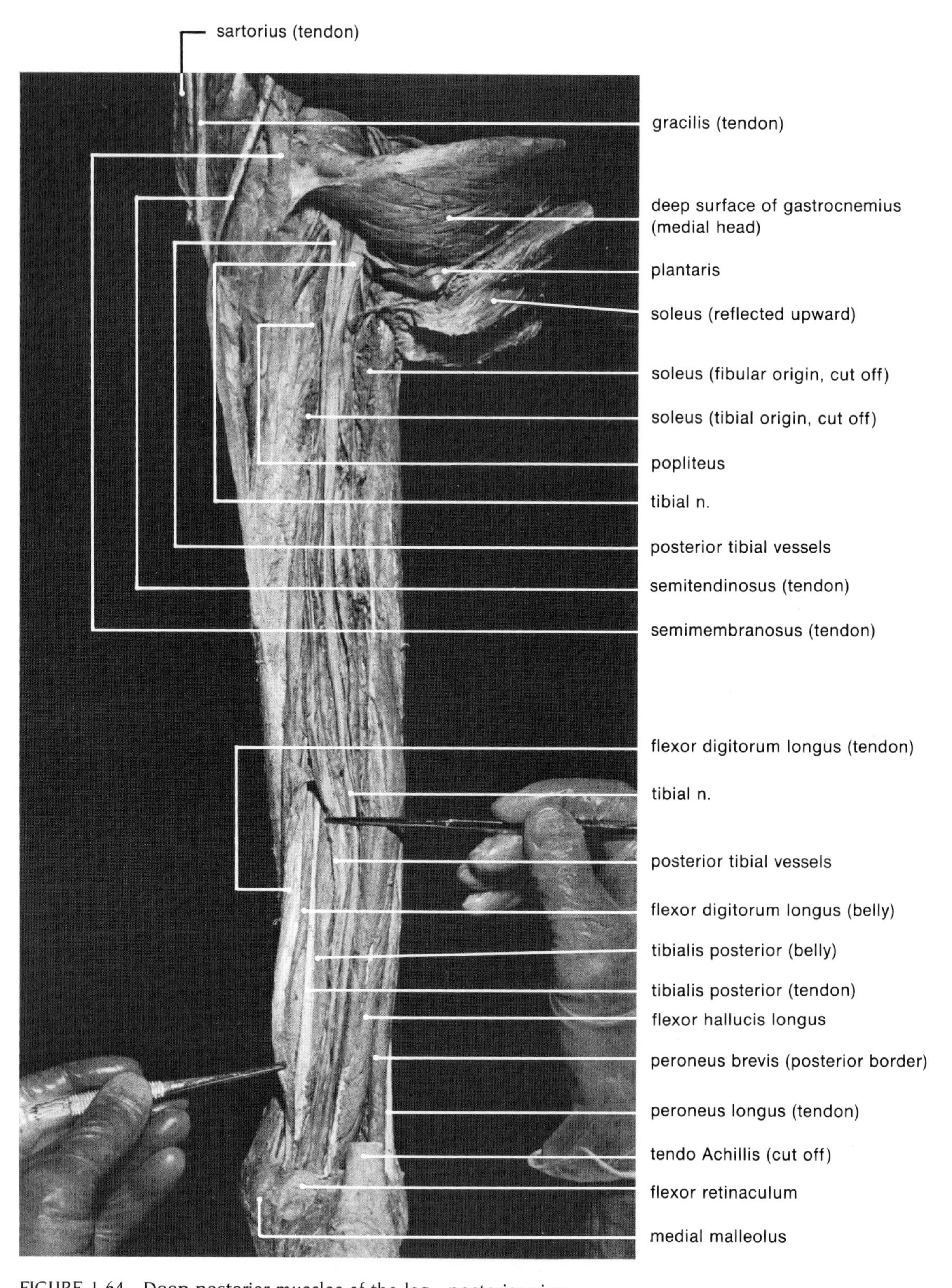

FIGURE 1-64 Deep posterior muscles of the leg—posterior view.
Note: The posterior tibial vessels and the tibial nerve have been drawn laterally by the upper probe.

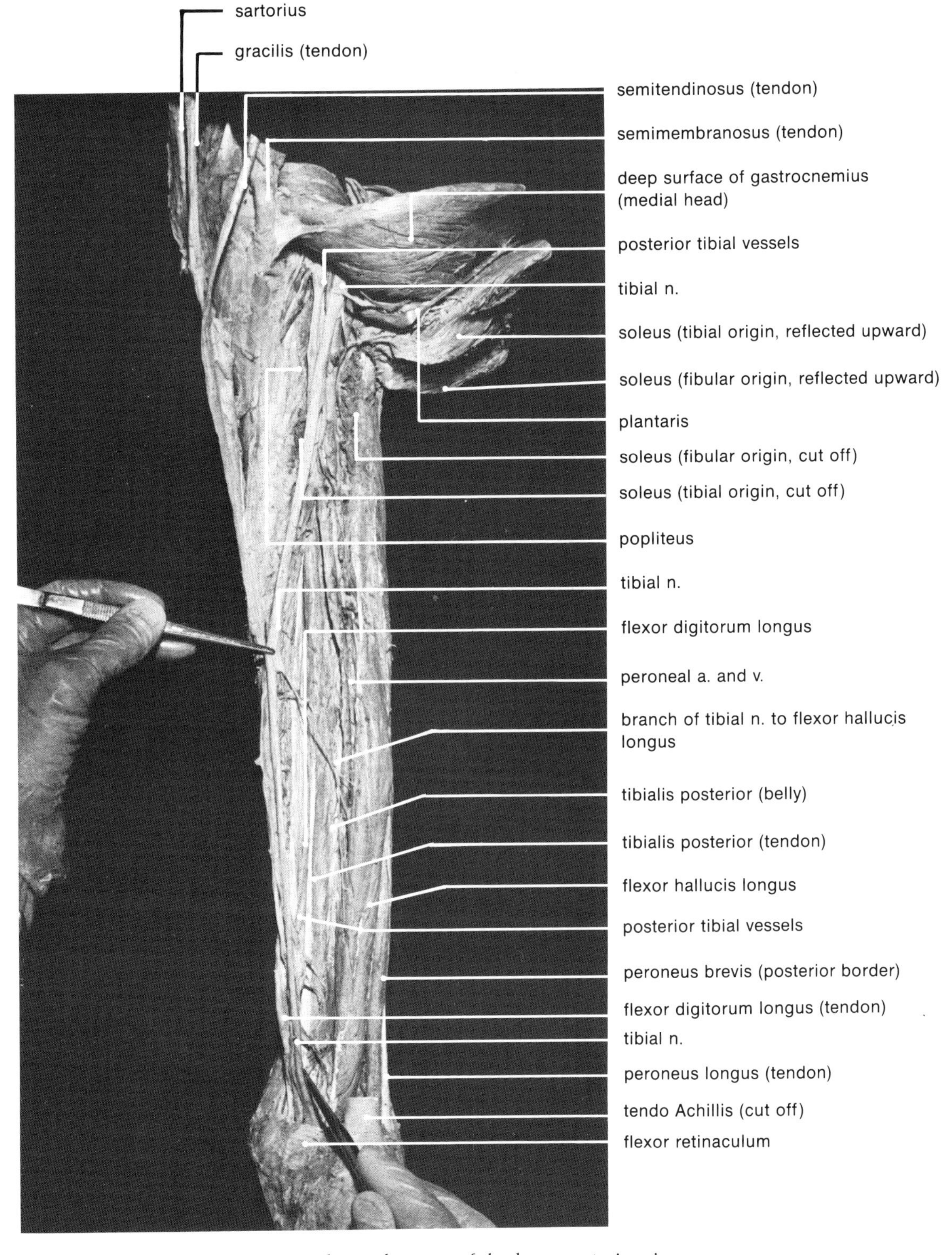

FIGURE 1-65 Deep posterior muscles and nerves of the leg—posterior view.
Note: The tibialis posterior muscle is displayed by drawing the posterior tibial vessels and the tibial nerve medially.

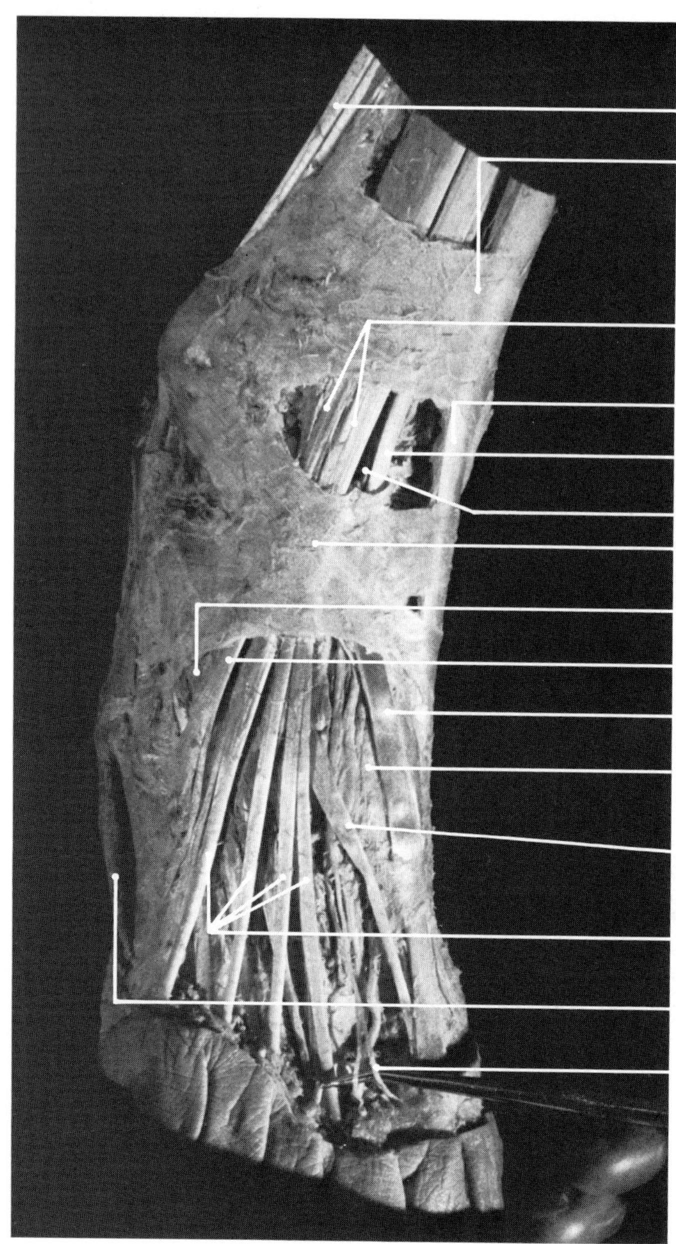

FIGURE 1-66 Foot and ankle—dorsal view.

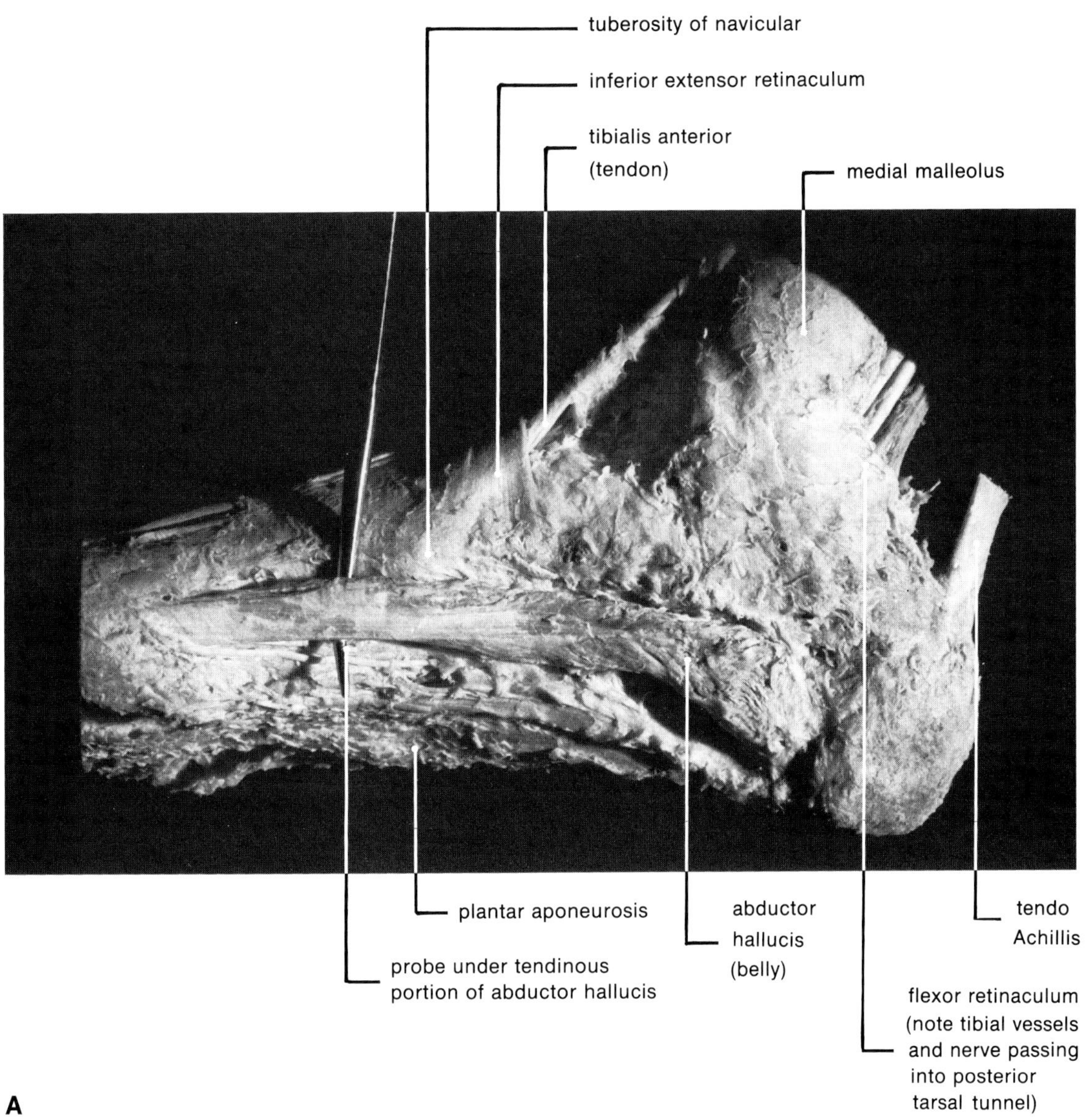

FIGURE 1-67 (A) Foot—medial view. (*Figure continues on next page.*)

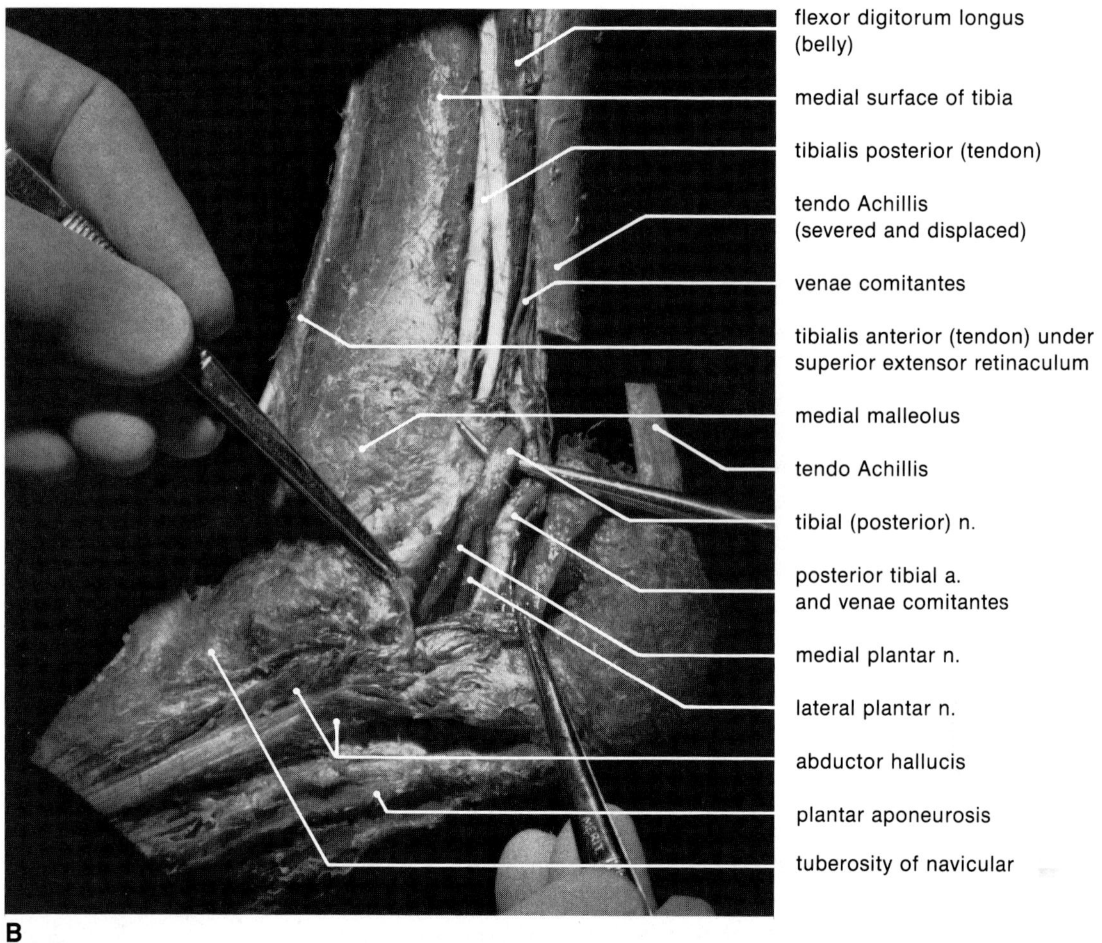

FIGURE 1-67 (B) Ankle region—medial view, contents of the tarsal tunnel displayed.
Note: The right forceps grasps the lower border of the rolled-back segment of the flexor retinaculum, which covers the tarsal tunnel. The left forceps grasps the lower border of the flexor retinaculum along the anterior wall of the tarsal tunnel. The tibial nerve divides into the medial and lateral plantar nerves at the mid-level of the tarsal tunnel in this specimen. The probe hooked under the main trunk of the tibial nerve crosses the reflected cover of the tarsal tunnel (flexor retinaculum) near its upper border.

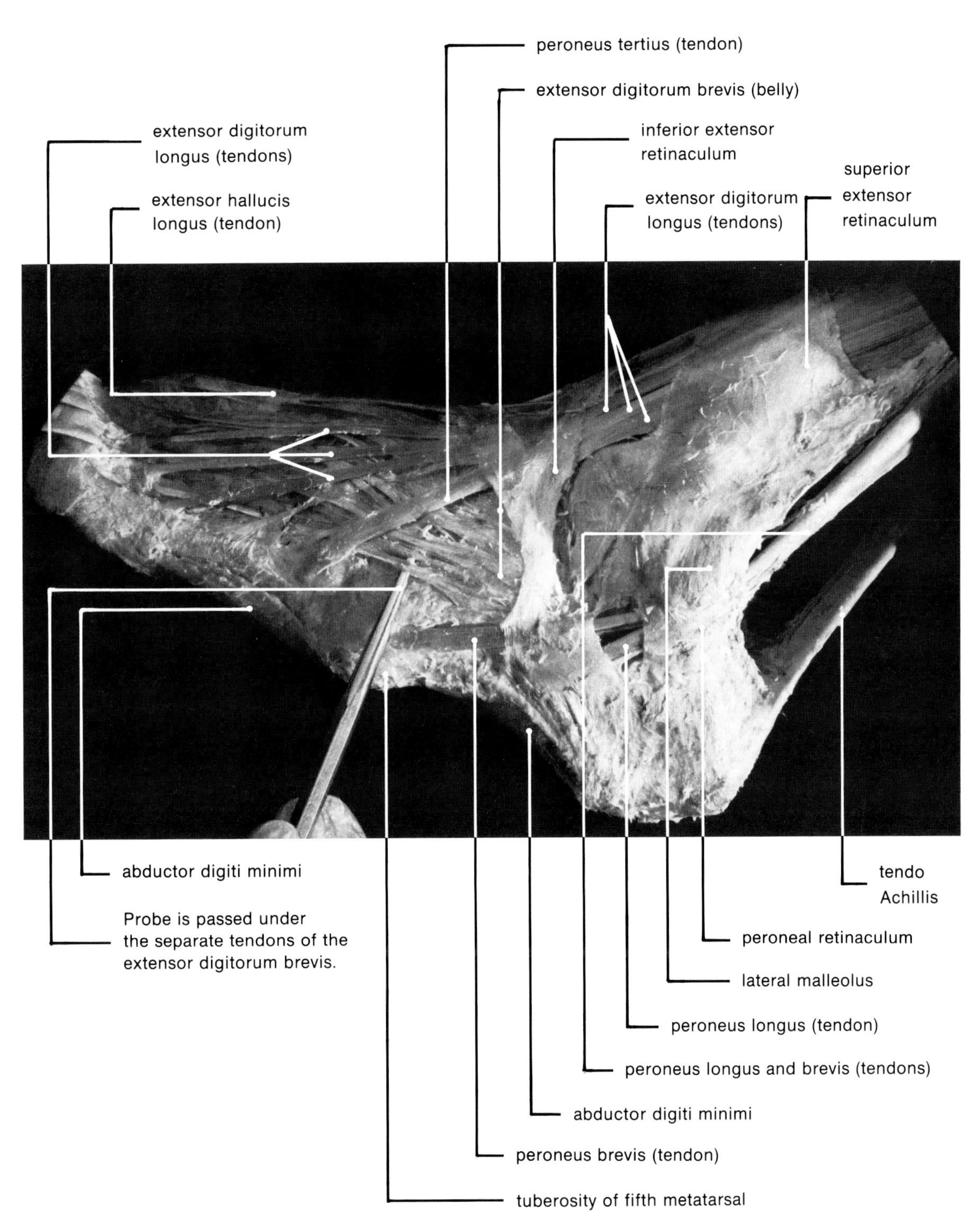

FIGURE 1-68 Left foot—lateral view.

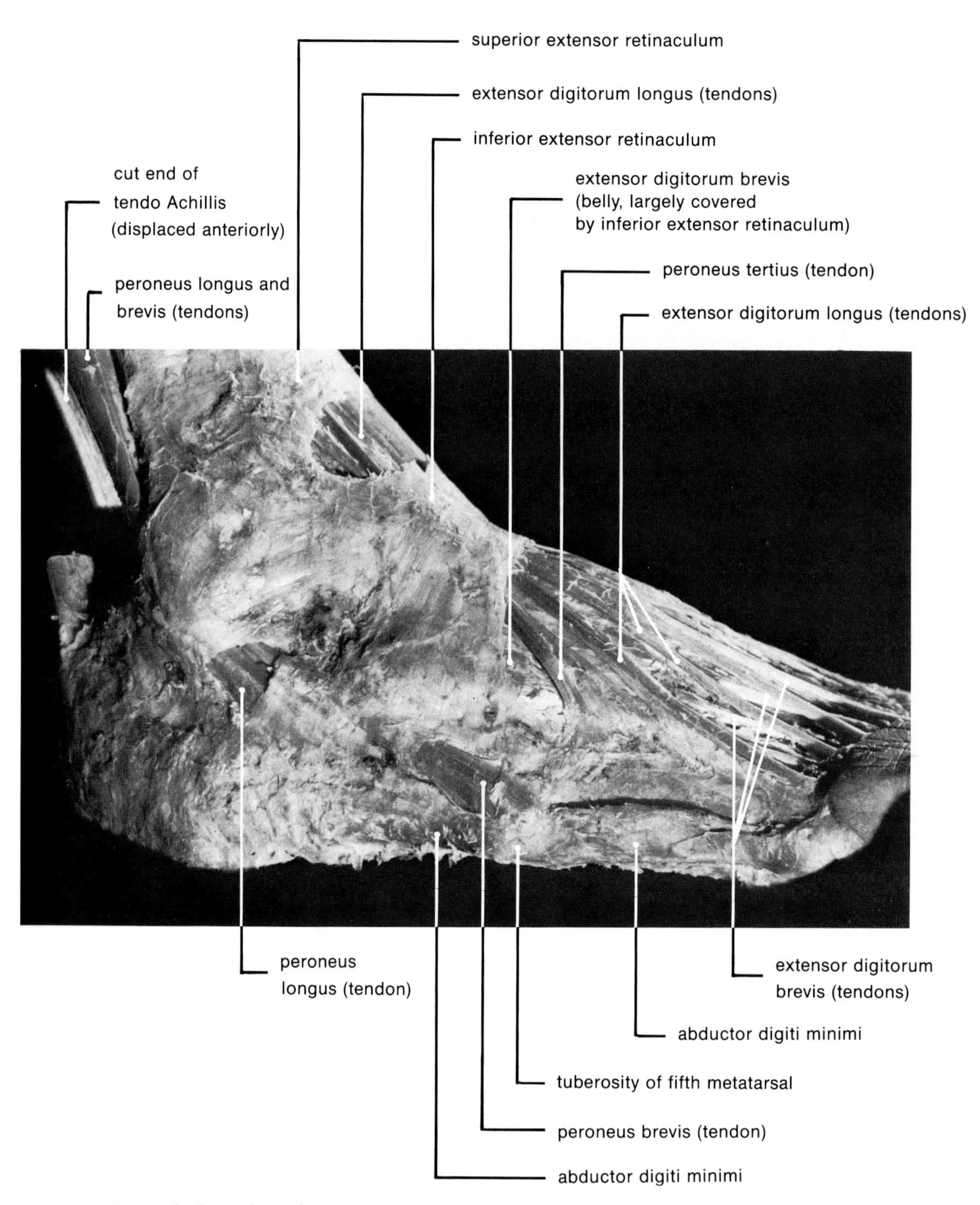

FIGURE 1-69 Right foot—lateral view.

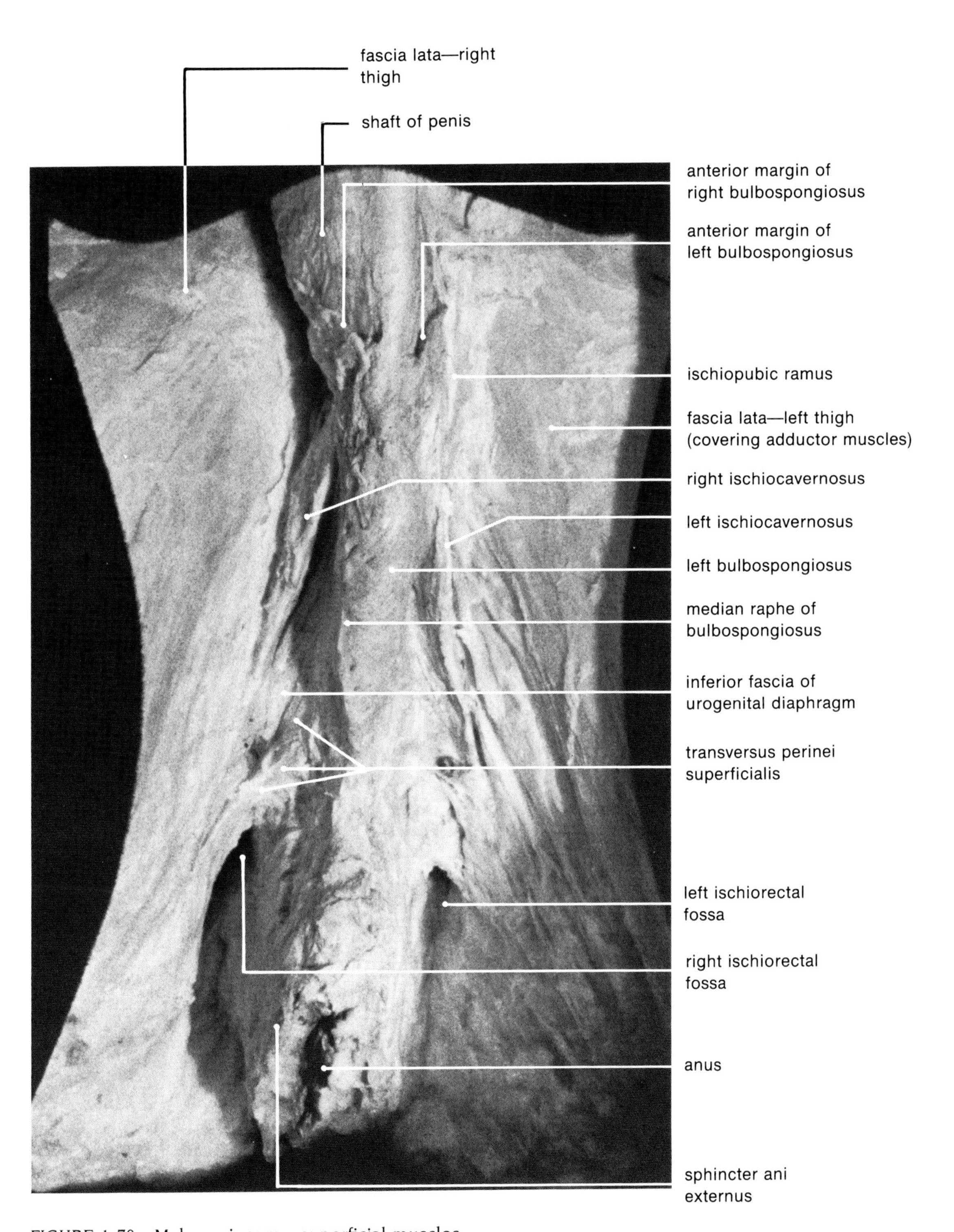

FIGURE 1-70 Male perineum—superficial muscles.

2
Clinical Anatomy

Jennifer Chu-Andrews
Robert J. Johnson

The purpose of this chapter is to teach the examiner to identify individual muscles. The basic principle used to identify muscles is to identify each muscle in the context of its action. By knowing the action of a muscle and making it contract, you can define the bordering indentations and can thus localize the muscle to be studied. If the muscle itself is not easily identifiable, the relationship of that muscle to adjacent prominent muscles will enable the examiner to locate it. For example, the brachioradialis in contraction is a very prominent muscle and can be used as a landmark to identify the extensor carpi radialis longus and brevis laterally and the pronator teres medially. Knowledge of the relationships of a muscle to prominent bony landmarks also aids in the localization of the muscle. This is especially important in the case of the deeper muscles, the actions of which cannot be readily palpated.

The chapter also deals with relaxing and minimally and maximally contracting the muscle. Knowledge of how to relax a muscle effectively follows from knowing the action of the muscle. For example, the flexor carpi ulnaris both flexes the wrist and deviates the wrist in the ulnar direction. To relax this muscle effectively, the examiner places the wrist joint in extension and radial deviation. Usually, effective relaxation of a muscle can be achieved by flexing the joint on which the muscle acts, if it acts to extend the joint, and by extending the joint, if the muscle acts to flex it. However, this position may actually stretch the agonist muscle, giving it a physiological advantage for contraction. Clinically, however, by stretching the muscle, the examiner makes it harder for the patient to contract even a few motor unit potentials (MUPs) unknowingly in response to pain from the needling.

Most muscles have more than a single action. By knowing the actions of a muscle, one can obtain either full maximum contraction or weak minimal contraction. For example, the tensor fasciae latae aids in flexion, abduction, and internal rotation of the hip. This muscle can be made to contract fully if at least two of the actions are called into play; that is, hip flexion and abduction or hip flexion and internal rotation. When minimal contraction is required, you must ensure that only single MUPs come into contraction. In the case of the tensor fasciae latae, minimal contraction can be obtained when the hip is partially flexed while being kept in external rotation. If the contraction still proves too strong, a gravity-eliminating position can be used with hip flexion or abduction alone to induce minimal contraction.

By repeating the process of muscle identification and isolation many times on normal muscles, you will become confident with this technique and will be able to transfer this knowledge to identify weak or paralyzed muscles. The same is true for palpation for grooves between the muscles and for prominent bony landmarks. If any doubt persists, low-threshold electrical stimulation through the needle inserted in the muscle causes the tendon of the muscle to contract in isolation and thus helps to identify the muscle.

The photographs in this chapter have been taken so that the muscle of interest is placed in the position best suited for examination in clinical electromyography (EMG). In some cases the photograph depicts just the patient, the anatomical landmarks, and the site for pin insertion. An accompanying inset shows the muscle of interest in relation to the surrounding muscles. The surrounding muscles have been made to contract for the insets. The position of the patient in the insets is the position best suited for eliciting contraction in the muscle of interest or in the surrounding muscles; it is not the position meant for EMG. The position of pin insertion is indicated by the pin itself or a line indicator.

Many patients are threatened by use of the word *needle*, and therefore in the accompanying text the word *pin* has been substituted. The instructions for the patient are written in nonmedical vocabulary, and the actual anatomical terms are given in parentheses.

You will obtain the most out of this chapter by referring to Chapter 1, Applied Anatomy. If clarification of the action of a muscle is needed, refer to the diagrams of the bony attachments of the muscles in the appendix. By visualizing the sites of origin and insertion of a given muscle, you will better be able to appreciate its action. The figure numbers of corresponding cadaver dissection photographs are cited at the beginning of most sections in this chapter.

MUSCLES SUPPLIED BY THE CRANIAL NERVES

Temporalis (*Fig.* 2-1; *see also Fig.* 1-9, A)

Action: Elevating the mandible and clenching and grinding the teeth (primarily done by the anterior part). Retracts the mandible after protrusion and after wide opening (done by the posterior part primarily).

Patient Position: Supine

Pin Insertion: Select a point 2.5 cm posterior to the lateral margin of the orbit and 2.5 cm above the upper border of the zygomatic arch. Insert the pin through the skin and the temporalis fascia into the muscle at this point.

Relaxation: Instruct the patient as follows: "Relax your jaw and let your mouth fall slightly open."

Contraction: *Minimal*: Instruct the patient as follows: "Bring your teeth together. Clench them very slightly."

Contraction: *Maximal*: Instruct the patient as follows: "Clench your teeth as tightly as you can."

Nerve Supply: Anterior and posterior deep temporal branches of the mandibular division of the trigeminal nerve

Root Supply: Motor root of the trigeminal nerve

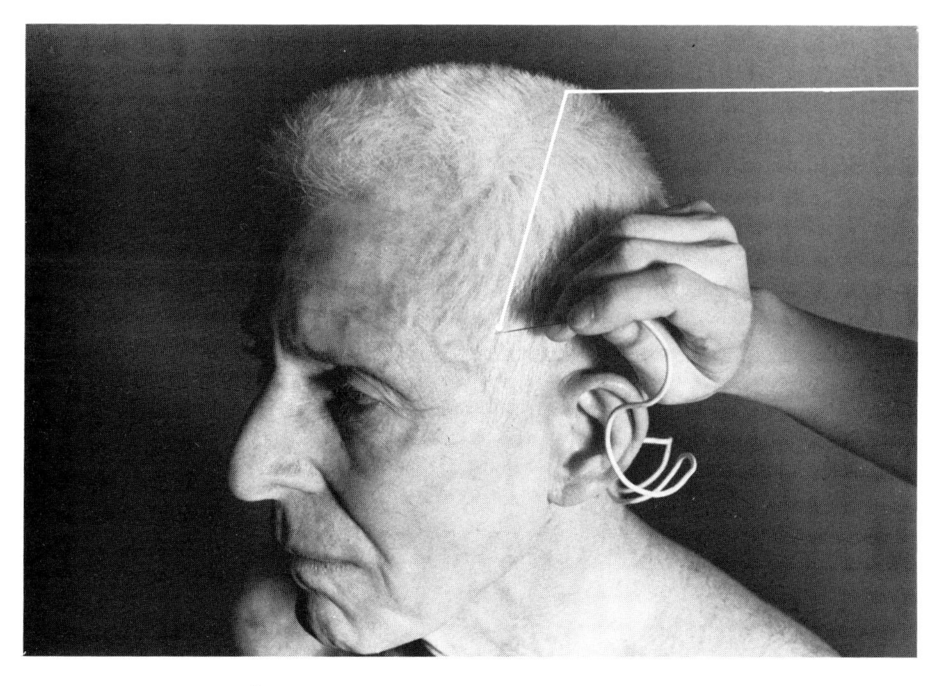

FIGURE 2-1 Temporalis.

Masseter (*Fig.* 2-2; *see also Fig.* 1-9)

Action: Elevates the mandible, clenches the teeth, and assists slightly in protracting the mandible.

Patient Position: Supine or sitting

Pin Insertion: Identify the angle of the mandible by palpation and instruct the patient to clench the teeth and then relax several times. The masseter can be felt easily at approximately 2 cm above the angle of the mandible. Insert the pin at this point.

Relaxation: Instruct the patient as follows: "Relax your jaws."

Contraction: *Minimal*: Instruct the patient as follows: "Clench your jaws slightly."

Contraction: *Maximal*: Instruct the patient as follows: "Clench your jaws together as tightly as you can."

Peripheral Nerve Supply: Masseteric branch of the mandibular division of the trigeminal nerve

Root Supply: Motor root of the trigeminal nerve

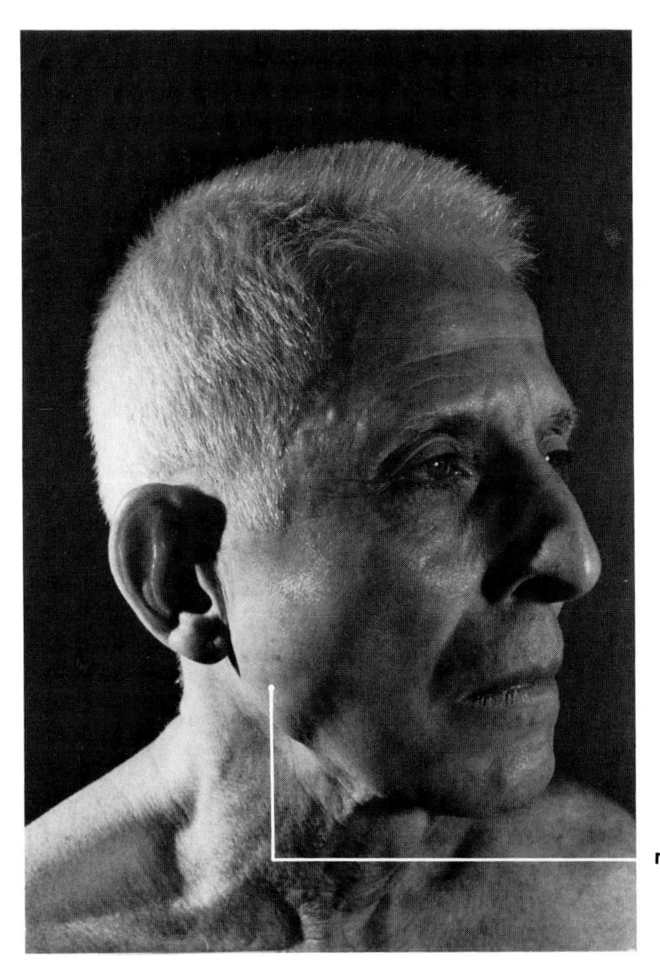

FIGURE 2-2 Masseter.

Internal (Medial) Pterygoid (*Fig.* 2-3; *see also Fig.* 1-9, B)

Action: Protraction and elevation of the mandible. Assists in deviating the chin to the opposite side.

Patient Position: Supine

Pin Insertion: Palpate the angle of the jaw and insert the pin just medial to the angle at a point 1.5 cm anterior to the angle. The pin passes through the sagittal plane at this point.

Relaxation: Instruct the patient as follows: "Relax your jaws. Let the upper and lower teeth part slightly."

Contraction: *Minimal*: Instruct the patient as follows: "Clench your teeth slightly."

Contraction: *Maximal*: Instruct the patient as follows: "Clench your teeth together as hard as you can."

Peripheral Nerve Supply: Pterygoid branch of the mandibular division of the trigeminal nerve

Root Supply: Motor root of the trigeminal nerve

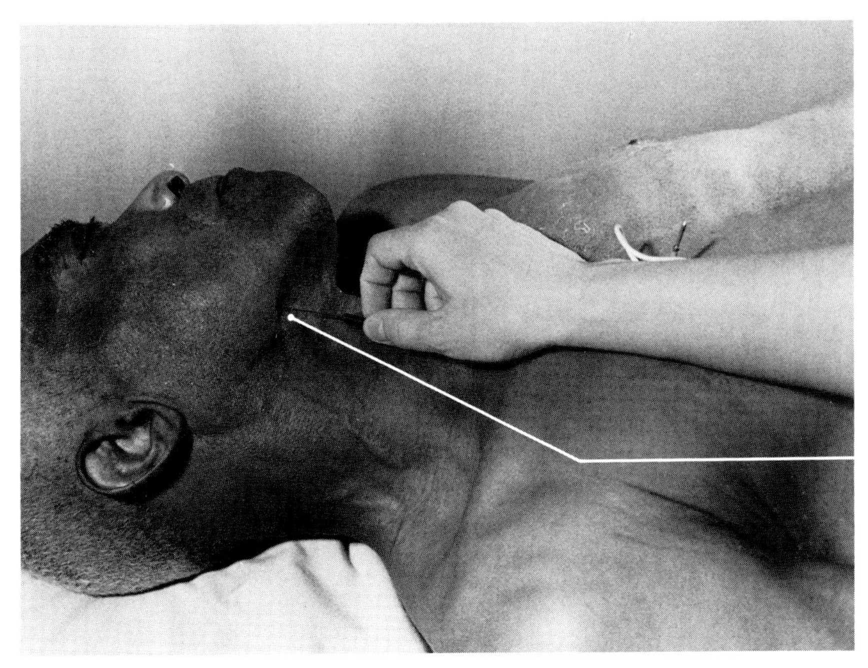

FIGURE 2-3 Internal (medial) pterygoid.

Auriculаris Posterior (*Fig. 2-4; see also Fig. 1-6*)

Action: Retraction of the ear

Patient Position: Lateral recumbent

Pin Insertion: Just posterior to the junction of the auricle with the mastoid portion of the temporal bone, in line with a firm tissue ledge, which is the tendinous end of the muscle. If the patient can contract the muscle, it may be felt to contract when your fingertip is laid flat against the skin behind the ear. Remember, the muscle is very thin and flat, and gentle pressure may be needed to palpate its contraction.

Relaxation: Relaxation should pose no problems, since the muscle is so seldom used that most people have not learned how to contract it.

Contraction: *Minimal*: Instruct the patient as follows: "Try to move your ear backward without touching it."

Contraction: *Maximal*: Instruct the patient as follows: "Try to move your ear backward as much as you can without touching it."

Peripheral Nerve Supply: Posterior auricular branch of the facial nerve

Root Supply: Facial nerve

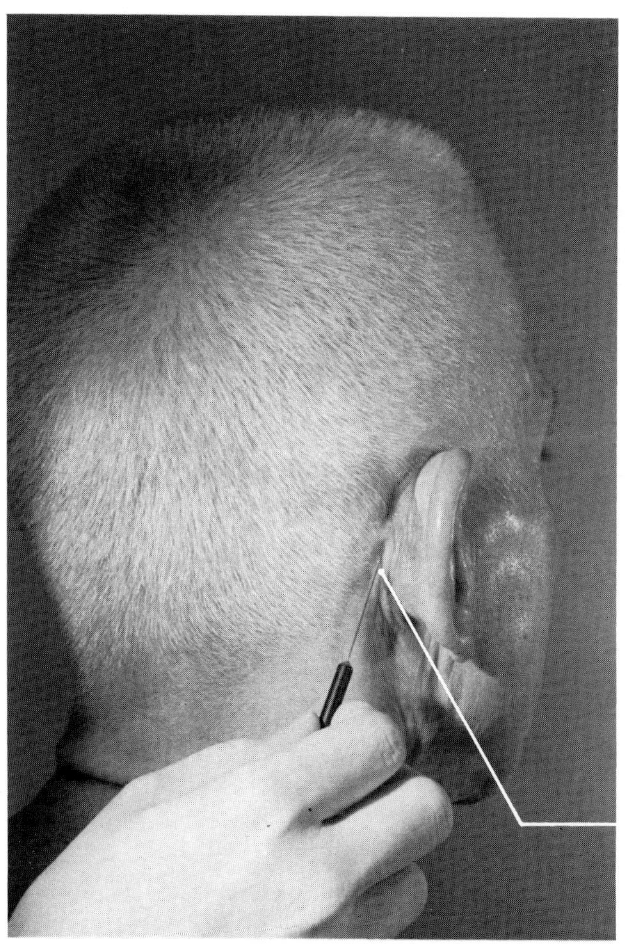

FIGURE 2-4 Auricularis posterior.

Frontalis (*Fig.* 2-5; *see also Appendix Fig.* 22)

Action: Raises the eyebrows
Patient Position: Supine
Pin Insertion: Into the wrinkled skin of the forehead as the patient raises his eyebrows. The pin should be approximately in line with the middle of the orbital aperture or with the middle of the eyebrow.
Relaxation: Instruct the patient as follows: "Relax your eyebrows."
Contraction: *Minimal*: Instruct the patient as follows: "Raise your eyebrow slightly."
Contraction: *Maximal*: Instruct the patient as follows: "Raise your eyebrow as if you would like to look at the ceiling. Try to wrinkle the skin above your eyebrow as much as you can."
Peripheral Nerve Supply: Temporal branch of the facial nerve
Root Supply: Facial nerve

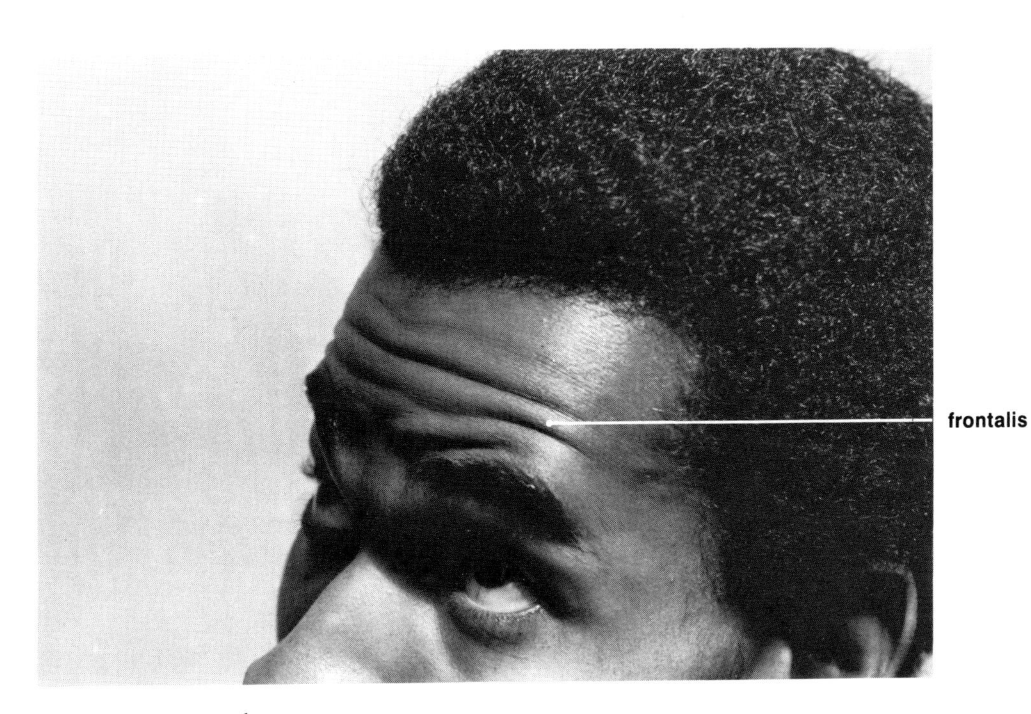

FIGURE 2-5 Frontalis.

Orbicularis Oculi (*Fig. 2-6; see also Figs. 1-1 and 1-2*)

Action: Closure of the eyelids

Patient Position: Supine

Pin Insertion: Into the skin wrinkles at the lateral corner of the eyelids, approximately 3 mm to 4 mm lateral to the bony margin of the orbit as the patient closes his eyes

Relaxation: Instruct the patient as follows: "Look up at the ceiling." (The eyes must be open for relaxation.)

Contraction: *Minimal*: Instruct the patient as follows: "Close your eyes very gently."

Contraction: *Maximal*: Instruct the patient as follows: "Shut your eyelids as tightly as you can."

Peripheral Nerve Supply: Temporal and zygomatic branches of the facial nerve

Root Supply: Facial nerve

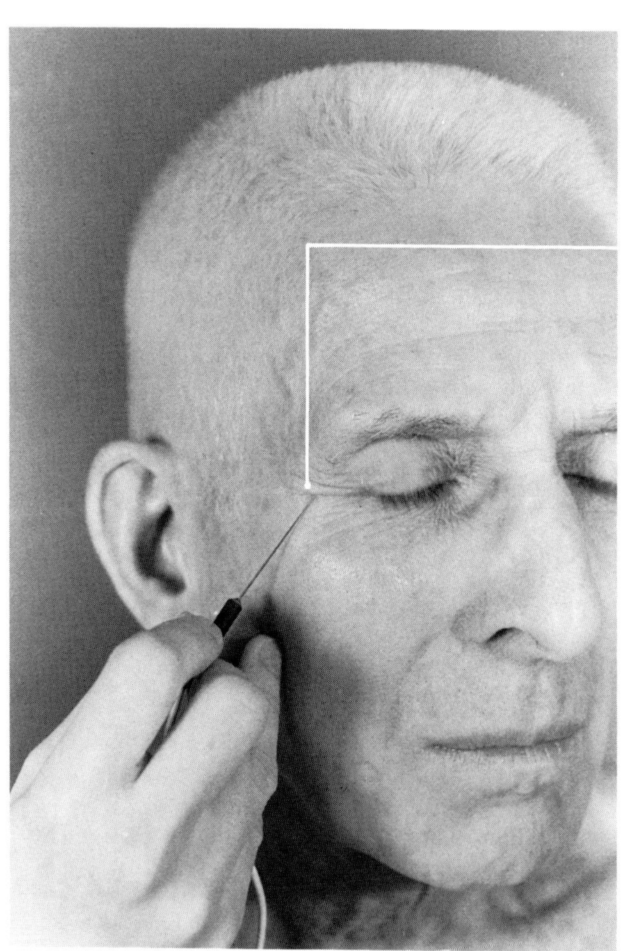

FIGURE 2-6 Orbicularis oculi.

Nasalis (*Fig. 2-7; see also Figs. 1-1 and 1-2*)

Action: Flaring of the ala of the nose with widening of the nasal aperture by the contraction of the transverse part of the nasalis. There is also a downward and slightly medial movement of the ala that is accomplished by the contraction of the alar part of the nasalis. This results in narrowing of the nostril. The two parts are together at the posterior end of the ala.

Patient Position: Supine or sitting

Pin Insertion: Into the posterior end of the lower border of the ala in the angle where the ala joins the skin of the upper lip. Here the point of the pin first passes through the levator labii superioris alaque nasi and then, slightly deeper, the fibers of the nasalis.

Relaxation: Instruct the patient as follows: "Relax your nostrils and breathe easily."

Contraction: *Minimal*: Instruct patient as follows: "Flare your nostril just slightly" (pars transversa), or "try to pull the outer side of your nostril downward" (pars alaris).

Contraction: *Maximal*: Instruct the patient as follows: "Flare your nostril as hard as you can," or "pull the outer side of your nostril downward as hard as you can."

Peripheral Nerve Supply: Zygomatic and upper buccal branches of the facial nerve

Root Supply: Facial nerve

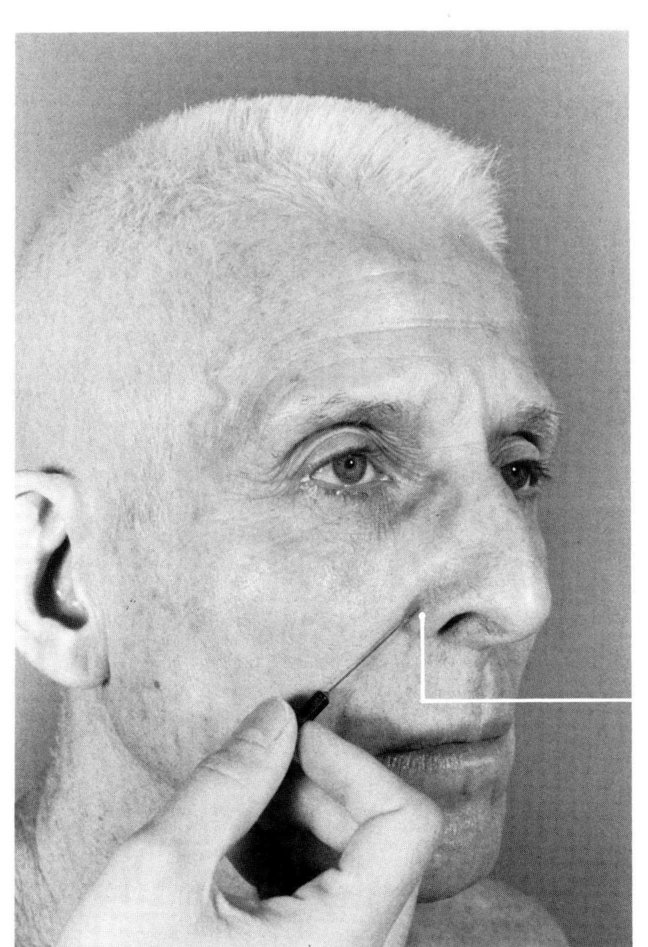

FIGURE 2-7 Nasalis.

Mentalis (*Fig.* 2-8; *see also Fig.* 1-8, B)

Action: Flattens the skin of the chin and raises and protrudes the lower lip, as when one blows through slightly parted lips.

Patient Position: Supine or sitting

Pin Insertion: Approximately 1 cm lateral to the midline of the chin and midway between the vermilion border of the lip and the lower border of the chin

Relaxation: Instruct the patient as follows: "Relax your lower lip."

Contraction: *Minimal*: Instruct the patient as follows: "Slightly separate your lips and blow gently through that space. Do not try to whistle, but keep the lips together."

Contraction: *Maximal*: Instruct the patient as follows: "Slightly separate your lips and blow strongly through the space. Do not try to whistle, but let me hear the air coming out."

Peripheral Nerve Supply: Mandibular branch and/or marginal mandibular branch of the facial nerve

Root Supply: Facial nerve

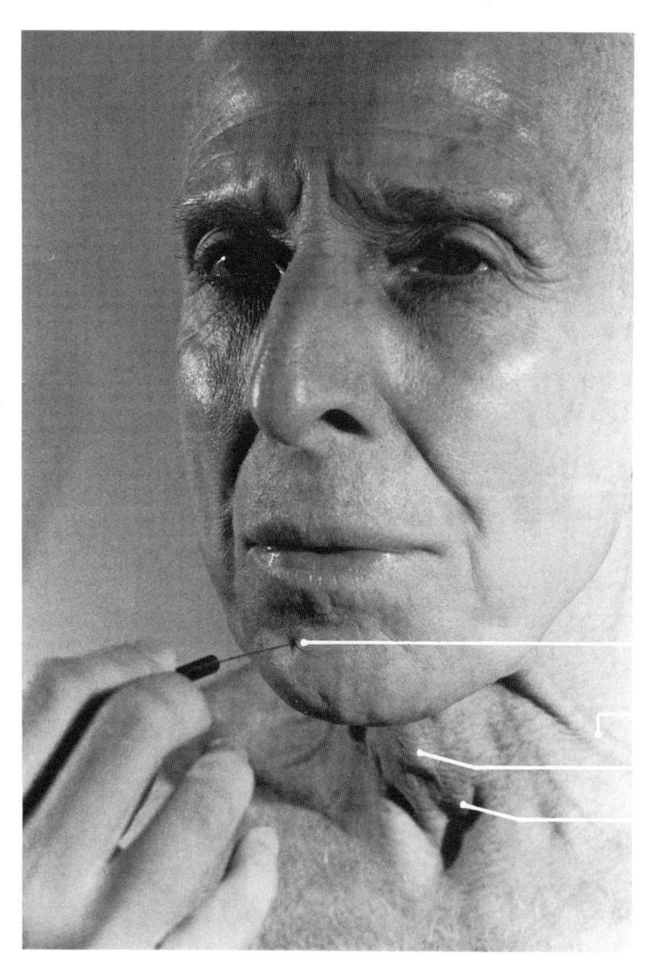

FIGURE 2-8 Mentalis.

Orbicularis Oris (*Fig. 2-9; see also Figs. 1-1 and 1-2*)

Action: Compression and protrusion of the lips. Closes the lips and pulls them against the teeth.
Patient Position: Supine
Pin Insertion: Approximately 5 mm below the vermilion border of the lateral portion of the lower lip
Relaxation: Instruct the patient as follows: "Relax your lips. Let them separate slightly."
Contraction: *Minimal*: Instruct the patient as follows: "Pout your lips slightly."
Contraction: *Maximal*: Instruct patient as follows: "Pout your lips as strongly as you can."
Peripheral Nerve Supply: Buccal and mandibular branches of the facial nerve
Root Supply: Facial nerve

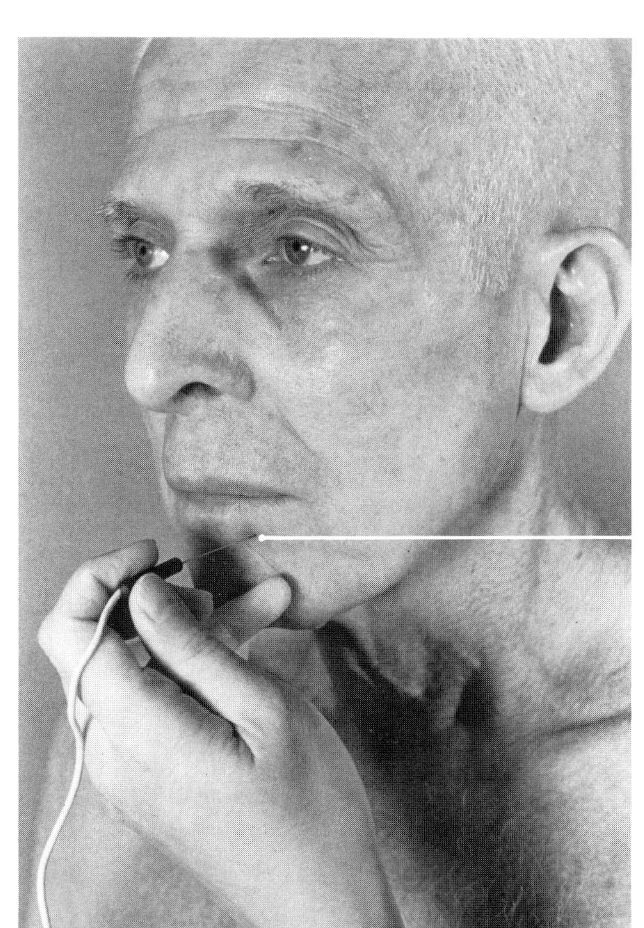

FIGURE 2-9 Orbicularis oris.

Platysma (*Fig.* 2-10; *see also Figs.* 1-1 *and* 1-2)

Action: Elevation of the skin of the lower neck anteriorly, with ridging or bridging out of the skin of the neck and depression of the lower jaw and lip

Patient Position: Supine or sitting

Pin Insertion: Into the raised skin folds of the neck seen when the muscle is contracted, midway between the chin and the clavicle. The muscle lies in the deepest layer of the superficial fascia.

Relaxation: Instruct the patient as follows: "Relax your jaw." (The neck may also be placed in passive flexion.)

Contraction: *Minimal*: Instruct the patient as follows: "Pull the corners of your mouth down just slightly."

Contraction: *Maximal*: Instruct the patient as follows: "Pull the corners of your mouth down as hard as you can. Fix your jaw and jut out your chin."

Peripheral Nerve Supply: Cervical branch of the facial nerve

Root Supply: Facial nerve

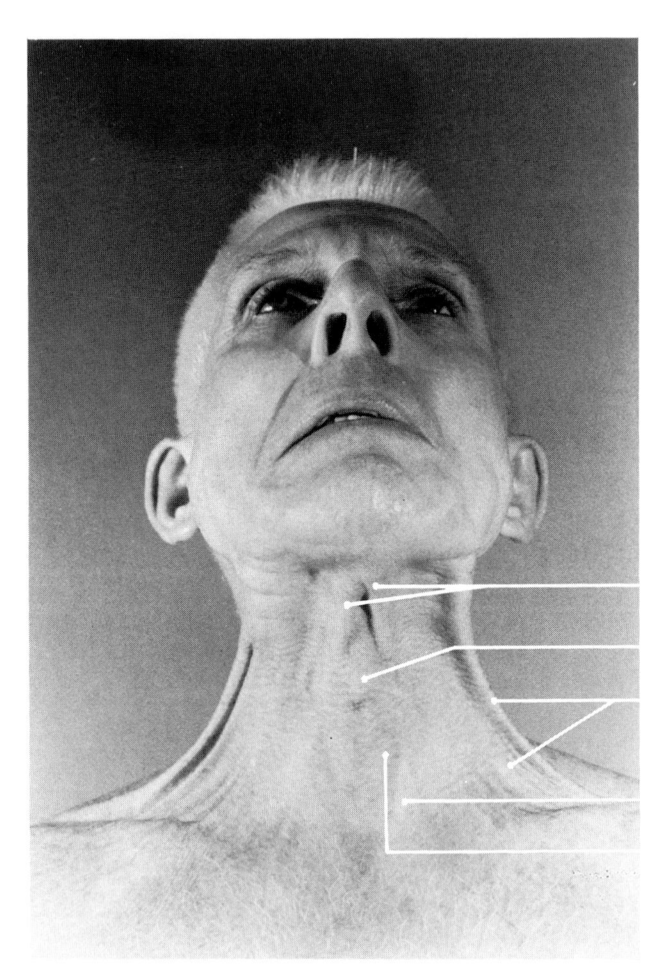

FIGURE 2-10 Platysma.

Cricothyroid (*Fig.* 2-11; *see also Fig.* 1-7)

Action: Produces elongation and increased tension of the vocal cords by approximation of the anterior arch of the cricoid cartilage toward the lower border of the thyroid cartilage (rotation occurring about a transverse axis through the cricothyroid joints).

Patient Position: Supine

Pin Insertion: Feel for the laryngeal prominence and draw the tip of your finger down along the midline of the thyroid cartilage until you feel the middle of the upper border of the arch of the cricoid cartilage. Insert the pin approximately 5 mm lateral to this midline point on either side.

Relaxation: Instruct the patient as follows: "Relax your neck and don't speak or swallow."

Contraction: *Minimal*: Instruct the patient as follows: "Make a gentle but high-pitched and continuously crooning 'eeeee' sound."

Contraction: *Maximal*: Instruct the patient as follows: "Make a stronger and more intensely high-pitched and continuously crooning 'eeeee' sound." The patient's total larynx may be abruptly elevated with this effort.

Peripheral Nerve Supply: External branch of the superior laryngeal nerve

Root Supply: Vagus nerve

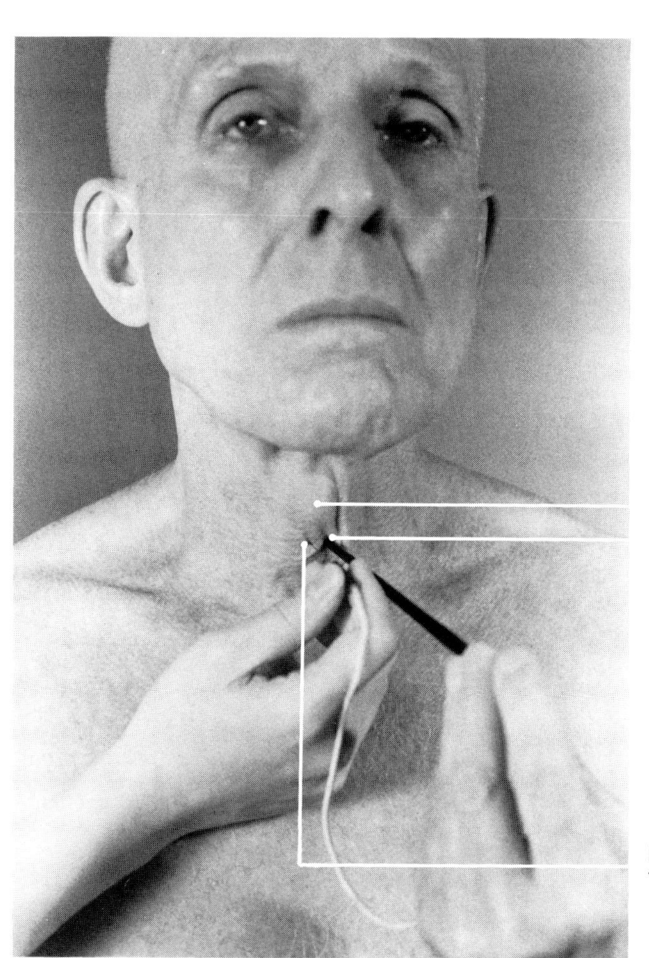

FIGURE 2-11 Cricothyroid.

Genioglossus (*Fig.* 2-12; *see also Fig.* 1-8)

Action: Protrusion and retraction of the tongue and depression of the central portion of the tongue. By unilateral action of the muscle, the genioglossus protrudes the tongue toward the opposite side.

Patient Position: Supine

Pin Insertion: Palpate the laryngeal prominence; just superior to this is the hyoid bone. By palpation, identify in the midline the midpoint between the hyoid bone and the posterior aspect of the anterior end of the mandible. Just above the latter is the genial spine (mental spine). Insert the pin 1 cm lateral to this midpoint between the hyoid and the genial spine on either side. The depth of insertion is determined by the appearance of crisp-sounding MUPs on protrusion of the tongue. The tip of the pin must pass through the mylohyoid and the geniohyoid muscles to reach the genioglossus. At least 2 cm of pin penetration is required to pass through the skin and fascia. In some cases the pin first penetrates the decussating fibers of the platysma as they cover the submental triangle.

The genioglossus may also be reached intraorally if pin penetration is kept well behind the frenulum of the tongue and below the broad body of the tongue. (Remember that the geniohyoid muscle, though supplied by a peripheral branch from the hypoglossal nerve, does not receive innervation from the root of the hypoglossal; its fibers come instead from the C1 spinal nerve root and merely travel their peripheral course in the hypoglossal nerve.)

Relaxation: Instruct the patient as follows: "Close your mouth and relax your tongue."

Contraction: *Minimal*: Instruct the patient as follows: "Show me the tip of your tongue."

Contraction: *Maximal*: Instruct the patient as follows: "Stick your tongue out as much as you can."

Peripheral Nerve Supply: Branches of the hypoglossal nerve

Root Supply: Hypoglossal nerve

Note: The lateral elements of the intrinsic muscles of the tongue can also be examined by inserting the pin into the lateral aspect of the tongue while the patient keeps the tongue protruded.

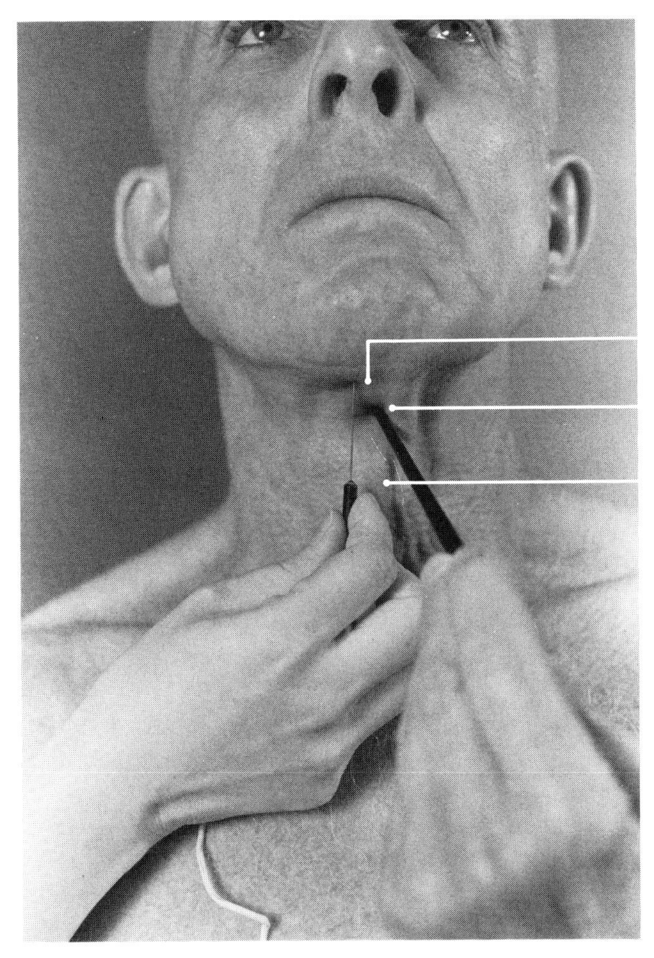

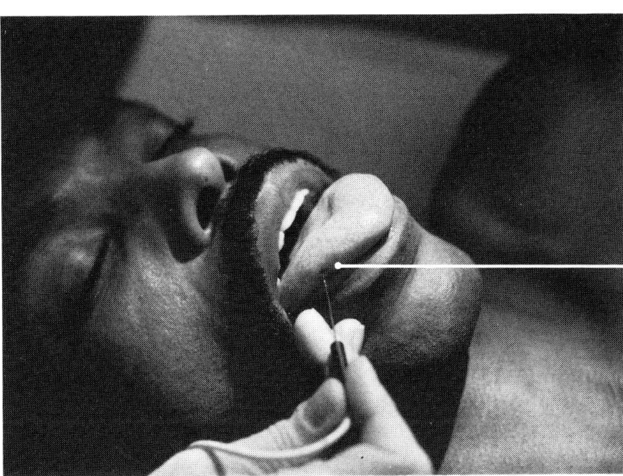

FIGURE 2-12 (*Top*) Genioglossus. (*Bottom*) Lateral muscles of the tongue.

MUSCLES OF THE NECK, TRUNK, AND PERINEUM

Muscles of the Neck

Sternocleidomastoid (*Fig.* 2-13; *see also Figs.* 1-9 *and* 1-16 *through* 1-18)

Action: Lateral bending of the neck and rotation of the face and chin to the opposite side and upward when acting unilaterally. When acting bilaterally, the two muscles are flexors of the head and neck. When the neck and head are fixed, the two sternocleidomastoids can raise the sternum and hence become accessory muscles of respiration.

Patient Position: Supine

Pin Insertion: If the right sternocleidomastoid is to be tested, instruct the patient as follows: "Turn your face to the left side and try to touch your right ear to your right shoulder." For examination of the left sterncleidomastoid, the face has to be turned to the right side with the patient attempting to touch his left ear to his left shoulder. The sternocleidomastoid is then seen to contract with these motions and can be grasped between the examiner's thumb and fingers. Insert the pin at about the junction of the upper and middle thirds of the muscle.

Relaxation: For testing the right sternocleidomastoid, instruct the patient as follows: "Lay your head back on the bed and turn your chin to the right" (rotation of the face and chin to the same side). For examination of the left sternocleidomastoid, the chin is rotated to the left.

Contraction: *Minimal*: For testing the right sternocleidomastoid, instruct the patient as follows: "Tilt your head slightly as if you want to touch your right ear to your right shoulder" (minimal lateral bending of the neck). For examination of the left sternocleidomastoid, the head is tilted slightly, with the patient attempting to touch his left ear to his left shoulder.

Contraction: *Maximal*: For examination of the right sternocleidomastoid, instruct the patient as follows: "Turn your chin strongly to the left and tilt your head sideways so that your right ear is brought toward your right shoulder. Now, don't let me push your chin toward the right" (maximal rotation of the face and chin to the opposite side against resistance, accompanied by lateral bending of the neck). For examination of the left sternocleidomastoid, the chin is turned strongly to the right, the head is tilted sideways, the patient attempts to touch his left ear to his left shoulder, and resistance is given to lateral neck bending.

Peripheral Nerve Supply: Spinal accessory nerve from spinal cord segments C1–C5 and by direct twigs from the cervical plexus (from C2 and C3)

Root Supply: C1–C5 nerve roots, mainly the C2 nerve root

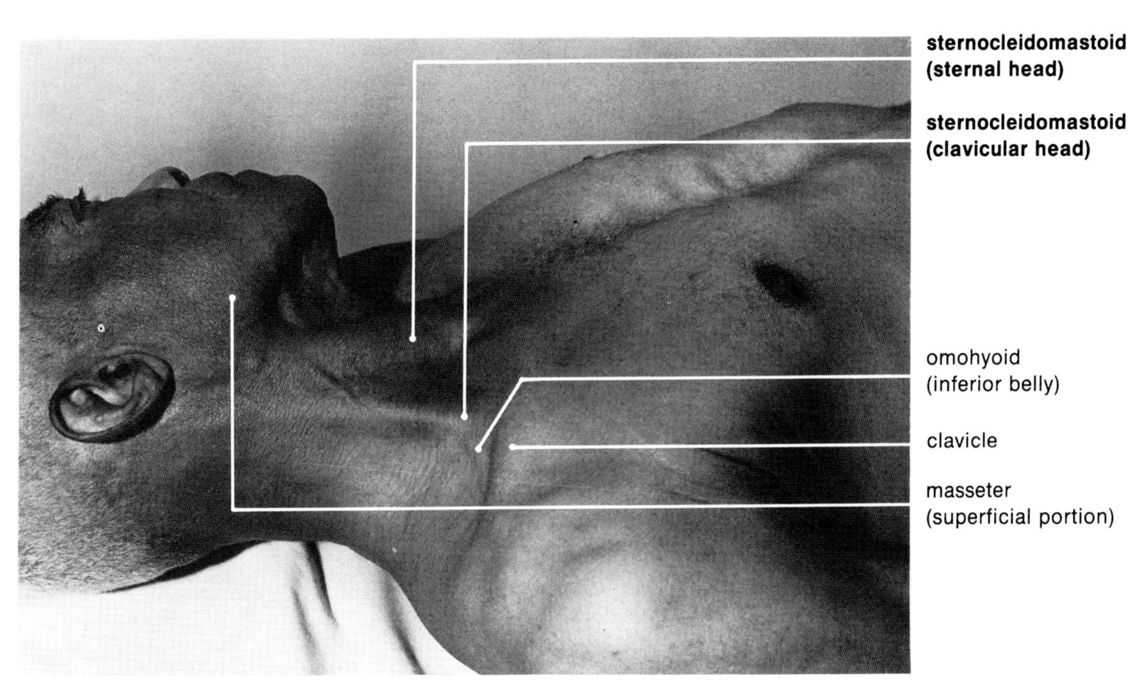

FIGURE 2-13 Sternocleidomastoid.
Note: The clavicular attachment of the clavicular head of the sternocleidomastoid is unusually far lateralward in this case.

Cervical Paraspinal Muscles (Deep or Intrinsic Muscles of the Neck) (*Fig.* 2-14; *see also Fig.* 1-14)

Action: Extension and lateral bending and rotation of the head and neck

Patient Position: Prone

Pin Insertion: Approximately 2 cm to 2.5 cm lateral to the spinous process of the cervical vertebrae

Relaxation: Instruct the patient to turn the face and chin to the side opposite that being examined. The neck may also be placed in lateral flexion toward the side being examined.

Contraction: *Minimal*: With the patient's head in the median position, instruct him as follows: "Lift your head up slightly" (minimal neck extension). If the contraction is too strong, a position midway between the median position of the head and the position used for relaxation may be employed.

Contraction: *Maximal*: With the patient's head placed in the median position, instruct him as follows: "Lift your head off the bed as high as you can as if you want to look up to the ceiling. Don't let me push your head down" (maximal neck extension against resistance).

Peripheral Nerve Supply: Medial and lateral branches of the posterior primary rami of the cervical nerves

Root Supply: Posterior primary rami of the cervical nerves. Insert the pin to reach the transverse process and withdraw slightly (1 mm to 2 mm) to examine the multifidus muscle, which gives better localization of the root supply. Extend the examination distally or proximally if negative findings are seen at corresponding levels. The multifidus segments in the neck are supplied by only the medial branches of the posterior primary rami of cervical nerves C3–C8.

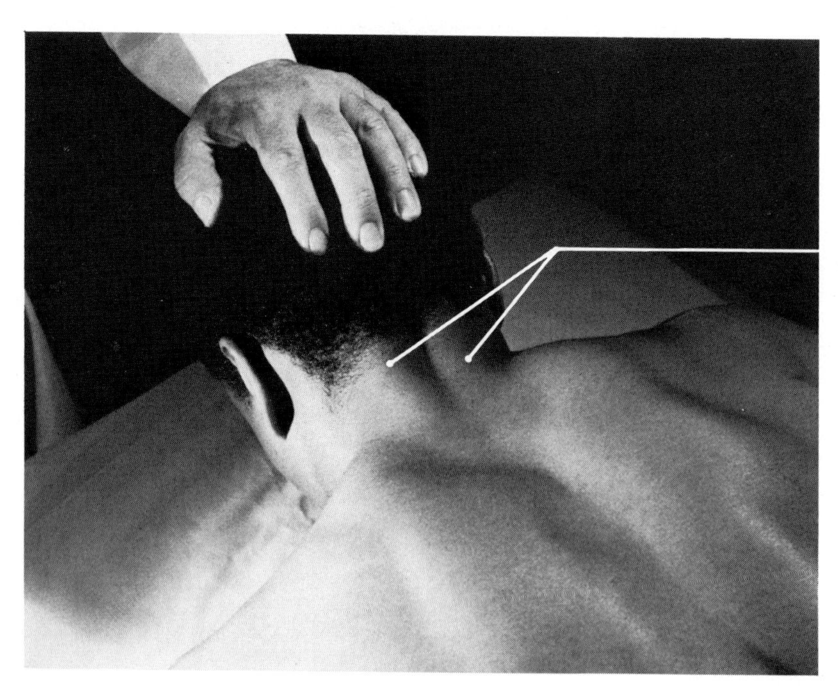

FIGURE 2-14 Cervical paraspinal muscles.

Muscles of the Trunk

Thoracic and Lumbosacral Paraspinal Muscles (*Fig.* 2-15; *see also Fig.* 1-14)

Action: Extend, laterally bend, and rotate the vertebral column. They also control forward flexon by play-out against gravity.

Patient Position: Prone

Pin Insertion: Approximately 2 cm to 3 cm lateral to the spinous processes of the vertebrae. Insert the pin to reach the transverse process and withdraw 1 mm to 2 mm for examination of the multifidus. If the pin is more superficial, the erector spinae will be examined.

Relaxation: The patient should be in the lateral recumbent position, and the side to be examined should be uppermost.

Contraction: *Minimal*: With the patient prone, instruct him to lift the opposite arm off the bed with the elbow in extension. If contraction is too strong, the examiner may instruct the patient to lift the arm on the side being examined. The outstretched arm should be close to the patient's head and ear so that the upper limb is extended in line with the body, thus making the paraspinal muscles fix the spine to serve as a base for the limb extension (actually extreme flexion). Abduction of the limb out to the side calls the trapezius into action rather than the paraspinal muscles.

Contraction: *Maximal*: Instruct the patient to lift the opposite arm and leg off the bed. Ensure that the outstretched arm is close to the patient's head and ear.

Peripheral Nerve Supply: Medial and lateral branches of the posterior primary rami of the spinal nerves

Root Supply: The erector spinae has an overlapping nerve root supply from the adjacent posterior primary rami of the spinal nerves. The multifidus usually has corresponding-level posterior primary rami supplying it. Feel for the posterior superior iliac spine and examine at that level for the S1 posterior primary rami supply. Allow approximately 2.5 cm per spinal nerve segment as you work proximally.

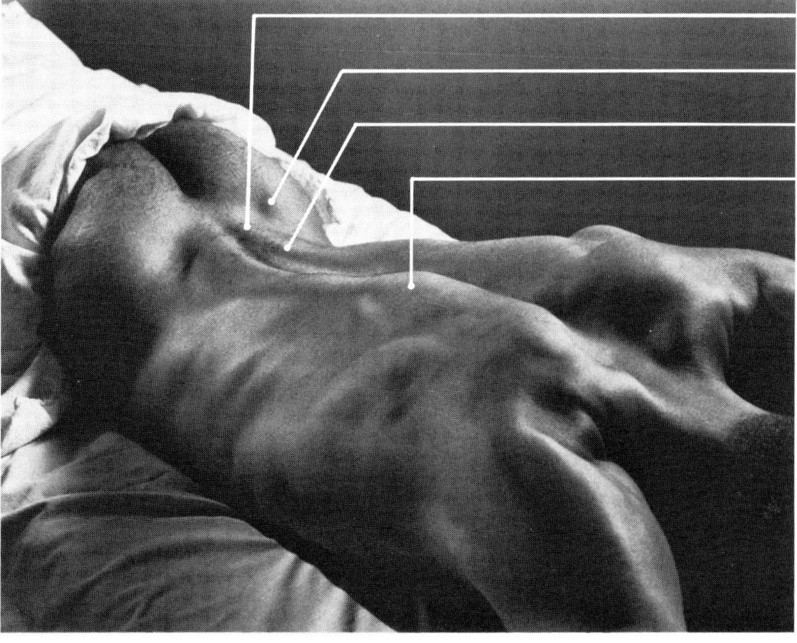

FIGURE 2-15 Thoracic and lumbosacral paraspinal muscles.

External Oblique (*Fig.* 2-16; *see also Fig.* 1-15)

Action: Compression of the abdomen and contraction in forced expiration. Bilateral action flexes the lumbar spine; unilateral action effects lateral bending. Acting with the contralateral internal oblique, the two muscles, working as a kinetic chain, cause turning or rotation of the torso.

Patient Position: Supine

Pin Insertion: Instruct the patient as follows: "Try to do a sit-up in such a manner that you can touch your right elbow with your left knee." The right external oblique will come into action. Insert the pin into the bulk of the muscle, staying just lateral to the vertical line of the anterior superior iliac spine of the ilium. The depth needed can be guided by the sound of the MUPs. Examination can also be done at the attachment of this muscle to the ribs; however, this region is harder to define, especially in obese patients and in women with pendulous breasts.

Relaxation: Instruct the patient as follows: "Relax your 'belly' muscles."

Contraction: *Minimal*: Instruct the patient as follows: "Try to act as if you would like to touch your right elbow to your left hip." If the shoulder blade comes off the table, the action may be sufficient. The correct amount of contraction can be ascertained by the appearance of the MUPs.

Contraction: *Maximal*: Instruct the patient as follows: "Contract your 'belly' muscles and try to touch your right elbow to your left hip." In older persons, if the shoulder blade comes off the table, the contraction is sufficient.

Peripheral Nerve Supply: Anterior primary rami of the lower six thoracic nerves

Root Supply: Nerve roots T6 through T12

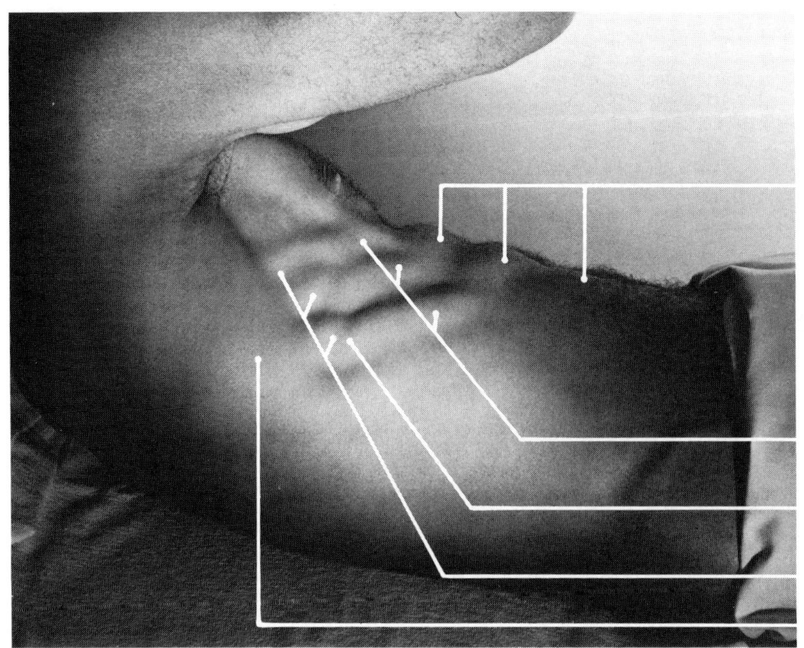

FIGURE 2-16 External oblique.

Rectus Abdominis (*Fig.* 2-17; *see also Fig.* 1-15)

Action: Flexion of the lumbar vertebral column and depression of the thoracic cage or costal margin. It stabilizes the pelvis in walking or running.

Patient Position: Supine

Pin Insertion: Instruct the patient to do a sit-up as follows: "Put your hands behind your head and try to lift your shoulder blades off the bed." The rectus abdominis will be seen to come into action. It is necessary to examine the muscle in contraction to be able to gauge the depth of needle insertion. This avoids injury to the peritoneum. Examination of only the lower segments is sufficient when examination of the thoracic roots is needed.

Relaxation: Instruct the patient to lie on his side. Choose the side on which he is lying for examination of the relaxed muscle.

Contraction: *Minimal*: With the patient supine, instruct him as follows: "Try to lift your shoulder blades just slightly off the bed."

Contraction: *Maximal*: Instruct the patient as follows: "Try to lift your shoulder blades off the bed, and try to do a sit-up." In older patients, it is sufficient just to have the shoulders lifted partially off the bed.

Peripheral Nerve Supply: The lower six or seven thoracic nerves

Root Supply: Nerve roots T6 through T12

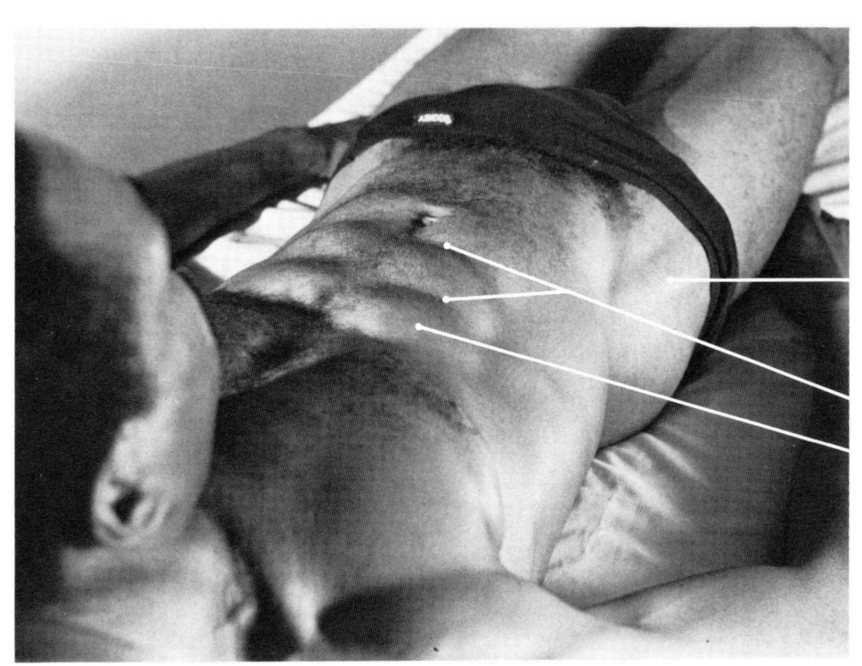

FIGURE 2-17 Rectus abdominis.

Bulbospongiosus (Bulbocavernosus) in the Male (*Fig.* 2-18; *see also Fig.* 1-70)

Action: Empties the urethra at the end of urination and during ejaculation and also aids in penile erection.

Patient Position: Supine, with the legs bent at the hips and knees and the thighs spread apart

Pin Insertion: Midway between the anus and the root of the scrotum, 1 cm lateral to the midline with the pin entering in the sagittal plane. The bulb of the penis may be palpated by moving the skin of the perineum from side to side along the midline while pressing firmly inward. Use the sounds of the MUPs as a guide for the depth of needle penetration.

Relaxation: Instruct the patient as follows: "Relax the muscles between your thighs."

Contraction: *Minimal*: Instruct the patient as follows: "Try to tighten all the muscles between your thighs very slightly."

Contraction: *Maximal*: Instruct the patient as follows: "Try to tighten all the muscles between your thighs as if to prevent urination or defecation."

Peripheral Nerve Supply: Perineal branches of the pudendal nerve

Root Supply: Nerve roots S2 through S4

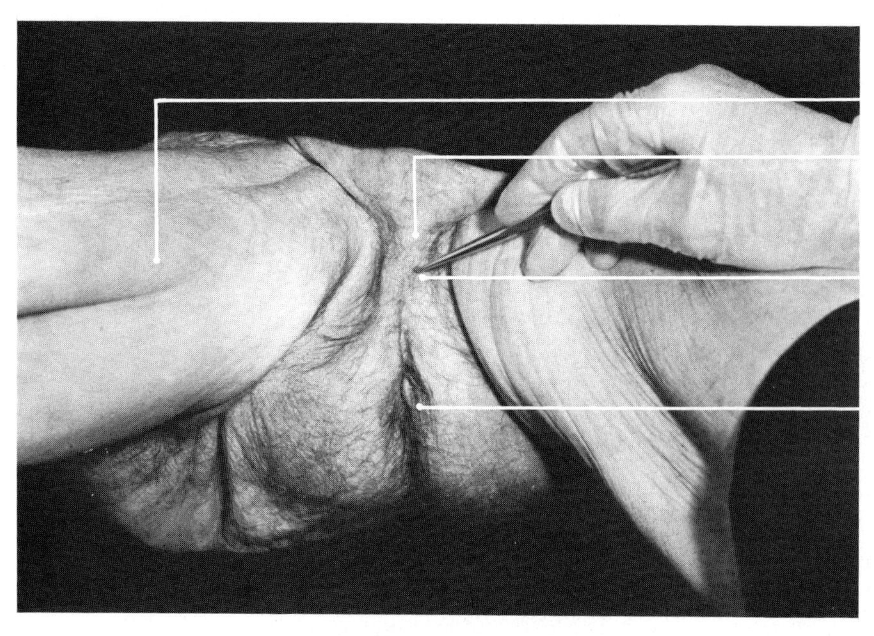

FIGURE 2-18 Bulbospongiosus (bulbocavernosus) in the male.
Note: Intact perineum of male cadaver

Bulbospongiosus (Bulbocavernosus) in the Female (*Fig.* 2-19)

Action: Slight constriction of the vaginal orifice; also, probably aids in erection of the clitoris by compression of the dorsal vein of the clitoris. The medial fibers of the pubococcygeus are more important than this muscle, however, in constricting the lower end of the vagina.

Patient Position: Supine, with the hips and knees flexed and the thighs spread apart

Pin Insertion: The level of pin penetration is lateral to the fossa navicularis, the depressed area between the posterior margin of the vaginal orifice and the posterior frenulum of the labia minora (fourchette). Insert the pin into the groove between the root of the labium minus and the medial aspect of the labium majus. The axis of needle entry should be slightly lateral. Listen for the sounds of the MUPs and observe for their appearance and the direction in which the sounds become crisp, for the muscle is very thin. This entry minimizes the likelihood of penetration into the bulb of the vestibule, which would lead to a hematoma. This is more likely to occur if the needle passes through the full thickness of the labium majus, since this is of variable thickness.

Relaxation: Instruct the patient as follows: "Relax the muscles between your thighs slightly."

Contraction: *Minimal*: Instruct the patient as follows: "Tighten the muscles between your thighs just slightly."

Contraction: *Maximal*: Instruct the patient as follows: "Tighten the muscles between your thighs as strongly as you can, as if to avoid urination or defecation."

Peripheral Nerve Supply: Perineal branches of the pudendal nerve

Root Supply: Nerve roots S2 through S4

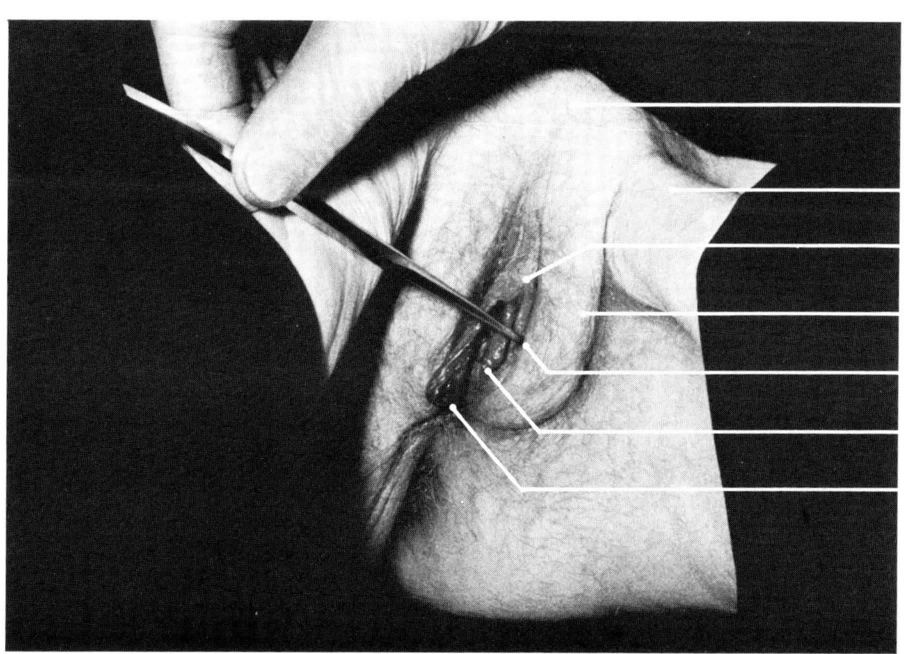

FIGURE 2-19 Bulbospongiosus (bulbocavernosus) in the female.
Note: Intact perineum of female cadaver. The tip of the probe is in the groove between the base of the labium minus and the base of the labium majus.

Muscles of the Perineum

Sphincter Ani Externus (*Fig.* 2-20; *see also* *Fig.* 1-70)

Action: Closure of the anal orifice

Patient Position: Supine, with the hips and knees flexed and the thighs spread apart

Pin Insertion: On the side to be examined, use the thumb of your left hand to press the skin and soft tissue lateral to the anal orifice inward (deeply) and lateral to reduce the funnelling effect of the perineal soft tissue. Insert the pin at the anteroposterior midlevel of the anus, at a point 2 cm lateral to the anal verge.

Relaxation: Instruct the patient as follows: "Relax the muscles between your thighs and especially the anus, the opening of your rectum."

Contraction: *Minimal*: Instruct the patient as follows: "Squeeze your anus just slightly."

Contraction: *Maximal*: Instruct the patient as follows: "Squeeze your anus as tightly as you can, as if you want to stop a bowel movement."

Peripheral Nerve Supply: Inferior rectal branches of the pudendal nerve and the perineal branch of S4

Root Supply: Nerve roots S2 through S4

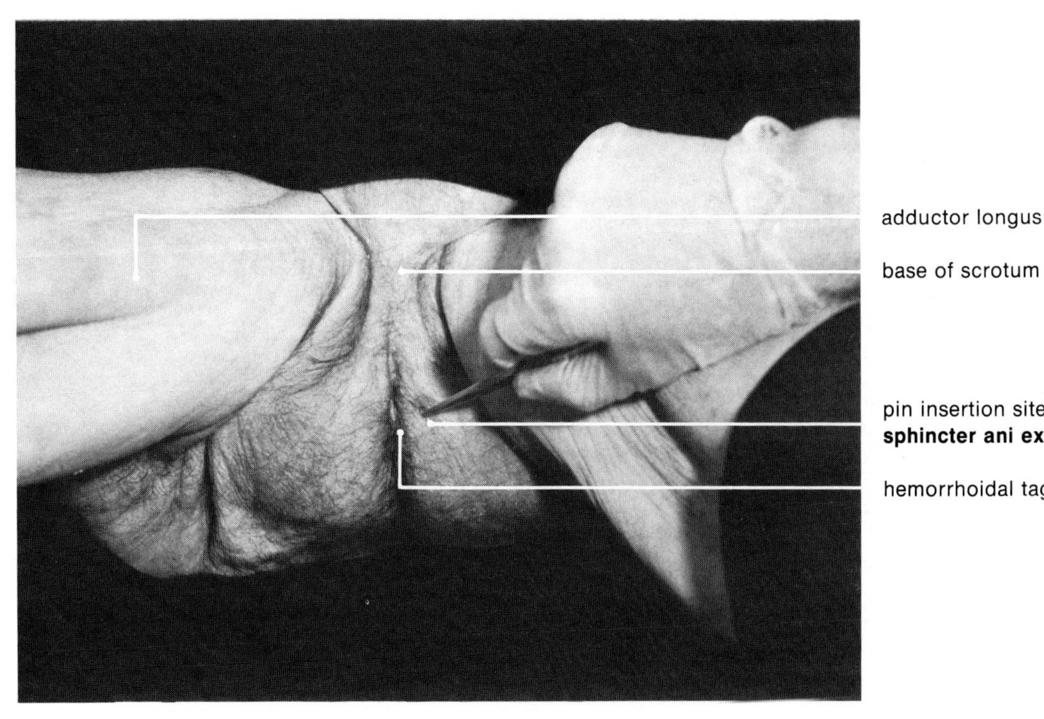

FIGURE 2-20 Sphincter ani externus.
Note: Intact perineum of male cadaver

MUSCLES OF THE SHOULDER GIRDLE AND CHEST WALL

Trapezius (Upper Portion) (*Fig.* 2-21; *see also Figs.* 1-10 *and* 1-11)

Action: Elevates the scapula.

Patient Position: Lateral recumbent

Pin Insertion: Instruct the patient as follows: "Shrug your shoulder toward your ear" (shoulder elevation). The ridge formed by the upper trapezius will be seen between the upper part of the neck and shoulder. Insert the pin into the most prominent part of the ridge, or at about the junction of middle and lateral thirds of the distance between the posterior base of the skull and the tip of the shoulder. The pin must be kept superficial; if deep, it may be in the supraspinatus.

Relaxation: Instruct the patient as follows: "Drop your shoulder down and relax your shoulder. Keep your arm close to your chest" (the shoulder is kept relaxed in the position of passive adduction).

(*Text continues on next page.*)

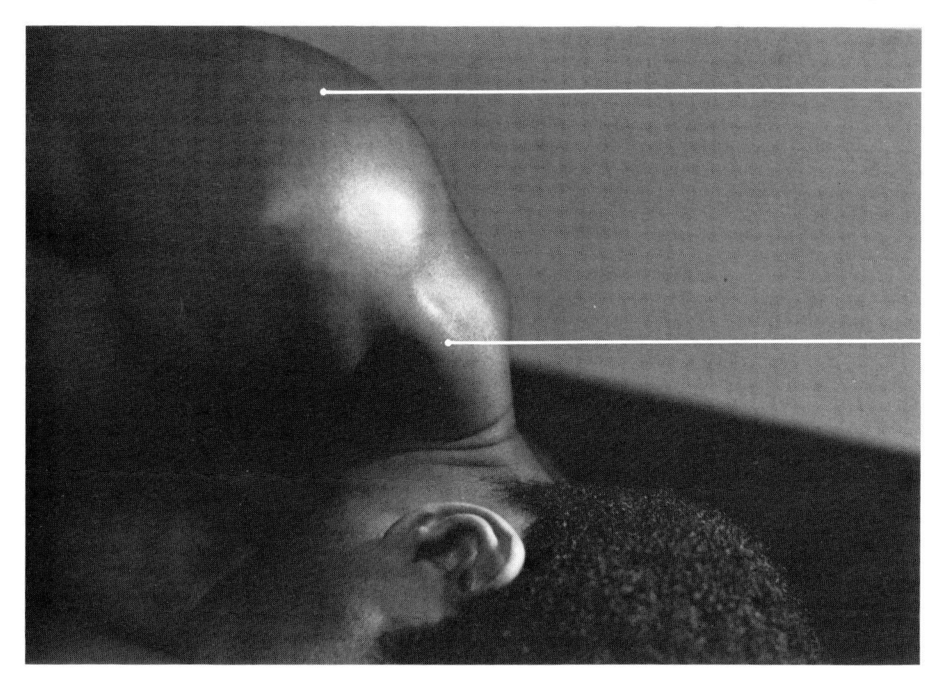

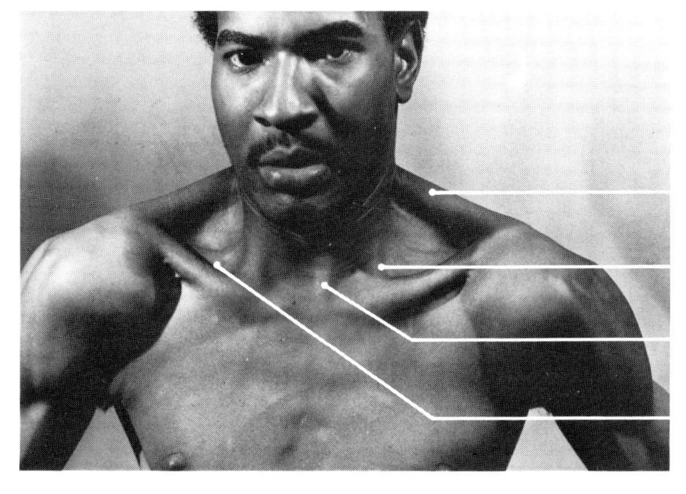

FIGURE 2-21 Trapezius (upper portion).

Trapezius (Upper Portion) *(Continued from previous page)*

Contraction: Minimal: Instruct the patient as follows: "Shrug your shoulder upward slightly" (minimal shoulder elevation).

Contraction: Maximal: Instruct the patient as follows: "Shrug your shoulder upward as if you want to touch the tip of your shoulder to your ear. Resist me when I push down on your shoulder." (Maximal shoulder elevation is obtained first, and then resistance is given.) If the patient is in the lateral recumbent position, apply inferior pressure on the tip of the shoulder in the sagittal plane.

Peripheral Nerve Supply: Spinal accessory nerve from C1 to C5, plus direct twigs from C3 and C4 via the cervical plexus. These latter twigs are both motor and sensory (proprioceptive).

Root Supply: Nerve roots C1 through C5 via the spinal accessory nerve; mainly nerve roots C3 and C4

Trapezius (Middle Portion) (*Fig.* 2-22; *see also Fig.* 1-10)

Action: Adducts and retracts the scapula.

Patient Position: Prone, with the forehead touching the surface of the examination bed. Place the shoulder in external rotation with the arm at 90° of abduction and the elbow at 90° of flexion.

Pin Insertion: Instruct the patient to lift the entire upper extremity off the bed with the arm and elbow positioned as described above. The bulk formed by the middle portion of the trapezius will be seen as it contracts. Identify it between the C7 and T3 vertebrae medially and the spine of the scapula laterally. Insert the pin between these points, but somewhat nearer to the vertebrae. The pin must be kept superficial, or it will be in the rhomboideus minor.

Relaxation: Instruct the patient to hang the entire upper extremity from the shoulder distally off the edge of the bed.

Contraction: *Minimal*: Instruct the patient as follows: "Brace your shoulder backward slightly" (minimal scapular adduction).

Contraction: *Maximal*: With the patient's arm and elbow kept in the position described under pin insertion, instruct the patient as follows: "Lift your arm and elbow up off the bed as high as you can. Don't let me push your shoulder down" (maximal scapular adduction and retraction). Apply downward pressure in the direction of shoulder flexion or scapular protraction, against the upper lateral edge of the scapula or against the acromion.

Peripheral Nerve Supply: Spinal accessory nerve via roots from segments C1 through C5

Root Supply: Mainly C3 and C4 nerve roots via the spinal accessory nerve plus direct twigs from the same segments through the cervical plexus

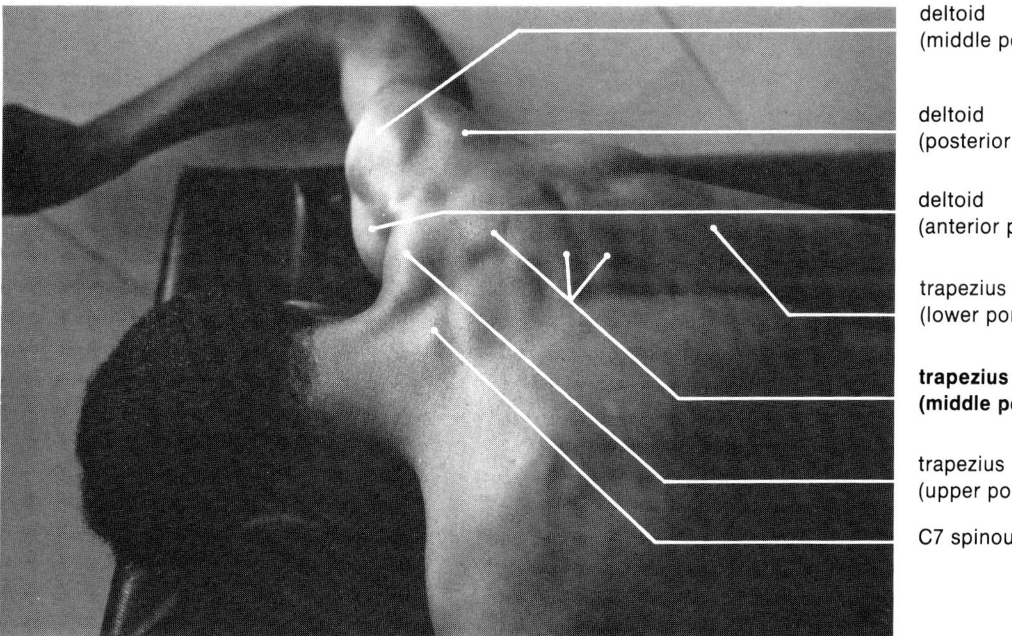

FIGURE 2-22 Trapezius (middle portion).

Trapezius (Lower Portion) (*Fig.* 2-23; *see also Fig.* 1-10)

Action: Depresses the medial border of the scapula (thus rotating the scapula when the upper fibers are elevating the lateral angle of the scapula).

Patient Position: Prone. The patient lies with his forehead touching the surface of the examination bed, keeping the outstretched limb in front of him, close to the side of his head as if he is ready to dive from a diving board.

Pin Insertion: Identify the lower trapezius as it contracts when the patient lifts his outstretched upper limb off the bed. The lower trapezius will be seen extending between the middle and lower thoracic vertebrae medially and the spine of the scapula laterally. Insert the pin between these two points, somewhat nearer to the vertebrae, about 2 cm to 5 cm lateral to the midthoracic vertebrae (T6–T8 level). Also use the inferior ridge of the lower trapezius as a guide and stay medial to this ridge.

Relaxation: Place the patient's entire upper extremity beside him, with the arm in adduction and the elbow extended alongside the thorax, or place the entire upper extremity from the shoulder distally hanging over the side of the bed.

Contraction: *Minimal*: With the shoulder slightly abducted and the elbow flexed, instruct the patient as follows: "Slightly lift the elbow off the bed."

Contraction: *Maximal*: With the patient's arm placed as described in patient position, instruct him as follows: "Lift your entire arm off the bed." Apply downward pressure in the direction of shoulder flexion, against the upper lateral portion of the scapula.

Peripheral Nerve Supply: Spinal accessory nerve from segments C1 through C5

Root Supply: Nerve roots C1 through C5, mainly C4 and C5 with some overlap or a mixture of nerve roots C3 and C4 via direct twigs from the cervical plexus

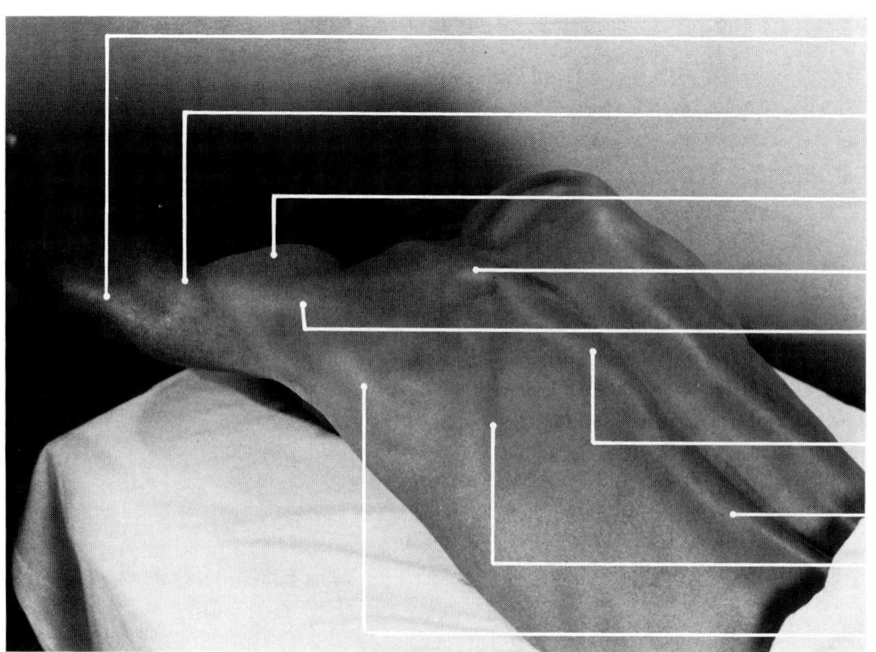

FIGURE 2-23 Trapezius (lower portion).

Levator Scapulae (*Fig. 2-24; see also Figs. 1-6 and 1-13*)

Action: Elevates the scapula.

Patient Position: Sitting or lateral recumbent position

Pin Insertion: To examine the right levator scapulae, have the patient shrug his right shoulder upward by action of the right upper trapezius. Also, have his face and chin turned to the left by action of the right sternocleidomastoid. For examination of the left levator scapulae, the patient should shrug his left shoulder up, and the face and chin should be turned to the right. The levator scapulae will be seen to come into action between the trapezius laterally and the sternocleidomastoid medially. Insert the pin into the most palpable bulk of the muscle, usually at about the junction of the middle and lower thirds of the muscle.

Relaxation: Instruct the patient as follows: "Drop your shoulder down and relax."

Contraction: *Minimal*: Instruct the patient as follows: "Shrug your shoulder up slightly toward your ear" (minimal shoulder elevation).

Contraction: *Maximal*: Instruct the patient as follows: "Shrug your shoulder up strongly toward your ear and don't let me push it down" (maximal shoulder elevation against resistance). Apply downward pressure on the shoulder.

Peripheral Nerve Supply: Direct twigs from spinal nerve roots C3 through C5 and variably from the dorsal scapular nerve (C5)

Root Supply: Nerve roots C3 through C5, mainly C3

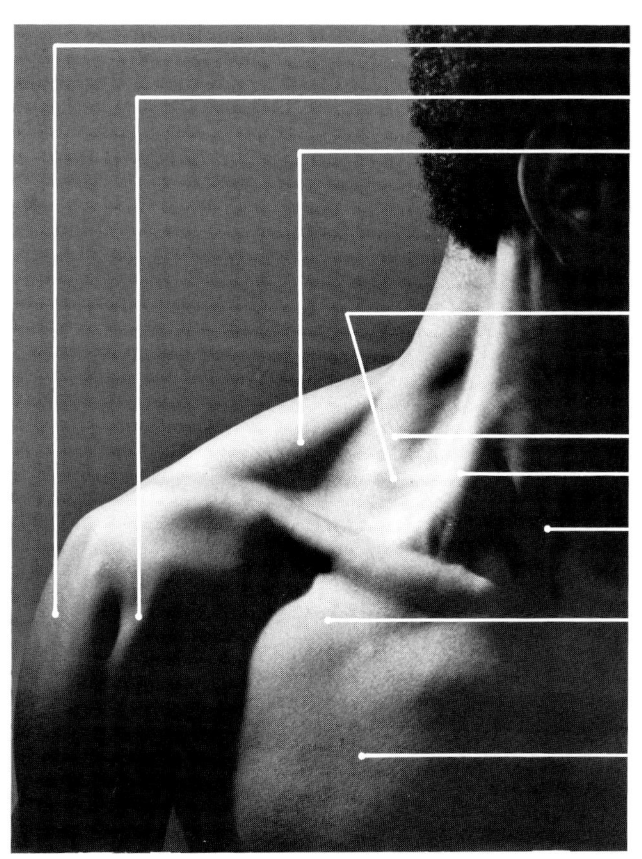

FIGURE 2-24 Levator scapulae.

Rhomboideus Major (*Fig. 2-25; see also Figs. 1-10 through 1-13*)

Action: Elevation and retraction of the scapula

Patient Position: Lateral recumbent or prone

Pin Insertion: Sit behind the patient and palpate the inferior angle and the adjacent portion of the medial border of the scapula. Then place the metacarpophalangeal joint of your left thumb against the inferior angle of the patient's scapula and push the upper part of the inferior or lateral edge of the lower trapezius medially. The tip of your left thumb will now lie at about the inferior border of the rhomboideus major. Insert the pin into the rhomboideus major by penetrating into the muscle just above the tip of your left thumb. This muscle is not covered by any other muscle in this region; however, since the pleura is underneath, caution must be used. Use the sounds of the MUPs for guidance in directing the needle. Do not go deeper if the MUP sounds become more distant. In most patients, not more than 2 cm of the pin needs to be inserted. In obese patients, palpation of the inferior angle and the medial border of the scapula may be difficult and can be facilitated by moving the patient's shoulder about.

Relaxation: (1) *Lateral Recumbent*: Position the patient's arm so that it is adducted at the side of his chest. The elbow is kept extended. (2) *Prone*: Have the patient hang the entire upper extremity from the shoulder distally over the side of the bed.

Contraction: *Minimal*: (1) *Lateral Recumbent*: Protract the patient's shoulder anteriorly and, with the arm abducted and the elbow slightly bent, have the patient place the palm of his hand on his hip. Instruct the patient as follows: "Press your palm slightly into your hip." (2) *Prone*: Position the patient's arm so that the shoulder is protracted anteriorly and the dorsum of the hand is on the patient's buttock. Instruct the patient as follows: "Lift your hand off the buttock very slightly."

Contraction: *Maximal*: (1) *Lateral recumbent*: Instruct the patient as follows: "Bend your elbow and push backward as though you would like to jab me with your elbow. Don't let me push

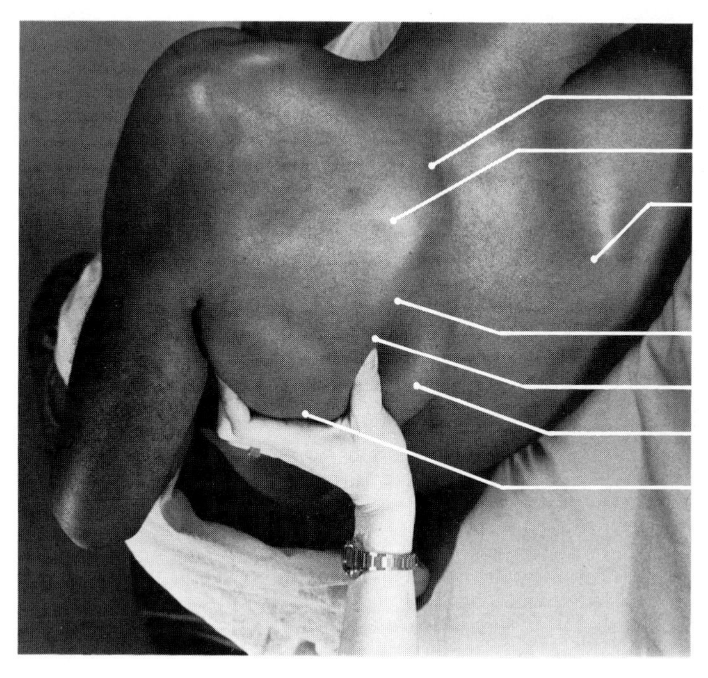

FIGURE 2-25 Rhomboideus major. (*Figure continues on facing page.*)

your elbow forward" (scapular retraction with arm kept in extension and the elbow kept in flexion). Apply resistence at the lower part of the arm and push forward in the direction of arm flexion. (2) *Prone*: Instruct the patient as follows: "Lift your hand off your buttock. Don't let me push your shoulder down" (maximum scapular retraction against resistance). Apply downward pressure over the scapula and shoulder area in the direction of scapular protraction.

Peripheral Nerve Supply: Dorsal scapular nerve from the anterior primary ramus of the C5 nerve root

Root Supply: C5 nerve root

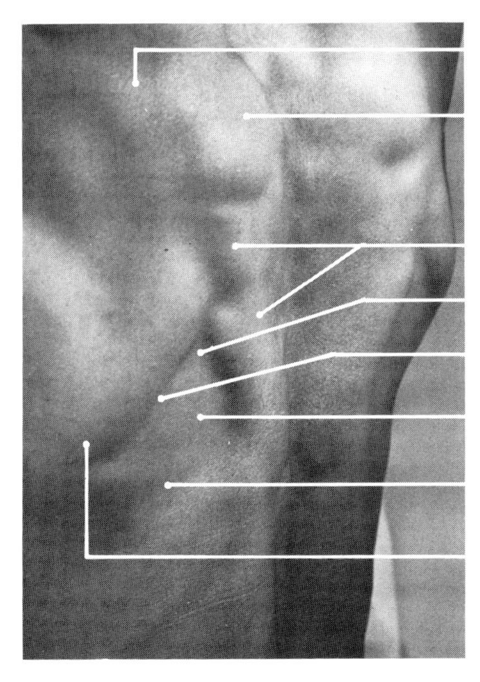

FIGURE 2-25 (*Continued*)

Rhomboideus Minor (*Fig.* 2-26; *see also Figs.* 1-6, 1-12, *and* 1-13)

Action: Scapular elevation and retraction
*Patient Position**
Pin Insertion: Feel for the medial end of the crest of the spine of the scapula and the C7 spinous process. Insert the pin midway between these two points. At least 2 cm of the pin should be inserted to ensure penetration through the middle trapezius, which overlies the rhomboideus minor.
*Relaxation**
*Contraction**
*Peripheral Nerve Supply**
*Root Supply**

* See rhomboideus major.

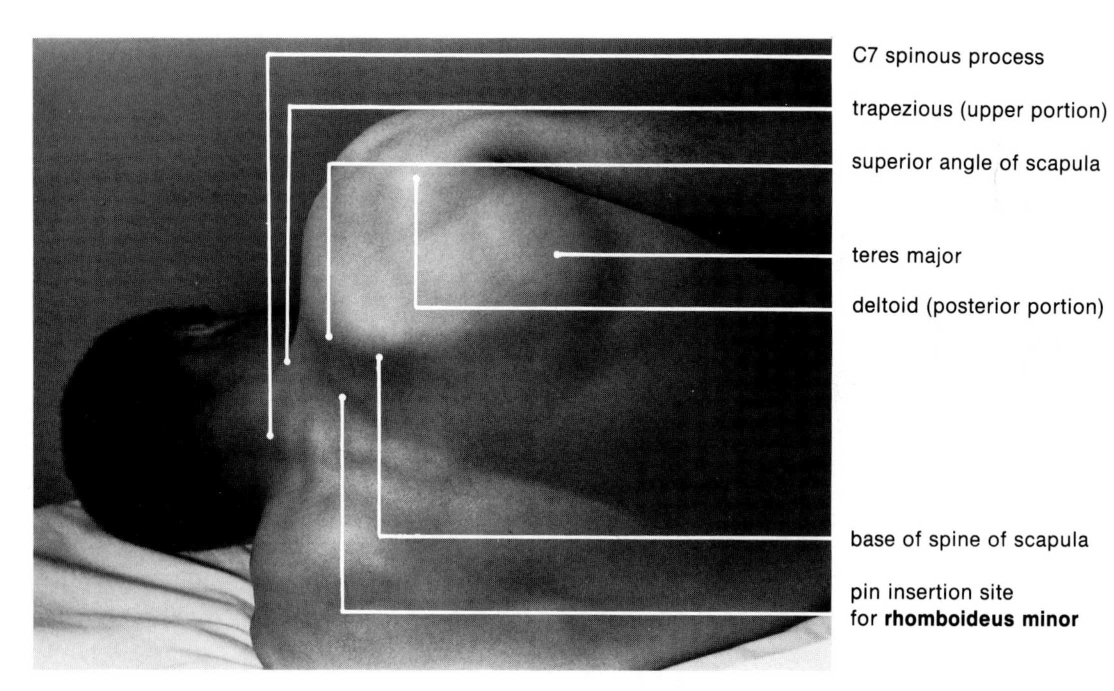

FIGURE 2-26 Rhomboideus minor.

Supraspinatus (*Fig.* 2-27; *see also* Figs. 1-6 *and* 1-13)

Action: Abduction of the arm

Patient Position: Lateral recumbent

Pin Insertion: Feel for the superior border of the spine of the scapula and insert the pin within 2 cm above this edge, at about the junction of the lateral two thirds and the medial third of the length of the spine of the scapula. Insert the pin until the periosteum is touched lightly, and withdraw the pin approximately 1 mm to 2 mm.

Relaxation: Place the patient's arm in adduction and internal rotation, with the elbow bent to 90° and the forearm across the patient's chest, or have patient lie prone or semiprone with the entire upper extremity hanging over the edge of the bed with the arm in internal rotation.

Contraction: *Minimal*: With the patient in the lateral recumbent position and the arm and forearm placed across the chest as described above under relaxation, instruct the patient as follows: "Lift your elbow slightly off the side of your chest" (abduction of the arm while the arm is kept in slight internal rotation). Occasionally ask the patient to "lift just your arm and elbow slightly off your chest." This motion initiates minimal contraction.

Contraction: *Maximal*: Position the patient's arm in 90° of abduction and the elbow at 90° of flexion. Apply pressure on the elbow in the direction of adduction.

Peripheral Nerve Supply: Suprascapular nerve from the upper trunk of the brachial plexus

Root Supply: Nerve roots C5 and C6, mainly C5

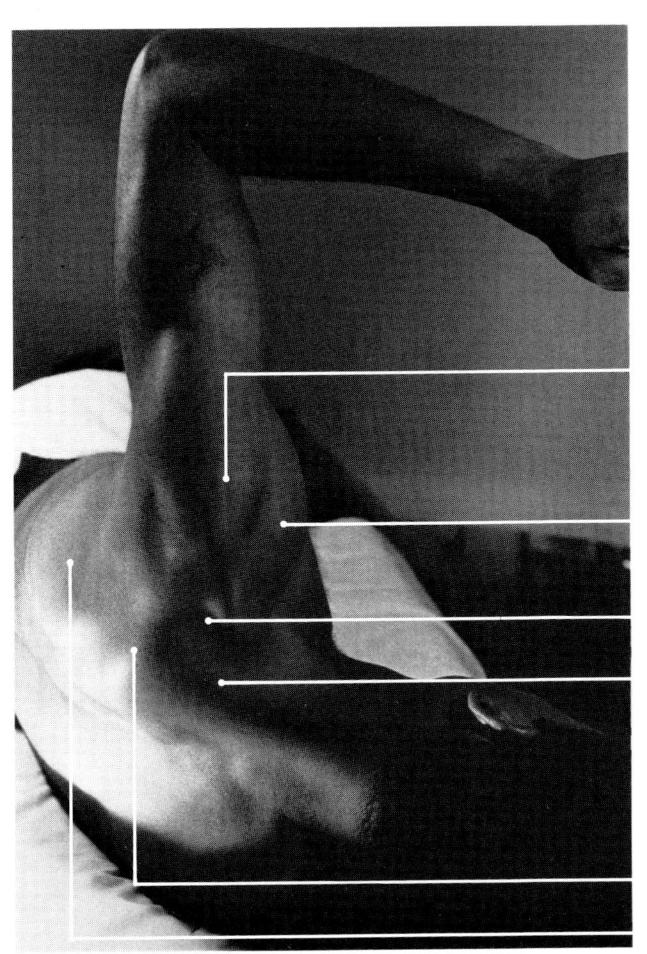

FIGURE 2-27 Supraspinatus.

Infraspinatus (*Fig.* 2-28; *see also Figs.* 1-10, 1-12, *and* 1-13)

Action: External rotation of the arm while in an adducted position

Patient Position: Lateral recumbent

Pin Insertion: Feel for a point along the inferior margin of the spine of the scapula that is 2.5 cm lateral to the medial end. From this point, move inferiorly for approximately 2.5 cm and insert the pin at this level. Alternatively, the lower trapezius and the teres major could be made to contract. The pin could be inserted between these two muscles to examine the infraspinatus, since this muscle is superficial in this region. Insert the pin until the periosteum is touched, and withdraw approximately 1mm to 2 mm.

*Relaxation**

Contraction: External rotation of the humerus while in an adducted position. If the humerus is in an abducted position, the deltoid will assist in external rotation, and maximal action of the infraspinatus will not be obtained.

*Peripheral Nerve Supply**

*Root Supply**

* See supraspinatus.

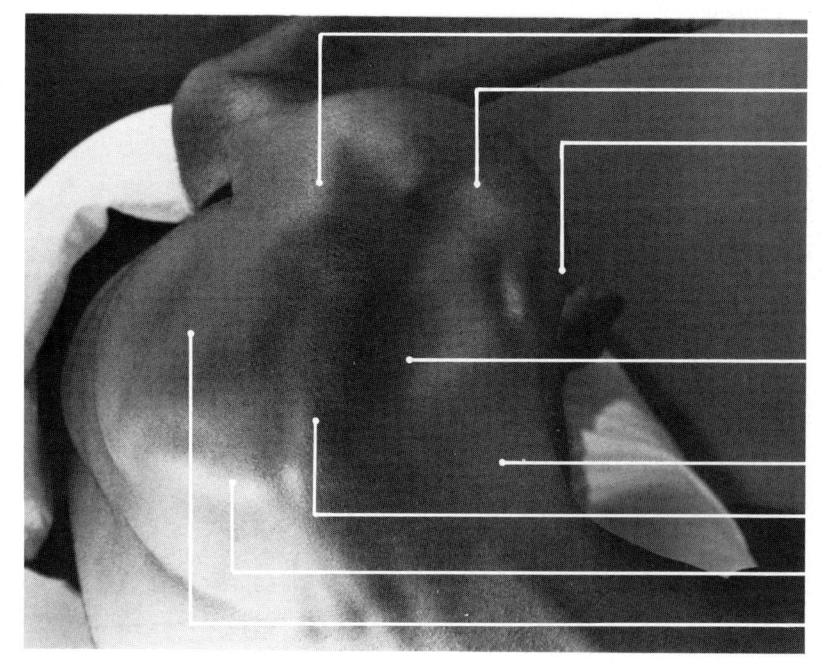

FIGURE 2-28 Infraspinatus.

Teres Major (*Fig. 2-29; see also Figs. 1-11 and 1-13*)

Action: Internal rotation, adduction, and extension of the arm

Patient Position: Lateral recumbent

Pin Insertion: Position the patient's arm in abduction and internal rotation, and stretch out the teres major by applying pressure at the elbow in the direction of flexion of the arm. The patient's resistance to the forward pressure of the examiner's hand causes the teres major to be easily identifiable at the lower lateral border of the scapula. Insert the pin approximately 5 cm superior to the inferior angle of the scapula and approximately 1 cm lateral to the lateral border of the scapula.

Relaxation: Instruct the patient as follows: "Put your arm against the side of your chest. Keep your elbow straight and try to relax" (arm in adduction and elbow in extension). The arm may also be placed passively into external rotation.

Contraction: *Minimal*: With the arm in abduction and internal rotation and the elbow in flexion, instruct the patient as follows: "Put your hand on your hip and press lightly" (minimal arm adduction).

Contraction: *Maximal*: With the patient's shoulder in abduction and internal rotation and the elbow in flexion, give resistance at the elbow as the patient tries to extend the arm.

Peripheral Nerve Supply: Lower subscapular nerve from the posterior cord of the brachial plexus

Root Supply: Nerve roots C5 and C6, mainly C6

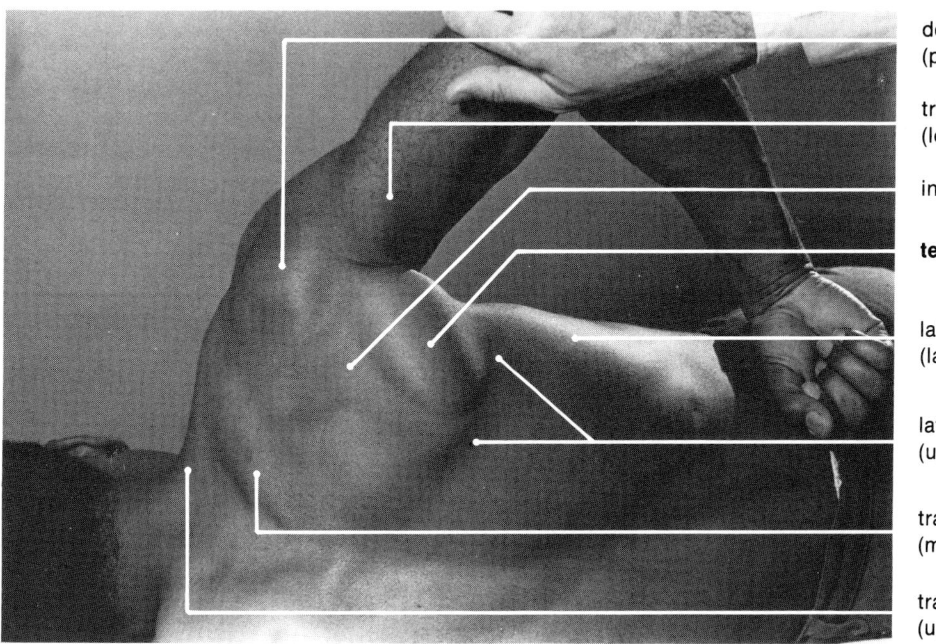

FIGURE 2-29 Teres major.

Teres Minor (*Fig. 2-30; see also Figs. 1-10 through 1-12 and 1-24*)

Action: External rotation of the arm

Patient Position: Lateral recumbent

Pin Insertion: Position the patient's arm in external rotation and define the lower edge of the posterior portion of the deltoid (elicit the action of this muscle as described later in this chapter) and the upper limit of the teres major by making this muscle contract as previously described. The teres minor is along the lateral edge of the scapula between these two muscles. At this region, feel for the lateral margin of the scapula and insert the pin approximately 1 cm lateral to this margin and approximately 1 cm below the lower edge of the posterior deltoid.

Relaxation: Position the patient's arm against his chest so that the arm is in adduction and the elbow is in extension.

Contraction: *Minimal*: With the patient's arm at the side of his chest and the elbow flexed to 90°, instruct him as follows: "Lift your forearm and hand slightly outward" (very minimal external rotation). Adjust the amount of contraction needed by slightly rotating the arm internally or externally.

Contraction: *Maximal*: Position the patient's shoulder in external rotation and apply downward pressure at the upper forearm in the direction of internal rotation. Ask the patient to resist.

Peripheral Nerve Supply: Axillary nerve from the posterior cord of the brachial plexus

Root Supply: Nerve roots C5 and C6, mainly C6

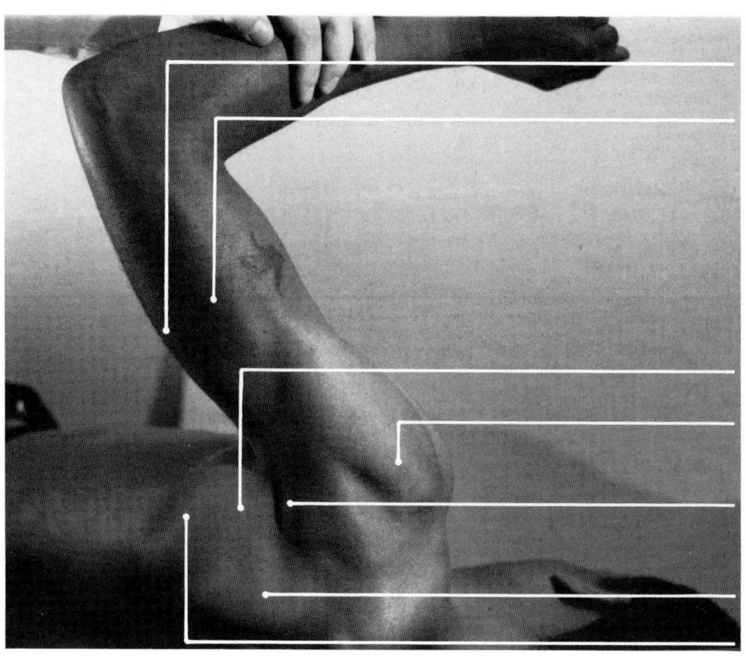

FIGURE 2-30 Teres minor.

Serratus Anterior (*Fig.* 2-31; *see also* Figs. 1-5 *and* 1-23)

Action: Rotation of the scapula about an anteroposterior axis so that the inferior angle moves laterally as in abduction of the arm. It also protracts the scapula, as in reaching forward, and it holds the scapula fixed to the chest, as when pushing against an object.

Patient Position: Lateral recumbent or supine

Pin Insertion: The serratus anterior will be seen to come into action as the patient presses his palms together with his arms outstretched in front of his chest. Palpate for the ribs of the digitations to be examined and straddle the rib with the middle and index fingers. The middle finger is used to guard the intercostal space above, and the index finger the intercostal space below. The examination is easier to do at the level of the 5th through 8th ribs, since the serratus anterior is not covered by any other muscle at this level. Insert the pin until the periosteum of the rib is touched gently and then withdraw approximately 1 mm to 2 mm. Examination is best done with the pin angled posteriorly into the muscle.

Relaxation: (1) *Lateral Recumbent Position*: Stand behind the patient and place his arm on your shoulder. The patient's scapula then will be retracted. Instruct the patient as follows: "Put the weight of your arm on my shoulder and relax it." The arm can also be placed overhead and extended. (2) *Supine Position*: The patient

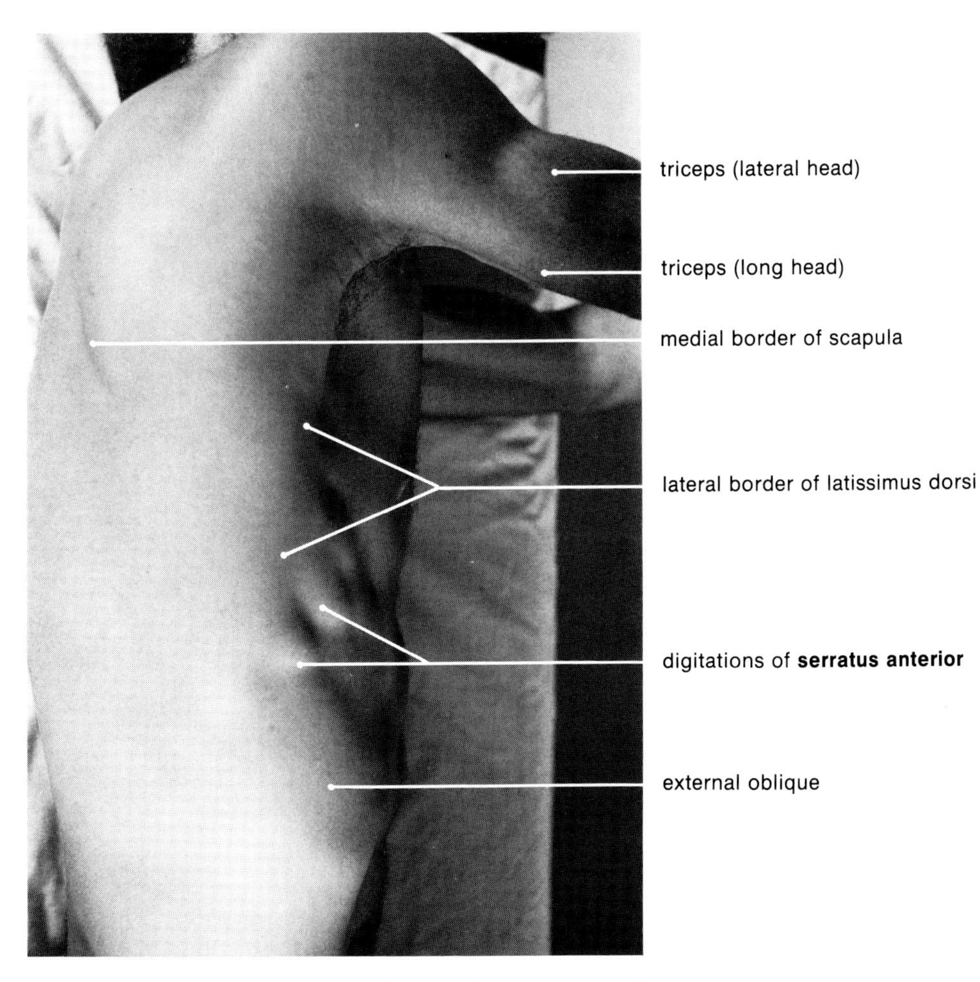

FIGURE 2-31 Serratus anterior. (*Figure continues on next page.*)

Serratus Anterior *(Continued from previous page)*

relaxes by placing the arm back on the bed, adducted and relaxed.

Contraction: Minimal: Instruct the patient as follows: "Lift your arm upward slightly" (minimal arm flexion).

Contraction: Maximal: Instruct the patient as follows: "Push both your arms forward strongly and press your palms together" (protraction of the shoulder against resistance). Apply resistance to arm flexion by pressing downward in the direction of arm extension.

Peripheral Nerve Supply: Long thoracic nerve, direct from the anterior primary rami of nerve roots C5 through C7

Root Supply: Nerve roots C5 through C7

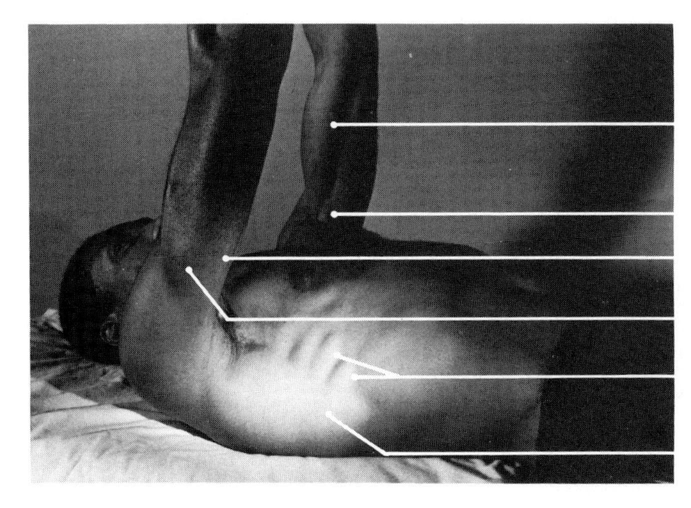

FIGURE 2-31 *(Continued)*

Latissimus Dorsi (*Fig.* 2-32; *see also Figs.* 1-10 *through* 1-13)

Action: Adduction, internal rotation, and extension of the arm

Patient Position: Lateral recumbent

Pin Insertion: For examination of the right latissimus dorsi, stand behind the patient and place the patient's right hand on your left shoulder. The patient's left hand can be placed on your right shoulder for examination of the left latissimus dorsi. Instruct the patient as follows: "Push your hand down into my shoulder" (arm adduction). The latissimus dorsi will be seen to come into action, forming part of the posterior wall of the axilla. The upper edge of the muscle can be seen when resistance is given to arm extension with the arm kept in abduction and internal rotation. Feel for the inferior angle of the scapula and insert the pin approximately 5 cm inferior to this angle.

Relaxation: Place the patient's arm at his side. If relaxation cannot be achieved in this position, place the patient's arm above his head so that the arm is abducted, flexed, and externally rotated. This position stretches out the muscle, but it will be more difficult for the patient to contract the muscle unknowingly in case of pain from needling.

Contraction: *Minimal*: Place the patient's arm in partial abduction and internal rotation and the elbow in partial flexion, with the palm placed on the hip. Instruct the patient as follows: "Push your palm slightly into your hip" (minimal arm adduction).

Contraction: *Maximal*: Have the patient's arm extended and abducted, and instruct the patient as follows: "Push your arm down onto my shoulder [shoulder adduction against resistance] while pushing backward with your arm" (shoulder extension against resistance). Apply pressure in the direction of shoulder abduction and shoulder flexion by giving resistance at the level of the lower arm.

Peripheral Nerve Supply: Thoracodorsal nerve (long subscapular nerve) from the posterior cord of the brachial plexus

Root Supply: Nerve roots C6 through C8

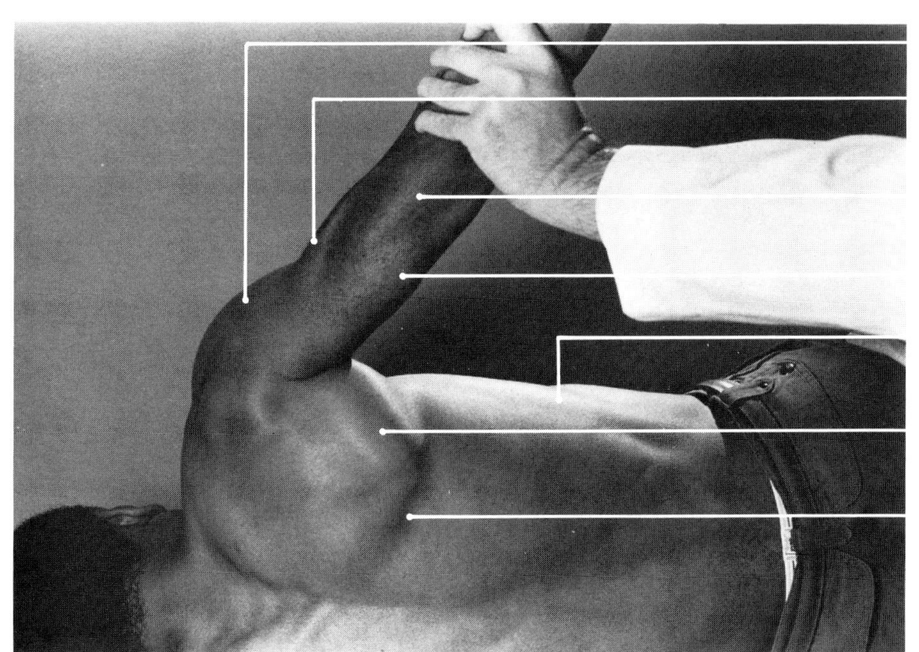

FIGURE 2-32 Latissimus dorsi.

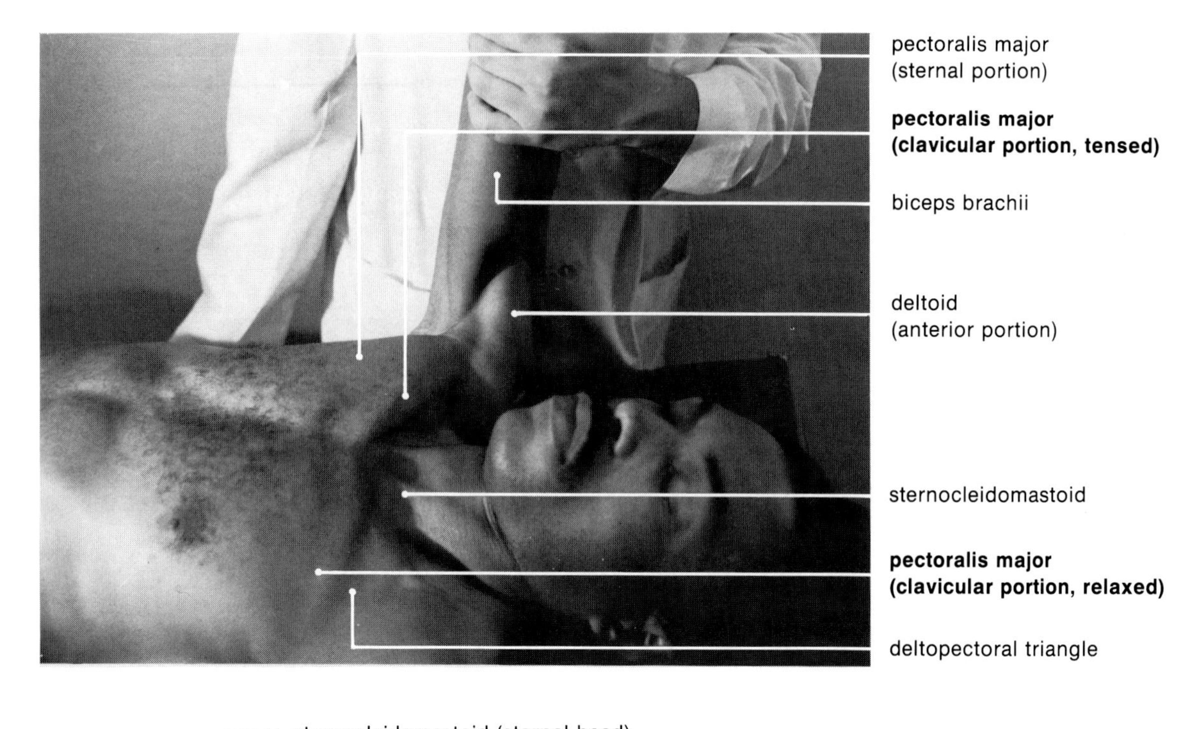

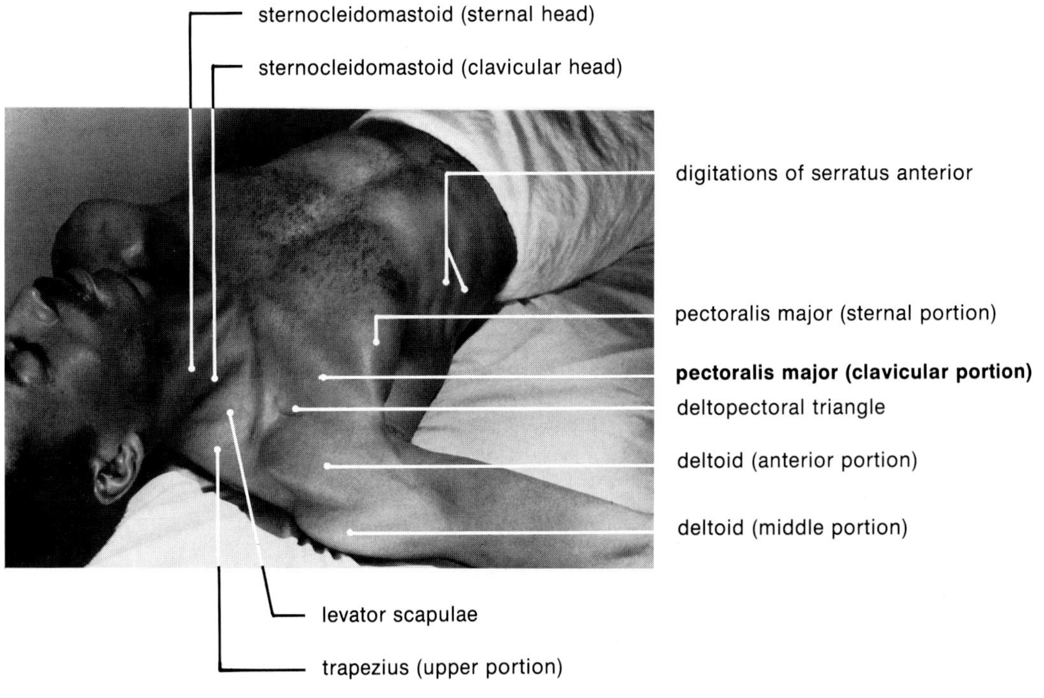

FIGURE 2-33 Pectoralis major (clavicular portion).

Pectoralis Major (*Figs. 2-33 and 2-34; see also Figs. 1-4 and 1-5*)

Action: Adduction and internal rotation of the arm

Patient Position: Supine

Pin Insertion: (1) *Clavicular Head (see Fig. 2-33)*: Locate a point 3 cm lateral to the medial end of the clavicle and insert the pin 2 cm inferior to this point. (2) *Sternal Head (see Fig. 2-34)*: Grasp the lower edge of the anterior axillary fold between your thumb and index finger, and insert the pin between the two.

Relaxation: Place the patient's arm against his side. If the patient cannot fully relax, position the arm in abduction and external rotation and place it on the bed above the patient's head. This stretches the muscle; however, it will be more difficult for the patient to contract the muscle unknowingly in case of pain from the needling.

Contraction: *Minimal*: Instruct the patient as follows: "Bend your elbow and draw your arm slightly downward toward your chest" (arm adduction).

Contraction: *Maximal*: Instruct the patient as follows: "Pull your arm strongly downward across your chest." Give resistance to adduction by applying pressure to the medial aspect of the lower arm in the direction of abduction.

Peripheral Nerve Supply: Clavicular portion: lateral pectoral nerve; sternal portion: lateral and medial pectoral nerves

Root Supply: Clavicular portion: roots C5 and C6; sternal portion: roots C7, C8, and T1

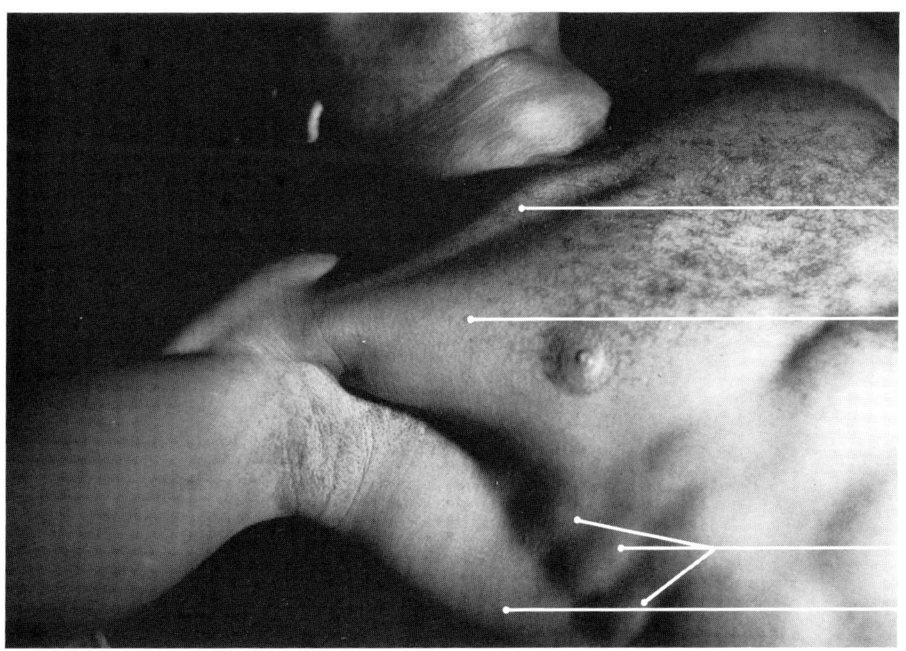

FIGURE 2-34 Pectoralis major (sternal portion).

MUSCLES OF THE ARM

Deltoid (Anterior or Clavicular Portion) *(Fig. 2-35; see also Figs. 1-21 and 1-22)*

Action: Primarily flexes the arm. Also assists in arm abduction by stabilizing the shoulder joint.

Patient Position: Supine

Pin Insertion: Instruct the patient as follows: "Lift your arm off the bed" (shoulder flexion). The anterior deltoid is easily identified between the deltopectoral groove medially and the middle deltoid laterally. Insert the pin medial to the groove that separates it from the middle deltoid approximately 2 cm to 4 cm distal to the lateral tip of the clavicle.

Relaxation: Place the patient's shoulder in the adducted position at the side of his chest with the posterior tip of the acromion completely flat against the bed.

Contraction: *Minimal*: Place the patient's forearm across his chest with the elbow flexed and the arm slightly abducted. Instruct patient as follows: "Slide your elbow in toward your chest" (minimal shoulder adduction). To initiate contraction, occasionally instruct the patient as follows: "Lift your elbow slightly off the bed" (minimal shoulder flexion).

Contraction: *Maximal*: Instruct the patient as follows: "Lift your arm up off the bed with your elbow straight, and don't let me push your arm down." (Give resistance to arm flexion with the patient's elbow kept in extension.) Apply downward pressure at the level of lower arm in the direction of shoulder extension.

Peripheral Nerve Supply: Axillary nerve from the posterior cord of the brachial plexus

Root Supply: Nerve roots C5 and C6, mainly C5

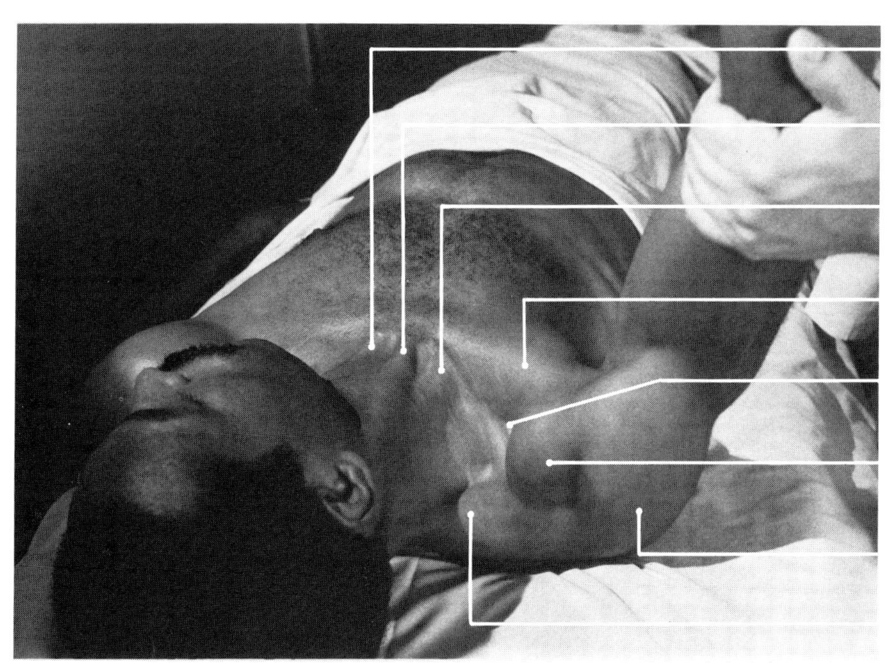

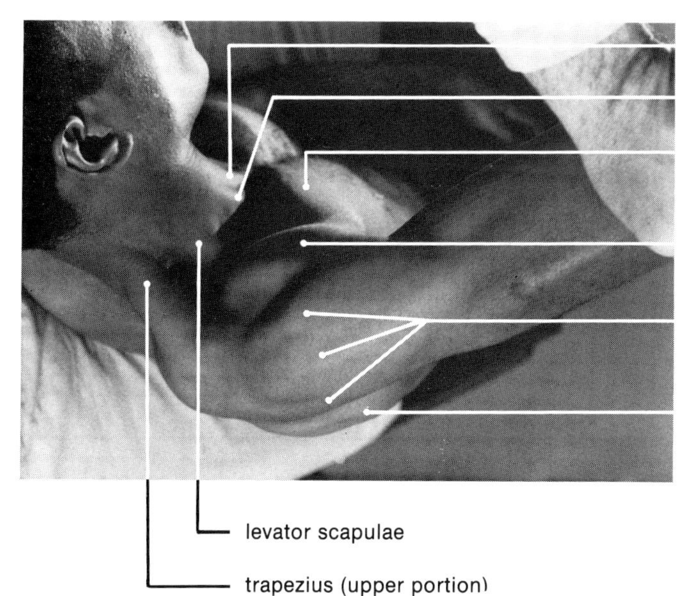

FIGURE 2-35 Deltoid (anterior portion).

Deltoid (Middle or Acromial Portion) (*Fig.* 2-36; *see also Figs.* 1-21 *and* 1-22)

Action: Abduction of the arm

Patient Position: Lateral recumbent

Pin Insertion: Position the patient's shoulder so that it is kept at 90° of abduction, with the elbow also flexed to 90°. You will be able to identify the multipennate middle portion of the deltoid between the anterior and posterior portions. Insert the pin medial to the groove that separates it from the posterior portion, approximately 2 cm to 4 cm distal to the lateral border of the acromion.

Relaxation: Position the patient's arm in adduction against the side of his chest. Keep the elbow extended.

Contraction: *Minimal*: With the patient's arm in adduction and the elbow slightly flexed, instruct the patient as follows: "Lift your elbow upward, away from your chest, just slightly" (minimal shoulder abduction).

Contraction: *Maximal*: With the patient's arm and elbow placed as described under pin insertion, instruct the patient as follows: "Lift your arm upward, away from your chest, as high as you can against my resistance, as if you want to touch your elbow to your ear" (maximum arm abduction with the elbow in flexion). Apply resistance at the level of the lower arm in the direction of shoulder adduction.

Peripheral Nerve Supply: Axillary nerve from the posterior cord of the brachial plexus

Root Supply: Nerve roots C5 and C6, C6 may be dominant.

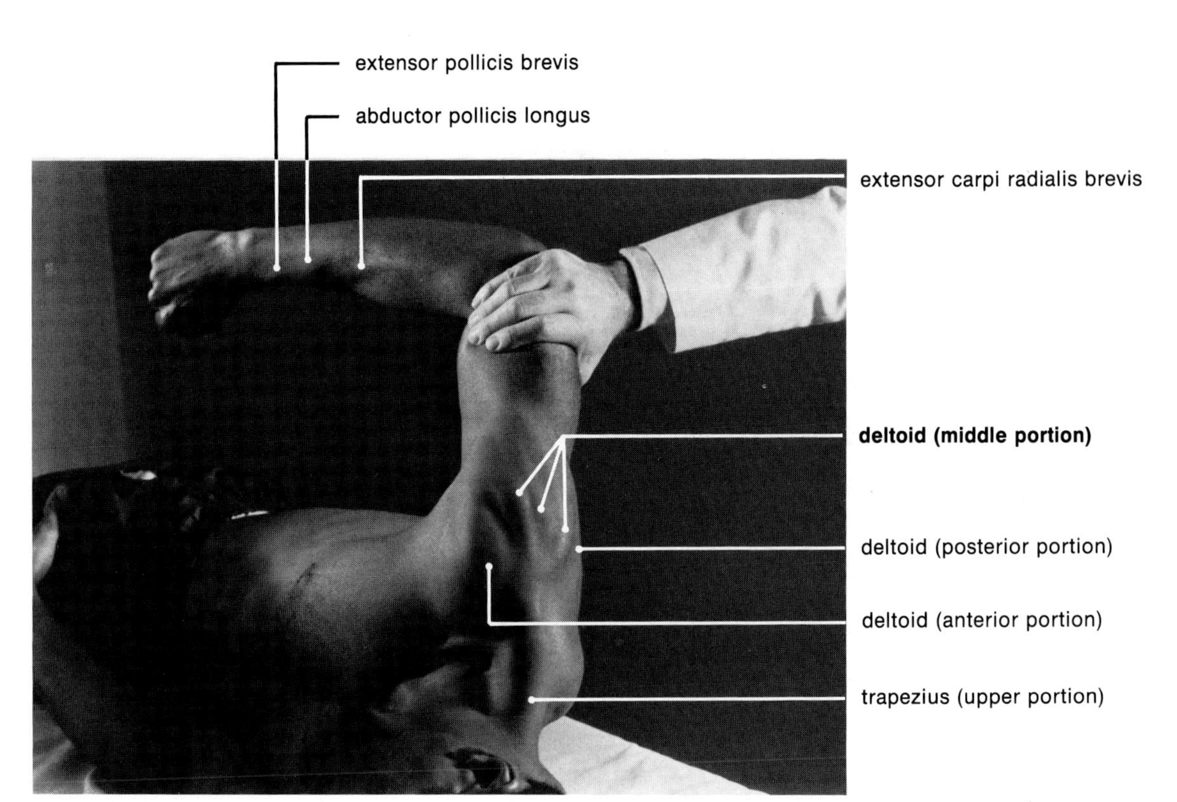

FIGURE 2-36 Deltoid (middle portion).

Deltoid (Posterior or Spinous Portion)

(*Fig. 2-37; see also Figs. 1-21 and 1-23*)

Action: Extension of the arm

Patient Position: Lateral recumbent

Pin Insertion: Instruct the patient as follows: "Push backward with your elbow bent" (arm extension with the elbow flexed). The posterior portion of the deltoid comes into action as the shoulder extends. Insert the pin posterior to the groove that separates it from the middle portion of the deltoid approximately 2 cm to 4 cm distal to the lateral border of the acromion.

Relaxation: Position the patient's arm in adduction against his side. If the patient is unable to relax, position the arm in flexion and adduction across his chest. This stretches the muscle; however, it will be more difficult for the patient to contract the muscle unknowingly in case of pain from the needling.

Contraction: *Minimal*: Instruct the patient as follows: "Keep your elbow bent and push it slightly backward" (minimal arm extension with the elbow kept in flexion).

Contraction: *Maximal*: Instruct the patient as follows: "Keep your elbow bent and push your elbow backward strongly" (maximal arm extension with the elbow in flexion). Apply resistance at the lower arm by pushing forward against it in the direction of shoulder flexion.

Peripheral Nerve Supply: Axillary nerve from the posterior cord of the brachial plexus

Root Supply: Nerve roots C5 and C6, mainly C6

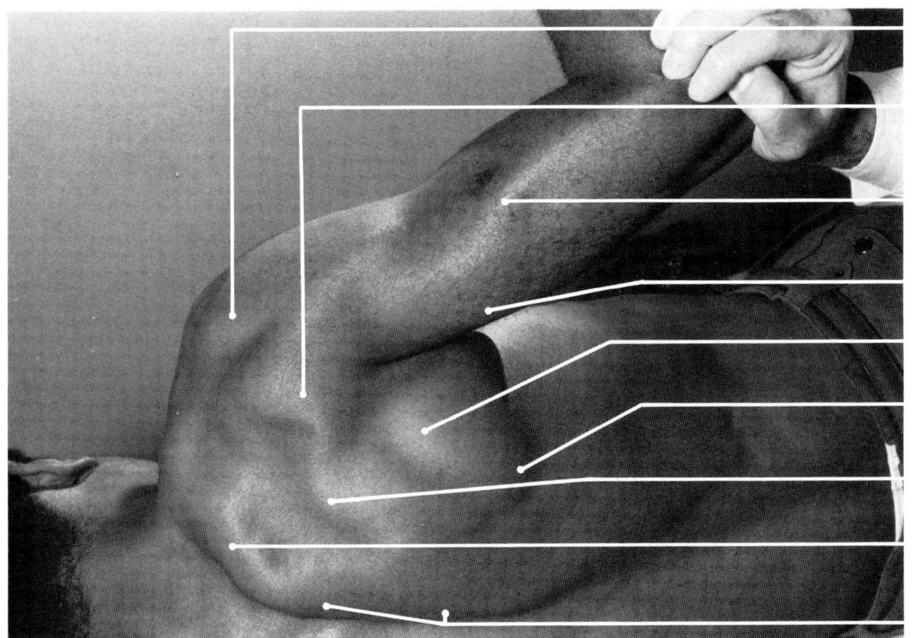

FIGURE 2-37 Deltoid (posterior portion).

Biceps Brachii (Long Head) (*Fig. 2-38; see also Figs. 1-19 and 1-20*)

Action: Flexion of the elbow, supination of the forearm, and, to a lesser degree, flexion of the shoulder joint

Patient Position: Supine

Pin Insertion: Feel for the central groove that separates the long and short heads of the biceps brachii. The groove is easily palpable if the muscle is kept at slight tension by flexing the elbow to about 45°. Lateral to this groove is the long head of the biceps brachii. Insert the pin at about the junction of the upper and middle thirds of the muscle.

Relaxation: Instruct the patient as follows: "Straighten your elbow and keep your palm down toward the bed" (elbow extension with the forearm in pronation).

Contraction: *Minimal*: Position the patient's forearm in midpronation with the elbow flexed to about 30° and the palm toward the bed. This will allow the elbow to be flexed further, with gravity partially or totally eliminated. If the contraction is so minimal that the sampling of the MUPs becomes limited, occasionally instruct the patient as follows: "Bend your elbow just a little more," and give one-finger resistance to elbow flexion to ensure contraction.

Contraction: *Maximal*: Fully supinate the patient's forearm and position the elbow at about 60° of flexion. Instruct the patient as follows: "Resist my trying to straighten your elbow, but don't try to bend your elbow up further" (elbow flexion against resistance). Apply downward pressure at the lower forearm in the direction of elbow extension.

Peripheral Nerve Supply: Musculocutaneous nerve from the lateral cord of the brachial plexus

Root Supply: Nerve roots C5 and C6, mainly C5

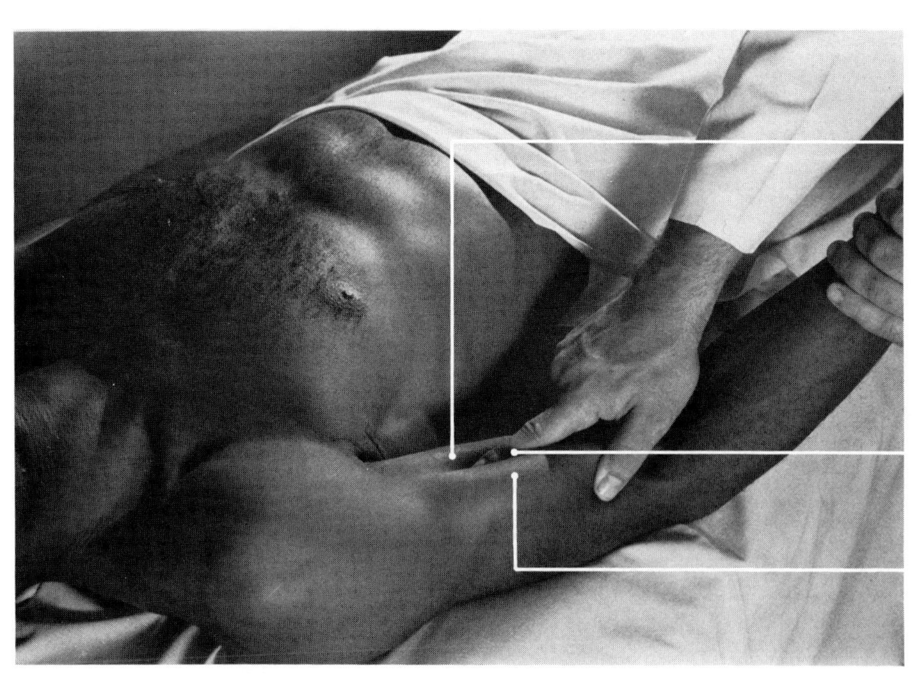

FIGURE 2-38 Biceps brachii (long head).

Biceps Brachii (Short Head) (*Fig.* 2-39; *see also* Figs. 1-19 *and* 1-20)

Action: Flexion of the elbow with the forearm supinated
Patient Position: Supine
Pin Insertion: Insert your index finger into the groove that separates the long and short heads of the biceps brachii. The groove is easily felt at the midline of the muscle with the muscle in slight contraction. Medial to this groove is the short head of the biceps brachii. Insert the pin approximately 2.5 cm medial to this groove at about the junction of the upper and middle thirds of the muscle.
*Relaxation**
*Contraction**
*Peripheral Nerve Supply**
Root Supply: Nerve roots C5 and C6, mainly C6

* See biceps brachii (long head).

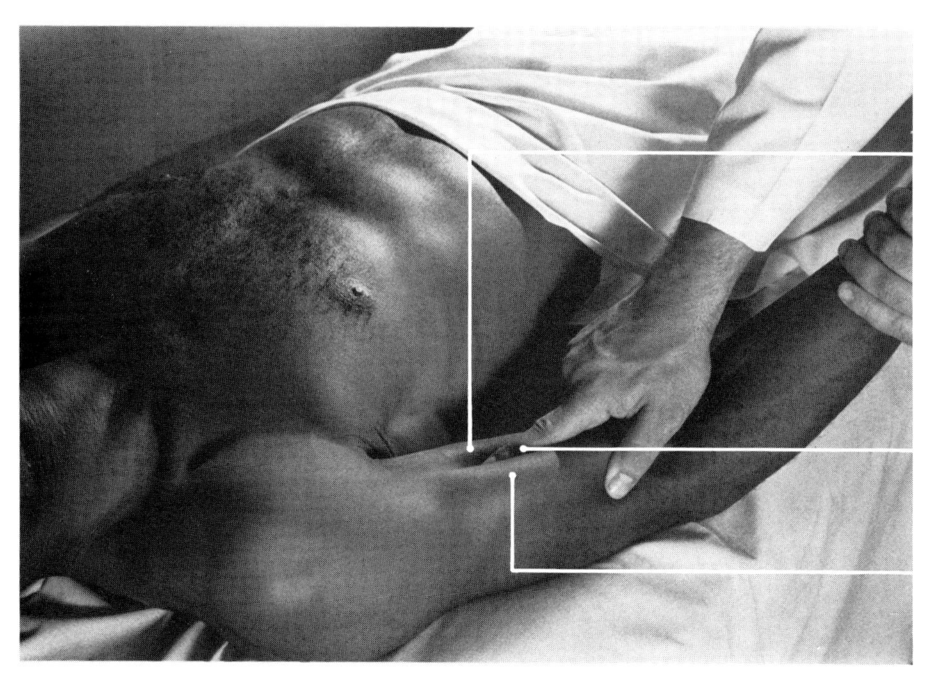

FIGURE 2-39 Biceps brachii (short head).

Coracobrachialis (*Fig.* 2-40; *see also* Figs. 1-19 *and* 1-20)

Action: Flexion and adduction of the arm

Patient Position: Supine

Pin Insertion: Position the patient's arm so that it is in 90° of flexion. Keep the elbow in full flexion with the forearm supinated. Give resistance by applying downward and lateral pressure at the lower part of the arm. The coracobrachialis will be seen to contract. It is at the upper third of the arm between the short head of the biceps brachii and the long head of the triceps and is best seen near the axilla. Insert the pin into the most prominent portion of the bulge of the muscle.

Relaxation: Position the patient's arm on the bed in abduction, making sure that the tip of the shoulder is lying flat on the bed.

Contraction: *Minimal*: With the patient's arm in abduction and the elbow flexed to about 45°, instruct the patient as follows: "Keep your arm resting on the bed and move or slide it in slightly toward your body" (minimal arm adduction without the factor of gravity).

Contraction: *Maximal*: With the patient's arm and elbow kept as in minimal contraction, instruct the patient as follows: "Keep your arm resting on the bed and move or slide it in forcefully against my hand so that you can bring your arm in toward the side of your body." Apply lateral resistance by pushing against the patient's elbow.

Peripheral Nerve Supply: Musculocutaneous nerve from the lateral cord of the brachial plexus

Root Supply: Nerve roots C6 and C7, mainly C6

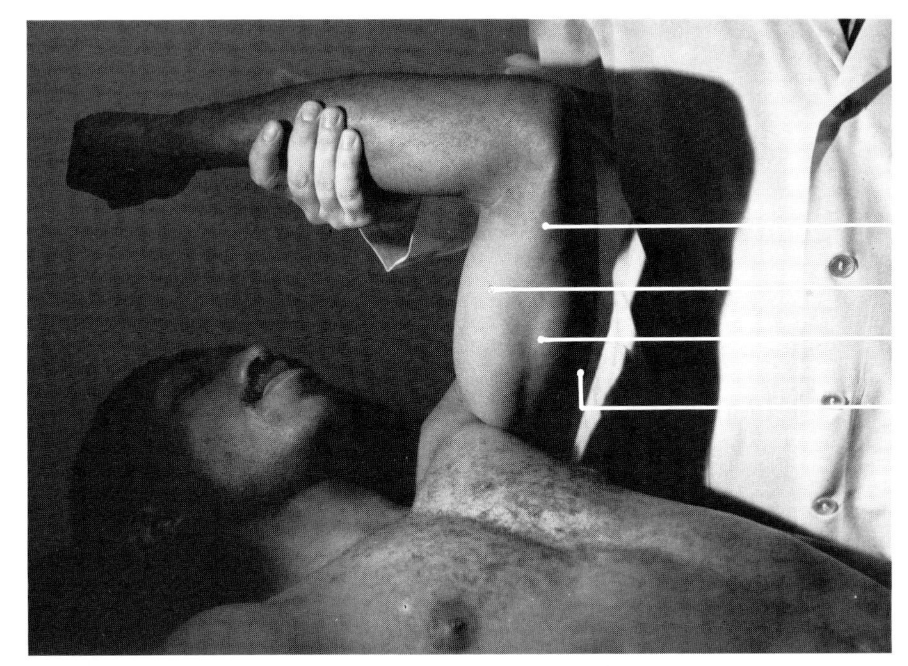

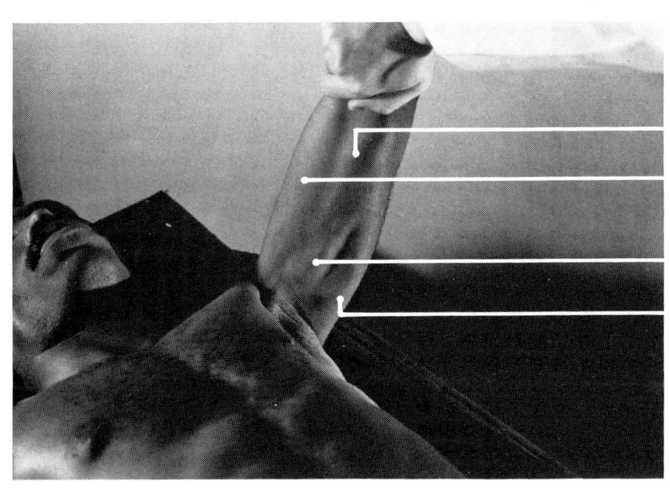

FIGURE 2-40 Coracobrachialis.

Brachialis (*Fig.* 2-41; *see also* *Figs.* 1-20 *through* 1-22)

Action: Flexion of the elbow

Patient Position: Supine

Pin Insertion: Get the biceps brachii to contract and feel for the lateral edge of the long head of this muscle. The brachialis will be seen to contract and can be identified between the long head of the biceps brachii anteriorly and the lateral head of the triceps posteriorly. Insert the pin into the brachialis at about the junction of the middle and lower thirds of the arm.

Relaxation: Instruct the patient as follows: "Keep your elbow straight and have the palm up facing the ceiling" (elbow in extension and forearm in supination).

Contraction: *Minimal*: Position the patient's forearm in midpronation so that its medial border is partially resting on the examination bed. Instruct the patient as follows: "Bend your elbow slightly" (minimal elbow flexion with gravity partially eliminated by support from the bed).

Contraction: *Maximal*: Position the patient's elbow in about 60° of flexion with the forearm supinated. The forearm can be in either supination or pronation, since the brachialis inserts into the ulna, but the pronated position puts the brachioradialis into stronger action and increases the mechanical advantage of the biceps brachii. Hence, this position reduces the load on the brachialis and forces the examiner to push harder without getting any better reaction from the brachialis. This will confuse the examiner as to the effort being made by the brachialis. Apply downward pressure to the lower forearm in the direction of elbow extension and instruct the patient as follows: "Don't let me push your forearm down" (resistance is given to forearm flexion).

Peripheral Nerve Supply: Musculocutaneous nerve plus a twig from the radial nerve to a small lateral and distal part of the brachialis (this twig is probably only sensory)

Root Supply: Nerve roots C5 and C6, mainly C6

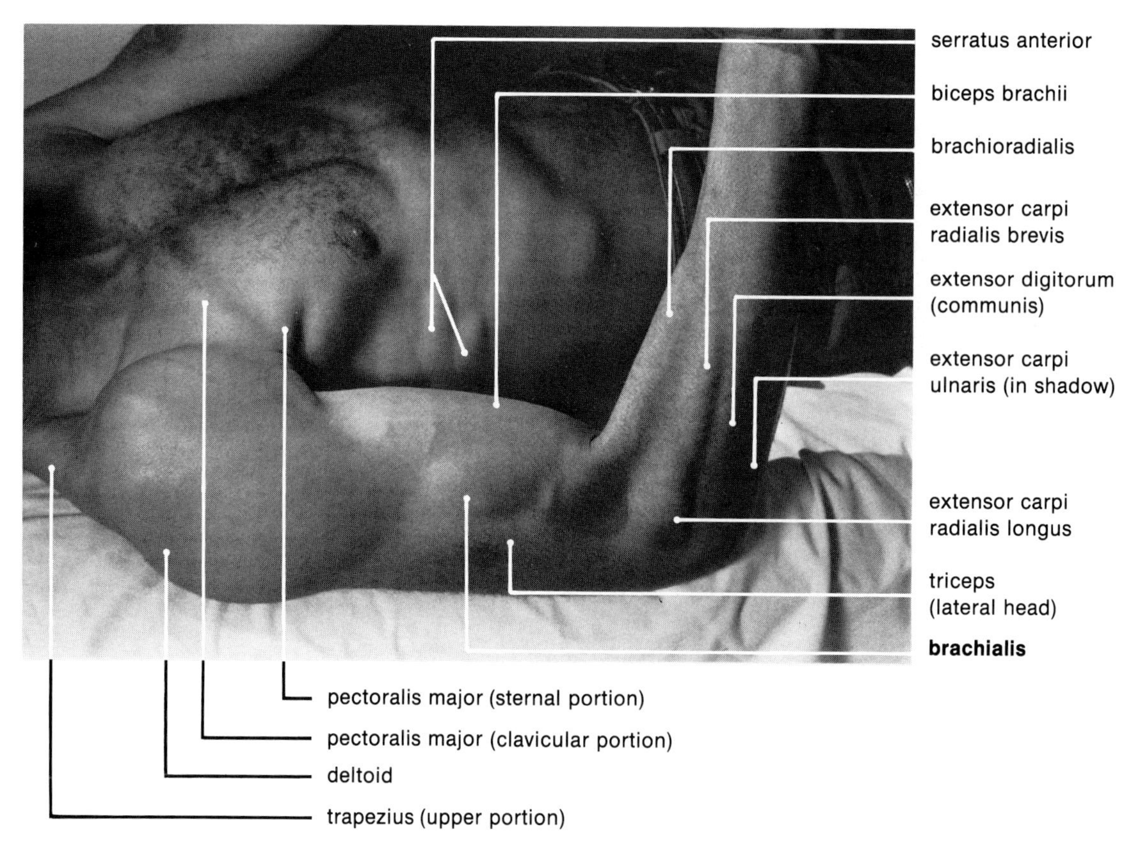

FIGURE 2-41 Brachialis.

Triceps (Lateral Head) (*Fig.* 2-42; *see also Figs.* 1-20 *through* 1-24)

Action: Extension of the elbow joint

Patient Position: Supine, with the arm at the side

Pin Insertion: Instruct the patient as follows: "Roll or rotate your arm and forearm inward so that your palm faces away from your body and your thumb is against the table. Now push your forearm out toward me with your elbow straight and stiff" (arm in internal rotation and adduction and elbow in extension). The lateral head of the triceps will be seen to come into action. Insert the pin lateral to the groove that marks the junction of the triceps with the aponeurotic tendon of insertion of the triceps, at the level of the junction of the middle and lower thirds of the arm.

Relaxation: Instruct the patient as follows: "Bend your elbow and put your forearm on your chest. Keep your elbow relaxed" (elbow in flexion).

Contraction: *Minimal*: Instruct the patient as follows: "Roll or rotate your arm and forearm inward, straighten your elbow, and push your forearm out toward me just a little." (With the arm in internal rotation and the elbow in passive extension, the patient attempts weak extension of the forearm on the arm.)

Contraction: *Maximal*: Instruct the patient as follows: "Roll or rotate your arm and forearm inward, straighten your elbow so that it will be straight and stiff, and push your forearm outward toward me as hard as you can" (arm in internal rotation and adduction and elbow in forceful extension). Have the patient lift his entire upper extremity off the bed, and apply resistance at the lower forearm in the direction of elbow flexion.

Peripheral Nerve Supply: Radial nerve as it lies in the radial sulcus

Root Supply: Nerve roots C6 through C8, mainly C7

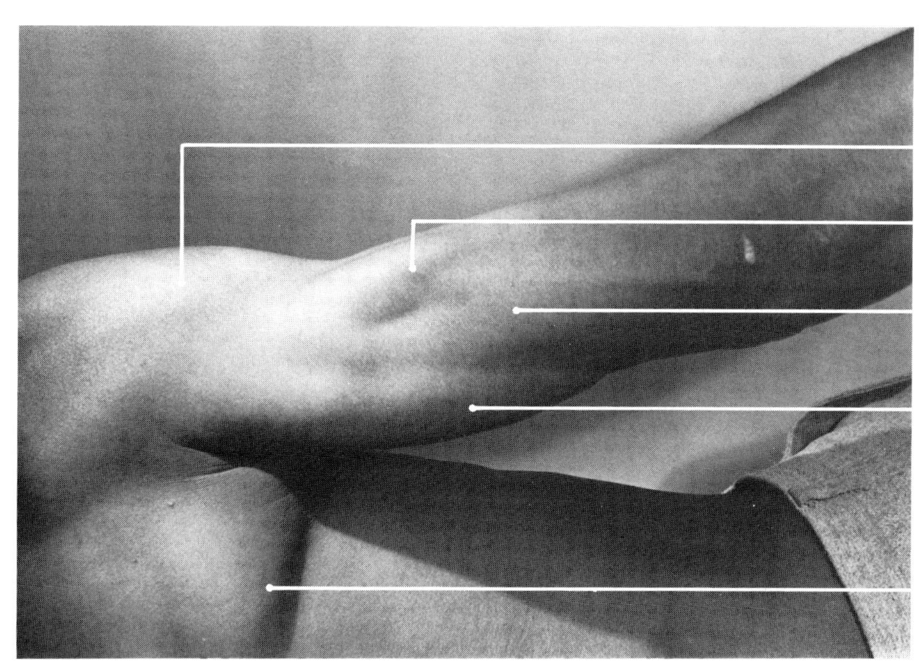

FIGURE 2-42 Triceps (lateral head).

Triceps (Medial Head) (*Fig.* 2-43; *see also Figs.* 1-23 *and* 1-24)

Action: Extension of the elbow joint

Patient Position: Lateral recumbent, with the arm against the side

Pin Insertion: Instruct the patient as follows: "Roll your arm inward and straighten your elbow" (arm in internal rotation and adduction and elbow in extension). Deep to the aponeurotic tendon of insertion of the triceps is the medial head of the triceps. Insert the pin through this tendon approximately 1 cm to 2 cm medial to the groove that marks its junction with the lateral head of the triceps.

*Relaxation**

*Contraction**

*Peripheral Nerve Supply**

Root Supply: Nerve roots C7 and C8

* See triceps (lateral head).

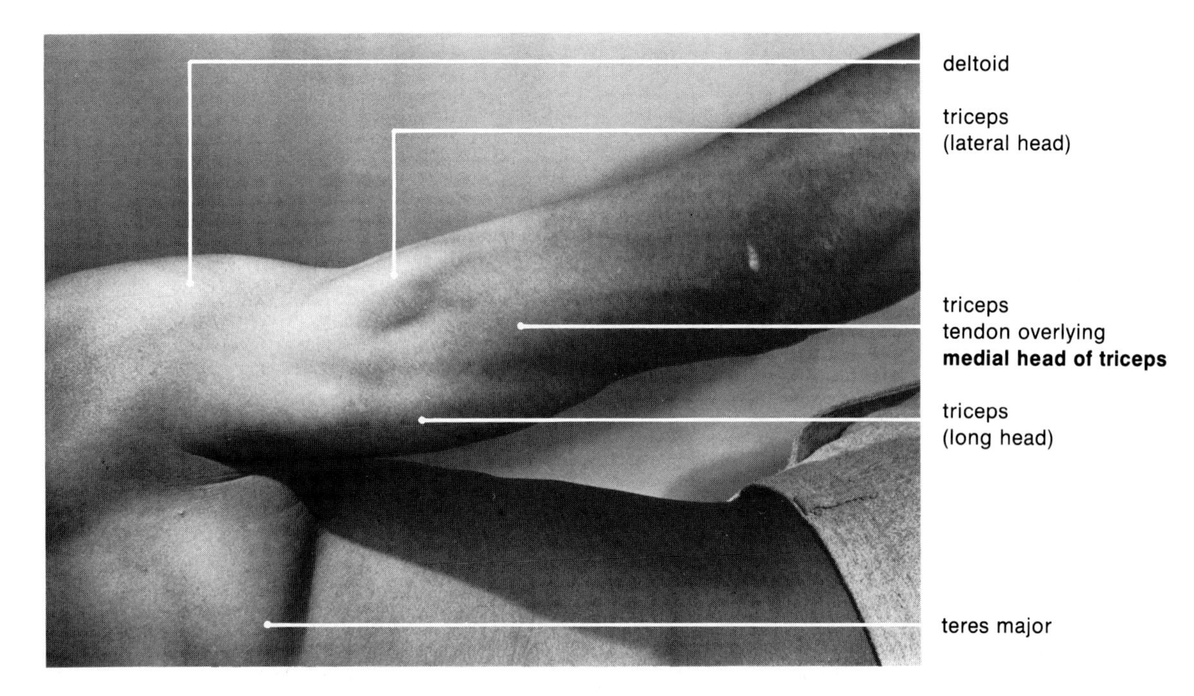

FIGURE 2-43 Triceps (medial head).

Triceps (Long Head) (*Fig. 2-44; see also Figs. 1-23 and 1-24*)

Action: Extension of the elbow joint

Patient Position: Lateral recumbent, with the arm against the side

Pin Insertion: Instruct the patient as follows: "Roll or rotate your arm inward and keep your elbow straight" (arm in internal rotation and adduction and elbow in extension). The long head of the triceps will be seen coming into action medial to the aponeurotic tendon of insertion of the triceps. Insert the pin into the muscle that forms the posteromedial bulge of the arm at about the junction of the upper and middle thirds of the arm.

*Relaxation**

*Contraction**

*Peripheral Nerve Supply**

Root Supply: Nerve roots C7 and C8

* See triceps (lateral head).

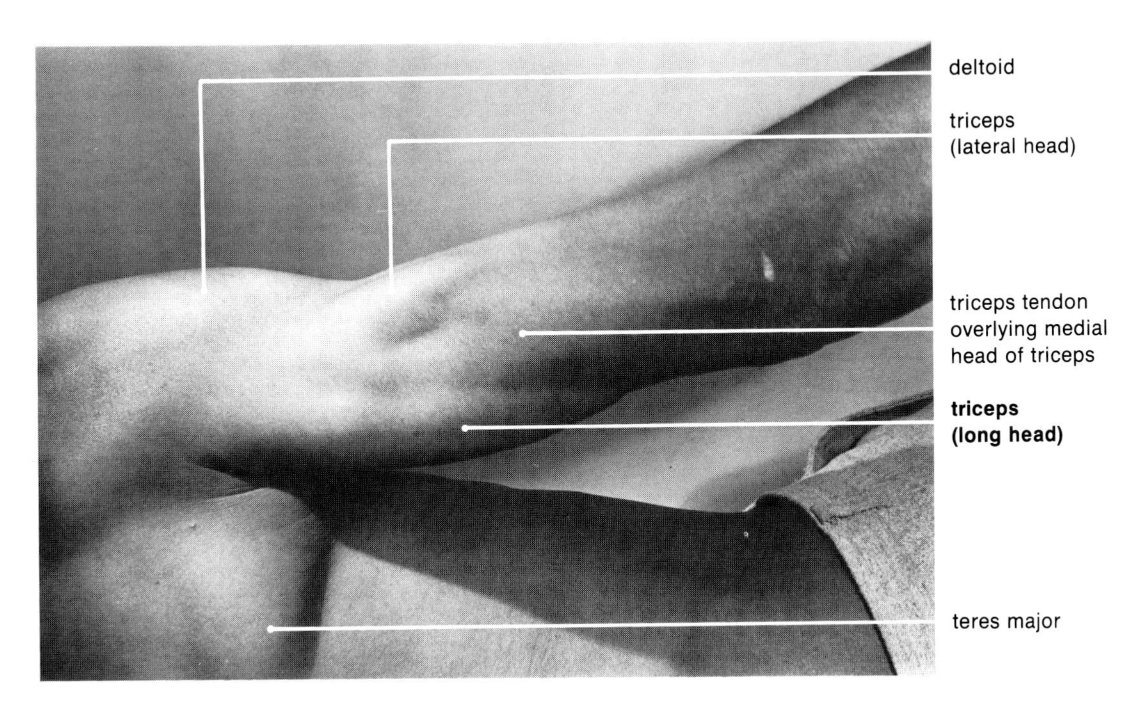

FIGURE 2-44 Triceps (long head).

MUSCLES OF THE POSTERIOR ASPECT OF THE FOREARM

Anconeus (*Fig.* 2-45; *see also* Figs. 1-33 *and* 1-38)

Action: Extension of the elbow joint
Patient Position: Lateral recumbent or supine
Pin Insertion: Palpate for the uppermost tip of the olecranon and identify a point approximately 1 cm distal. Palpate the lowermost tip of the lateral epicondyle and identify a point 1 cm distal to it. Insert the pin about midway between these two points.
*Relaxation**
*Contraction**
*Peripheral Nerve Supply**
*Root Supply**

* See triceps (lateral head).

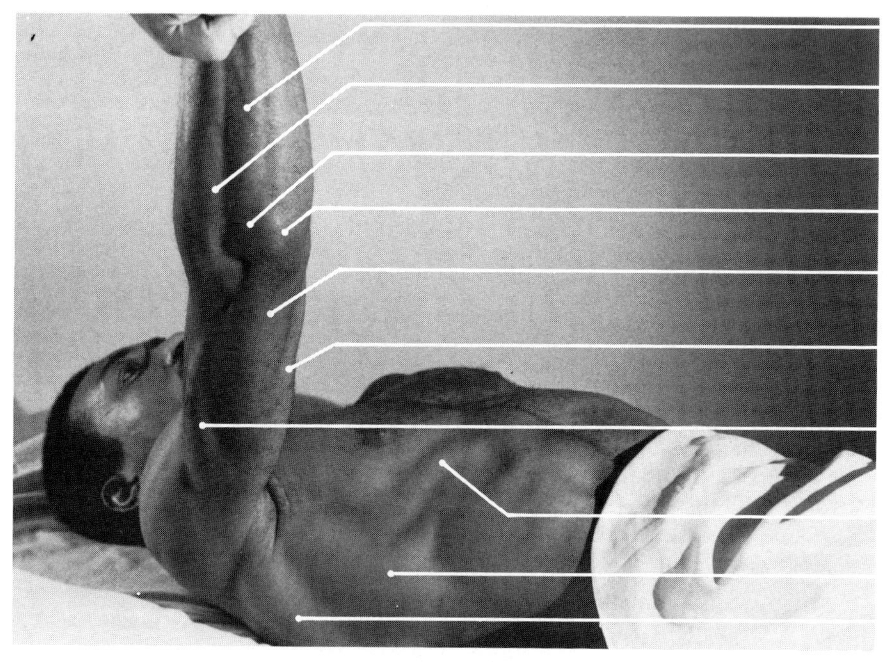

FIGURE 2-45 Anconeus.

Brachioradialis (*Fig. 2-46; see also Figs. 1-32 and 1-36*)

Action: Flexion of the elbow with the forearm in midpronation

Patient Position: Supine

Pin Insertion: With the patient's forearm placed in midpronation, instruct the patient as follows: "Bend your elbow and don't let me push your hand down" (resistance is given to elbow flexion). Apply pressure just above the wrist in the direction of elbow extension. The brachioradialis will be seen as a prominent ridge from the lower arm to the upper forearm. Insert the pin into the ridge at about the junction of the upper and middle thirds of the forearm.

Relaxation: Instruct the patient as follows: "Straighten your elbow and relax." The forearm should be either fully supinated or fully pronated.

Contraction: *Minimal*: Place the patient's arm in abduction and internal rotation and the forearm in midpronation. This position allows the elbow to flex with gravity reduced or eliminated because the forearm is resting on the bed. Instruct the patient as follows: "Bend your elbow slightly" (minimal elbow flexion). Give resistance at the lower forearm with one-finger pressure to maintain or initiate minimal contraction.

Contraction: *Maximal*: With the patient's forearm in midpronation and the elbow flexed to 60° against gravity (the forearm not against the bed), instruct the patient as follows: "Bend your elbow strongly and don't let me push your hand down." Apply resistance to elbow flexion above the wrist level in the direction of elbow extension.

Peripheral Nerve Supply: Radial nerve

Root Supply: Nerve roots C5 and C6, mainly C6

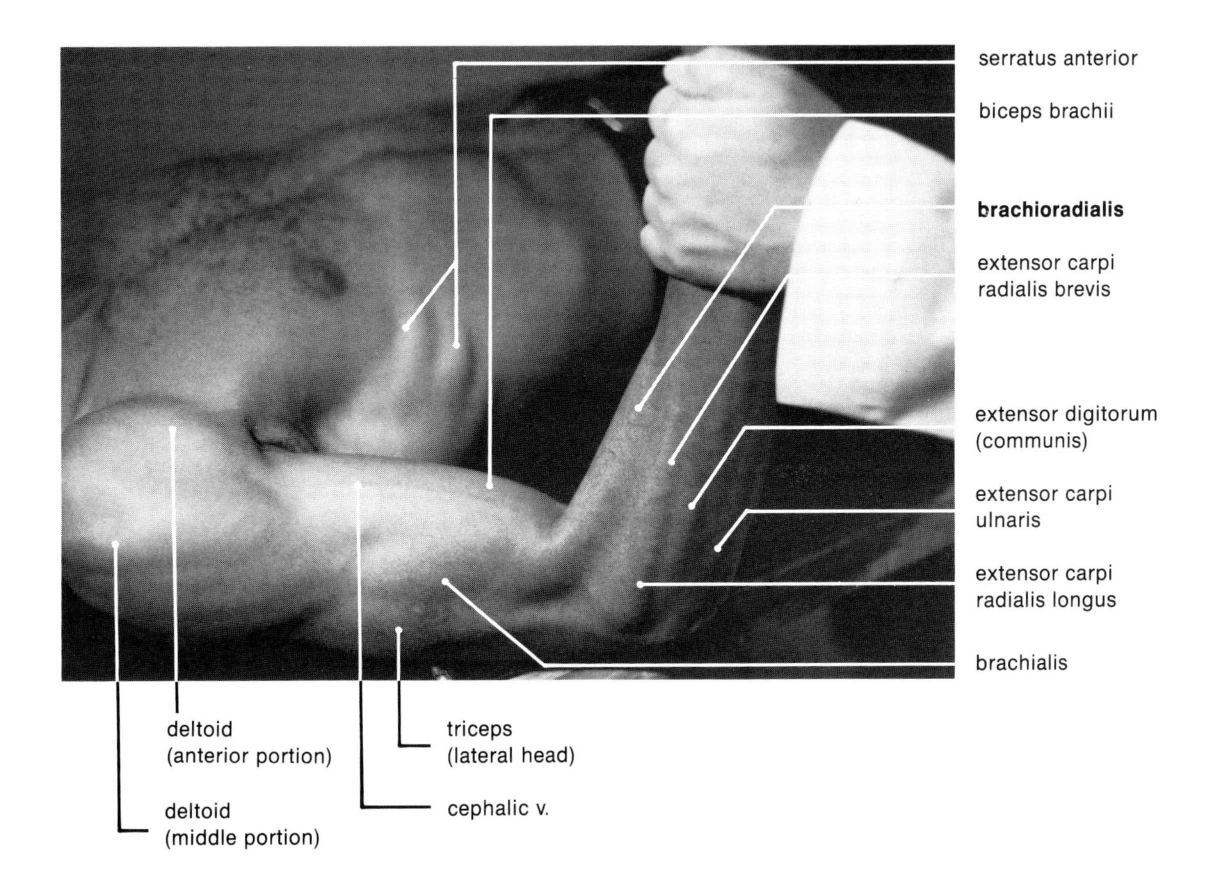

FIGURE 2-46 Brachioradialis.

Extensor Carpi Radialis Longus (*Fig.* 2-47; *see also* Figs. 1-32, 1-33, *and* 1-36)

Action: Wrist extension and radial deviation

Patient Position: Supine, forearm pronated

Pin Insertion: Bring out the brachioradialis as previously described and define its medial and lateral edges. At the elbow level, the first muscle lateral to the uppermost lateral edge of the brachioradialis is the extensor carpi radialis longus. You can define its edges by asking the patient to make a fist and lift his hand upward (wrist extension). It is a small, round-bellied muscle. Insert the pin approximately 1 cm below the lower tip of the lateral epicondyle, making sure that the pin is inserted lateral to the upper lateral edge of the brachioradialis. Direct the pin upward and laterally.

Relaxation: Instruct patient as follows: "Hang your wrist and forearm over the edge of the bed and relax your wrist" (passive wrist flexion).

Contraction: *Minimal*: Position the patient's partially pronated forearm so that its medial border is lying on the bed in the gravity-eliminating position and the dorsal surface of the forearm is facing you. Instruct the patient as follows: "Bend your hand or wrist slightly backward toward me" (wrist extension without the factor of gravity).

Contraction: *Maximal*: Position the patient's forearm in pronation. Instruct the patient as follows: "Make a fist and lift your hand or wrist upward toward your face. Now don't let me push your hand down" (maximal wrist extension against gravity and against resistance). Apply pressure on the dorsum of the hand in the direction of wrist flexion.

Peripheral Nerve Supply: A branch of the radial nerve that enters the muscle just above, or at, the elbow level

Root Supply: Nerve roots C6 and C7, mainly C6

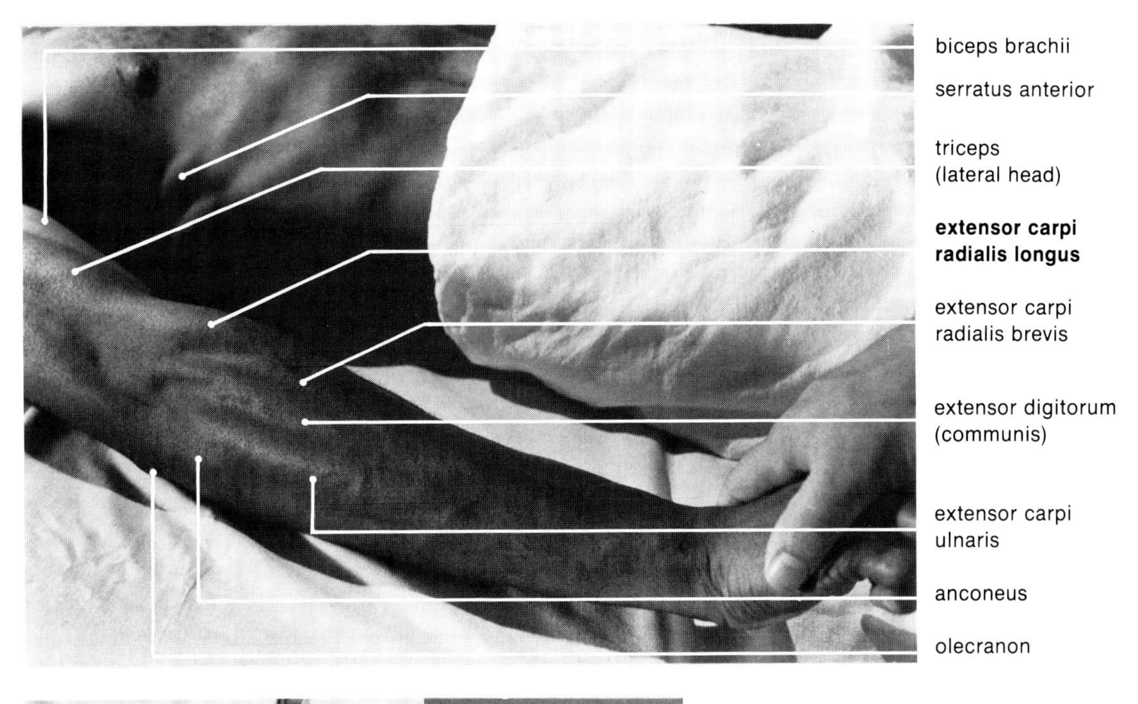

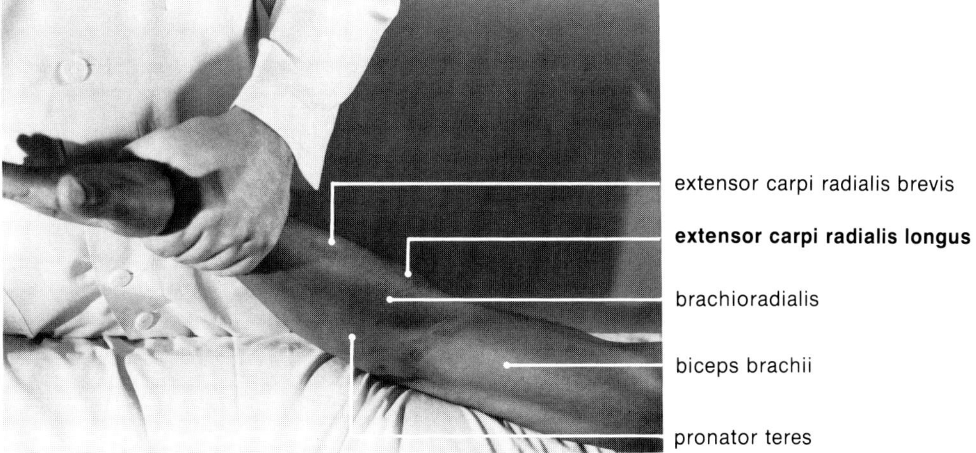

FIGURE 2-47 Extensor carpi radialis longus.

Extensor Carpi Radialis Brevis (*Fig.* 2-48; *see also Figs.* 1-32, 1-33, *and* 1-36)

Action: Wrist extension

Patient Position: Supine, with the forearm pronated

Pin Insertion: Bring out the brachioradialis and define its lateral edge, and instruct the patient to extend his wrist. The extensor carpi radialis brevis will be seen to come into action lateral to the lateral edge of the midportion of the brachioradialis. Its belly extends further distally than does the belly of the extensor carpi radialis longus. Insert the pin at the level of the junction of the upper and middle thirds of the forearm.

Relaxation: Instruct the patient as follows: "Hang your wrist and forearm over the edge of the bed and relax it" (passive wrist flexion).

Contraction: *Minimal*: Position the patient's forearm with its medial border on the bed so that the dorsal surface faces you. Instruct the patient as follows: "Bend your hand or wrist backward toward me just slightly" (wrist extension without the factor of gravity).

Contraction: *Maximal*: Position the patient's forearm in the pronated position. Instruct the patient as follows: "Lift your hand upward toward your face and don't let me push your hand down" (maximum wrist extension against gravity and resistance). Apply pressure on the dorsum of the hand in the direction of wrist flexion.

Peripheral Nerve Supply: A twig from the deep branch of the radial nerve at the level of the elbow joint and before piercing the supinator. It often receives a second twig from the posterior interosseous nerve, which is the continuation of the deep branch of the radial nerve after it has pierced the supinator.

Root Supply: Nerve roots C6 and C7 and occasionally C8, but mainly C6

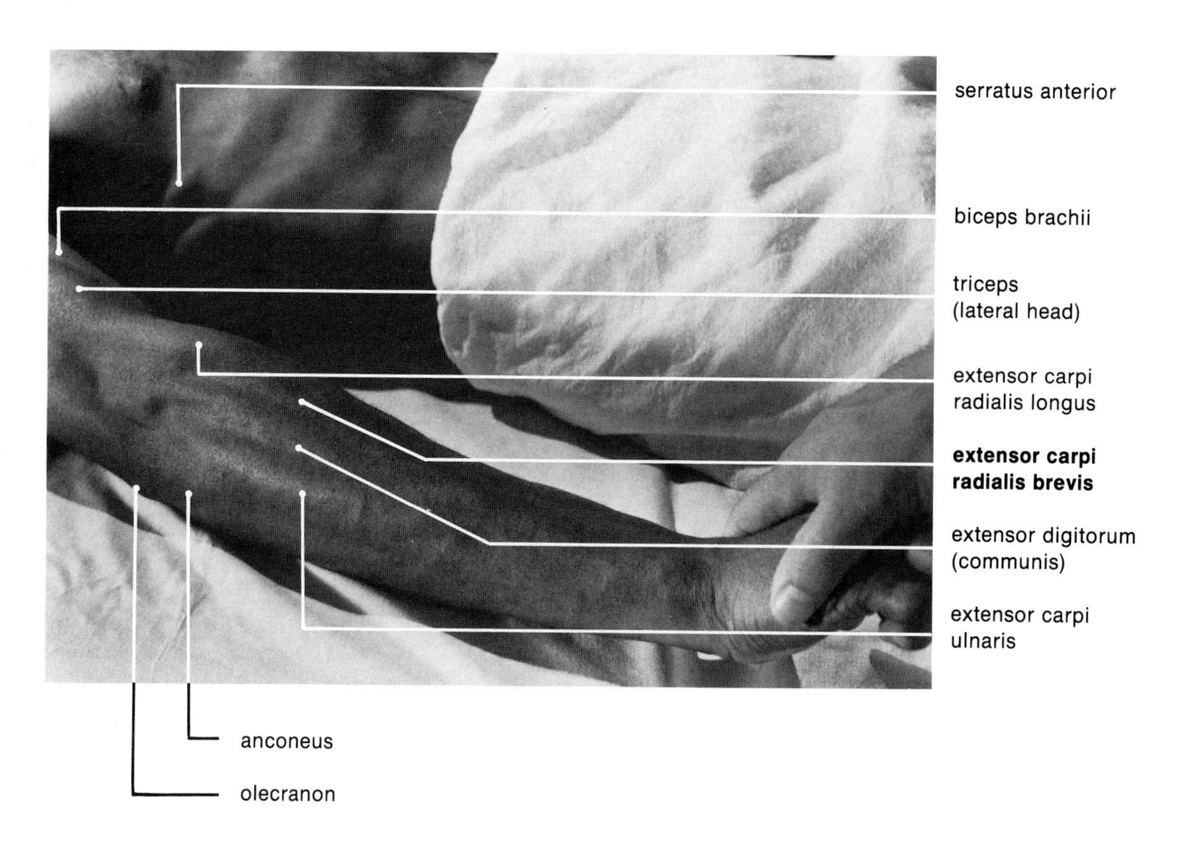

FIGURE 2-48 Extensor carpi radialis brevis.

Supinator (*Fig. 2-49; see also Figs. 1-34 and 1-35*)

Action: Supination of the forearm

Patient Position: Supine, forearm pronated

Pin Insertion: Instruct the patient as follows: "Turn your hand upward and then downward so that the palm faces up toward the ceiling and down toward the floor, alternately" (alternate supination and pronation). While the patient does this, feel for the head of the radius. Insert the pin approximately 3 cm distal to the radial head through the tendinous origin of the extensor digitorum (communis). Touch the periosteum of the radius lightly and withdraw the pin 1 mm to 2 mm.

Relaxation: Instruct the patient as follows: "Turn your hand over so that the palm faces the bed" (pronation).

Contraction: *Minimal*: Place the patient's forearm in midpronation and instruct the patient as follows: "Turn your hand over slightly so that the palm faces the ceiling" (minimal supination).

Contraction: *Maximal*: Place the patient's forearm in full supination with the elbow in slight flexion. Instruct the patient as follows: "Keep your palm facing up toward the ceiling, and don't let me twist your hand down" (supination against resistance). Apply rotatory pressure on the hand in the direction of pronation.

Peripheral Nerve Supply: Deep branch of the radial nerve (posterior interosseous nerve)

Root Supply: Nerve roots C5 and C6, mainly C6

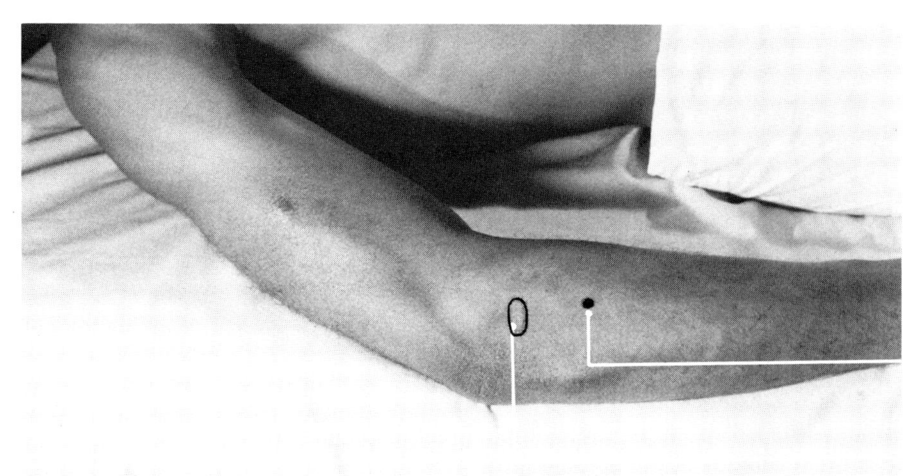

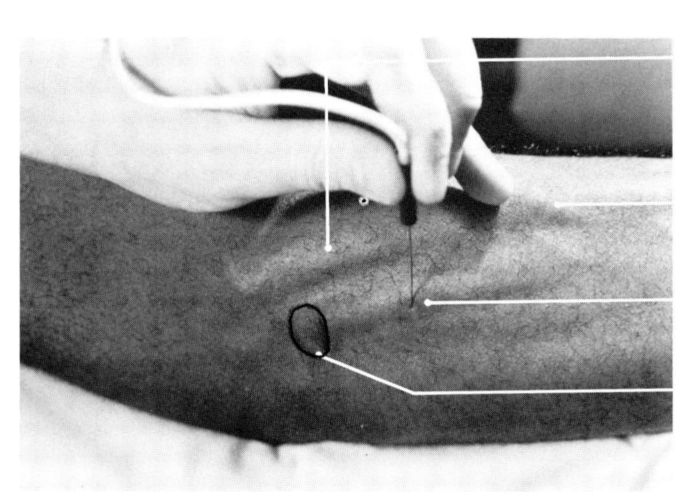

FIGURE 2-49 Supinator.

Extensor Digitorum (Communis) (*Fig.* 2-50; *see also Figs.* 1-32, 1-33, 1-36, *and* 1-37)

Action: Extends the metacarpophalangeal joints and assists in extending the interphalangeal joints.

Patient Position: Supine, forearm pronated

Pin Insertion: Feel for the dorsal border of the ulna and slide your fingers toward the dorsal aspect of the forearm. The first muscle to be palpated is the extensor carpi ulnaris. Feel for the lateral edge of this muscle, and there will be a groove that separates this muscle from the next prominent muscle, the extensor digitorum (communis) and its subsidiary, the extensor digiti minimi. Identify the extensor digitorum (communis) by instructing the patient as follows: "Lift your middle finger up and down" (extension and flexion of the middle finger at the metacarpophalangeal joint). Place your fingers over this muscle and you will feel the muscle contract and relax as the patient moves his middle finger. Insert the pin at about the junction of the upper and middle thirds of the forearm.

Relaxation: Instruct the patient as follows: "Hang your wrist and hand over the edge of the bed and totally relax your fingers and knuckles" (passive flexion of the metacarpophalangeal joints).

Contraction: *Minimal*: Instruct the patient as follows: "Lift your middle finger up very slightly" (minimal extension of the metacarpophalangeal joint of the third digit). If contractions are too strong, the forearm can be placed on its medial border so that the dorsal surface of the forearm faces you. Instruct the patient as follows: "Move your middle finger slightly outward toward me" (extension of the metacarpophalangeal joint of the third digit without the factor of gravity).

Contraction: *Maximal*: Instruct the patient as follows: "Lift all your fingers up so that your knuckles are straight and spread your fingers wide. Don't let me push your fingers down" (extension of the metacarpophalangeal joints against gravity and against resistance).

Peripheral Nerve Supply: Posterior interosseous nerve

Root Supply: Nerve roots C7 and C8, mainly C7

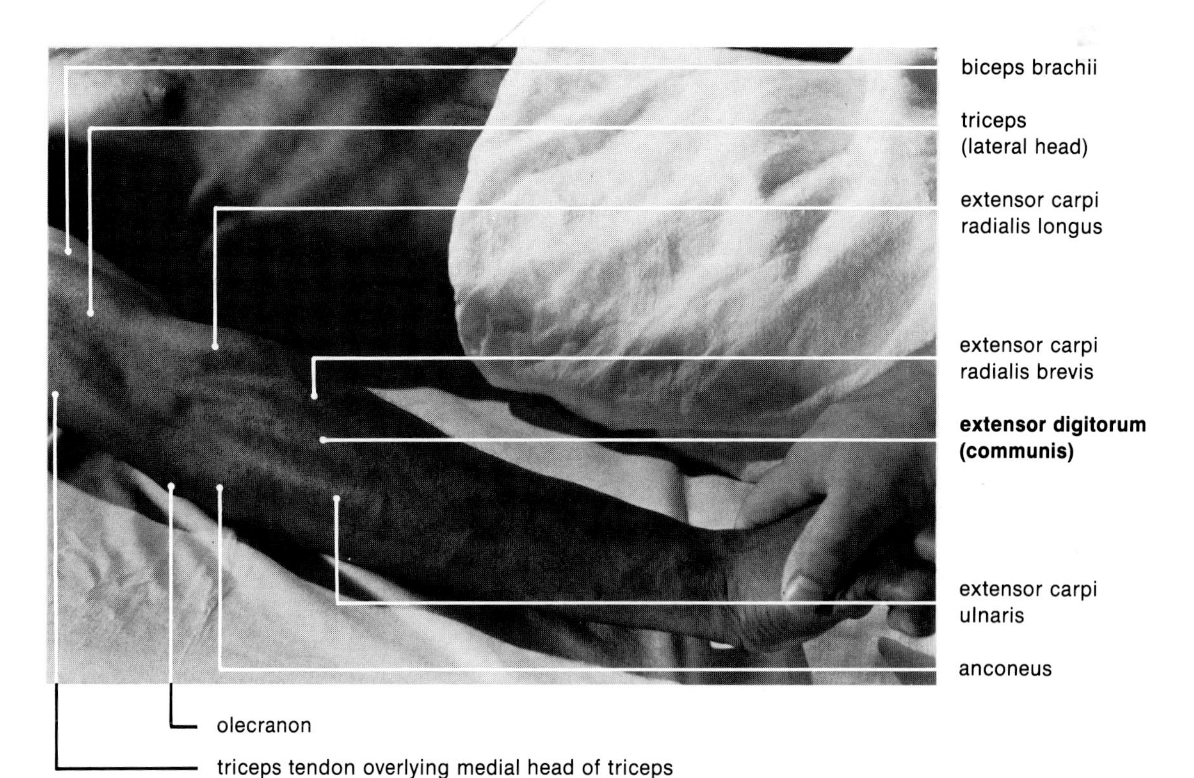

FIGURE 2-50 Extensor digitorum (communis).
Note: The metacarpophalangeal joints must be kept in extension, and the wrist should be kept in neutral position for examination of the extensor digitorum (communis) (see Fig. 2-51).

Extensor Digiti Minimi (*Fig.* 2-51; *see also* *Figs.* 1-36 *and* 1-37)

Action: Extension of the metacarpophalangeal joint of the fifth digit

Patient Position: Supine, forearm pronated

Pin Insertion: Feel for the ulna and slide your finger dorsally. The first muscle that you will palpate is the extensor carpi ulnaris. The groove between this muscle and the extensor digitorum reveals a narrow slip of muscle that can be seen contracting and relaxing as the patient extends and flexes the metacarpophalangeal joint of the fifth digit.

Relaxation: Instruct the patient as follows: "Try to relax your little finger, especially at the knuckle joint." The fingers may be placed in passive flexion at the metacarpophalangeal and interphalangeal joints of the little finger.

Contraction: *Minimal*: Instruct the patient as follows: "Lift your little finger up very slightly."

Contraction: *Maximal*: Instruct the patient as follows: "Lift your finger up as strongly as you can." Resistance is given at about the middle of the dorsum of the proximal phalanx of the fifth digit in the direction of flexion.

Peripheral Nerve Supply: Posterior interosseous nerve from the radial nerve

Root Supply: Nerve roots C7 and C8, mainly C7

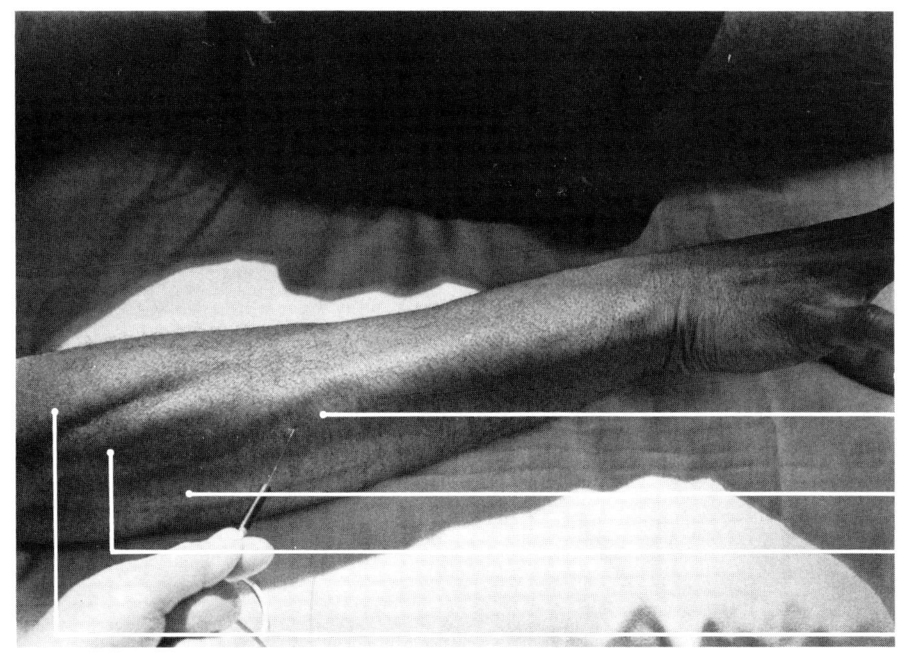

FIGURE 2-51 Extensor digiti minimi.

Extensor Carpi Ulnaris (*Fig.* 2-52; *see also Figs.* 1-32, 1-33, 1-36, *and* 1-37)

Action: Extension of the wrist joint, ulnar deviation of the hand, and fixation of the wrist for a strong grip

Patient Position: Supine, forearm pronated

Pin Insertion: Feel for the prominent dorsal border of the ulna, and slide your fingers dorsally. The first muscle to be palpated is the extensor carpi ulnaris. Insert the pin into the muscle at about the junction of the upper and middle thirds of the forearm.

Relaxation: Instruct the patient as follows: "Hang your wrist and hand over the table edge and relax your wrist" (passive wrist flexion).

Contraction: *Minimal*: Place the patient's forearm in the gravity-eliminating position so that it is lying on its medial border and the dorsal surface faces you. Instruct the patient as follows: "Bend your hand slightly toward me" (wrist extension without the factor of gravity). Occasionally, slight resistance may be given to wrist extension to initiate or maintain contraction.

Contraction: *Maximal*: Position the patient's forearm in pronation and instruct the patient as follows: "Lift your hand up as far backward as you can, spread your fingers, and don't let me push your hand down" (maximum wrist extension against resistance). Apply pressure on the dorsum of the hand in the direction of wrist flexion.

Peripheral Nerve Supply: Posterior interosseous nerve

Root Supply: Nerve roots C7 and C8, mainly C7

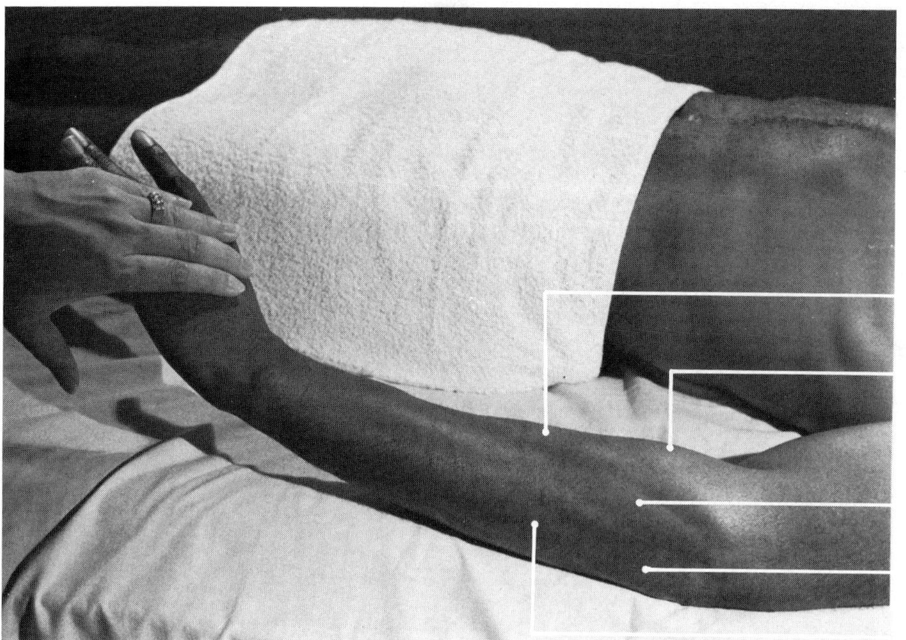

FIGURE 2-52 Extensor carpi ulnaris.

Abductor Pollicis Longus (*Fig. 2-53; see also Figs. 1-31 through 1-33 and 1-35 through 1-37*)

Action: Abduction and extension of the carpometacarpal joint of the thumb

Patient Position: Supine, forearm pronated

Pin Insertion: Instruct the patient as follows: "Lift your hand up and pull your thumb outward and away from your index finger" (abduction of the thumb at the carpometacarpal joint). Palpate for the belly of the muscle in the lower third of the forearm, in line with the web space of the thumb and index fingers. Two small bulges will be felt at that level. The more proximal bulge is that of the belly of the abductor pollicis longus.

Relaxation: Place the pronated forearm and wrist flat on the bed and position the thumb at the side of the index finger (thumb adduction).

Contraction: *Minimal*: Instruct the patient as follows: "Move your thumb slightly away from your index finger" (minimal thumb abduction).

Contraction: *Maximal*: Instruct the patient as follows: "Lift your wrist up and move your thumb away from your index finger. Don't let me push it back toward your index finger" (resistance is given to thumb abduction and extension). Apply pressure at the middle of the first metacarpal bone in the direction of adduction, and flexion, in the plane of the palm.

Peripheral Nerve Supply: Posterior interosseous nerve

Root Supply: Nerve roots C7 and C8, mainly C7

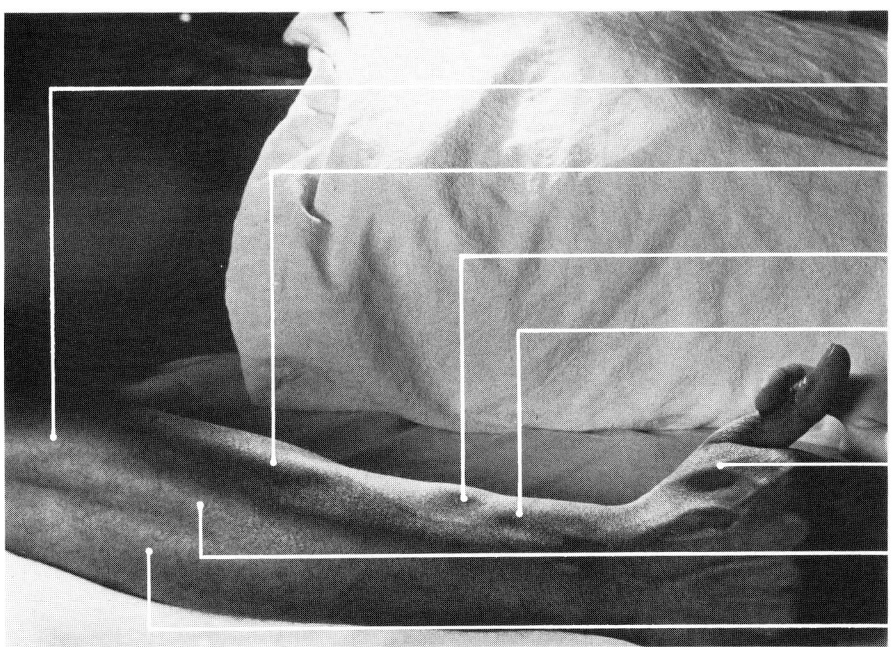

FIGURE 2-53 Abductor pollicis longus.

Extensor Pollicis Brevis (*Fig.* 2-54; *see also Figs.* 1-31 *through* 1-33 *and* 1-35 *through* 1-37)

Action: Extension of the metacarpophalangeal joint of the thumb

Patient Position: Supine, forearm pronated

Pin Insertion: Instruct the patient as follows: "Lift your wrist up slightly, keep the knuckle joint of your thumb straight, and pull your thumb away from the rest of the hand. Now relax your thumb and pull it away from the hand again" (extension and flexion of the thumb at the metacarpophalangeal joint of the thumb). As the patient does this several times, you will be able to feel for the belly of the muscle at the lower third of the forearm, which is the more distal of the two bulges in this region (the upper or proximal bulge is the belly of the abductor pollicis longus). Insert the pin into the more distal bulge, in line with the web space of the thumb and index finger, for examination of the extensor pollicis brevis.

Relaxation: Place the metacarpophalangeal and interphalangeal joints of the patient's thumb in passive flexion.

Contraction: *Minimal*: Instruct the patient as follows: "Keep the knuckle joint of your thumb straight and pull your thumb slightly away from the rest of the hand" (minimal thumb extension at the metacarpophalangeal joint).

Contraction: *Maximal*: Instruct the patient as follows: "Keep the knuckle joint of the thumb straight and pull your thumb away from the rest of the hand as far as you can. Don't let me push your thumb against the rest of your hand" (resistance is given to maximal thumb extension at the metacarpophalangeal joint). Give one-finger pressure at about the middle of the proximal phalanx of the thumb.

Peripheral Nerve Supply: Posterior interosseous nerve

Root Supply: Nerve roots C7 and C8, mainly C7

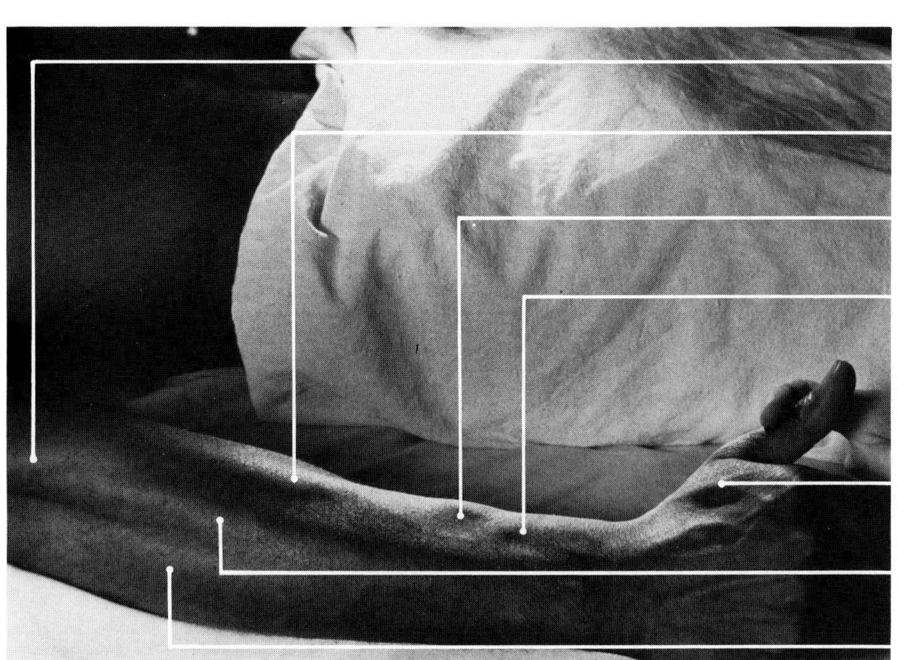

FIGURE 2-54 Extensor pollicis brevis.

Extensor Pollicis Longus (*Fig.* 2-55; *see also Figs.* 1-32 *and* 1-36)

Action: Extension of the distal and proximal phalanges of the thumb, with extension and slight lateral rotation of the first metacarpal

Patient Position: Supine, forearm pronated

Pin Insertion: Instruct the patient as follows: "Pull your thumb backward and away from your hand so that the tip of the thumb points toward your face. Now relax and pull it back up again" (extension and flexion of the interphalangeal, metacarpophalangeal, and carpometacarpal joints of the thumb). As the muscle contracts and relaxes, you will be able to identify the belly of the muscle by palpating approximately 3 cm above the wrist joint, in line with the web space of the index and middle fingers. Insert the pin at this point. This point is at the apex of the angle formed between the extensor pollicis brevis and the tendons of the extensor digitorum (communis), both of which are palpable on action. The point is approximately 2.5 cm directly proximal to the dorsal tubercle of Lister (on the radius), around which the tendon of the extensor pollicis longus angles like a rope on a pulley.

Relaxation: Place the metacarpophalangeal and interphalangeal joints of the patient's thumb in passive flexion.

Contraction: *Minimal*: Instruct the patient as follows: "Keep your thumb joints straight and pull your thumb back slightly toward your face (minimal extension of the distal phalanx of the thumb).

Contraction: *Maximal*: Instruct the patient as follows: "Keep your thumb joints straight and pull your thumb backward as hard as you can. Don't let me bend your thumb down" (resistance is given to maximal extension of the thumb at the interphalangeal joint). Apply pressure at the distal phalanx of the thumb in the direction of flexion.

Peripheral Nerve Supply: Posterior interosseous nerve

Root Supply: Nerve roots C7 and C8, mainly C7

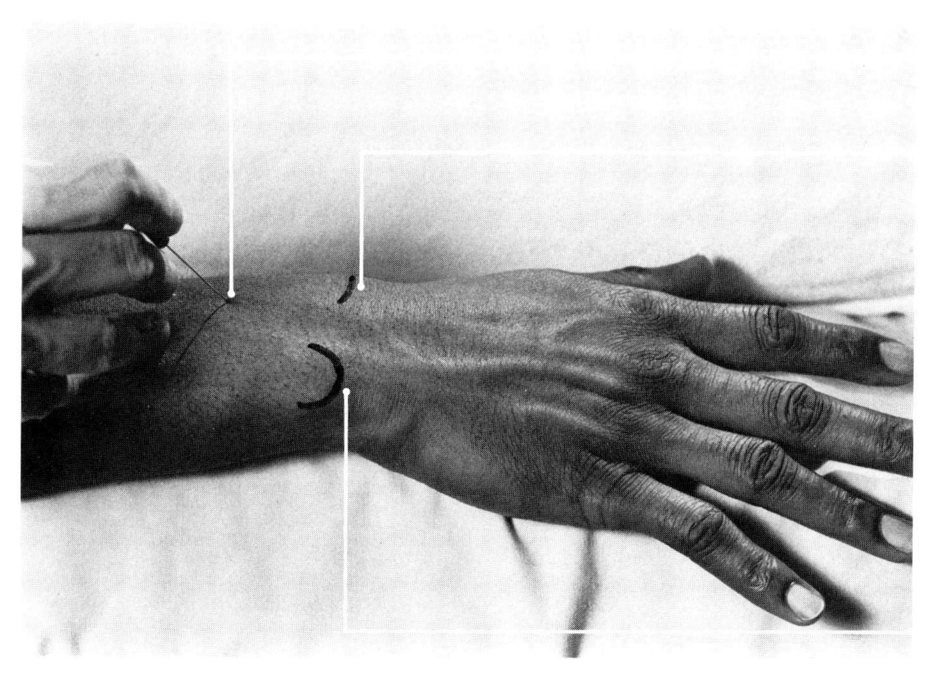

FIGURE 2-55 Extensor pollicis longus.

Extensor Indicis (*Fig. 2-56; see also Figs. 1-33 and 1-37*)

Action: Extension of the metacarpophalangeal joint of the index finger

Patient Position: Supine, forearm pronated

Pin Insertion: Feel for the proximal edge of the head of the ulna and insert the pin approximately 2.5 cm proximally, in line with the lateral aspect of the ulnar head. Instruct the patient as follows: "Lift your index finger up and down" (flexion and extension of the metacarpophalangeal joint of the index finger). You will be able to feel the muscle belly of the extensor indicis contract and relax as the patient does this. Insert the pin at the apex of the angle between the extensor carpi ulnaris and the extensor digiti minimi, the tendons of which are easily palpable here.

Relaxation: Instruct the patient as follows: "Hang your wrist over the edge of the bed and relax your index finger" (passive flexion of the index finger).

Contraction: *Minimal*: Instruct the patient as follows: "Lift your index finger up slightly" (minimal extension of the index finger).

Contraction: *Maximal*: Instruct the patient as follows: "Lift your index finger upward toward your face as far as you can and don't let me push it down" (resistance is given to maximum extension of the metacarpophalangeal joint of the index finger). Apply one-finger pressure on the proximal phalanx of the index finger in the direction of flexion.

Peripheral Nerve Supply: The posterior interosseous nerve, by a distal branch

Root Supply: Nerve roots C7 and C8, mainly C7

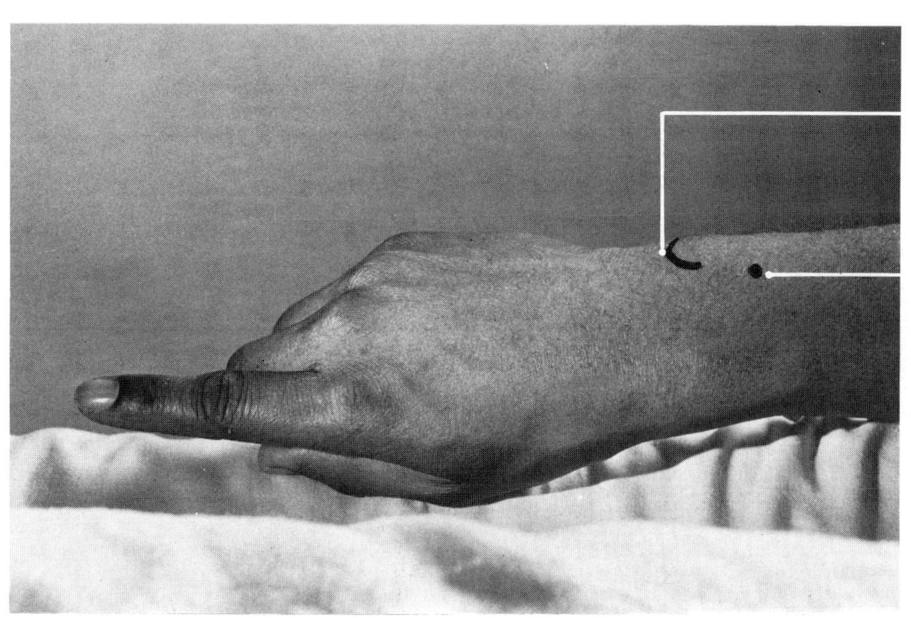

FIGURE 2-56 Extensor indicis.

MUSCLES OF THE ANTERIOR ASPECT OF THE FOREARM

Pronator Teres (*Fig.* 2-57; *see also Figs.* 1-25 *and* 1-26)

Action: Pronation of the forearm

Patient Position: Supine, forearm in midpronation

Pin Insertion: Bring out the brachioradialis, which will form the upper edge of the V of the antecubital fossa. The medial edge of the V is formed by the lateral edge of the pronator teres. This muscle can be seen when resistance is given to elbow flexion at the same time that forearm pronation is being achieved. Insert the pin into the muscle approximately 2.5 cm distal to the elbow crease and direct the pin upward and medially.

Relaxation: Position the patient's forearm on its medial border in midpronation and instruct the patient to relax.

Contraction: *Minimal*: Position the patient's forearm in pronation and instruct the patient as follows: "Press the end of your thumb lightly into the bed" (minimal pronation). The pressure of the thumb pressing into the bed initiates and maintains the firing of single MUPs for minimal contraction.

Contraction: *Maximal*: Position the forearm in pronation and instruct the patient as follows: "Keep your forearm in this position with your palm down toward the floor. Don't let me turn your palm away from this position" (resistance is given to forearm pronation). Give resistance by forcefully attempting to turn the patient's hand in the direction of supination.

Peripheral Nerve Supply: From the median nerve by a branch that commonly arises just before this nerve passes between the two heads of the pronator teres

Root Supply: Nerve roots C6 and C7, mainly C6, but may often have C7 root dominance

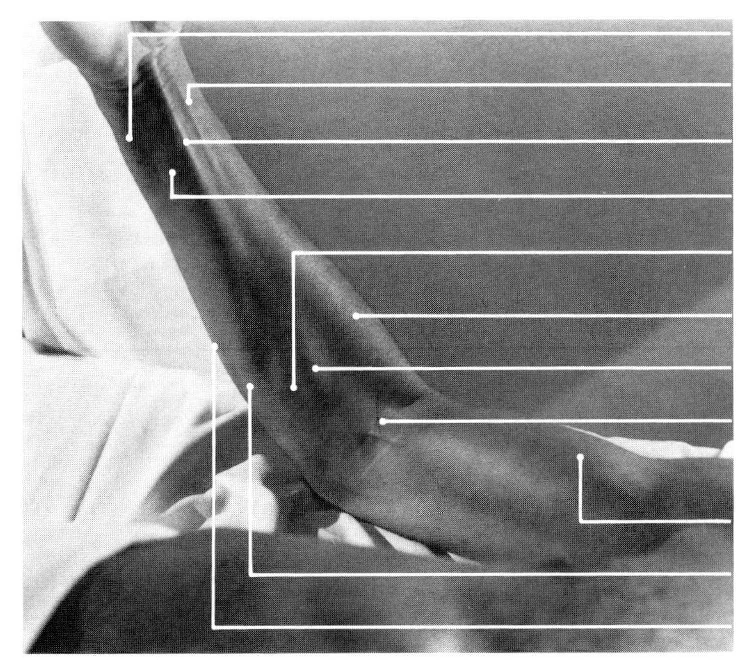

FIGURE 2-57 Pronator teres.

Flexor Carpi Radialis (*Fig. 2-58; see also Figs. 1-25 through 1-27*)

Action: Flexion and radial deviation of the wrist joint

Patient Position: Supine

Pin Insertion: Place the patient's forearm on its medial border in midpronation and give resistance to wrist flexion. The tendon of the flexor carpi radialis is the most lateral of the three prominent tendons on the ventral surface of the lower forearm. Follow this tendon proximally along the forearm toward the medial epicondyle and insert the pin along this line at the junction of the upper and middle thirds of the forearm.

Relaxation: Supinate the forearm and keep the wrist in extension and slight ulnar deviation.

Contraction: *Minimal*: Keep the patient's forearm on its medial border in midpronation and instruct the patient as follows: "Bend your wrist slightly toward your body" (minimal wrist flexion without the factor of gravity). You may occasionally give slight resistance to wrist flexion to initiate or maintain contraction. This can be done by asking the patient to push his fingers slightly against the side of his body, with the wrist and forearm kept in the position described above.

Contraction: *Maximal*: Keep the forearm in the same position and instruct the patient as follows: "Keep your fingers straight and bend your wrist strongly toward your body. Resist me when I try to straighten your wrist" (resistance is given to maximal wrist flexion). Apply pressure at the midpalm in the direction of wrist extension.

Peripheral Nerve Supply: Median nerve

Root Supply: Nerve roots C6 through C8, mainly C7

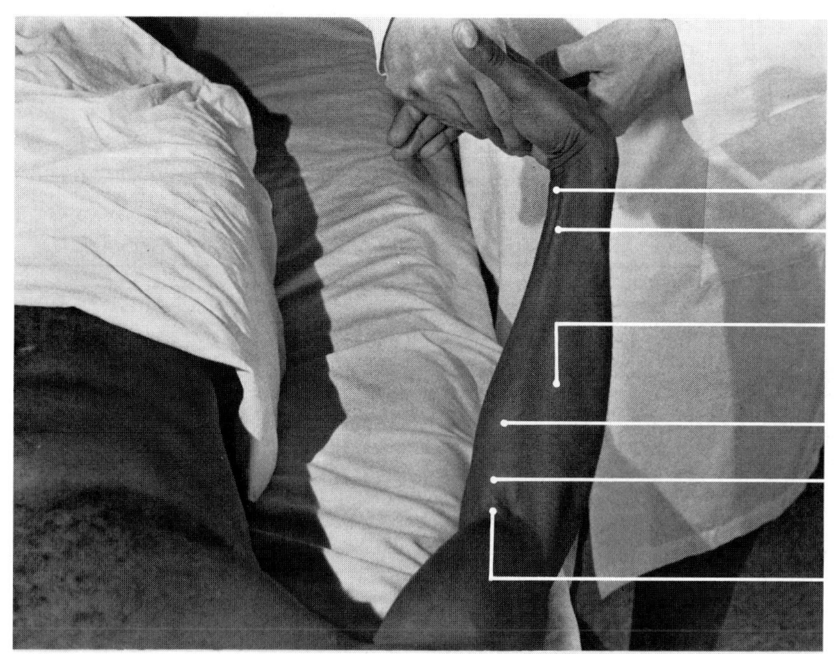

FIGURE 2-58 Flexor carpi radialis.

Flexor Digitorum Superficialis (Sublimis) *(Fig. 2-59; see also Figs. 1-26 and 1-27)*

Action: Flexion of the proximal interphalangeal joints of the medial four digits

Patient Position: Supine, forearm supinated

Pin Insertion: Instruct the patient as follows: "Make a fist and then open it. Do this several times" (finger flexion, with particular attention to obtaining maximal flexion at the proximal interphalangeal joints). As the patient does this several times, the tendons of the flexor digitorum superficialis will be seen to come into action as a bulge between the tendon of the palmaris longus laterally and the tendon of the flexor carpi ulnaris medially in the lower third of the forearm. Follow this bulge proximally and insert the pin at about the junction of the upper and middle thirds of the forearm, in the long, narrowing angle between the muscle bellies of the palmaris longus laterally and the flexor carpi ulnaris medially. The radial head of the flexor digitorum superficialis is also exposed on the radial side of the flexor carpi radialis, but here it tends to be too thin to be entered with certainty by the point of the pin.

Relaxation: Instruct the patient as follows: "Straighten out your fingers and relax" (passive finger extension, especially at the proximal interphalangeal joints).

Contraction: *Minimal*: Instruct the patient as follows: "Bend your fingers just slightly" (minimal flexion at the proximal interphalangeal joints).

Contraction: *Maximal*: Instruct the patient as follows: "Hook your fingers strongly around my fingers and don't let me straighten your fingers out" (resistance is given to maximum finger flexion at the proximal interphalangeal joints). Ensure that the distal interphalangeal joints are kept extended. If stronger force is needed, the patient may be instructed to make a fist while the needle is kept superficial to ensure its placement in the flexor digitorum superficialis.

Peripheral Nerve Supply: Median nerve

Root Supply: Nerve roots C7, C8, and T1, mainly C8

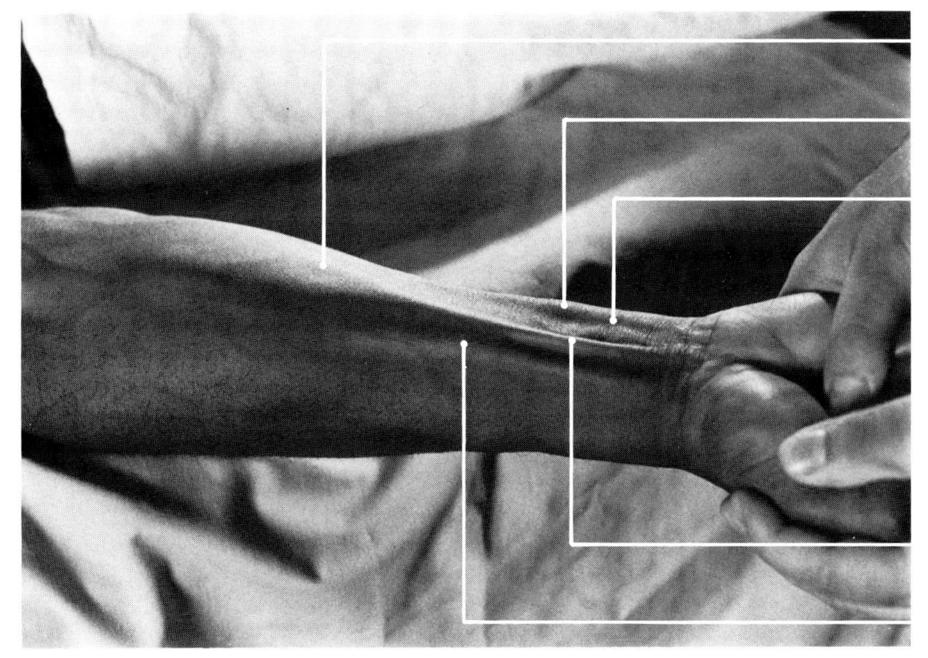

FIGURE 2-59 Flexor digitorum superficialis (sublimis).

Flexor Carpi Ulnaris (*Fig.* 2-60; *see also* Figs. 1-26 *through* 1-29)

Action: Flexion of the wrist joint and ulnar deviation at the wrist

Patient Position: Supine, forearm supinated

Pin Insertion: Instruct the patient as follows: "Bend your hand upward and draw it inward toward your body without moving your forearm" (wrist flexion with ulnar deviation). Give resistance to ulnar deviation and grasp the belly of the flexor carpi ulnaris between your thumb and index finger by following the tendor proximally. Insert the pin at about the junction of the upper and middle thirds of the forearm.

Relaxation: With the patient's forearm in supination, instruct the patient as follows: "Hang your wrist over the edge of the bed and relax" (passive wrist extension). You may also position the wrist in radial deviation.

Contraction: *Minimal*: Instruct the patient as follows: "Bend your wrist up slightly toward your face" (minimal wrist flexion).

Contraction: *Maximal*: Instruct the patient as follows: "Bend your wrist up strongly, keep your fingers spread apart, and don't let me push your wrist down" (maximal wrist flexion). You will get the best results when resistance is also given in the direction of radial abduction by applying pressure at the medial border of the hand. The pin should be inserted perpendicular to the skin and muscle.

Peripheral Nerve Supply: Ulnar nerve

Root Supply: Nerve roots C7 and C8, mainly C8

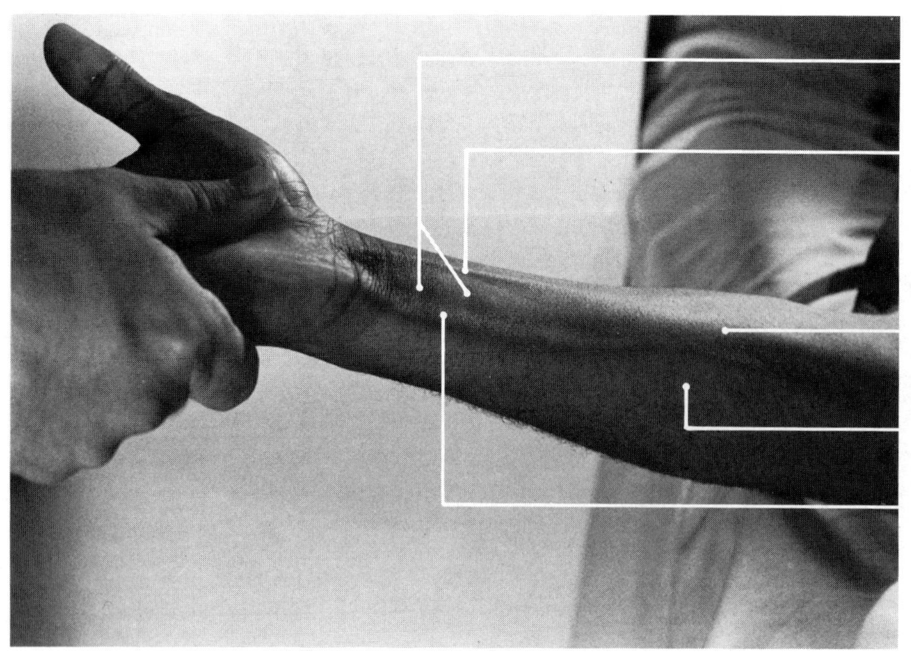

FIGURE 2-60 Flexor carpi ulnaris.

Flexor Digitorum Profundus (*Fig.* 2-61; *see also Fig.* 1-28)

Action: Primarily flexion of the distal interphalangeal joints of the medial four digits, but it also helps to flex every one of the joints across which its tendons pass.

Patient Position: Supine, forearm pronated

Pin Insertion: Feel for the medial surface of the ulna and slide your index finger ventrally. The belly of the muscle can be identified on palpation through the thin aponeurotic ulnar origin of the flexor carpi ulnaris as it contracts and relaxes. Instruct the patient as follows: "Make a fist and then straighten out your fingers. Do that several times." Insert the pin into the muscle at about the junction of the upper and middle thirds of the forearm. The needle must pierce the aponeurosis of the flexor carpi ulnaris, after which it encounters the fibers of the medial two slips of the flexor digitorum profundus. If the needle is inserted passing laterally in the coronal plane and tangential to the anterior surface of the ulna to a depth of 1.5 cm, the muscle fibers to the lateral two slips will be encountered.

Relaxation: Instruct the patient as follows: "Straighten out your fingers and keep them relaxed."

Contraction: *Minimal*: Instruct the patient as follows: "Bend the tips of your fingers slightly" (minimal flexion of the distal interphalangeal joints).

Contraction: *Maximal*: Instruct the patients as follows: "Bend the tips of your fingers as strongly as you can. Don't let me straighten them out" (resistance is given to maximal flexion of the distal interphalangeal joints of the digits). Apply resistance on the palmar aspect of the distal phalanges of the fingers in the direction of extension.

Peripheral Nerve Supply: Ulnar nerve

Root Supply: Nerve roots C8 and T1, mainly C8. The medial half of the muscle (for the little and ring fingers) is typically supplied by the ulnar nerve from C8 and T1. The lateral half of the muscle (for the middle and index fingers) is supplied by fibers from nerve roots C7, C8, and T1 via the anterior interosseous branch of the median nerve. However, there is considerable variation in the precise amount supplied by each nerve and in the degree of anastomosis between the two nerves in the forearm (Martin-Gruber anastomoses).

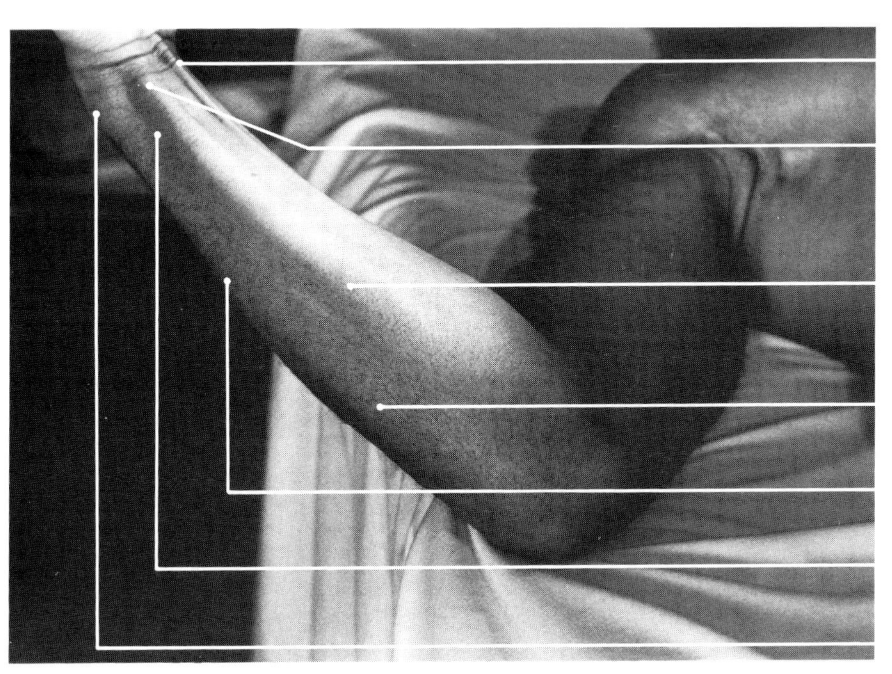

FIGURE 2-61 Flexor digitorum profundus.

Flexor Pollicis Longus (*Fig.* 2-62; *see also Fig.* 1-28)

Action: Flexion of the distal phalanx of the thumb

Patient Position: Supine, forearm supinated

Pin Insertion: Instruct the patient as follows: "Bend the tip of your thumb and then straighten it out and relax. Do that several times" (flexion and extension of the interphalangeal joint of the thumb). The belly of the muscle will be felt to contract and relax as you palpate at about the junction of the middle and lower thirds of the forearm by placing your four fingers at this level. Insert the pin at this level between the tendons of the brachioradialis laterally and the flexor carpi radialis medially. Do not insert the pin above this level because the variably developed radial head of the flexor digitorum superficialis often overlies the flexor pollicis longus down to this level. When inserting the pin, touch the periosteum of the radius gently and withdraw the pin 1 mm to 2 mm to ensure that it is in the flexor pollicis longus.

Relaxation: Instruct the patient as follows: "Straighten your thumb out and relax" (passive extension of the interphalangeal joint of the thumb).

Contraction: *Minimal*: Instruct the patient as follows: "Bend the tip of your thumb slightly" (minimal flexion of the distal phalanx of the thumb).

Contraction: *Maximal*: Instruct the patient as follows: "Bend the tip of your thumb strongly and don't let me straighten it out" (resistance is given to maximal flexion of the distal phalanx of the thumb). Apply pressure on the palmar surface of the distal phalanx of the thumb in the direction of extension.

Peripheral Nerve Supply: Anterior interosseous nerve branch of the median nerve

Root Supply: Nerve roots C8 and T1, mainly C8

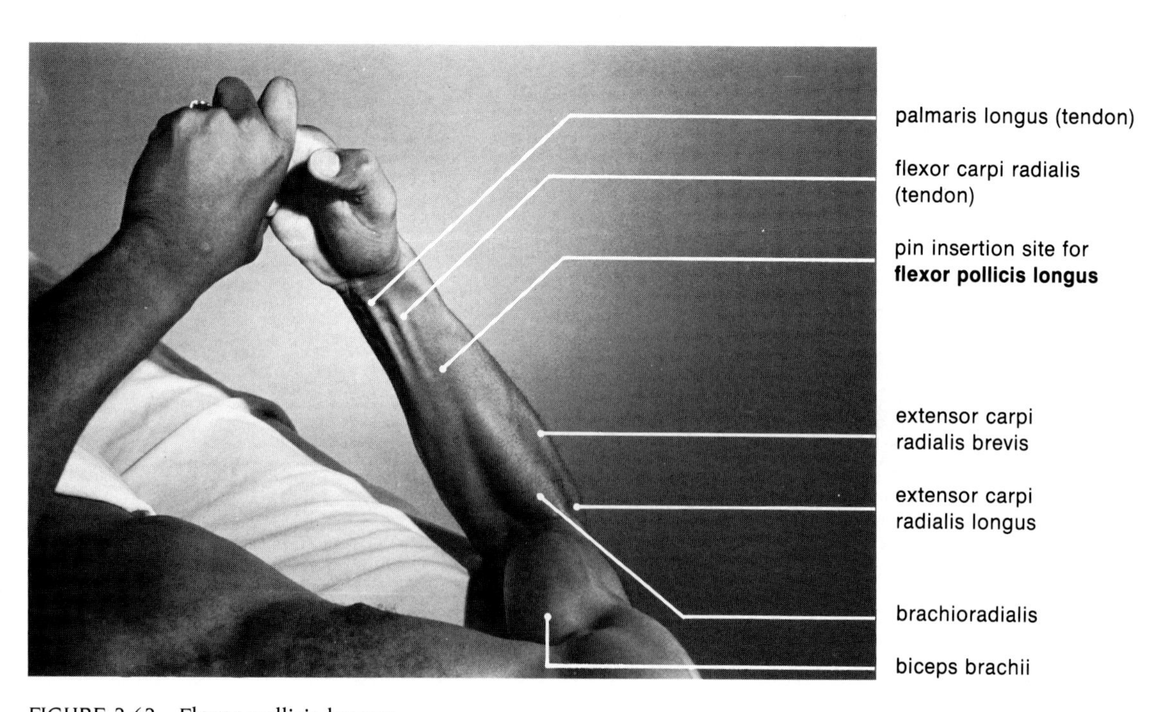

FIGURE 2-62 Flexor pollicis longus.

Pronator Quadratus (*Fig. 2-63; see also Figs. 1-28 and 2-61*)

Action: Pronation of the forearm

Patient Position: Supine, forearm supinated

Pin Insertion: Feel for the tendon of the flexor carpi ulnaris and insert the pin posterior and medial to it approximately 2 cm proximal to the prominence of the head of the ulna. Direct the pin laterally (radially) and slightly proximally so that it passes across the anterior (palmar) surface of the ulna.

Relaxation: Instruct the patient as follows: "Turn your forearm over so that your palm faces up toward the ceiling" (supination).

Contraction: *Minimal*: Instruct the patient as follows: "Turn your forearm over just slightly so that your palm faces toward you partially" (partial pronation).

Contraction: *Maximal*: Instruct the patient as follows: "Turn your hand and forearm so that your palm faces the floor. Don't let me twist your hand so that your palm faces upward" (resistance is given to maximal pronation). Apply resistance by giving pressure at the proximal portion of the hand in the direction of supination.

Peripheral Nerve Supply: Anterior interosseous nerve branch from the median nerve

Root Supply: Nerve roots C8 and T1, mainly C8

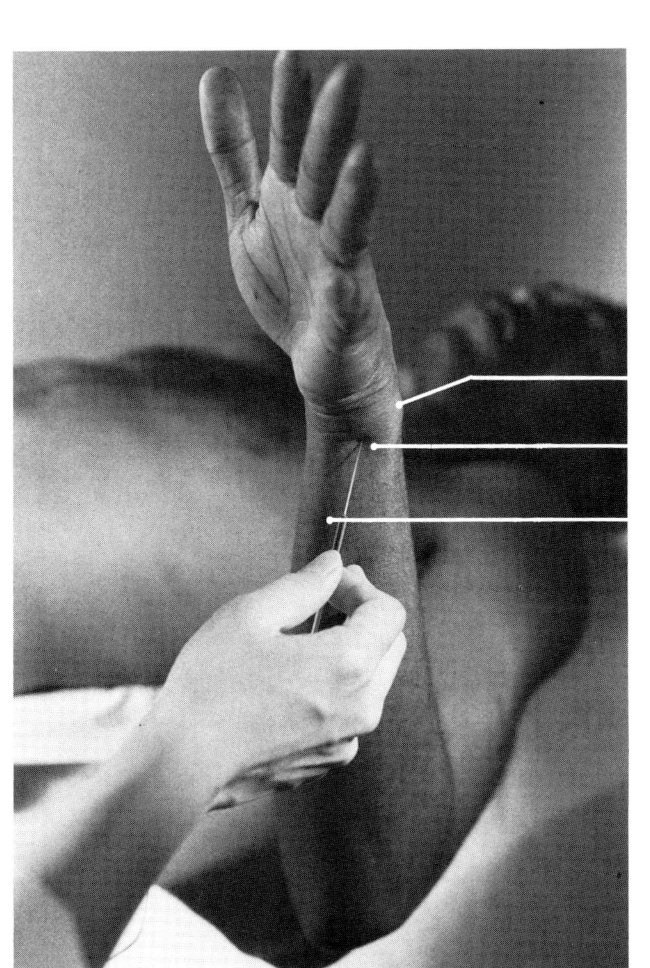

FIGURE 2-63 Pronator quadratus.

Note: The direction of the physician's hand and the direction of the pin in this figure are arranged so as not to block the reader's view and to illustrate the point of pin insertion and the position of the forearm for examining this muscle. Actually, the pin should be directed transversely across the forearm, or even somewhat proximally, as it passes across the ulna, to ensure that it enters the lower border of the pronator quadratus. The latter is rather oblique and higher on the ulnar side. See Figure 2-61 for the level of pin insertion for this muscle.

MUSCLES OF THE HAND

Opponens Pollicis (*Fig.* 2-64; *see also Figs.* 1-26, 1-27, 1-29, *and* 1-30)

Action: Draws the first metacarpal bone forward and medially so that the pad of the distal phalanx of the thumb can be brought against the pad of the distal phalanges of the other fingers.

Patient Position: Supine, forearm supinated

Pin Insertion: Feel for the midpoint of the first metacarpal bone. The opponens pollicis is the first muscle on this bone as your finger slides around toward the palmar aspect.

Relaxation: Instruct the patient as follows: "Relax your thumb and lay it flat on the bed" (thumb placed in passive extension).

Contraction: *Minimal*: Instruct the patient as follows: "Act as if you want to touch the tip of your thumb to the other fingers" (minimal thumb opposition).

Contraction: *Maximal*: Instruct the patient as follows: "Bring the tip of your thumb against another finger and push them together strongly. Don't let me spread them apart" (maximal thumb opposition with resistance applied at the first metacarpal bone in the direction of thumb extension).

Peripheral Nerve Supply: Recurrent branch of the median nerve. In approximately three fourths of cases a twig from the ulnar nerve also supplies the muscle.[2–4]

Root Supply: Nerve roots C8 and T1, mainly C8

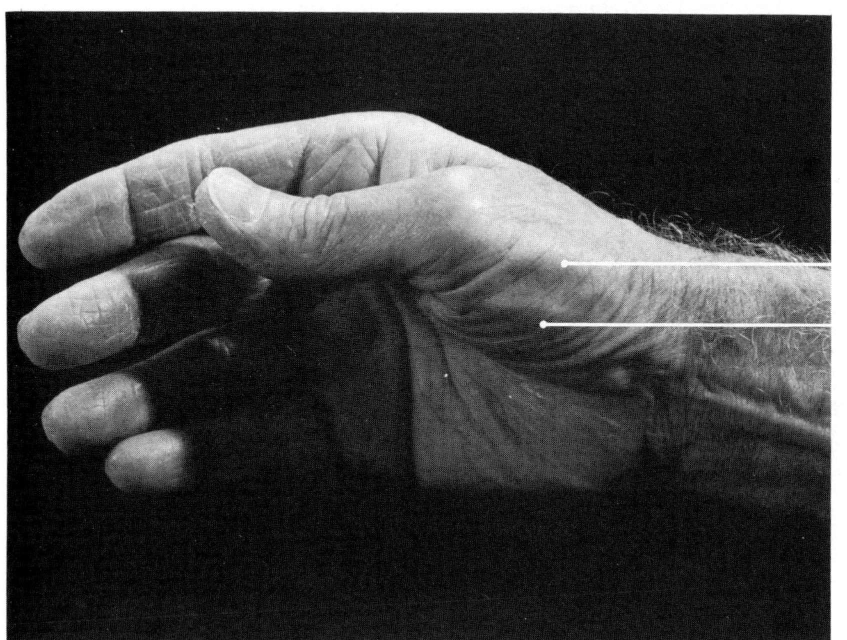

FIGURE 2-64 Opponens pollicis.

Abductor Pollicis Brevis (*Fig.* 2-65; *see also Figs.* 1-26, 1-27, 1-29, *and* 1-30)

Action: Abduction of the thumb

Patient Position: Supine, forearm supinated

Pin Insertion: Instruct the patient as follows: "Lift your thumb and point it toward the ceiling. Keep the back of your hand on the bed." Ensure that the thumb is in abduction by placing it at 90° to the plane of the palm. Then palpate the first metacarpal bone and slide the palpating finger around toward the palmar side. The first muscle encountered will be a narrow strip of the most superficial fibers of the opponens pollicis. A longitudinal groove separates the opponens pollicis from the abductor pollicis brevis. The latter muscle is along a line between the scaphoid and the base of the proximal phalanx of the thumb. Insert the pin near the midpoint of the muscle.

Relaxation: This muscle can be made to relax by placing the patient's thumb in the plane of the palm, with the metacarpophalangeal and interphalangeal joints of the thumb in slight passive flexion.

Contraction: *Minimal*: Instruct the patient as follows: "Lift your thumb up slightly" (minimal abduction of the thumb).

Contraction: *Maximal*: Instruct the patient as follows: "Point your thumb up toward the ceiling and don't let me push it down" (the thumb is kept at 90° to the plane of the palm, and the examiner applies pressure at about the tip of the proximal phalanx of the thumb in the direction of adduction, that is, toward the plane of the palm).

Peripheral Nerve Supply: Recurrent branch of the median nerve

Root Supply: Nerve roots C8 and T1, mainly C8

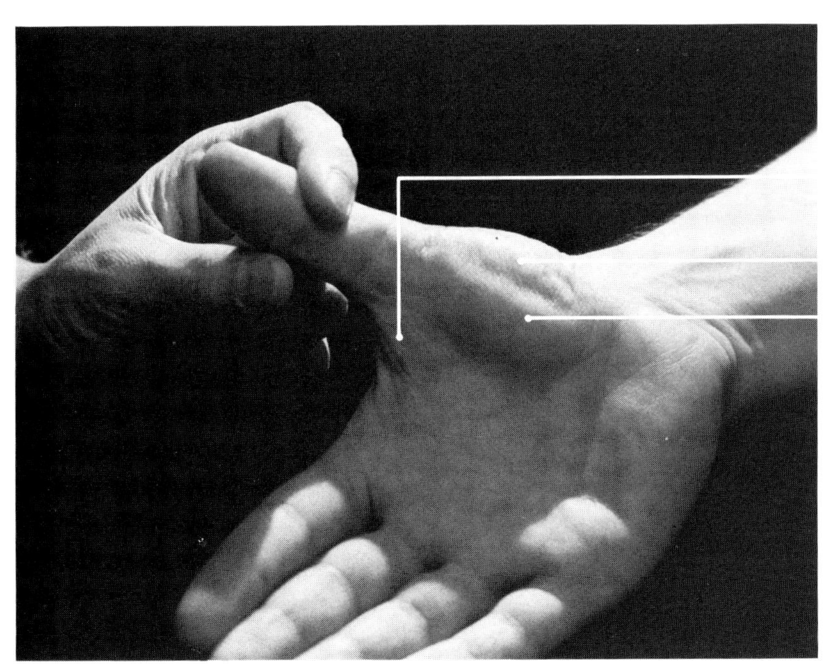

FIGURE 2-65 Abductor pollicis brevis.

Flexor Pollicis Brevis (*Fig.* 2-66; *see also Figs.* 1-26, 1-27, 1-29, *and* 1-30)

Action: Flexion of the thumb at the metacarpophalangeal joint

Patient Position: Supine, forearm supinated

Pin Insertion: First define the borders of the abductor pollicis brevis as previously described. Palpate this muscle between your thumb and index fingers. The next muscle medial to the medial border of the abductor pollicis brevis is the flexor pollicis brevis. It is a flat muscle, and pin insertion is done after instructing the patient as follows: "Bend your thumb at the knuckle and bring it across the palm" (flexion of the thumb at the proximal phalanx in the plane of the palm). With superficial pin insertion, the superficial head of the flexor pollicis brevis can be examined. If the pin insertion is deeper (1.5 cm), the deep head can be examined.

Relaxation: Instruct the patient as follows: "Straighten your thumb out and lay it flat on the bed" (the thumb is extended at the metacarpophalangeal joint in the plane of the palm). The interphalangeal joint may be placed in passive flexion.

Contraction: *Minimal*: Instruct the patient as follows: "Bend your thumb just slightly at the knuckle" (minimal flexion of the thumb at the level of the metacarpophalangeal joint).

Contraction: *Maximal*: Instruct the patient as follows: "Bend your thumb at the knuckle and bring the thumb across the palm. Don't let me push your thumb back" (maximal flexion at the metacarpophalangeal joint of the thumb). Give resistance at the distal end of the proximal phalanx in the direction of extension.

Peripheral Nerve Supply: Recurrent branch of the median nerve to the superficial head and a branch of the ulnar nerve to the deep head. However, there is much variability in the innervation and even in the existence of the deep head.[1]

Root Supply: Nerve roots C8 and T1, mainly C8

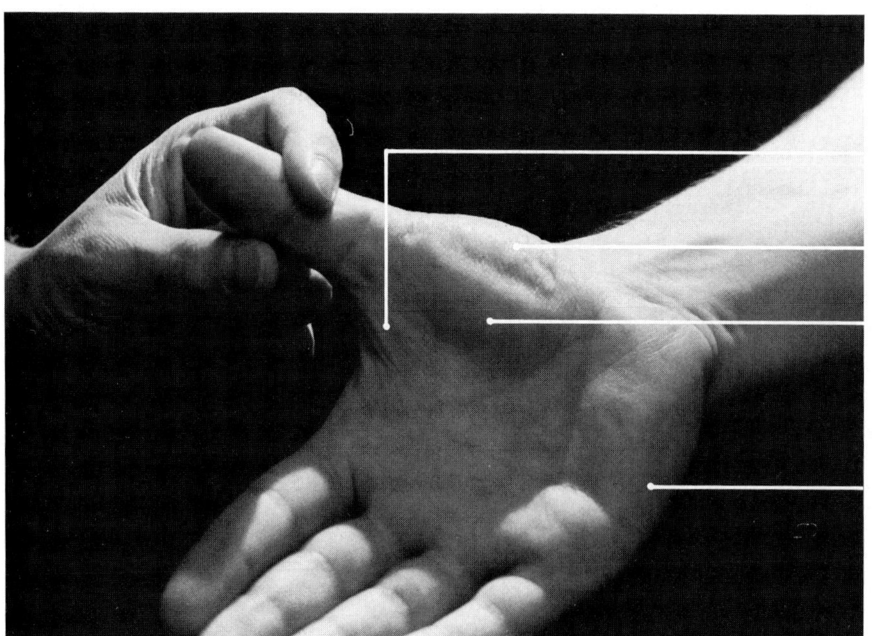

FIGURE 2-66 Flexor pollicis brevis.

Adductor Pollicis (*Fig. 2-67; see also Fig. 1-29*)

Action: Adduction of the thumb

Patient Position: Supine, forearm in midpronation

Pin Insertion: Define the lateral edge of the first dorsal interosseous muscle by asking the patient to point his index finger toward the ceiling. Insert the pin into the free skinfold anterior to the lateral edge of the first dorsal interosseous muscle, directing the pin toward the palmar aspect of the base of the first metacarpal bone. To ensure that the pin is in the adductor pollicis and not in the first dorsal interosseous, check for the appearance of MUPs on adduction of the thumb but not on abduction of the index finger.

Relaxation: Instruct the patient as follows: "Spread your thumb out and relax it" (passive abduction of the thumb). You may also place the metacarpophalangeal and interphalangeal joints of the patient's thumb in passive flexion.

Contraction: *Minimal*: Instruct the patient as follows: "Bring your thumb in slightly toward the side of the index finger" (minimal adduction of the thumb).

Contraction: *Maximal*: Instruct the patient as follows: "Bring your thumb in toward the side of the index finger and don't let me spread them apart" (maximal adduction of the thumb). Apply pressure at the distal tip of the proximal phalanx of the thumb in the direction of abduction.

Peripheral Nerve Supply: Deep branch of the ulnar nerve

Root Supply: Nerve roots C8 and T1, mainly T1

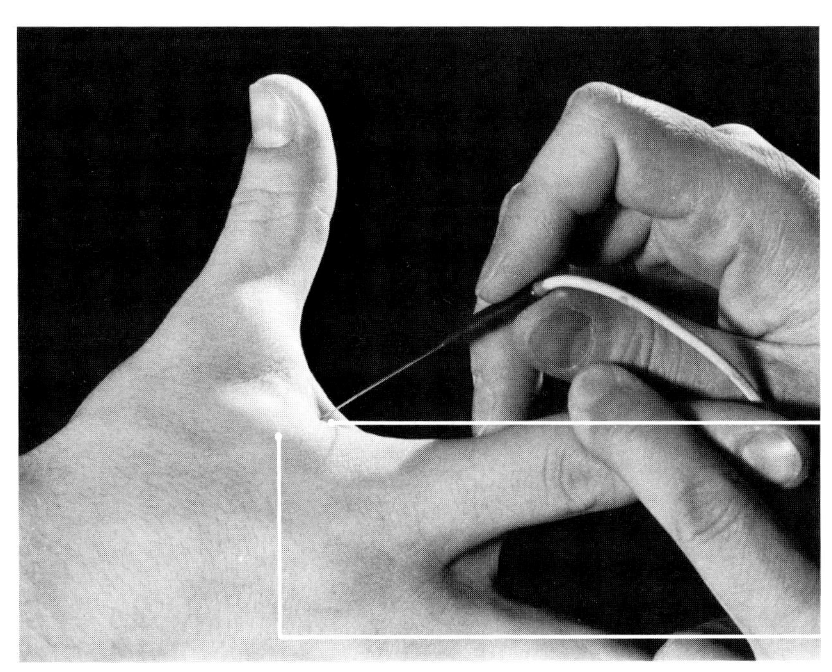

FIGURE 2-67 Adductor pollicis.

Dorsal Interossei (*Figs.* 2-68 *and* 2-69; *see also* *Figs.* 1-31 *and* 1-39)

Action: There are four dorsal interosseous muscles. The first abducts the index finger toward the thumb, the second abducts the middle finger toward the index finger, the third abducts the middle finger toward the ring finger, and the fourth abducts the ring finger toward the little finger. Thus, all are abductors of the fingers away from the middle finger. In addition, they flex the metacarpophalangeal joints and extend the interphalangeal joints.

Patient Position: Supine, forearm pronated or in midpronation

Pin Insertion: *First Dorsal Interosseous*: With the patient's forearm in midpronation, instruct the patient as follows: "Lift your index finger and point it toward the ceiling over your opposite shoulder" (abduction of the index finger). Insert the pin into the bulk of the muscle. *Second to Fourth Dorsal Interossei*: With the patient's forearm kept in pronation, feel for the distal portion of the shafts ("neck") of the metacarpal bones, just proximal to the heads, and insert the pin in this region in the intermetacarpal spaces. The second dorsal interosseous is examined in the intermetacarpal space between the index and middle fingers. The third dorsal interosseous is examined between the middle and ring fingers. The fourth dorsal interosseous is examined between the ring and little fingers.

Relaxation: Instruct the patient as follows: "Relax your fingers; don't spread them apart" (fingers are kept in passive adduction).

Contraction: *Minimal*: Instruct the patient as follows: "Spread your fingers slightly" (minimal abduction of the fingers).

Contraction: *Maximal*: Instruct the patient as follows: "Spread your fingers strongly" (maximal abduction of the fingers). Apply pressure in the direction of adduction against the side of the proximal phalanx of the finger to be examined.

Peripheral Nerve Supply: Deep branch of the ulnar nerve

Root Supply: Nerve roots C8 and T1, mainly T1

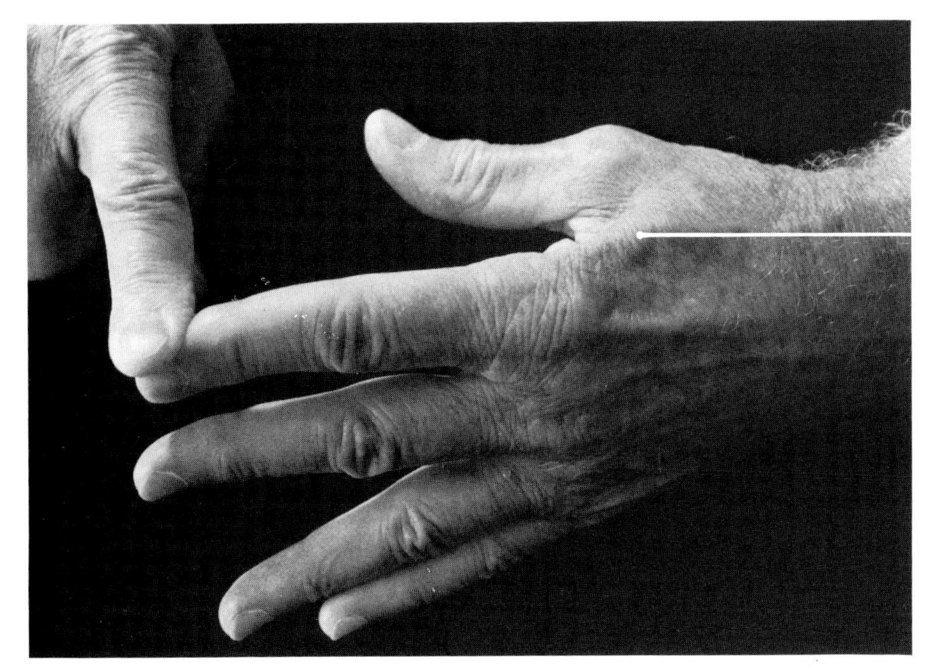

FIGURE 2-68 First dorsal interosseous.

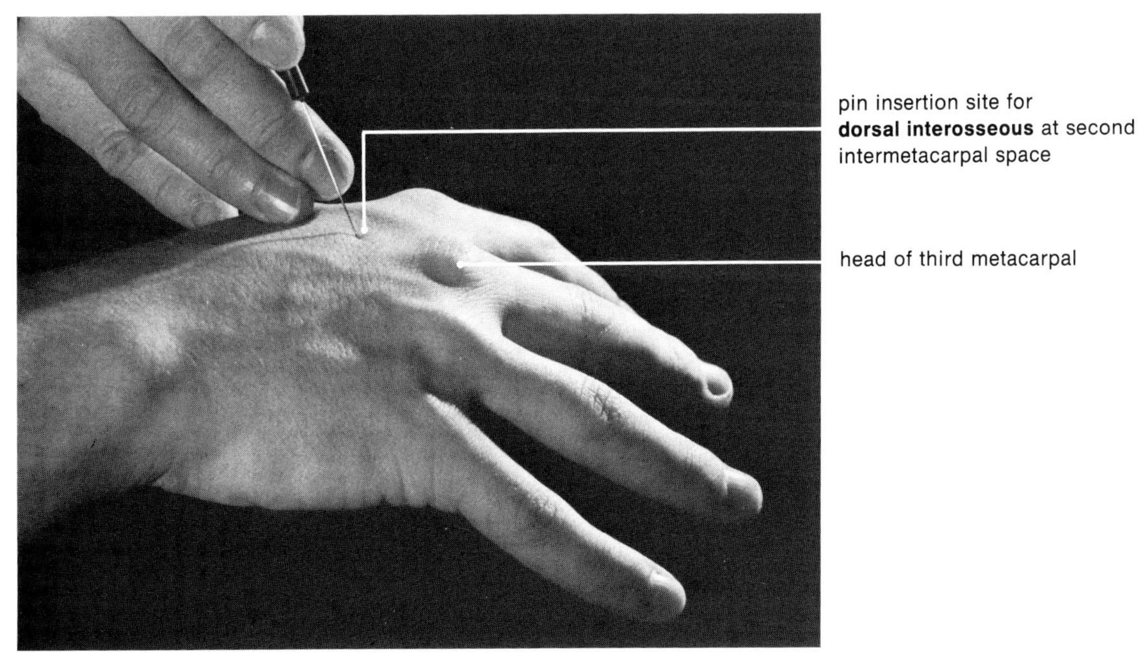

FIGURE 2-69 Dorsal interossei.

Palmar Interossei (*Fig.* 2-70)

Action: There are three palmar interossei. The first and second bring the index finger and ring finger, respectively, toward the middle finger. The third brings the little finger toward the ring finger. Thus, all are adductors of the fingers toward the middle finger. They also flex the proximal phalanges and extend the middle and distal phalanges by means of their insertion into the dorsal aponeurosis.

Patient Position: Supine, forearm supinated

Pin Insertion: Feel for the interspaces between the second and third metacarpals, the third and fourth metacarpals, and fourth and fifth metacarpals for examination of the first, second, and third palmar interossei, respectively. Insert the pin at about the junction of the middle and distal thirds of the palm while instructing the patient to adduct the finger toward the midline. The point of insertion should be just between the proximal and distal transverse flexion crease of the palm. Follow the sounds of the MUPs to gauge the direction and depth of needle penetration.

Relaxation: Instruct the patient as follows: "Spread your fingers and relax." You may position the patient's fingers in partial flexion at all joints.

Contraction: *Minimal*: Depending on which palmar interosseous muscle is being examined, instruct the patient as follows: "Bring your finger in slightly toward the middle finger" (minimal adduction of the finger to be examined).

Contraction: *Maximal*: Instruct the patient as follows: "Press your fingers tightly against each other. Don't let me spread them apart" (maximal adduction of the finger to be examined).

Peripheral Nerve Supply: Deep branch of the ulnar nerve

Root Supply: Nerve roots C8 and T1, mainly T1

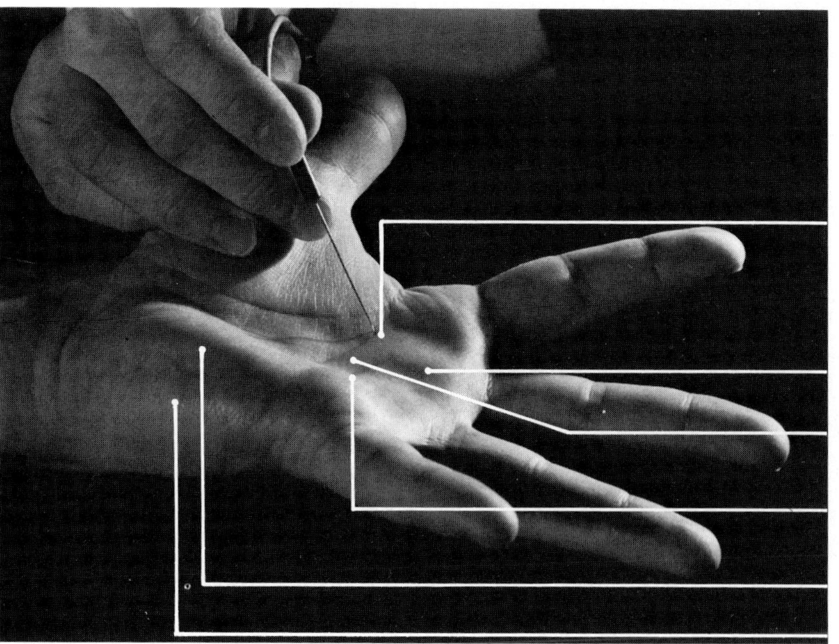

FIGURE 2-70 Palmar interossei.

Lumbricals (*Fig.* 2-71; *see also Fig.* 1-29)

Action: Extension of the interphalangeal joints and flexion of the metacarpophalangeal joints of the fingers

Patient Position: Supine, forearm supinated

Pin Insertion: Feel for the distal part of the shaft ("neck") of the metacarpal bones just proximal to the head and insert the pin in this region at a level slightly proximal to the distal transverse flexion crease of the palm. The first and second lumbricals are examined on the radial aspect of the second and third metacarpal "necks." The third lumbrical is examined at the region between the "necks" of the third and fourth metacarpal bones. The fourth lumbrical is examined between the "necks" of the fourth and fifth metacarpal bones. The lumbricals are deep to the palmar aponeurosis and in the plane of the tendons of the flexor digitorum profundus, from which they arise.

Relaxation: Instruct the patient as follows: "Relax your fingers." Place the proximal and distal interphalangeal joints of the patient's fingers in passive flexion and the metacarpophalangeal joints in passive extension.

Contraction: *Minimal*: Instruct the patient as follows: "Straighten your fingers slightly" (minimal extension of the interphalangeal joints of the fingers).

Contraction: *Maximal*: Instruct the patient as follows: "Straighten your fingers strongly and don't let me bend them" (maximal extension of the interphalangeal joints of the fingers). Apply resistance on the dorsal aspect of the middle and distal phalanges in the direction of flexion.

Peripheral Nerve Supply: Lateral two lumbricals, median nerve (variable); medial two lumbricals, ulnar nerve (variable)

Root Supply: Nerve roots C8 and T1, mainly T1

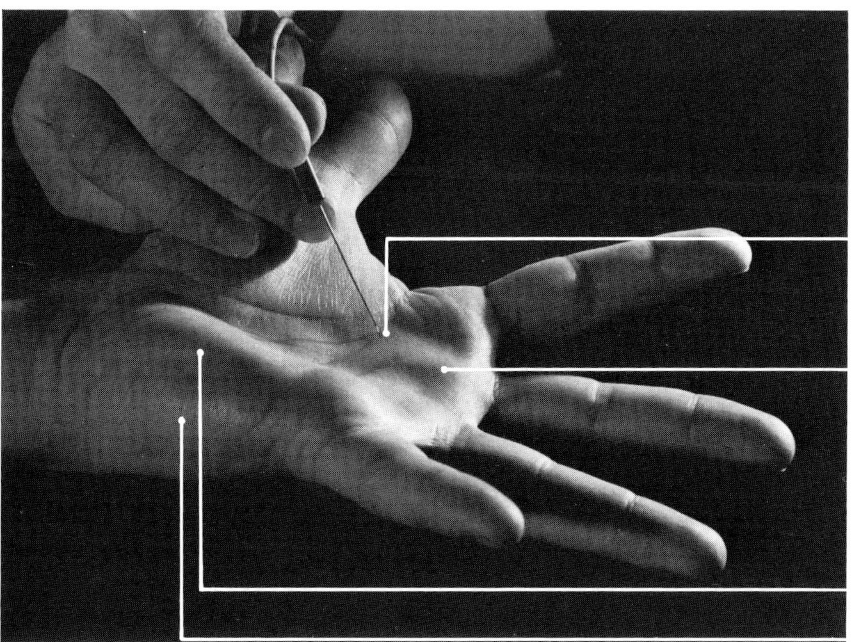

FIGURE 2-71 Lumbricals.

Abductor Digiti Minimi (*Fig. 2-72; see also Figs. 1-26, 1-27, 1-29, and 1-30*)

Action: Abduction of the fifth digit and flexion of the metacarpophalangeal joint with some assistance to extension of the interphalangeal joints

Patient Position: Supine, forearm supinated

Pin Insertion: Feel for the medial edge of the fifth metacarpal bone, and slide the palpating finger palmarward. The first muscle felt is the abductor digiti minimi. It is a bulky muscle, and the edges can be defined by abduction of the fifth digit. Insert the pin into the bulk of the muscle.

Relaxation: Instruct the patient as follows: "Relax your little finger." Place the patient's fifth metacarpophalangeal and interphalangeal joints in passive flexion.

Contraction: *Minimal*: Instruct the patient as follows: "Spread your little finger slightly away from the others" (minimal abduction of the fifth digit).

Contraction: *Maximal*: Instruct the patient as follows: "Spread your little finger out away from the others as strongly as you can" (maximal abduction of the fifth digit). Give resistance at the distal end of the proximal phalanx of the fifth digit in the direction of adduction.

Peripheral Nerve Supply: Ulnar nerve

Root Supply: Nerve roots C8 and T1, mainly T1

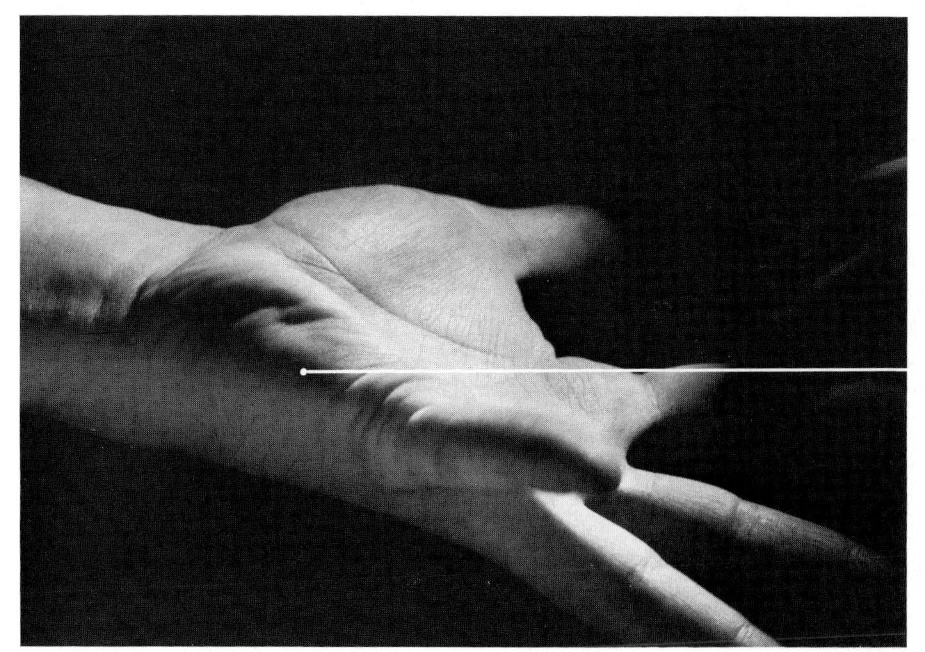

FIGURE 2-72 Abductor digiti minimi.

Flexor Digiti Minimi Brevis (*Fig.* 2-73; *see also Figs.* 1-26, 1-27, 1-29, *and* 1-30)

Action: Flexion of the proximal phalanx of the fifth digit, plus slight flexion of the carpometacarpal joint

Patient Position: Supine, forearm supinated

Pin Insertion: Define the abductor digiti minimi. Grasp its edges between your thumb and forefingers, and the next muscle lateral to it on the palmar aspect is the flexor digiti minimi brevis. It is in line with the hook of the hamate. Insert the pin near the midpoint of the muscle.

Relaxation: Instruct the patient as follows: "Relax your little finger." Place the little finger in passive extension at the metacarpophalangeal joint.

Contraction: *Minimal*: Instruct the patient as follows: "Bend your little finger slightly at the knuckle joint" (minimal flexion at the metacarpophalangeal joint of the fifth digit).

Contraction: *Maximal*: Instruct the patient as follows: "Bend your little finger strongly at the knuckle joint and don't let me straighten it" (maximal flexion of the fifth digit at the metacarpophalangeal joint). Try to extend the little finger by giving resistance to flexion at the distal end of the proximal phalanx.

Peripheral Nerve Supply: Deep branch of the ulnar nerve

Root Supply: Nerve roots C8 and T1, mainly T1

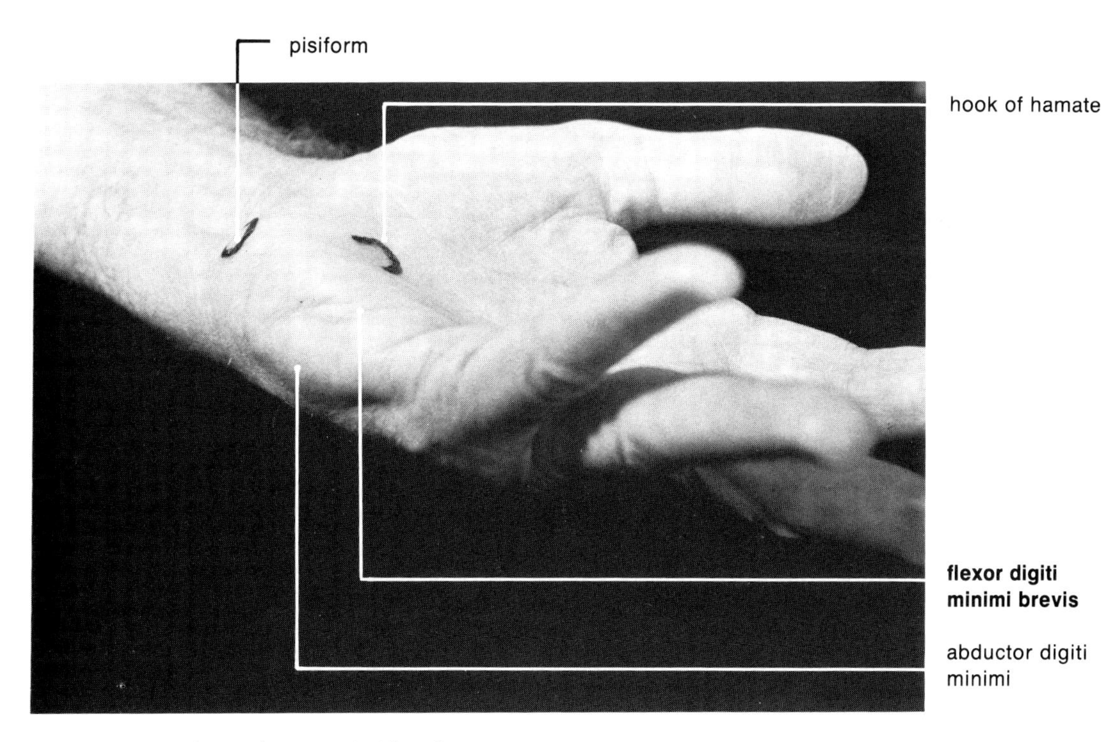

FIGURE 2-73 Flexor digiti minimi brevis.

Opponens Digiti Minimi (*Fig.* 2-74; *see also Figs.* 1-26, 1-27, 1-29, *and* 1-30)

Action: Flexion and lateral rotation of the fifth metacarpal at the carpometacarpal joint. It enables the fifth digit to be brought toward the thumb by drawing the fifth metacarpal bone forward, thus deepening the hollow of the palm.

Patient Position: Supine, forearm supinated

Pin Insertion: Feel for a point 1 cm distal to the hook of the hamate and lateral to the lateral edge of the flexor digiti minimi. Insert the pin at this point. The tendons of the flexor digitorum profundus and superficialis to the little finger make a palpable cord when taut. The opponens digiti minimi is immediately medial to this cord.

Relaxation: Instruct the patient as follows: "Straighten your little finger" (fifth digit is kept in passive extension).

Contraction: *Maximal*: Instruct the patient as follows: "Try to bring your little finger toward your thumb" (minimal opposition of the fifth digit).

Contraction: *Maximal*: Instruct the patient as follows: "Touch the tip of your little finger to the tip of your thumb. Don't let me spread them apart" (maximal opposition of the fifth digit). Apply pressure on the fifth metacarpal bone toward the plane of the palm (*i.e.*, dorsally).

Peripheral Nerve Supply: Deep branch of the ulnar nerve

Root Supply: Nerve roots C8 and T1, mainly T1

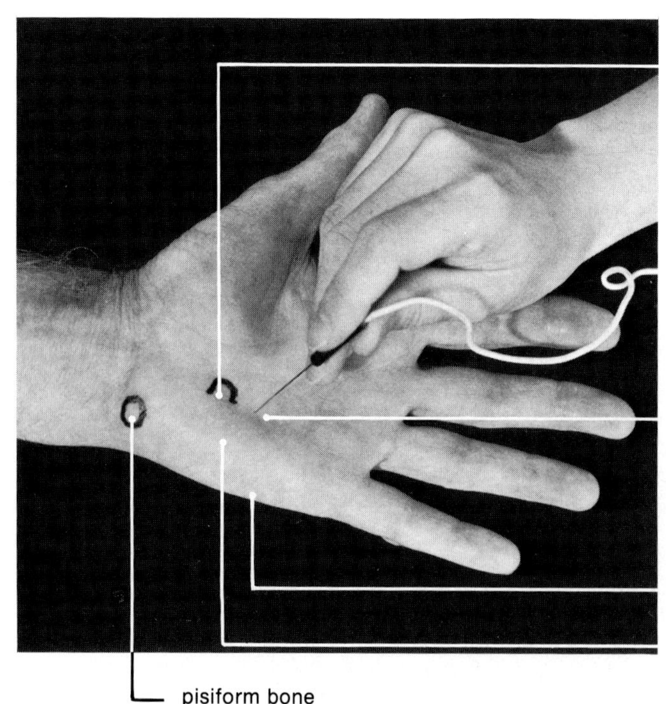

FIGURE 2-74 Opponens digiti minimi.

MUSCLES OF THE PELVIC GIRDLE AND HIP

Iliopsoas (*Fig.* 2-75; *see also Figs.* 1-45 *through* 1-47)

Action: Flexion of the hip joint

Patient Position: Supine

Pin Insertion: Define the sartorius by having the patient flex and externally rotate his thigh. Insert the pin medial to the medial edge of the upper end of the sartorius. The pin will be mainly in the iliacus portion of the iliopsoas. Ensure that the pin is lateral to the pulsation of the femoral artery (palpate this artery against the head of the femur).

Relaxation: Instruct the patient as follows: "Keep your hip joint straight, spread your leg outward at the thigh, and relax" (extension and abduction of the hip joint). Place the thigh in passive external rotation.

Contraction: *Minimal*: Instruct the patient as follows: "Bend your hip slightly" (minimal hip flexion). Place the thigh in external rotation. You may instruct the patient to flex the hip in the gravity-eliminating position, with the patient in a partially lateral recumbent position. *Maximal*: Instruct the patient as follows: "Bend your hip and knee and lift your heel off the bed" (flexion of the hip and knee against gravity). Place the hip joint in the neutral position and give resistance at the lower thigh in the direction of hip extension.

Peripheral Nerve Supply: Branches from the ventral rami of lumbar nerves L1, L2, and L3 for the psoas and branches from the femoral nerve for the iliacus.

Root Supply: Nerve roots L1, L2, L3, and sometimes L4 for psoas major, L2 and L3 via femoral nerve for iliacus

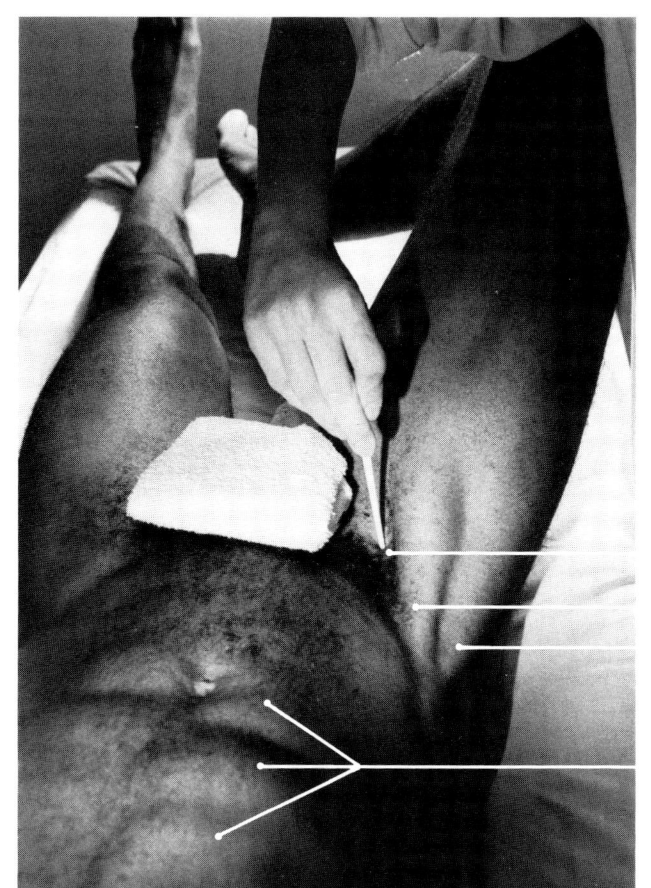

FIGURE 2-75 Iliopsoas.

Tensor Fasciae Latae (*Fig. 2-76; see also Figs. 1-45, 1-46, and 1-51*)

Action: Assists in internal rotation and abduction of the hip. In conjunction with the gluteus maximus and through the iliotibial band, it tethers the pelvis on the head of the femur when one is standing on the single ipsilateral leg. It stabilizes the knee joint on the lateral side via the iliotibial band. It gives slight assistance in flexion of the thigh but becomes more active when the leg is extended on the flexed thigh simultaneously, owing to the somewhat anterior attachment of the iliotibial band on the lateral tibial condyle.

Patient Position: Supine

Pin Insertion: Feel for a point approximately 5 cm inferior to the lower edge of the anterior superior iliac spine and insert the pin approximately 2.5 cm lateral to this point.

Relaxation: Instruct the patient as follows: "Roll your thigh outward and relax it." Rotate the thigh into passive external rotation.

Contraction: *Minimal*: Instruct the patient as follows: "Roll your thigh outward and bend your hip and knee" (with hip placed in external rotation to ensure minimal contraction, the patient is instructed to flex his hip and knee.) You may also instruct the patient as follows: "Lift your heel off the bed and then rest it back on the bed." This action usually initiates contraction. If too much contraction is obtained, the hip can be placed into more external rotation; if contraction is insufficient, the hip can be rolled back into more internal rotation.

Contraction: *Maximal*: Instruct the patient as follows: "Roll your thigh inward, keep your knee straight, and lift your leg straight up." (With hip in internal rotation and the knee in extension, the patient is instructed to flex his hip.) Give resistance to hip flexion by applying pressure just above the knee.

Peripheral Nerve Supply: Superior gluteal nerve

Root Supply: Nerve roots L4 and L5, mainly L5, but L4 may dominate.

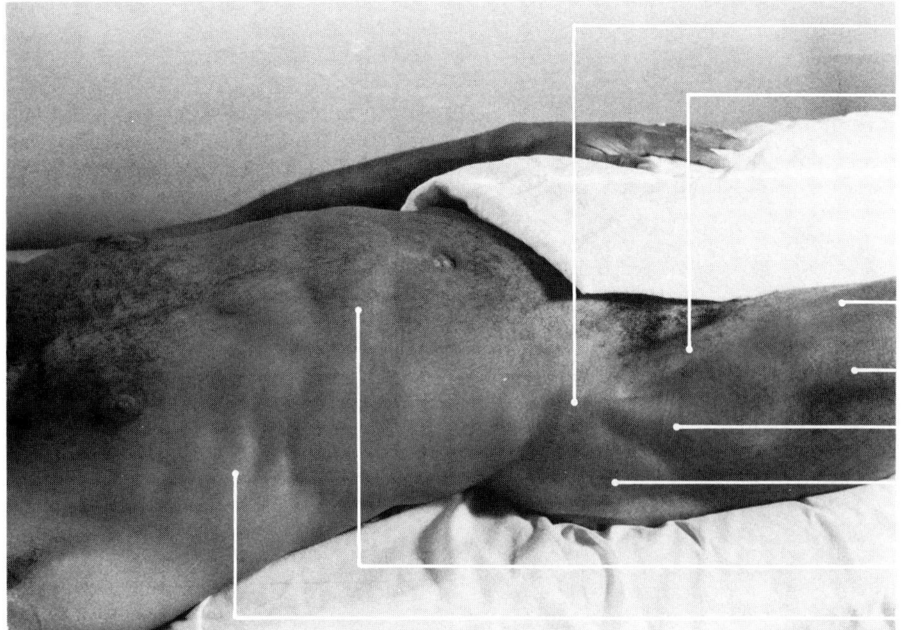

FIGURE 2-76 Tensor fasciae latae.

Gluteus Medius (*Fig.* 2-77; *see also Figs.* 1-41 *through* 1-43 *and* 1-51)

Action: Abduction and internal rotation of the thigh. In walking, it pulls the ilium toward the greater trochanter, thus preventing dropping of the unsupported side of the pelvis.

Patient Position: Lateral recumbent

Pin Insertion: Feel for the tubercle of the iliac crest or the highest point of the iliac crest and the greater trochanter and insert the pin along the line between these two points at about the level of the anterior superior iliac spine. The muscle is entered immediately deep to a tough fascial covering layer.

Relaxation: Place the upper part of the patient's hip at approximately 30° to 45° of hip flexion with the thigh adducted.

(*Text and figure continue on next page.*)

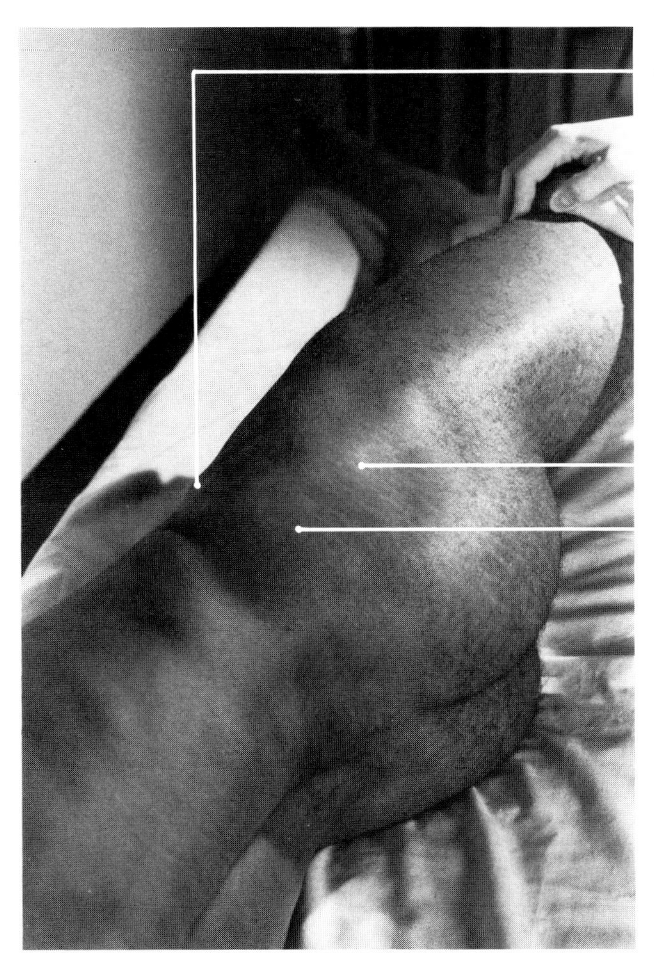

FIGURE 2-77 Gluteus medius.

Gluteus Medius *(Continued from previous page)*

Contraction: *Minimal*: Place the upper part of the patient's hip at approximately 30° to 45° of flexion and instruct the patient as follows: "Lift your thigh slightly off the bed" (minimal hip abduction).

Contraction: *Maximal*: Keep the upper part of the patient's hip in hyperextension with the knee in extension and instruct the patient as follows: "Lift your thigh off the bed" (maximal hip abduction). Apply pressure at the lower part of the thigh in the direction of hip adduction.

Peripheral Nerve Supply: Superior gluteal nerve

Root Supply: Nerve roots L4, L5, and S1, mainly L5

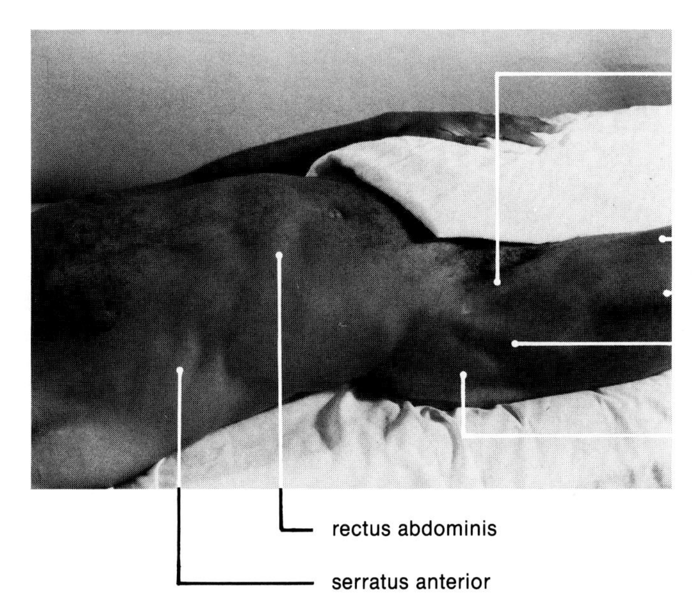

FIGURE 2-77 *(Continued)*

Gluteus Minimus (*Fig.* 2-78; *see also* 1-42)

Action: Abduction and internal rotation of the thigh

Patient Position: Lateral recumbent

Pin Insertion: Feel for the tubercle of the iliac crest and the greater trochanter. Insert the pin midway between these two points. The gluteus minimus is deep to the gluteus medius, which must be pierced to reach the gluteus minimus. A 5-cm pin electrode is usually required. The anterior part of the gluteus medius is thinner than the gluteus minimus in the same area, but it is best to reach bone gently and then withdraw 5 mm.

*Relaxation**

*Contraction**

*Peripheral Nerve Supply**

*Root Supply**

* See gluteus medius.

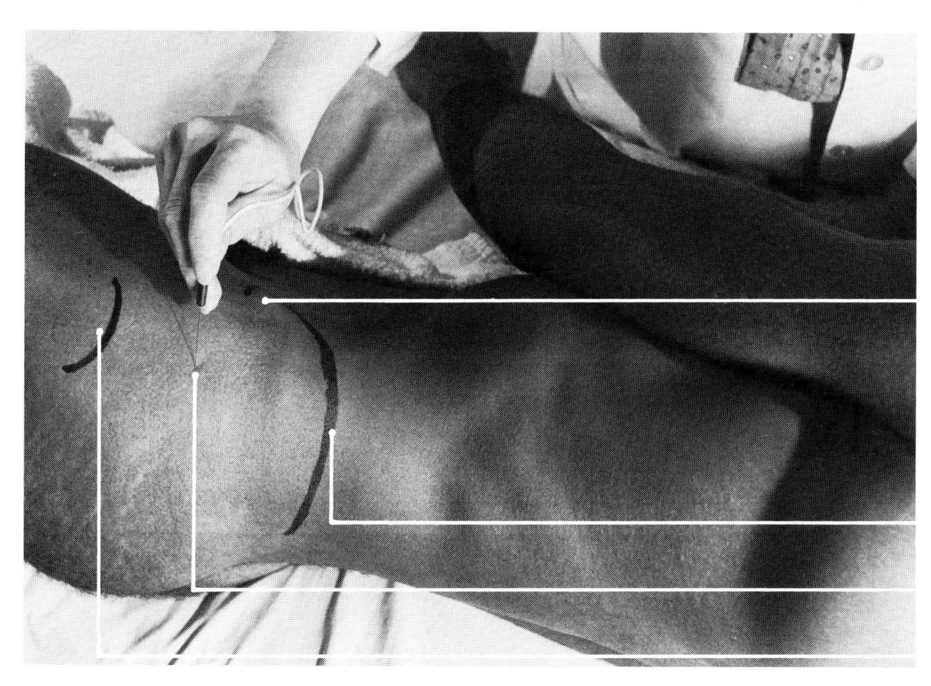

FIGURE 2-78 Gluteus minimus.

Gluteus Maximus (*Fig. 2-79; see also Figs. 1-50 and 1-51*)

Action: Extension of the hip joint, external rotation of the thigh, and extension of the torso on the fixed lower limbs, as in straightening upright from a bent-over position.

Patient Position: Prone

Pin Insertion: Approximately 2.5 cm inferior and lateral to the superior end of the intergluteal cleft. The least amount of subcutaneous tissue is encountered on penetration at this site.

Relaxation: Instruct the patient as follows: "Spread your thighs apart, flatten your buttocks, and relax" (hips are kept in slight abduction to relax the gluteus maximus).

Contraction: Minimal: Instruct the patient as follows: "Squeeze your buttocks together slightly" (minimal bearing-down action).

Contraction: Maximal: Instruct the patient as follows: "Squeeze your buttocks together strongly" (maximal bearing-down action). The strongest contraction can be obtained by instructing the patient as follows: "Bend your knee and lift it off the bed" (hip extension with knee in flexion). Give resistance at the lower thigh in the direction of hip flexion.

Peripheral Nerve Supply: Inferior gluteal nerve

Root Supply: Nerve roots L5, S1, and S2, mainly S1

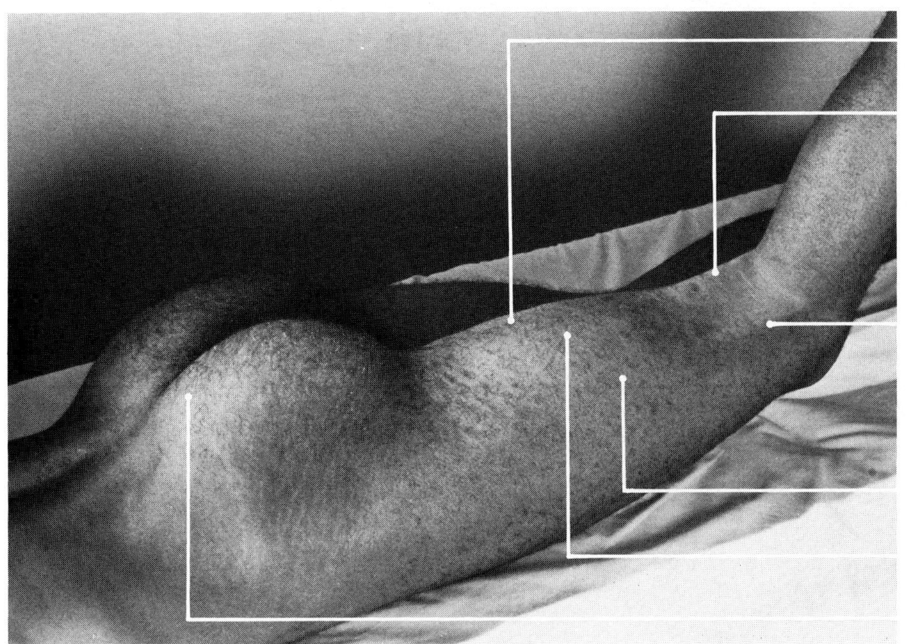

FIGURE 2-79 Gluteus maximus.
Note: The best pin insertion site for the gluteus maximus is approximately 2.5 cm lateral and 2.5 cm inferior to the uppermost level of the intergluteal cleft. At this site the pin encounters the least amount of subcutaneous tissue.

Piriformis (*Fig.* 2-80; *see also* Figs. 1-41 *through* 1-43)

Action: Lateral rotation of the extended thigh, abduction of the flexed thigh

Patient Position: Prone

Pin Insertion: Feel for the inferior tip of the coccyx and the posterior superior iliac spine. Midway between these two points, draw an imaginary line to connect the uppermost edge of the greater trochanter. This line passes along the lower margin of the piriformis. Insert the pin approximately 1 cm to 2 cm superior to this line at about the midpoint of this line.

Relaxation: Instruct the patient as follows: "Roll your leg and foot inward toward the other foot and relax" (hip in internal rotation).

Contraction: *Minimal*: Instruct the patient as follows: "Bend your knee and point it slightly outward" (knee in flexion and hip in slight external rotation).

Contraction: *Maximal*: Instruct the patient as follows: "Bend your knee, turn it outward, and lift it off the bed" (knee in flexion, hip in external rotation, and knee lifted against gravity). Forceful external rotation of the thigh is the essential action desired.

Peripheral Nerve Supply: Twigs from the ventral rami of spinal nerves L5, S1, and S2

Root Supply: Nerve roots L5, S1, and S2, mainly S1

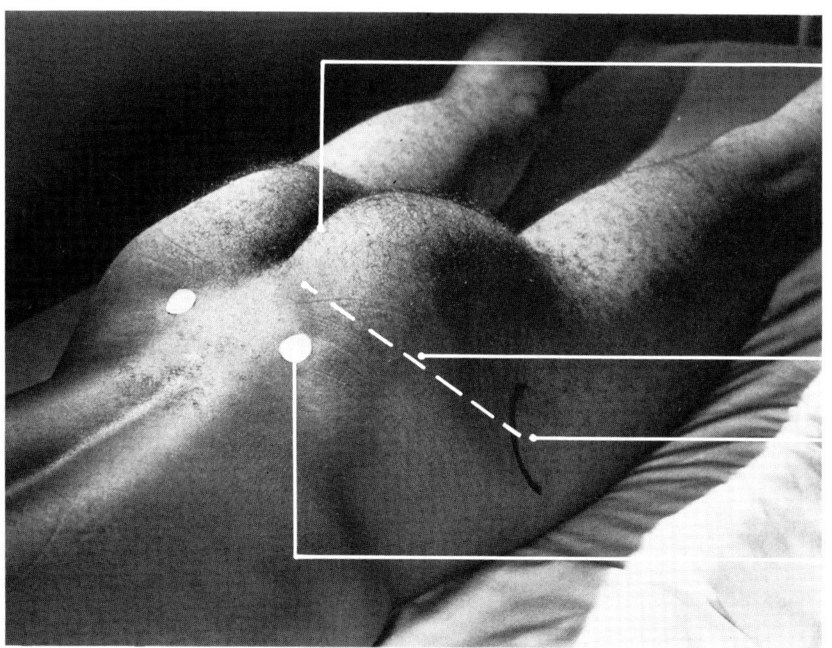

FIGURE 2-80 Piriformis.
Note: The lower border of the piriformis is obtained by drawing a line medially from the upper limit of the greater trochanter to bisect a line drawn from the tip of the coccyx to the posterior superior iliac spine on the same side.

MUSCLES OF THE ANTERIOR AND MEDIAL ASPECTS OF THE THIGH

Sartorius (*Fig.* 2-81; *see also Figs.* 1-45 *through* 1-47)

Action: Flexion and external rotation of the hip joint, flexion of the knee joint

Patient Position: Supine

Pin Insertion: Instruct the patient as follows: "Bend your hip and knee and put this heel on your other knee" (flexion of the hip and knee joints with external rotation of the hip joint). The prominent belly of the sartorius can be traced to its distal attachment from the anterior superior iliac spine. Hold the edges of the muscle between your thumb and index finger and insert the pin into the upper third of the muscle.

Relaxation: Instruct the patient as follows: "Put your hip and knee down on the bed and relax your thigh muscles" (hip and knee placed in extension). You can also rotate the hip into passive internal rotation.

Contraction: *Minimal*: Instruct the patient as follows: "Bend your hip and knee slightly" (minimal flexion of the hip and knee joint).

Contraction: *Maximal*: Instruct the patient as follows: "Bend your hip and knee, roll the knee outward, and lift your heel off the bed. Don't let me push your thigh down toward the bed." (The patient is instructed to flex his hip and knee with the hip placed in external rotation. He then lifts his heel off the bed. This will bring about maximal contraction of the sartorius.) Apply resistance at the lower thigh in the direction of hip extension.

Peripheral Nerve Supply: Femoral nerve

Root Supply: Nerve roots L2 and L3, mainly L2

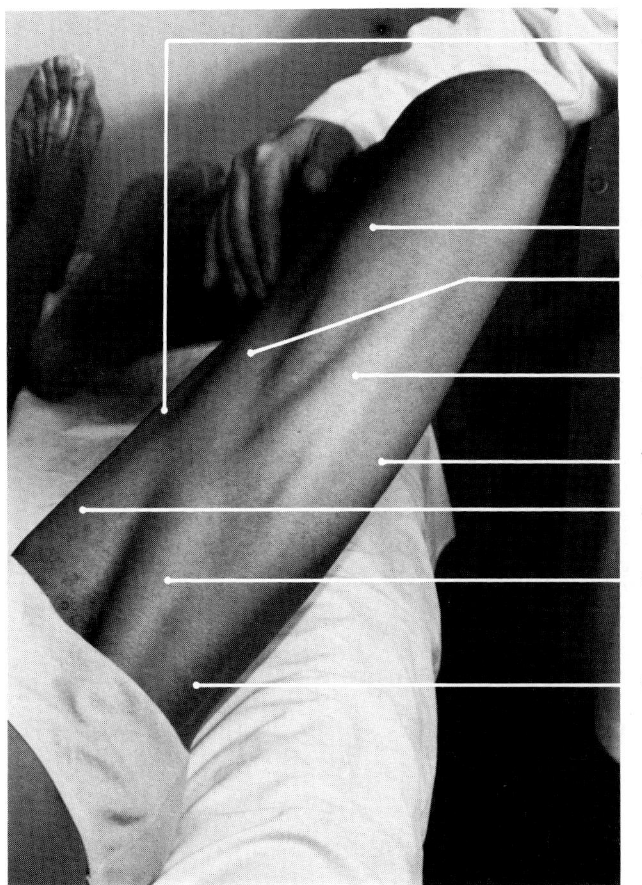

FIGURE 2-81 Sartorius.

Rectus Femoris (*Fig. 2-82; see also Figs. 1-45 through 1-47*)

Action: Extension of the knee joint and flexion of the hip joint

Patient Position: Supine

Pin Insertion: Instruct the patient as follows: "Keep your knee straight and push the back of it down into the bed" (extension of the knee joint). A firm muscle will be seen to come into action at about the middle of the thigh. This is the rectus femoris. Insert the pin into the muscle at about the junction of the lower and middle thirds of the thigh.

Relaxation: Instruct the patient as follows: "Bend your hip and knee slightly" (flexion of the hip and knee joints).

Contraction: Minimal: Instruct the patient as follows: "Press the back of your knee slightly into the bed" (minimal isometric contraction of the muscle).

Contraction: Maximal: Instruct the patient as follows: "Press the back of your knee strongly into the bed and make your knee very stiff" (maximal isometric contraction of the muscle).

Peripheral Nerve Supply: Femoral nerve

Root Supply: Nerve roots L2, L3, and L4, mainly L3

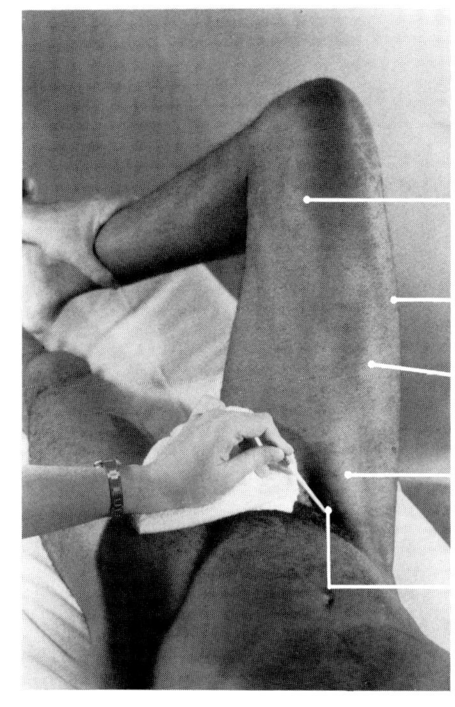

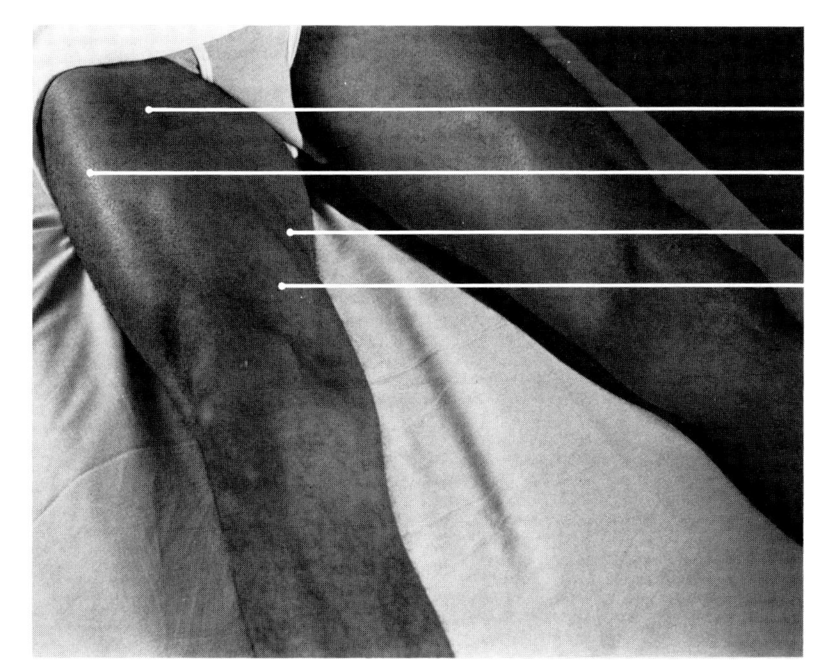

FIGURE 2-82 Rectus femoris.

Vastus Lateralis (*Fig.* 2-83; *see also Figs.* 1-45 *and* 1-46)

Action: Extension of the knee joint

Patient Position: Supine

Pin Insertion: Instruct the patient as follows: "Push your knee down into the bed and tighten your thigh" (isometric contraction of the muscle). The vastus lateralis will be seen to bulge out at the anterolateral aspect of the thigh. Insert the pin into the muscle at about the junction of the middle and lower thirds of the thigh, staying anterior to the shallow groove between this muscle and the iliotibial tract.

Relaxation: Instruct the patient as follows: "Bend your knee and relax your thigh muscles" (flexion of the knee joint). You may rotate the patient's hip into passive external rotation.

Contraction: *Minimal*: Instruct the patient as follows: "Push the back of your knee slightly into the bed and slightly tighten your thigh."

Contraction: *Maximal*: Instruct the patient as follows: "Push the back of your knee strongly into the bed and strongly tighten your thigh" (maximal isometric contraction of the muscle). You may also instruct the patient as follows: "Keep your knee straight and lift your heel off the bed" (with the knee in extension, the patient is instructed to flex the hip). Give resistance at the lower leg in the direction of knee flexion.

Peripheral Nerve Supply: Femoral nerve

Root Supply: Nerve roots L2, L3, and L4, mainly L4

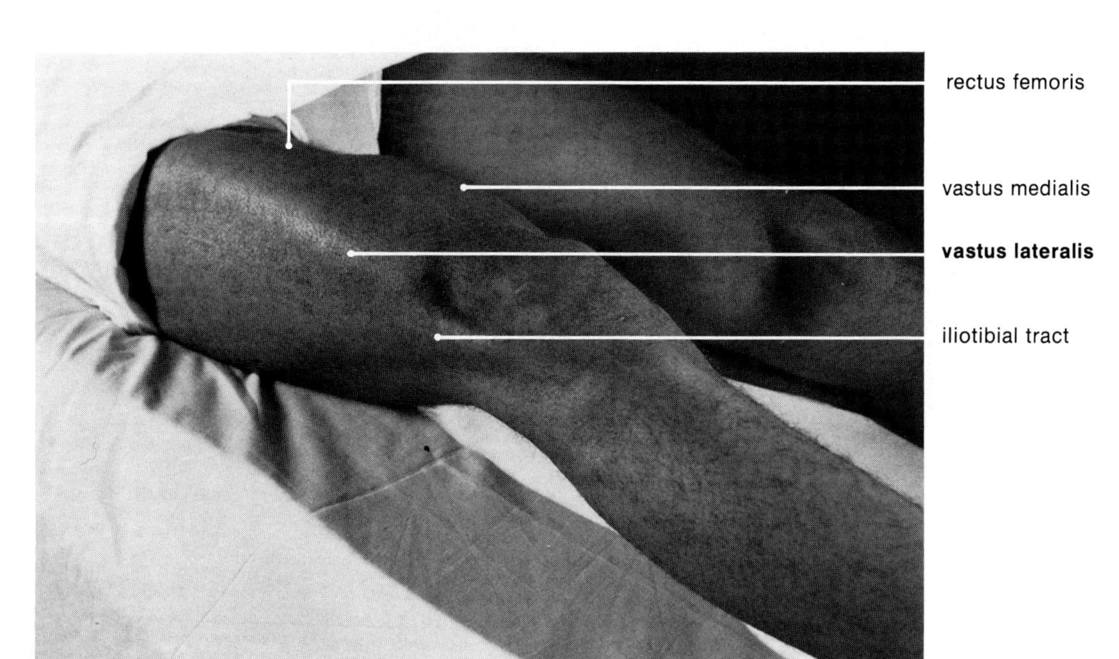

FIGURE 2-83 Vastus lateralis.

Vastus Medialis (*Fig.* 2-84; *see also Figs.* 1-45 *through* 1-47)

Action: Extension of the knee joint

Patient Position: Supine

Pin Insertion: Instruct the patient as follows: "Push your knee down into the bed and slightly tighten your thigh" (isometric contraction of the muscle). The distal portion of the vastus medialis will be seen to come into action at the medial aspect of the knee as a firm, round muscle. Insert the pin into the bulk of the muscle.

*Relaxation**

*Contraction**

*Peripheral Nerve Supply**

*Root Supply**

* See vastus lateralis.

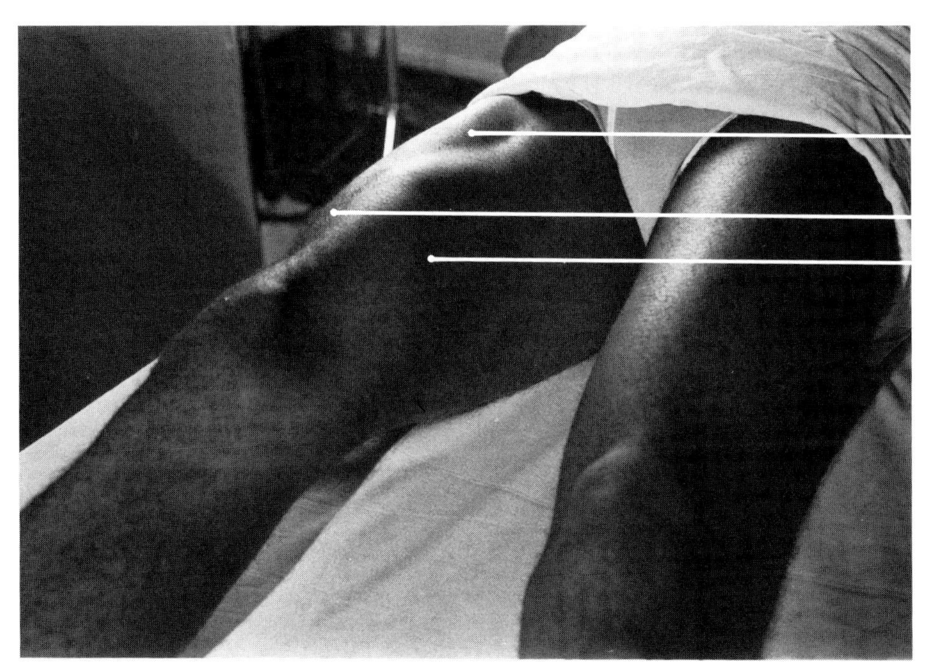

FIGURE 2-84 Vastus medialis.

Adductor Longus (*Fig. 2-85; see also Figs. 1-45 through 1-47*)

Action: Adduction and probably medial rotation of the thigh. It flexes the thigh when it is extended and extends the thigh when it is flexed. During walking, it prevents the torso from falling toward the ipsilateral side when the opposite leg is off the ground.

Patient Position: Supine

Pin Insertion: Instruct the patient as follows: "Bend your hip and knee and lift your heel off the bed." (The hip and knee are placed in flexion, and the patient is instructed to lift his heel off the bed.) A firm, long muscle stretching from the pubic crest to about the middle of the thigh will be seen and felt on the inner aspect of the thigh. This is the adductor longus. Insert the pin at about the junction of the upper and middle thirds of the thigh.

Relaxation: Instruct the patient as follows: "Put your hip and knee flat on the bed and relax" (hip and knee placed in extension). You may also place the hip into passive abduction and external rotation.

Contraction: *Minimal*: Instruct the patient as follows: "Bend your hip and knee slightly" (minimal flexion of the hip and knee joint). Also place the hip in external rotation.

Contraction: *Maximal*: Instruct the patient as follows: "Bend your hip and knee and lift your heel off the bed. Don't let me push your thigh away from your other thigh." (The hip and knee are kept in flexion, and the patient is instructed to lift his heel off the bed, a motion that will initiate strong contraction of the adductor longus muscle.) Give resistance at the lower thigh in the direction of hip abduction and extension.

Peripheral Nerve Supply: Anterior division of the obturator nerve

Root Supply: Nerve roots L2, L3, and L4, mainly L3

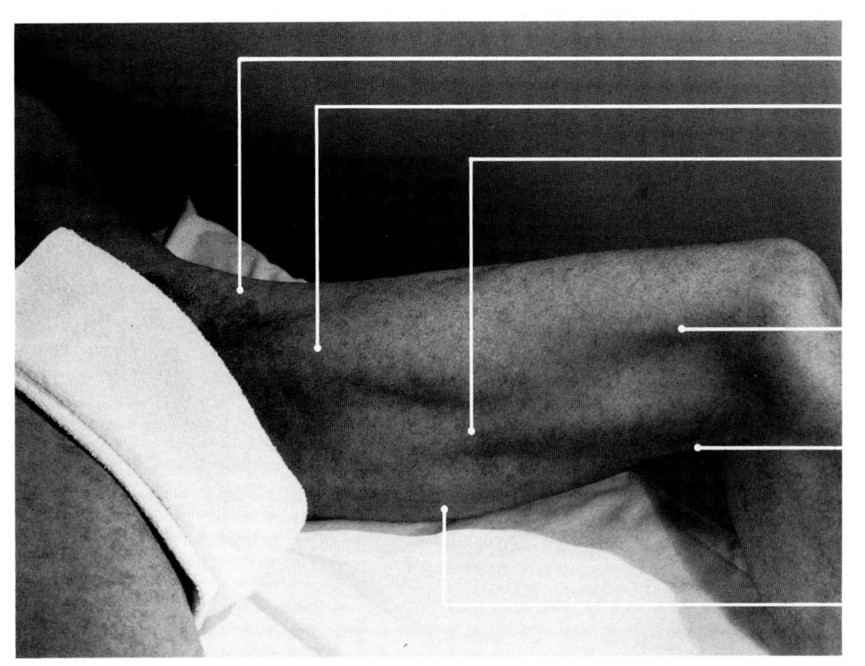

FIGURE 2-85 Adductor longus.

Gracilis (*Fig.* 2-86; *see also* Figs. 1-45 *through* 1-49)

Action: Flexion of the knee and internal rotation of the leg when the knee is flexed to 90°. It assists in adduction of the thigh. While one is standing on one leg, as in walking, it helps to tether the torso in a balanced position on the head of the femur.

Patient Position: Supine or prone

Pin Insertion: Instruct the patient as follows: "Bend your knee" (flexion of the knee joint). A strong, cordlike tendon will stand out at the most posteromedial aspect or corner of the knee joint. Follow this tendon, and this will lead to the belly of the gracilis. As you proceed to palpate the gracilis more proximally, you can trace the origin of this muscle to the ventral aspect of the body of the pubis.

Relaxation: Instruct the patient as follows: "Straighten your knee joint and spread your thigh to the outside." (The patient is instructed to extend his knee and abduct his hip joint.) You should also ensure that the hip is in external rotation.

Contraction: *Minimal*: Instruct the patient as follows: "Bend your knee slightly" (minimal flexion of the knee joint). You can also place the patient in a lateral recumbent position.

Contraction: *Maximal*: If the patient is supine, instruct him as follows: "Keep your knee bent and don't let me straighten it." If the patient is prone, instruct him as follows: "Bend your knee, turn your toes in toward the other foot, and don't let me push your knee down." (The patient is instructed to flex his knee with the leg in internal rotation.) Apply resistance to knee flexion at about the middle of the leg in the direction of knee extension.

Peripheral Nerve Supply: Anterior division of the obturator nerve

Root Supply: Nerve roots L2 and L3, mainly L2

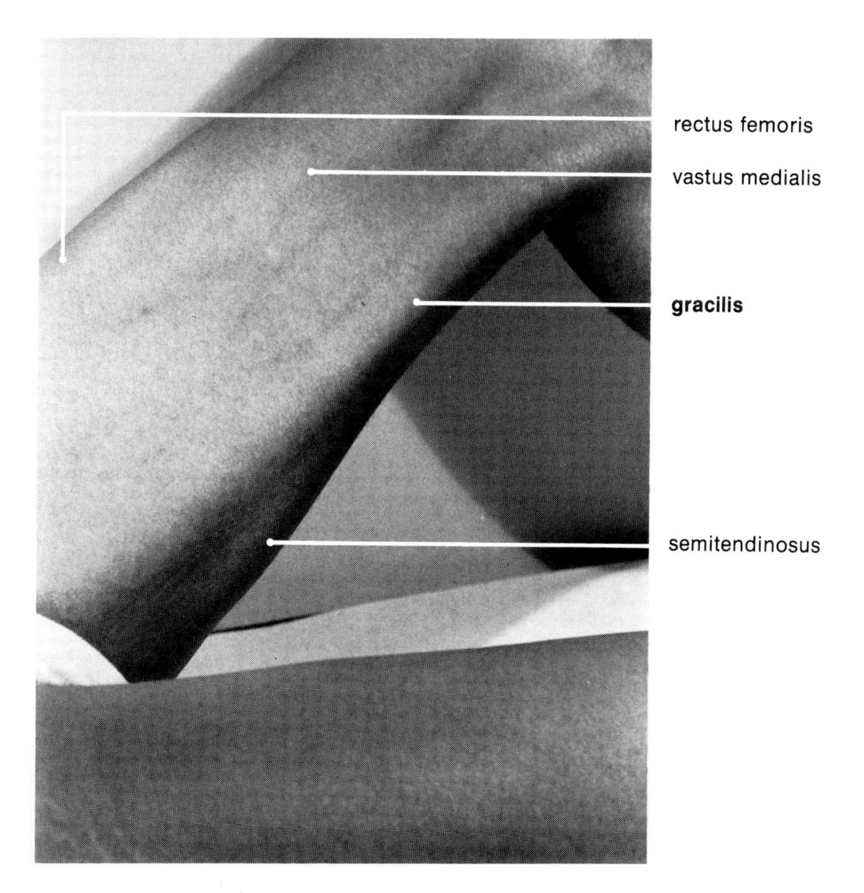

FIGURE 2-86 Gracilis.

MUSCLES OF THE POSTERIOR ASPECT OF THE THIGH

Adductor Magnus (*Fig. 2-87; see also Figs. 1-48 and 1-49*)

Action: Adduction of the thigh. Acting from the femur, it prevents excessive lateral sway of the torso by stabilizing the pelvis when one is walking. It is also active during flexion and medial rotation of the thigh.

Patient Position: Prone

Pin Insertion: Palpate for the belly of the gracilis as previously described and follow this muscle proximally. Just lateral (or posterior) to the lateral (or posterior) edge of the upper third of the gracilis is the belly of the adductor magnus. This superficial portion is primarily the ischial or ischiocondylar part of the adductor magnus, which is innervated by the sciatic nerve. The rest of the muscle, which inserts into the linea aspera, is supplied by the obturator nerve. Insert the pin into the muscle in the region of the upper third of the thigh.

Relaxation: Instruct the patient as follows: "Spread your thighs and relax" (hip abduction).

Contraction: *Minimal*: Instruct the patient as follows: "Bring your thigh in slightly" (minimal hip adduction).

Contraction: *Maximal*: Instruct the patient as follows: "Bring your thigh in strongly against my hand. Don't let me push your thigh away" (maximal hip adduction against resistance). Apply pressure at the lower third of the thigh in the direction of hip abduction.

Peripheral Nerve Supply: Posterior branch of the obturator nerve and the tibial part of the sciatic nerve

Root Supply: Nerve roots L2 through L4 via the posterior branch of the obturator nerve; L4 nerve root via the tibial part of the sciatic nerve

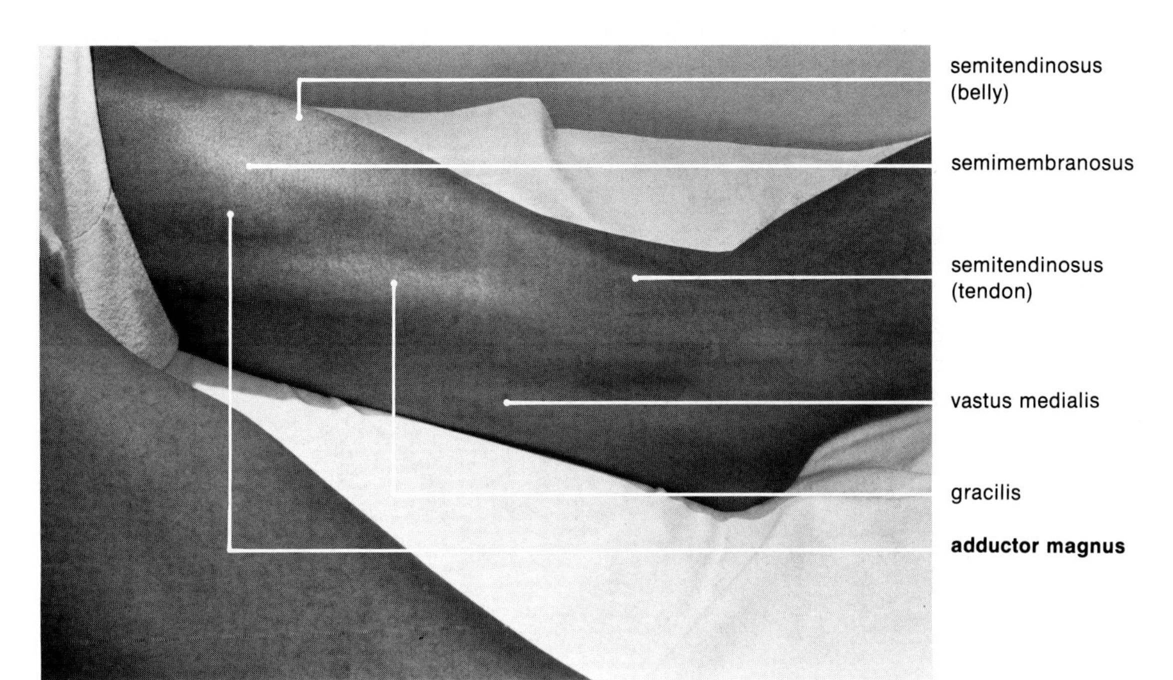

FIGURE 2-87 Adductor magnus.

Semitendinosus and Semimembranosus (*Fig.* 2-88; *see also* Figs. 1-48 *through* 1-50)

Action: Flexion of the knee joint and internal rotation of the leg when the knee is partially flexed. When acting from below on the fixed leg, the muscles are extensors of the hip joint, pulling the pelvis into an upright or extended position after bending forward.

Patient Position: Prone, ankle hanging off the edge of the bed

Pin Insertion: Instruct the patient as follows: "Bend your knee and turn your forefoot or toes in toward the other foot" (knee flexion with the leg in internal rotation). The very firm, taut tendon of the semitendinosus will be seen to stand out at the bend of the knee. Follow this tendon proximally, and it will be seen to lead to the ischial tuberosity. Insert the pin into the bulk of the muscle at about the junction of the upper and middle thirds of the thigh to examine the semitendinosus. At about the same level, define the medial edge of the semitendinosus and insert the pin medial to this edge to examine the semimembranosus.

Relaxation: Instruct the patient as follows: "Straighten your knee and relax it" (extension of the knee joint). You may position the leg in external rotation.

Contraction: *Minimal*: Instruct the patient as follows: "Bend your knee up slightly" (minimal knee flexion). The patient can also be placed in the lateral recumbent position to eliminate gravity to ensure firing of only a few MUPs.

Contraction: *Maximal*: Instruct the patient as follows: "Bend your knee, turn your forefoot or your toes in toward the other foot, and don't let me push your leg down" (flexion of the knee joint with the leg in internal rotation). The knee should be kept at about 30° to 60° of knee flexion, and resistance is given to knee flexion by applying pressure at about the junction of the middle and lower thirds of the leg.

Peripheral Nerve Supply: A branch from the tibial division of the sciatic nerve

Root Supply: Nerve roots L5, S1, and S2, mainly L5

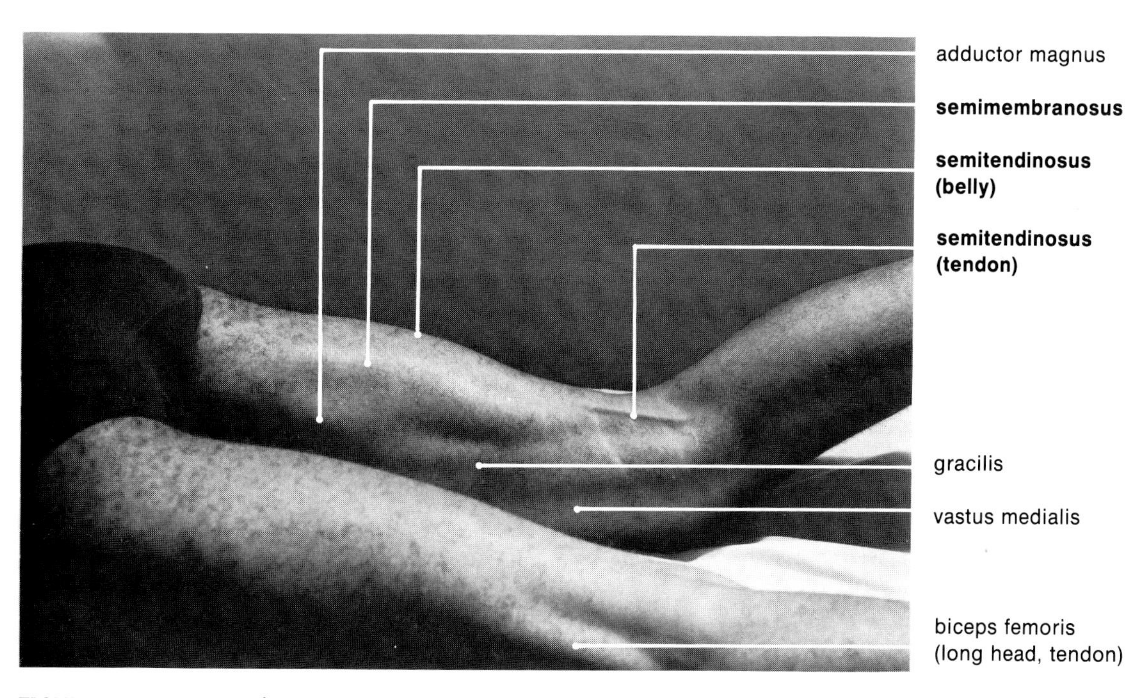

FIGURE 2-88 Semitendinosus and semimembranosus.

Biceps Femoris (Long Head) (*Fig.* 2-89; *see also* Figs. 1-48 *through* 1-51)

Action: Extends the hip joint when acting from below with the leg fixed. Flexion of the knee joint and external rotation of the leg on the thigh when the knee is partially flexed, but if the foot is fixed on the ground, the thigh and pelvis will be rotated internally when the knee is flexed and the biceps femoris (long head) contracts.

Patient Position: Prone, with the ankle hanging off the edge of the bed

Pin Insertion: Instruct the patient as follows: "Bend your knee and turn your forefoot or your toes outward, away from the other foot." The tendon of the long head of the biceps femoris will be seen at the lateral aspect of the bend of the knee, and it will be felt to lead distally toward the head of the fibula. Follow the tendon proximally toward the belly of the muscle. You may reconfirm the belly of the long head of the biceps femoris by defining the semitendinosus as previously described. Insert the pin approximately 2.5 cm lateral to the lateral edge of the semitendinosus, near the junction of the upper and middle thirds of the thigh. This point should be along a line connecting the ischial tuberosity and the tendon of the long head of the biceps femoris.

Relaxation: Instruct the patient as follows: "Straighten your knee and relax" (extension of the knee joint). Make sure that the leg is internally rotated.

Contraction: *Minimal*: Instruct the patient as follows: "Bend your knee slightly" (minimal flexion of the knee joint). The patient may be positioned in the lateral recumbent position to eliminate the effects of gravity.

Contraction: *Maximal*: Instruct the patient as follows: "Bend your knee, turn your forefoot or your toes outward away from the other foot, and don't let me straighten your knee" (knee flexion with the leg in external rotation). Flex the knee to about 30° to 60° and give resistance to knee flexion at about the junction of the middle and lower thirds of the leg.

Peripheral Nerve Supply: A branch from the tibial division of the sciatic nerve

Root Supply: Nerve roots L5, S1, and S2, especially S1

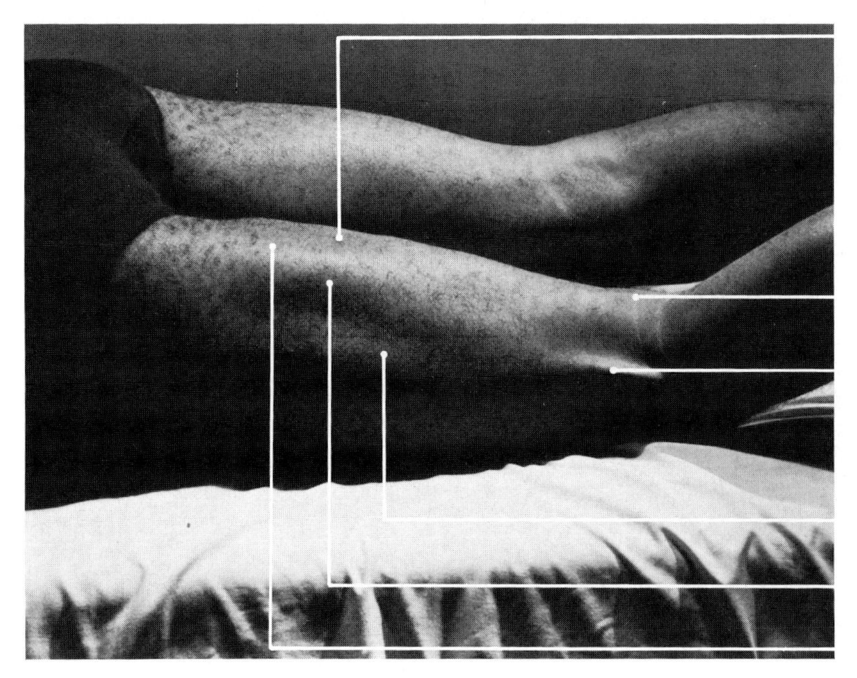

FIGURE 2-89 Biceps femoris (long head).

Biceps Femoris (Short Head) (*Fig. 2-90; see also Figs. 1-50 and 1-51*)

Action: Flexion of the knee joint and external rotation of the leg with the knee partially flexed

Patient Position: Prone, ankle hanging off the edge of the bed

Pin Insertion: Feel for the tendon of the long head of the biceps femoris as previously described. Insert the pin just medial or lateral to this tendon approximately 5 cm above the bend of the knee.

Relaxation: Instruct the patient as follows: "Straighten your knee and relax" (extension of the knee joint).

Contraction: *Minimal*: Instruct the patient as follows: "Bend your knee slightly" (minimal flexion of the knee joint).

Contraction: *Maximal*: Instruct the patient as follows: "Bend your knee, turn your forefoot or your toes away from the other foot, and don't let me push your knee down" (knee flexion with the leg in external rotation). Keep the knee at about 30° to 60° of flexion and give resistance to knee flexion by applying pressure at about the junction of the middle and lower thirds of the leg in the direction of knee extension.

Peripheral Nerve Supply: A branch from the common peroneal division of the sciatic nerve

Root Supply: Nerve roots L5, S1, and S2, mainly L5

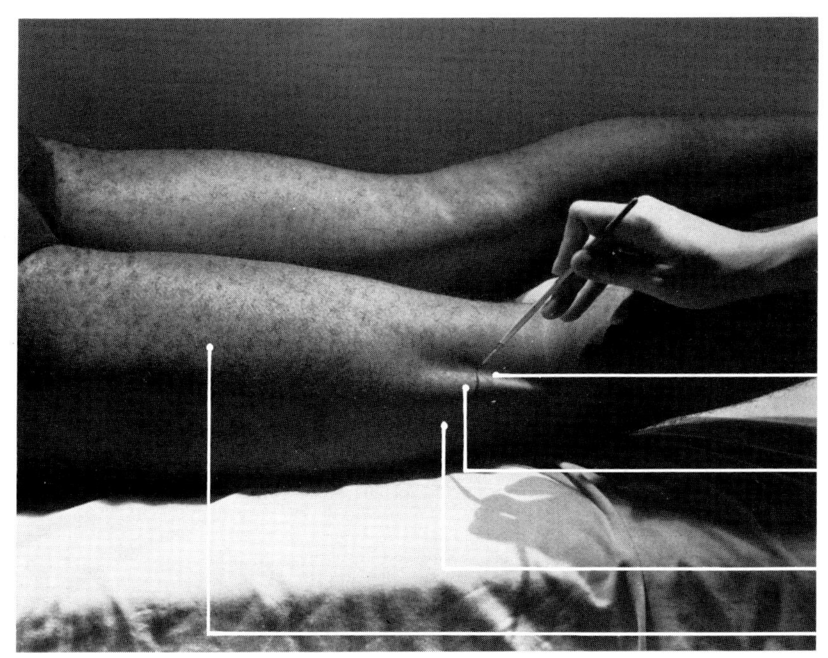

FIGURE 2-90 Biceps femoris (short head).

MUSCLES OF THE ANTERIOR AND LATERAL ASPECTS OF THE LEG

Tibialis Anterior (*Fig. 2-91; see also Figs. 1-54 through 1-57*)

Action: Dorsiflexion and inversion of the foot

Patient Position: Supine, foot resting on the bed

Pin Insertion: Instruct the patient as follows: "Bend your hip and knee and pull your forefoot upward toward your head. Now, turn the sole inward, toward the other foot." (The patient is instructed to flex his hip and knee and dorsiflex his ankle, with the foot in inversion.) The prominent tendon of the tibialis anterior will be seen to stand out, and if the tendon is followed proximally, the muscle belly of the tibialis anterior can be felt. It is the first muscle lateral to the anterior border of the tibia. Insert the pin approximately 1 cm to 2 cm lateral to this border, at about the junction of the upper and middle thirds of the leg.

Relaxation: Instruct the patient as follows: "Put your hip and knee down and relax your ankle (hip and knee in extension and ankle in passive plantar flexion). You may also passively place the patient's foot into eversion to stretch the muscle further.

Contraction: *Minimal*: Instruct the patient as follows: "Pull your forefoot up slightly" (minimal dorsiflexion of the ankle). The hip and knee are best kept in extension.

Contraction: *Maximal*: Instruct the patient as follows: "Bend your hip and knee and pull your forefoot up toward you. Now, turn the sole of your foot in toward the other foot. Don't let me push your foot down." (The patient is instructed to flex the hip and knee with the ankle in dorsiflexion and the foot in inversion.) Give resistance to full dorsiflexion by applying pressure on the dorsomedial aspect of the foot in the direction of plantar flexion.

Peripheral Nerve Supply: Deep peroneal nerve

Root Supply: Nerve roots L4 and L5, mainly L5, but L4 may dominate

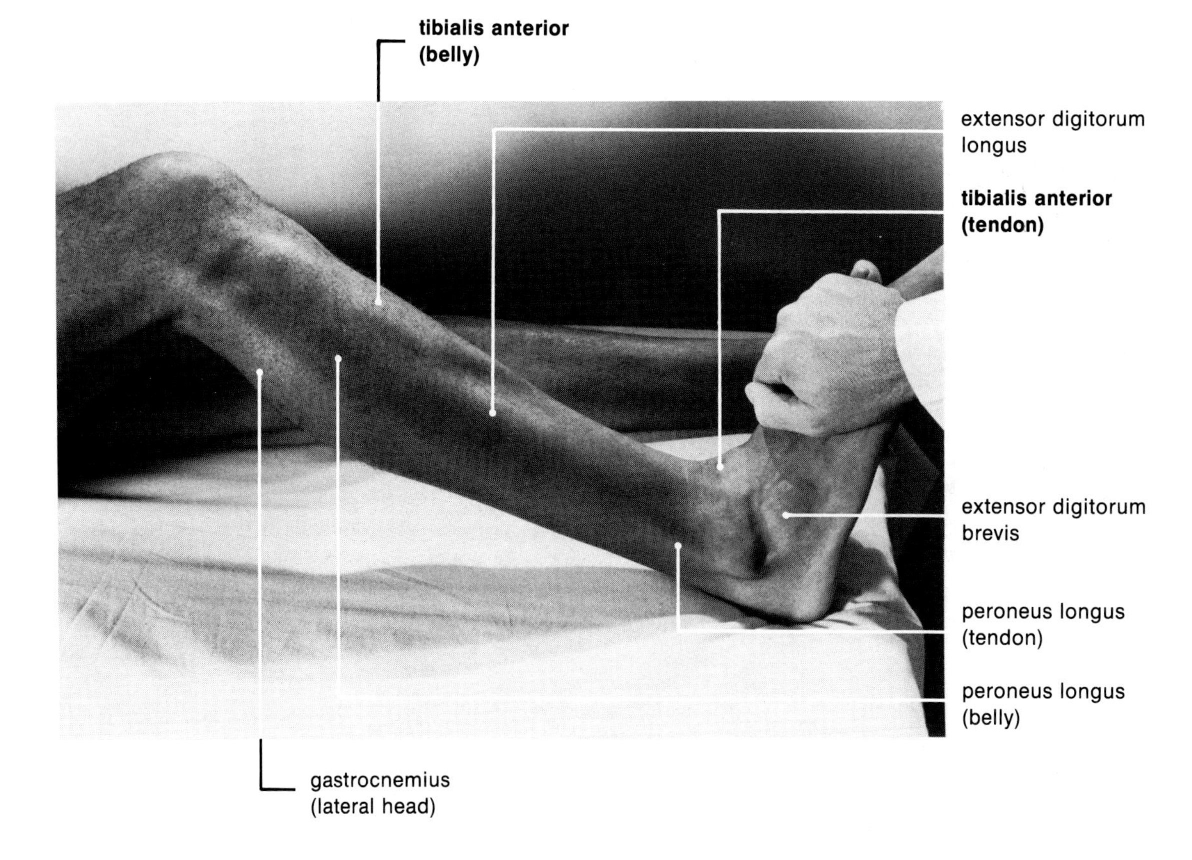

FIGURE 2-91 Tibialis anterior.

Extensor Digitorum Longus (*Fig.* 2-92; *see also* Figs. 1-54 *through* 1-57)

Action: Extension of the metatarsophalangeal joints. Assists in extension of the interphalangeal joints of the lateral four toes and in dorsiflexion of the ankle.

Patient Position: Supine, heel resting on the bed

Pin Insertion: Instruct the patient as follows: "Bend your hip and knee and pull your forefoot and toes upward toward your head" (flexion of the hip and knee joint with the ankle in full dorsiflexion). The flat, long belly of the extensor digitorum longus will be seen to stand out prominently in the lower third of the leg, lateral to the tendon of the tibialis anterior. It is not covered by any muscle at this level. Insert the pin into the muscle at about the junction of the middle and lower thirds of the leg or at approximately 15 cm (6 in) from the lower border of the malleoli.

Relaxation: Instruct the patient as follows: "Put your thigh and leg down and relax your leg and toes" (hip and knee in extension and ankle and toes in passive plantar flexion).

Contraction: *Minimal*: Instruct the patient as follows: "Lift your toes up slightly" (minimal extension of the toes at the metatarsophalangeal joints). The hip and knee are best kept in extension.

Contraction: *Maximal*: Instruct the patient as follows: "Bend your hip and knee and lift your toes strongly up toward you" (flexion of the hip and knee joints with full dorsiflexion of the toes and ankle). Give resistance to full dorsiflexion of the ankle by applying pressure on the dorsum of the foot and toes in the direction of plantar flexion.

Peripheral Nerve Supply: Deep peroneal nerve

Root Supply: Nerve roots L5 and S1, mainly L5

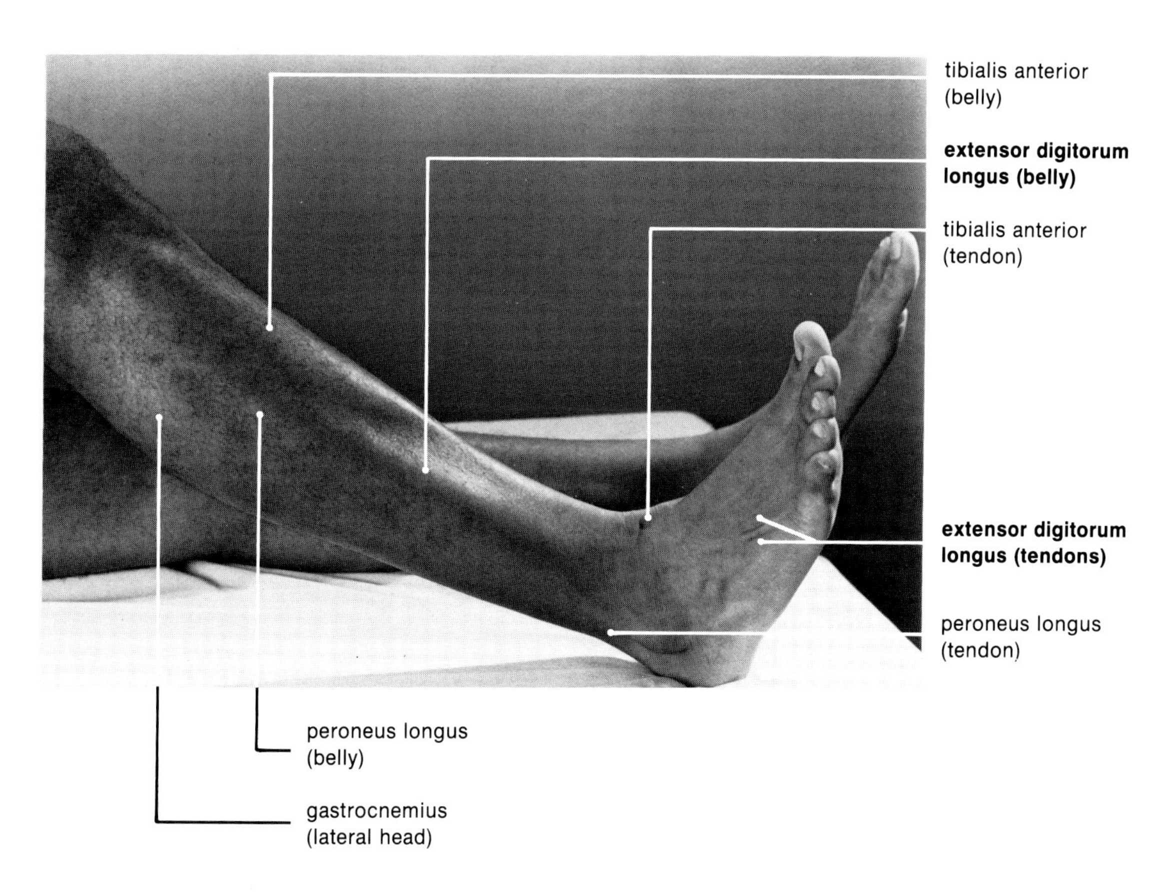

FIGURE 2-92 Extensor digitorum longus.

Extensor Hallucis Longus (*Fig.* 2-93; *see also Figs.* 1-54, 1-55, *and* 1-57)

Action: Extension of the distal and proximal phalanges of the great toe

Patient Position: Supine, foot resting on the bed

Pin Insertion: Feel for a point on the tendon of the tibialis anterior approximately 15 cm (6 in) from the lower border of the malleoli. At the lateral edge of this tendon is the groove that separates it from the belly of the extensor digitorum longus. Insert the pin into this groove to reach the extensor hallucis longus. Insert the pin approximately three quarters of its 37-mm length. Instruct the patient as follows: "Let me know if there is too much discomfort. Don't jerk your foot, because that will make the examination more uncomfortable."

Relaxation: Instruct the patient as follows: "Relax your big toe." (The great toe is kept in neutral position or in passive plantar flexion.)

Contraction: *Minimal*: Instruct the patient as follows: "Pull your big toe up slightly" (minimal extension of the great toe). Support the metatarsophalangeal joint of the great toe from the plantar aspect to avoid inadvertent relaxation or jerky contractions, especially in the direction of plantar flexion. Examination of this muscle is quite painful, since the pin must be inserted deeply.

Contraction: *Maximal*: Instruct the patient as follows: "Lift your big toe up strongly" (maximal extension of the big toe). Continue to support the metatarsophalangeal joint of the big toe. You may give resistance on the dorsum of the distal phalanx of the big toe.

Peripheral Nerve Supply: Deep peroneal nerve

Root Supply: Nerve roots L5 and S1, mainly L5

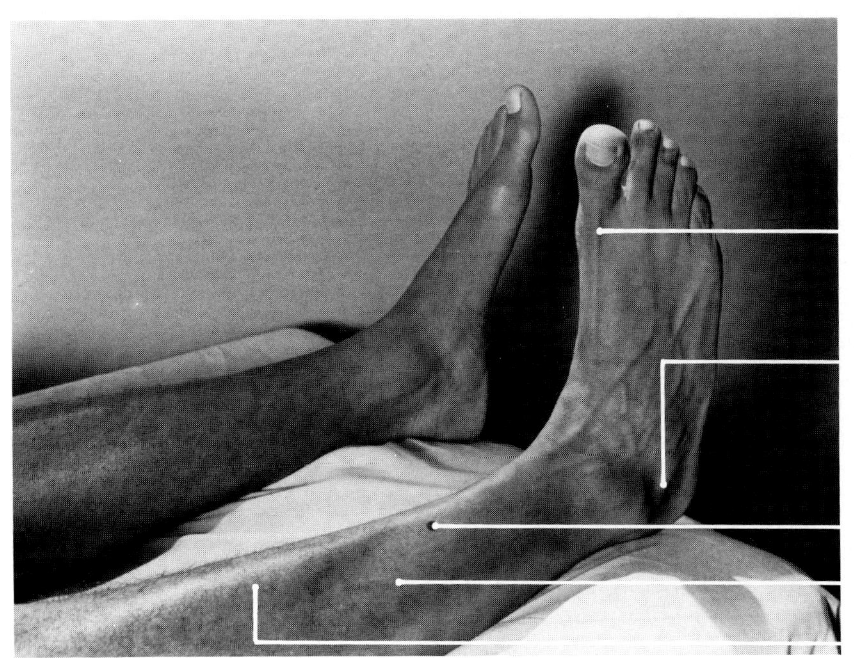

FIGURE 2-93 Extensor hallucis longus.

Peroneus Tertius (*Fig. 2-94; see also Fig. 1-54*)

Action: Dorsiflexion and eversion of the foot. This muscle is a part of the extensor digitorum longus but may be somewhat separated from the latter. It is inserted into the base of the fifth metatarsal rather than into the phalanges of the toes.

Patient Position: Supine

Pin Insertion: At the junction of the proximal three fourths and the distal fourth of the leg approximately 1.5 cm lateral to the tendon of the extensor digitorum longus and anterior to the palpable surface of the fibula. It may be reached even more distally between the superior and inferior extensor retinacula, where its belly may be palpable as the first muscle mass anterior to the lateral malleolus. Forceful eversion of the foot may help to make it more palpable at this site. This is a useful muscle to test when there is a need to examine muscles supplied by the deep peroneal nerve in the distal fourth of the leg, as in fractures in this region.

Relaxation: Instruct the patient as follows: "Relax your ankle." The foot may be placed in plantar flexion and inversion.

Contraction: *Minimal*: Instruct the patient as follows: "Lift your foot up slightly" (minimal dorsiflexion of the ankle).

Contraction: *Maximal*: Position the foot in dorsiflexion and instruct the patient as follows: "Keep your ankle in this position and don't let me push it down." Apply pressure on the dorsum of the foot in the direction of plantar flexion and inversion.

Peripheral Nerve Supply: Deep peroneal nerve

Root Supply: Nerve roots L5 and S1, mainly L5

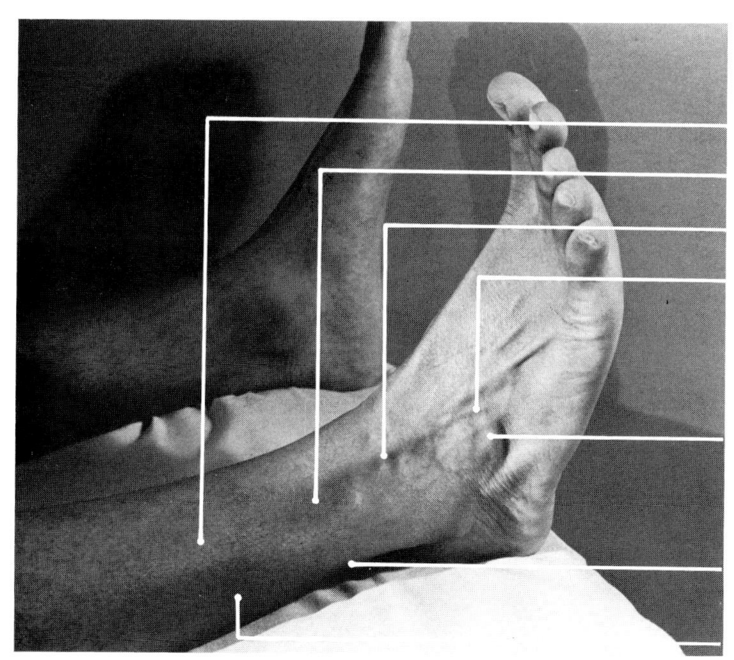

FIGURE 2-94 Peroneus tertius.

Peroneus Longus (*Fig. 2-95; see also Figs. 1-52 through 1-54, 1-56, and 1-57*)

Action: Eversion of the foot and depression of the first metatarsal bone. It also aids in plantar flexion of the foot.

Patient Position: Supine, heel resting on the bed

Pin Insertion: Instruct the patient as follows: "Push your forefoot downward and turn the sole of your foot outward. Press the big toe down especially" (plantar flexion of the foot and eversion and depression of the first metatarsal). The tendon of the peroneus longus will be seen to stand out at the lateral aspect of the ankle. Follow the tendon proximally toward the belly of the muscle. Insert the pin at about the junction of the upper and middle thirds of the leg. Stay anterior to the groove that separates the peroneus longus from the soleus.

Relaxation: Instruct the patient as follows: "Relax your ankle" (ankle is kept in the neutral position). You may position the foot passively into inversion.

Contraction: *Minimal*: Instruct the patient as follows: "Push your forefoot down slightly" (minimal plantar flexion of the foot).

Contraction: *Maximal*: Instruct the patient as follows: "Push your forefoot down strongly and turn the sole of your foot outward, away from the other foot. Push your big toe down especially" (maximal plantar flexion of the foot with eversion and depression or strong plantar flexion of the first metatarsal). Give resistance to full eversion by applying pressure at the lateral border of the forefoot in the direction of inversion.

Peripheral Nerve Supply: Superficial peroneal nerve

Root Supply: Nerve roots L5 and S1, mainly S1

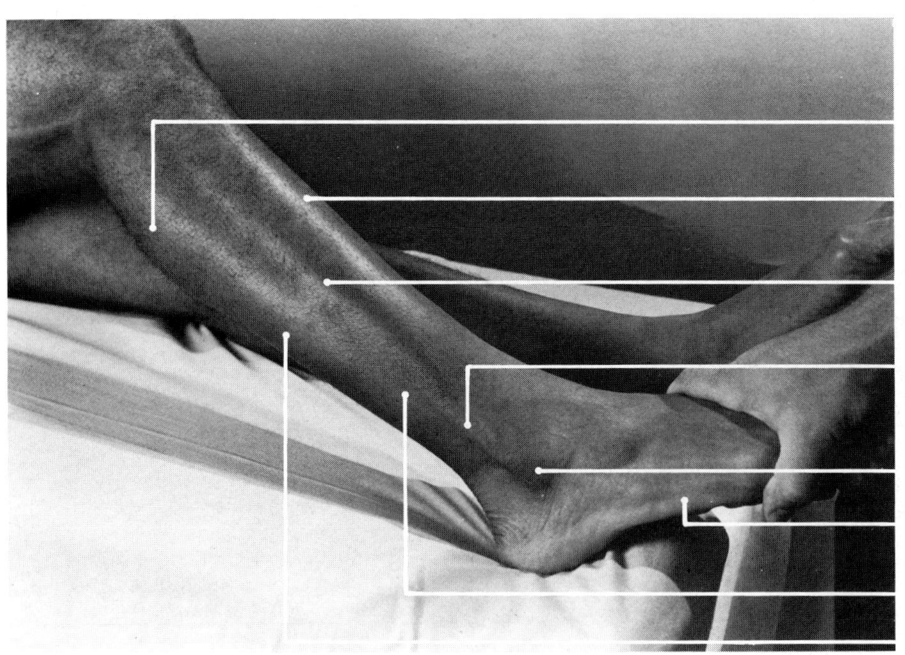

FIGURE 2-95 Peroneus longus.

Peroneus Brevis (*Fig.* 2-96; *see also Figs.* 1-52, 1-53, 1-56, *and* 1-61)

Action: Plantar flexion and eversion of the foot
Patient Position: Supine, heel resting on the bed
Pin Insertion: Elicit the action of the peroneus longus as previously described. Insert the pin just anterior or posterior to the tendon of the peroneus longus at the junction of the lower and middle thirds of the leg.
Relaxation: Instruct the patient as follows: "Relax your ankle" (ankle is kept in neutral position). You may push the patient's foot into passive dorsiflexion.
Contraction: *Minimal*: Instruct the patient as follows: "Push your foot down slightly" (minimal plantar flexion of the foot).
Contraction: *Maximal*: Instruct the patient as follows: "Push your foot down strongly and turn the sole of your foot outward" (plantar flexion of the foot with eversion).
Peripheral Nerve Supply: Superficial peroneal nerve
Root Supply: Nerve roots L5 and S1, mainly S1

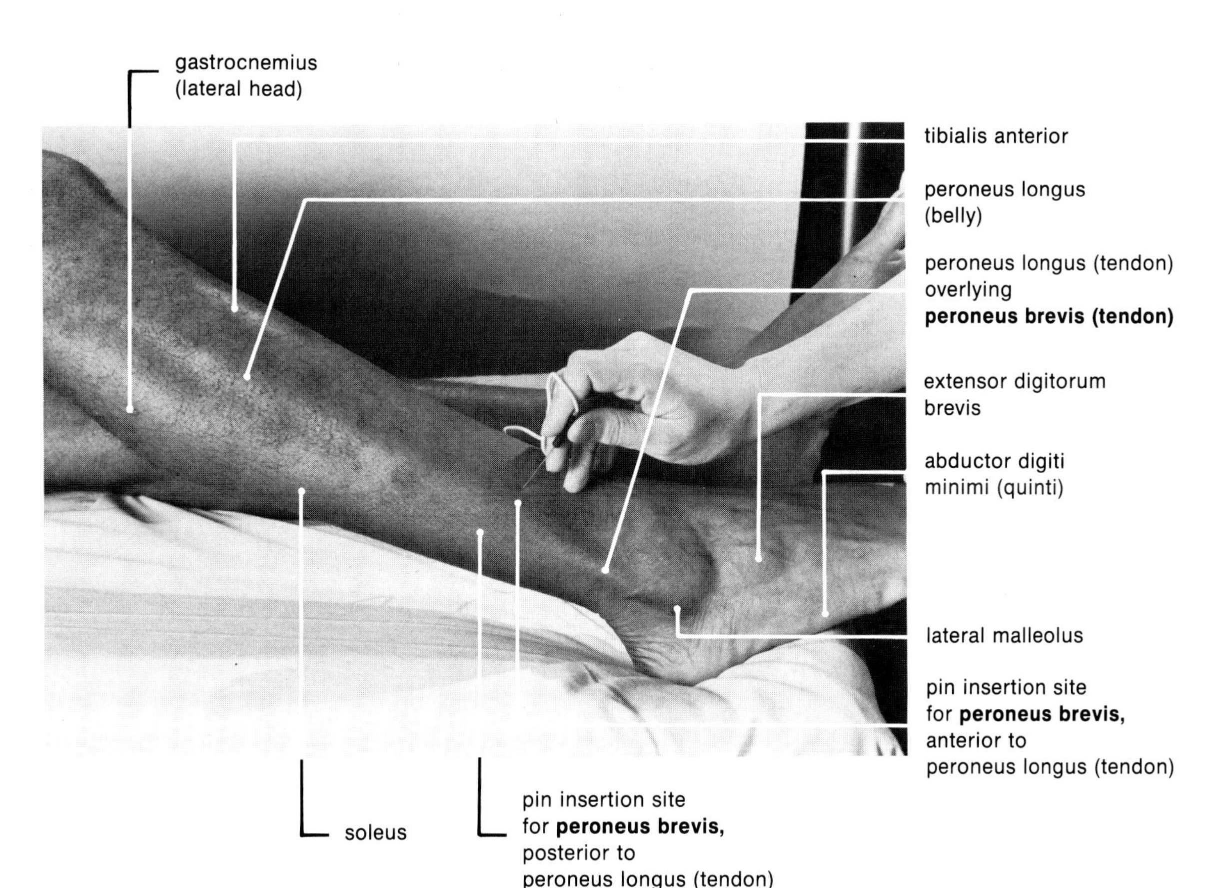

FIGURE 2-96 Peroneus brevis.

MUSCLES OF THE POSTERIOR AND MEDIAL ASPECTS OF THE LEG

Gastrocnemius (Medial Head) (*Fig.* 2-97; *see also* Figs. 1-48, 1-49, 1-52, *and* 1-60)

Action: Plantar flexion of the foot and assistance in flexion of the knee

Patient Position: Prone, ankle off the edge of the bed

Pin Insertion: Instruct the patient as follows: "Push your foot down against my hand and point your toes as if you would like to stand on the tips of your toes" (plantar flexion of the foot, the examiner stands at the foot of the bed to apply resistance to plantar flexion). The belly of the medial gastrocnemius will be seen to come into contraction on the medial aspect of the leg. Insert the pin into the muscle at about the upper third of the bulging belly of the muscle.

Relaxation: Instruct the patient as follows: "Relax your ankle" (ankle is placed in neutral position). You may position the patient's leg so that it lies on its lateral aspect.

Contraction: *Minimal*: Instruct the patient as follows: "Point your toes gently as if you would like to stand on the tips of your toes" (minimal plantar flexion of the foot). You may stand at the foot of the bed and give slight resistance to plantar flexion by applying pressure at the ball of the foot. This is occasionally needed to initiate or maintain minimal contraction.

Contraction: *Maximal*: Instruct the patient as follows: "Push your foot strongly against my hand, and point your toes as hard as you can against my hand. Act as if you want to stand on the tips of your toes" (maximal plantar flexion of the foot against resistance). Stand at the foot of the bed and apply pressure with both hands against the ball of the foot in the direction of dorsiflexion. Pressure exerted with two hands is needed, since this is a very strong muscle.

Peripheral Nerve Supply: Tibial nerve

Root Supply: Nerve roots S1 and S2, mainly S1

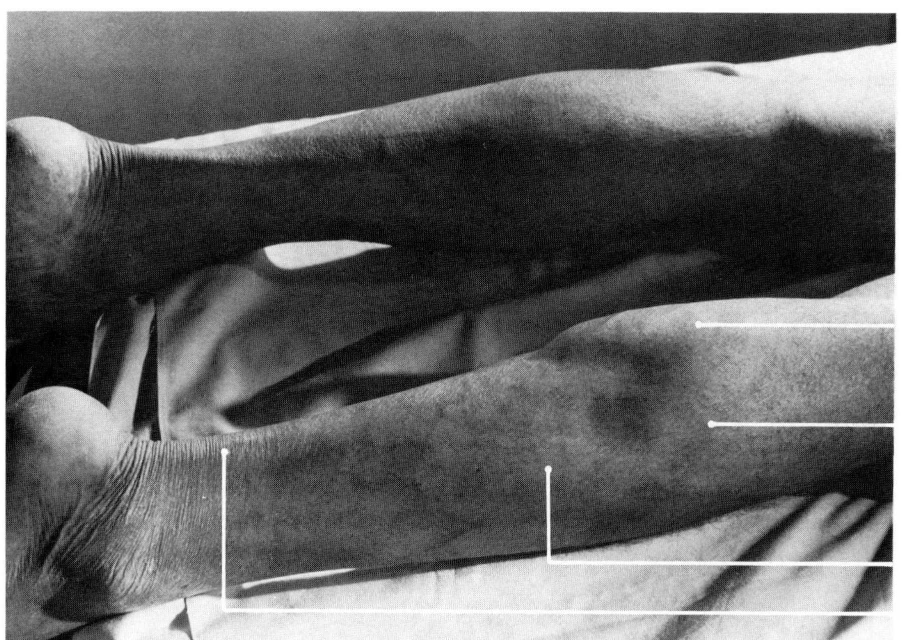

FIGURE 2-97 Gastrocnemius (medial head).

Gastrocnemius (Lateral Head) (*Fig.* 2-98; *see also* Figs. 1-48, 1-49, 1-52, 1-53, *and* 1-60)

Action: Plantar flexion of the foot

Patient Position: Prone, ankle off the edge of the bed

Pin Insertion: Instruct the patient as follows: "Push your foot against my hand and point your toes as if you would like to stand on the tips of your toes" (plantar flexion of the foot, the examiner stands at the foot of the bed to apply resistance to plantar flexion). The belly of the lateral gastrocnemius will be seen to contract at the lateral aspect of the leg. Insert the pin into the muscle at about the upper third of the bulging muscle belly.

Relaxation: Instruct the patient as follows: "Relax your ankle" (ankle is placed in neutral position). You may also rotate the leg so that it lies on its medial aspect.

Contraction: *Minimal*: Instruct the patient as follows: "Point your toes very gently as if you would like to stand on the tips of your toes" (minimal plantar flexion of the foot). You may give slight resistance to plantar flexion by applying pressure at the ball of the foot. This is occasionally needed to initiate or maintain minimal contraction.

Contraction: *Maximal*: Instruct the patient as follows: "Push your foot out strongly against my hand and point your toes hard as if you would like to stand on the tips of your toes" (maximal plantar flexion of the foot against resistance). Stand at the foot of the bed and apply pressure with both hands at the ball of the foot in the direction of dorsiflexion. Pressure exerted by two hands is needed, since this is a very strong muscle.

Peripheral Nerve Supply: Tibial nerve

Root Supply: Nerve roots S1 and S2, mainly S1

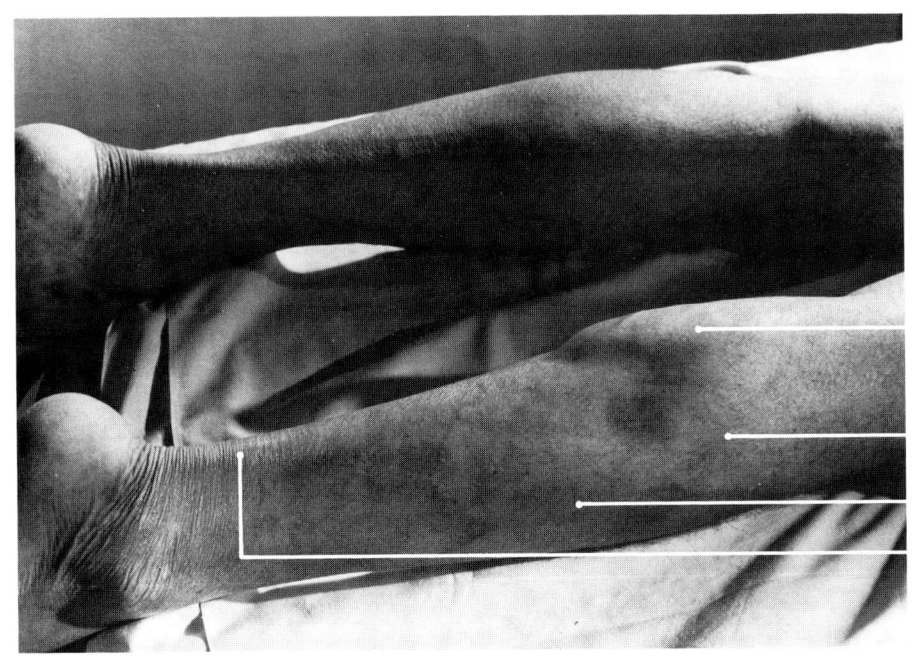

FIGURE 2-98 Gastrocnemius (lateral head).

Soleus (*Fig.* 2-99; *see also* Figs. 1-52, 1-53, 1-58, *and* 1-59)

Action: Plantar flexion of the foot

Patient Position: Prone, ankle off the edge of the bed

Pin Insertion: Instruct the patient as follows: "Push your foot out against my hand and point your toes as if you would like to stand on the tips of your toes" (plantar flexion of the foot; the examiner stands at the foot of the bed to apply reistance to plantar flexion). The belly of the soleus can be seen on either side of the Achilles tendon. The muscle can be examined medial or lateral to this tendon, but the examination is easier if done lateral to the tendon. Insert the pin into the muscle just posterior to the groove that separates it from the peroneus longus and brevis, at a level slightly below the lower margin of the lateral head of the gastrocnemius.

Relaxation: Instruct the patient as follows: "Relax your ankle" (ankle is placed passively into neutral position).

Contraction: *Minimal*: Instruct the patient as follows: "Point your toes out gently as if you would like to stand on the tips of your toes" (minimal plantar flexion of the foot). You may give slight resistance to plantar flexion by applying pressure against the ball of the foot. This is occasionally needed to initiate or maintain minimal contraction.

Contraction: *Maximal*: Instruct the patient as follows: "Push your foot strongly against my hand and point your toes as if you would like to stand on the tips of your toes" (maximal plantar flexion of the foot). The knee also may be kept in slight flexion. Stand at the foot of the bed and apply pressure with both hands at the ball of the foot in the direction of dorsiflexion. Pressure exerted with both hands is needed, since this is a very strong muscle.

Peripheral Nerve Supply: Tibial nerve

Root Supply: Nerve roots S1 and S2, mainly S1

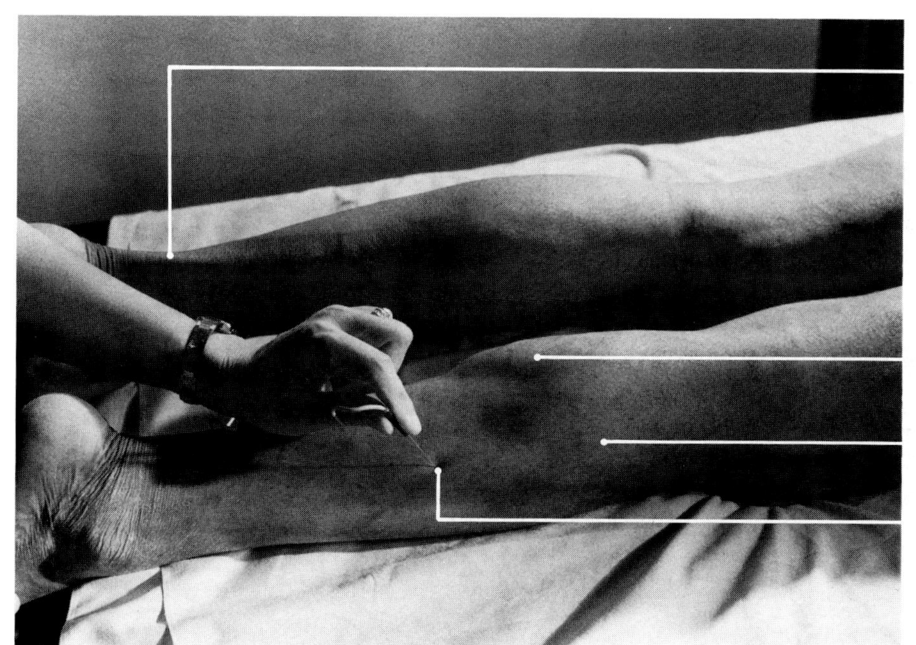

FIGURE 2-99 Soleus.

Tibialis Posterior (*Fig. 2-100; see also Figs. 1-64 and 1-65*)

Action: Inversion and plantar flexion of the foot

Patient Position: Prone, ankle hanging off the edge of the bed

Pin Insertion: Same for the flexor digitorum longus. This is at the level of the middle and lower thirds of the leg and within 1 cm medial to the medial border of the tibia. The pin should pass tangential to the posterior surface of the tibia in the coronal plane. The flexor digitorum longus must be pierced; however, at this level the muscle is very narrow along its origin from the tibia, and the tibialis posterior has moved more medially. The pin should be kept tangential to the posterior surface of the tibia in the coronal plane. It must be inserted approximately 3 cm to reach the tibialis posterior. In most legs the soleus will be missed if the needle stays close to the posterior surface of the tibia and passes laterally.

Relaxation: Instruct the patient as follows: "Relax your foot and ankle." The patient's leg may be placed on its lateral border.

Contraction: *Minimal*: Instruct the patient as follows: "Turn your foot inward slightly toward the other foot."

Contraction: *Maximal*: Instruct the patient as follows: "Turn your foot inward strongly toward the other foot. Don't let me turn it outward." Apply resistance at midfoot in the direction of eversion.

Peripheral Nerve Supply: Posterior tibial nerve

Root Supply: Nerve roots L5 and S1, mainly L5

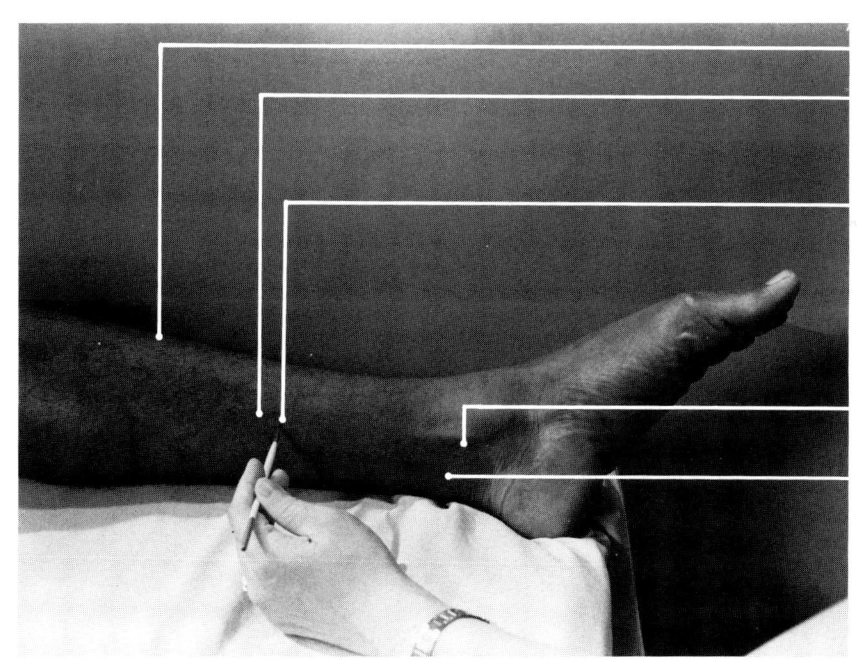

FIGURE 2-100 Tibialis posterior.

Flexor Digitorum Longus (*Fig.* 2-101; *see also Figs.* 1-58, 1-62, *and* 1-63)

Action: Flexion of the interphalangeal and metatarsophalangeal joints of the lateral four toes. It also assists in plantar flexion of the foot.

Patient Position: Supine, ankle resting on the bed

Pin Insertion: Instruct the patient as follows: "Bend your toes down as if you wanted to pick up very small marbles with them" (flexion of the interphalangeal and metatarsophalangeal joints of the lateral four toes). Palpate the medial border of the tibia and insert the pin within 1 cm of this border at about the junction of the middle and lower thirds of the leg or approximately 15 cm (6 in) above the lower border of the malleoli. In most legs these two methods of locating the vertical level of penetration yield about the same position.

Relaxation: Instruct the patient as follows: "Relax your toes" (toes are kept in neutral position).

Contraction: *Minimal*: Instruct the patient as follows: "Curl your toes slightly" (minimal flexion of the interphalangeal and metatarsophalangeal joints of the toes).

Contraction: *Maximal*: Instruct the patient as follows: "Curl your toes strongly as if you wanted to grip very small marbles" (maximal flexion of the interphalangeal and metatarsophalangeal joints of the toes). In addition, you may instruct the patient as follows: "Turn the sole of your foot in toward the other foot" (inversion of the foot).

Peripheral Nerve Supply: Posterior tibial nerve

Root Supply: Nerve roots L5, S1, and S2, mainly L5, but S1 may dominate.

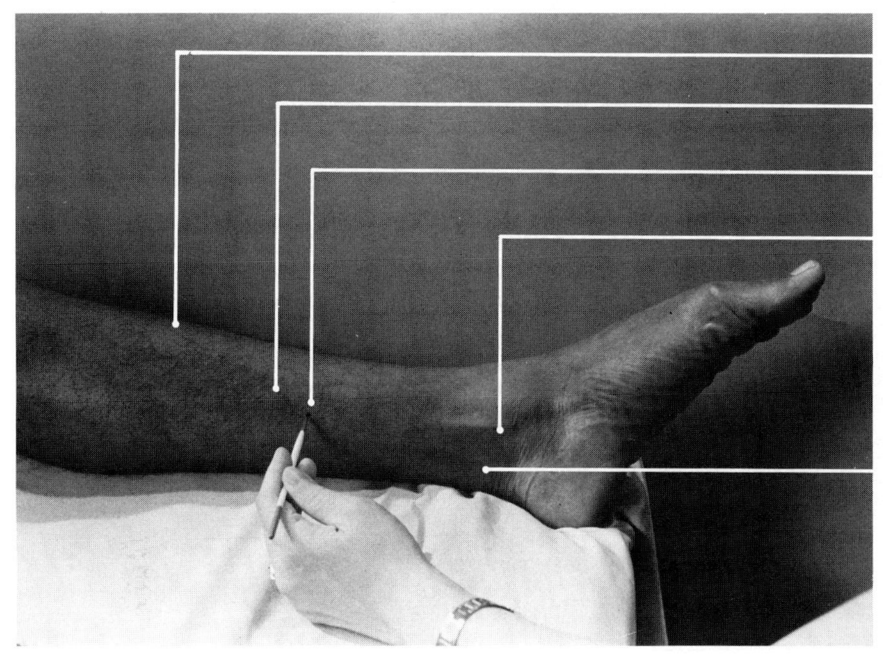

FIGURE 2-101 Flexor digitorum longus.

Popliteus (*Fig.* 2-102; *see also* Figs. 1-62 *through* 1-65)

Action: Rotates the tibia medially on the femur or the femur laterally on the tibia, depending on which is fixed. Assists in flexion of the knee, particularly at the "unlocking" of full extension. Also resists forward slippage of the femoral condyles on the tilted tibial condyles when one is crouched.

Patient Position: Supine

Pin Insertion: Locate the level of pin insertion by feeling for the posterior border of the medial tibial condyle. Insert the pin where the posterior border of the tibial condyle narrows to its junction with the shaft. Keep the pin in the coronal plane across the posterior surface of the tibia and fibula. As the needle passes laterally parallel to that plane, change its direction to a more anterior approach to enter the popliteus. The popliteus is usually entered after a depth of 1.5 cm beyond the medial border of the tibia has been reached.

Relaxation: Instruct the patient as follows: "Keep your knee straight and flat against the bed. Try to relax it."

Contraction: *Minimal*: Instruct the patient as follows: "Straighten your knee fully; now bend it slightly."

Contraction: *Maximal*: Instruct the patient as follows: "Bend your leg at the hip and knee. Now put your heel on the bed and pull the heel toward you." Resist knee flexion by giving resistance against the heel.

Peripheral Nerve Supply: Tibial nerve

Root Supply: Nerve roots L4, L5, and S1, mainly L5

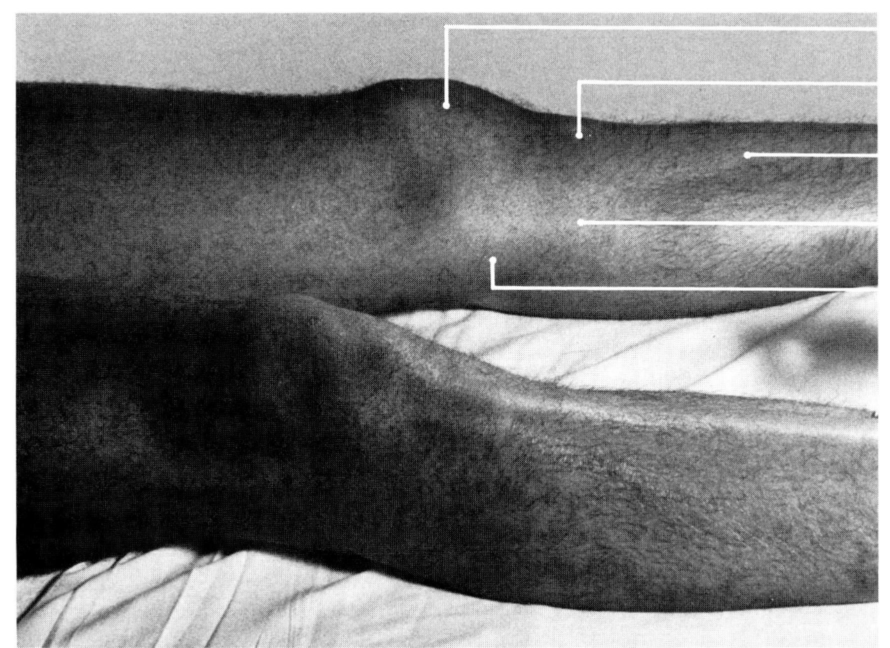

FIGURE 2-102 Popliteus.

MUSCLES OF THE FOOT

Abductor Hallucis (*Fig.* 2-103; *see also Fig.* 1-67)

Action: Abduction of the great toe at the metatarsophalangeal joint and aiding flexion at this joint

Patient Position: Supine, ankle and heel resting on the bed

Pin Insertion: Feel for the tuberosity of the navicular and insert the pin approximately 1 cm inferior and 1 cm to 2 cm posterior to this point. This will be just anterior to an imaginary line drawn through the anterior margin of the medial malleolus.

Relaxation: Instruct the patient as follows: "Relax your big toe."

Contraction: *Minimal*: Instruct the patient as follows: "Move your big toe outward slightly away from the others" (minimal abduction of the great toe).

Contraction: *Maximal*: Instruct the patient as follows: "Move your big toe out and away from the other toes. Don't let me push it back toward them" (maximal abduction of the great toe). Most patients are unable to isolate the action of the abductor hallucis, and the following instruction may be given: "Bring your forefoot in toward my hand" (adduction of the forefoot against resistance in the direction of abduction).

Peripheral Nerve Supply: Medial plantar nerve from the tibial nerve

Root Supply: Nerve roots S1 and S2, mainly S2

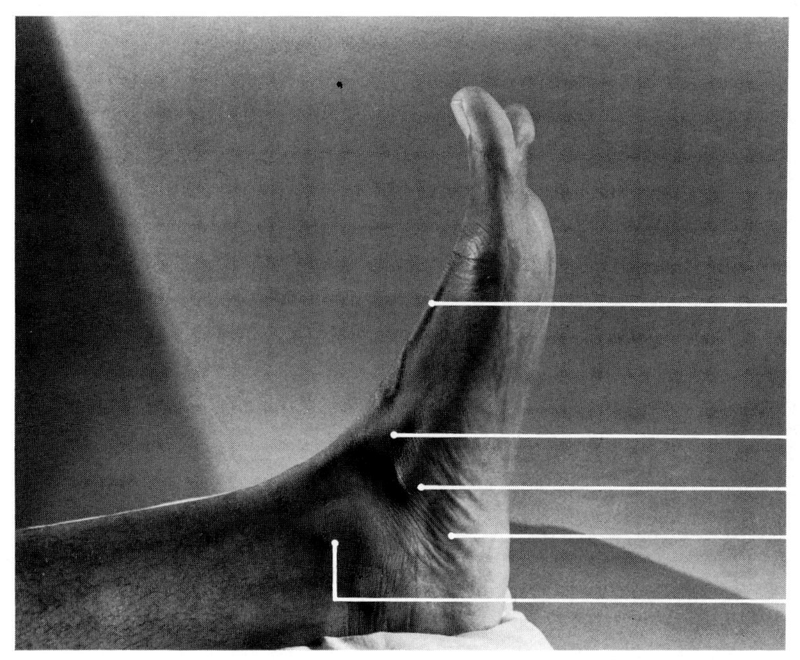

FIGURE 2-103 Abductor hallucis.

Abductor Digiti Minimi (Quinti) (*Fig.* 2-104; *see also* Figs. 1-68 *and* 1-69)

Action: Abduction and some degree of flexion of the fifth digit

Patient Position: Supine, ankle resting on the bed

Pin Insertion: Feel for the tuberosity of the fifth metatarsal and insert the pin anterior to this point at about the junction of the plantar and dorsal skin.

Relaxation: Instruct the patient as follows: "Relax your little toe."

Contraction: *Minimal*: Instruct the patient as follows: "Move your little toe outward slightly" (minimal abduction of the fifth digit).

Contraction: *Maximal*: Instruct the patient as follows: "Push your little toe outward strongly against my hand" (abduction of the fifth digit against resistance). Many patients will be unable to do this, and the patient may be instructed as follows: "Push your forefoot out toward my hand" (abduction of the forefoot against resistance in the direction of adduction).

Peripheral Nerve Supply: Lateral plantar nerve

Root Supply: Nerve roots S2 and S3, mainly S2

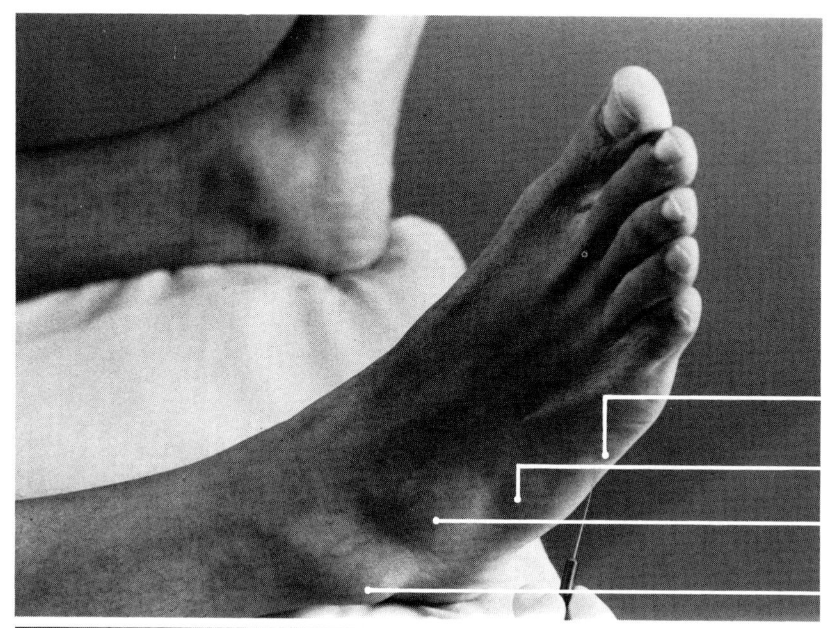

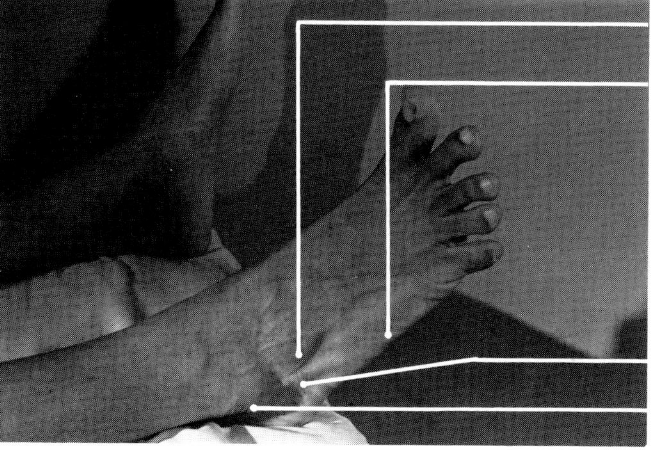

FIGURE 2-104 Abductor digiti minimi (quinti).

Dorsal Interossei (*Fig.* 2-105; *see also Fig.* 1-66)

Action: Abduction of the digits away from the axis of the second toe

Patient Position: Supine, ankle and heel resting on the bed

Pin Insertion: In the intermetatarsal spaces from the dorsal aspect

Relaxation: Instruct the patient as follows: "Relax your toes" (toes are kept in passive adduction).

Contraction: *Minimal*: Instruct the patient as follows: "Spread your toes out slightly" (minimal abduction of the toes).

Contraction: *Maximal*: Instruct the patient as follows: "Spread your toes out as strongly as you can" (maximal abduction of the toes). You may use your thumb and forefinger to span the patient's great and little toes, offering some resistance to abduction. Although this does not test the functions of the dorsal interossei, it quickly shows the patient what motion is wanted.

Peripheral Nerve Supply: By branches from the lateral plantar nerve via the tibial nerve

Root Supply: Nerve roots S2 and S3, mainly S2

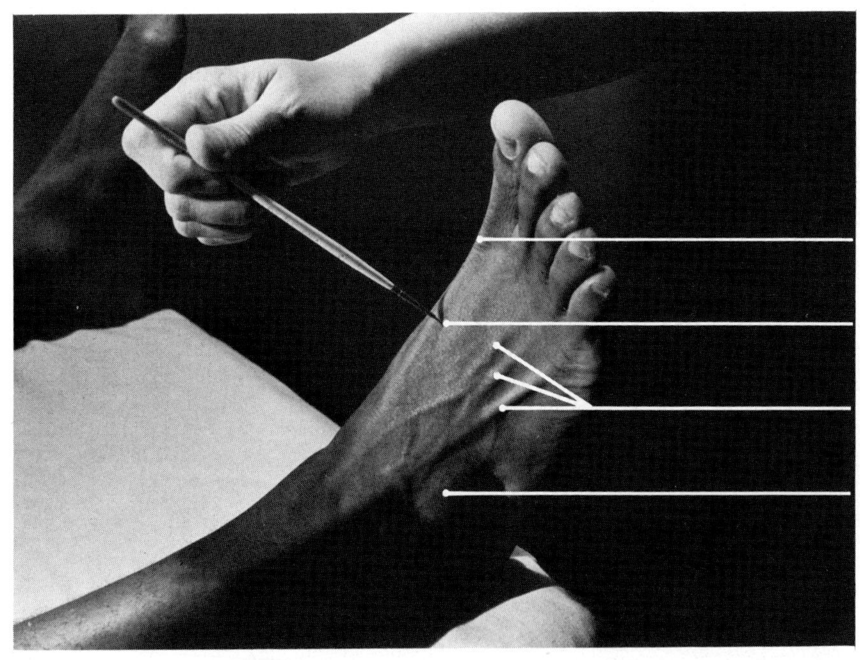

FIGURE 2-105 Dorsal interossei.

Extensor Digitorum Brevis (*Fig.* 2-106; *see also* *Figs.* 1-66, 1-68, *and* 1-69)

Action: Extension of the metatarsophalangeal joints of the first, second, third, and fourth toes. Also draws these toes somewhat laterally.

Patient Position: Supine, ankle and heel resting on the bed

Pin Insertion: Instruct the patient as follows: "Pull your toes up toward you" (extension of the toes at the metatarsophalangeal joints). The round belly of the extensor digitorum brevis will be seen lateral to the most lateral tendon of the extensor digitorum longus and anterior to and below the lateral malleolus. It is about the size of a silver dollar. Insert the pin into the bulk of the muscle.

Relaxation: Instruct the patient as follows: "Relax your toes" (toes are kept in neutral position).

Contraction: *Minimal*: Instruct the patient as follows: "Pull your toes up slightly" (minimal extension of the toes at the metatarsophalangeal joints).

Contraction: *Maximal*: Instruct the patient as follows: "Pull your toes up toward you as strongly as you can. Don't let me push them down" (maximal extension of the toes at the metatarsophalangeal joints against resistance). Give resistance at about the base of the proximal phalanges of the toes.

Peripheral Nerve Supply: Deep branch of the peroneal nerve

Root Supply: Nerve roots L5 and S1, mainly L5

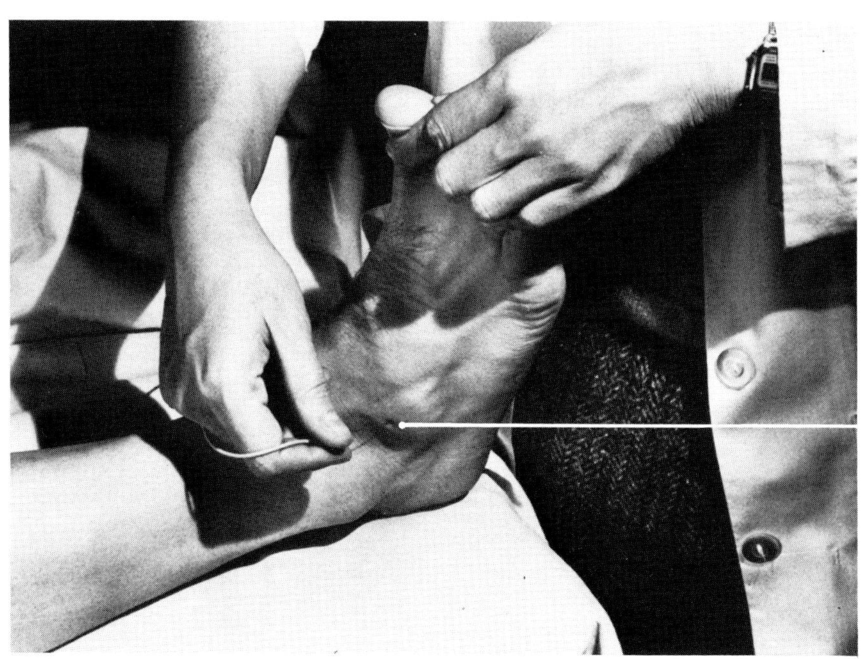

FIGURE 2-106 Extensor digitorum brevis.

REFERENCES

1. Day MH, Natier JR: The two heads of flexor pollicis brevis. J Anat 95:123–130, 1961
2. Forrest WJ: Motor innervation of human thenar and hypothenar muscles in 25 hands: A study combining EMG and percutaneous nerve stimulation. Can J Surg 19:196–199, 1967
3. Harness D, Sekeles E: The double anastomotic innervation of thenar muscles. J Anat 109:461–466, 1971
4. Harness D, Sekeles E, Chaco J: The double motor innervation of the opponens pollicis muscle: An electromyographic study. J Anat 117:329–331, 1974

BIBLIOGRAPHY

Anderson JE: Grant's Atlas of Anatomy, 7th ed. Baltimore, Williams & Wilkins, 1978

Appleton AB, Hamilton WJ, Simon G: Surface and Radiological Anatomy, 2nd ed. Baltimore, Williams & Wilkins, 1946

Basmajian JV: Muscles Alive, 4th ed. Baltimore, Williams & Wilkins, 1978

Brunnstrom S: Clinical Kinesiology, 3rd ed. Philadelphia, FA Davis, 1972

Daniels L, Worthingham C: Muscle Testing: Techniques of Manual Examination, 3rd ed. Philadelphia, WB Saunders, 1972

Delagi EF, Perotto A: Anatomic Guide for the Electromyographer: The Limbs, 2nd ed. Springfield, IL, Charles C Thomas, 1980

Goodgold J: Anatomical Correlates of Clinical Electromyography, 1st ed. Baltimore, Williams & Wilkins, 1975

Goss CM (ed): Gray's Anatomy, 29th ed. Philadelphia, Lea & Febiger, 1973

Hamilton WJ, Simon G, Hamilton SGI: Surface and Radiological Anatomy for Students and General Practitioners, 5th ed. Cambridge, England, Heffer, 1971

Hollinshead WH: Functional Anatomy of the Limbs and Back, 3rd ed. Philadelphia, WB Saunders, 1969

Hoppenfeld S: Orthopaedic Neurology: A Diagnostic Guide to Neurologic Levels. Philadelphia, JB Lippincott, 1977

Kendall FP, McCreary EK: Muscles: Testing and Function, 3rd ed. Baltimore, Williams & Wilkins, 1983

Lockhart RD: Living Anatomy, 5th ed. London, Faber & Faber, 1959

McMinn RMH, Hutchings RT: Color Atlas of Human Anatomy. Chicago Year Book Medical Publishers, 1983

Medical Research Council Memorandum No. 45: Aids to the Examination of the Peripheral Nervous System. London, Her Majesty's Stationery Office, 1976

Quiring DP: In Warfel JH (ed): The Head, Neck, and Trunk: Muscles and Motor Points, 2nd ed. Philadelphia, Lea & Febiger, 1960

Quiring DP: In Warfel JH (ed): The Extremities, 2nd ed. Philadelphia, Lea & Febiger, 1960

Rasch PJ, Burke RK: Kinesiology and Applied Anatomy, 5th ed. Philadelphia, Lea & Febiger, 1974

Rohen JW, Yokochi C: Color Atlas of Anatomy, 1st ed. New York, Igaku-Shoin, 1983

Royce J: Surface Anatomy. Philadephia, FA Davis, 1973

Sharrard WJW: The segmental innervation of the lower limb muscles in man. Ann R Coll Surg Eng 35:106, 1964

Spalteholz W: Hand-Atlas of Human Anatomy, 7th ed, Vols. 1 and 3. Philadelphia, JB Lippincott, 1937

Steindler A: Kinesiology of the Human Body under Normal and Pathological Conditions. Springfield, IL, Charles C Thomas, 1955

Part Two
CLINICAL ELECTRODIAGNOSIS

3
Principles of Electrodiagnostic Consultation

Jennifer Chu-Andrews

This chapter is meant as an aid to performing quality electrodiagnostic studies that will help toward an accurate diagnosis. For information on detailed studies and theoretical discussions, the reader is referred to standard textbooks on electrodiagnosis and clinical neurophysiology.

The electrodiagnostic examination helps in localizing dysfunction along lower motor neurons. Electrodiagnostic examination is therefore indicated when a disease process must be localized to the level of the anterior horn cell, root, plexus, peripheral nerve, neuromuscular junction, or muscle. To some extent the examination also identifies pathology attributable to upper motor neurons.[3]

As in all aspects of clinical medicine, a step-by-step approach, beginning with the history, a related clinical examination, and collection of any ancillary laboratory or roentgenologic data, is helpful in planning the method of electrodiagnostic examination. It is important to remember that the electrodiagnostic examination is an extension of the clinical examination. The best aid toward an accurate diagnosis is an open mind that will assimilate data during the course of the examination. It is important not to limit the examination because of preconceived ideas or diagnoses. The electrodiagnostic examination should not be terminated in cases in which the clinical impression is not confirmed. The examination should instead be carried out thoroughly to obtain what may be an unexpected solution to a complicated problem.

GENERAL PRINCIPLES

Always get a concise history of the problem for which the patient was referred. A visual examination of the degree and pattern of muscular atrophy, supplemented by a quick physical examination for strength, sensation, tone, and reflex changes, may alert you to search for diffuse pathology as opposed to a localized lesion.

Patients should be told at the time that the appointment is made that they should not wear jewelry or skin lotion when they come for their test. Prior to the procedure, explain the examination to the patient in simple terms. Many laboratories use preprinted forms that explain the nature and purpose of the test. A few additional words to the patient help convey the message that you care, and assist in developing a good rapport. Indicate the following to the patient: "In the first part of the test, a small electrical stimulation is done to see how your nerves conduct, relative to your age and height. In the second part, a small pin electrode is used to see how your muscles perform. Should any undue discomfort occur, tell me rather than moving or pulling away, since a sudden movement may cause more discomfort. The pin and muscle should move in coordinated fashion. If the pin causes too much discomfort, it can be moved in another direction or reinserted at another site." This brief explanation usually helps allay the patient's anxiety so that he is better able to cooperate.

Have the patient change into a gown so that

the examination can be extended as needed, unhampered by tight clothing. This will also enable you to note any old scars or other pathology normally covered by clothing. The electromyographic (EMG) examination is best done with the patient lying down.

Watch the patient for any untoward reactions during the examination. Some patients may complain of dizziness or lightheadedness. If a patient complains of dizziness or lightheadedness, or if he feels cold and clammy and looks pale, stop the test for a few minutes.

Observe for inappropriate responses. Some patients may demonstrate a jerky or cogwheeling motion to a given resistance, which may indicate a functional problem.

Examination of children may be difficult. We have found it beneficial to have parents in the examination room, since they can usually assist in allaying the child's anxiety. Others have found it essential to examine the child without the presence of parents.[1] It may also be helpful when examining children to tell them that the examination has to be done and that there can be no negotiation. Other techniques that you can try include pinching the child's skin to detract his attention from the pin and inserting the pin concurrently. You can hold the pin in such a way that the child is not aware of its presence before the skin insertion. Children may also be less fearful of you if you are not wearing a white coat.

Machinery must be carefully grounded and thoroughly checked by the hospital clinical engineering department. Calibration signals must be checked by the electromyographer before each investigation so that accuracy in the measurement of amplitudes and durations can be achieved. The shape of the calibration signal is useful as an indication of the filter settings. You should therefore be familiar with the shape of the square wave as it passes through the various standard filter settings.

Needles and surface electrodes must be checked frequently for usability and cleanliness. Needle tips should be examined under a light microscope from time to time. Concentric needle tips can be sharpened with an Arkansas stone. Bent needles and monopolar needles with retracted or perforated Teflon coatings should be discarded.[5] All needles must be autoclaved prior to the EMG examination.

There are relatively few contraindications to EMG examination. These include bleeding diathesis, coagulation disorders, blood dyscrasias, systemic infections, active inflammation in the regions to be examined, diseased heart valves, and prosthetic heart valves. Edema, whether due to active or chronic inflammation or to lymphatic blockage as seen following mastectomy, is also a contraindication to EMG. Needles are best discarded if they have been used on patients with transmissable infections, for example, viral hepatitis, acquired immune deficiency syndrome, or Jakob-Creutzfeldt disease. Nerve conduction studies must not be done in the patient with an indwelling cardiac catheter or a central venous pressure line.[2] These studies must be performed with care in the patient with a pacemaker, and proper grounding must be done.[4]

An occasional complication of EMG examination is a hematoma at the site of pin insertion. This can be avoided if you withdraw the needle as soon as you see oozing of blood around it. Apply pressure at the site of the needle puncture. Pneumothorax is an uncommon, but more serious, problem. It can be caused by improper needling of certain muscles, such as the rhomboideus major and minor and the serratus anterior, and can be avoided by good knowledge of surface anatomy. During the needling, use the audio to monitor whether the pin is getting closer to the active motor units.

PRINCIPLES FOR NERVE CONDUCTION STUDIES

Nerve conduction studies must be performed as part of the examination and are usually performed prior to EMG. Their purpose is to diagnose the presence of diffuse or focal lesions of peripheral nerves, to localize the site of maximum pathology, and to assess the severity of nerve damage. The study should also determine whether the damage is to the myelin, the axons, or both.

Electrical Stimulation

Electrical stimulation is usually done with a hand-held bipolar stimulator. In commercially available equipment the cathode and anode are usually separated by a fixed distance of 2 cm to 3 cm. Monopolar stimulation can be done by using a needle as a cathode and placing it close to or on a nerve trunk. The anode is a surface electrode or another needle placed subcutaneously. The anode is placed away from the nerve, usually within a few centimeters of the cathode. Needle stimulation requires less stimulus intensity than does surface stimulation. It is used when the nerve is difficult to stimulate because of obesity, thickened skin, or the deep location of the nerve, as in cervical or lumbosacral root stimulations. The conduction velocity obtained with monopolar stimulation differs from that of surface stimulation using a bipolar stimulator.[17]

Stimulation is usually done with either a constant-current or a constant-voltage stimulator. Constant-voltage stimulators are more readily available. These stimulators deliver a square pulse wave. The amount of current delivered to the nerve changes with skin impedance (resistance to current flow), since the voltage is fixed. With constant-current stimulators, the voltage changes according to skin impedance to keep the amount of current delivered constant. This type of stimulation is slightly more painful. Stimulation is usually done with a stimulus duration of 0.05 msec to 1 msec and voltage of 150 V to 300 V or current of 20 mA to 40 mA. The stimulus is delivered through an isolation transformer to ensure safety and to reduce the amount of stimulus artifact.

The stimulation is done with the cathode closer than the anode to the recording electrode. If the anode and cathode are reversed and a weak stimulus is used, the latency may increase by approximately 0.5 msec, since the cathode is farther away from the recording electrode.

Supramaximal stimulation is used for nerve conduction studies. Maximal current is defined as the smallest stimulating current that will produce a compound muscle action potential (CMAP) of maximal amplitude and shortest latency. Supramaximal current is 25% above maximal. A stronger stimulus strength may cause unnecessary pain. The current may also spread to adjacent nerves or muscles, and this will contaminate the recordings. If the stimulation is done with submaximal stimulus, longer latencies and lower amplitudes will be obtained.

Sitmulus artifacts, common with strong stimulation, can be reduced by placing the ground electrode between the stimulus and the recording electrode. The ground electrode should usually be placed closer to the recording electrode than to the stimulating electrode. Using the smallest stimulus that is supramaximal also reduces stimulus artifacts. Cleansing the skin with alcohol or ether will help. A piece of sandpaper or paper towel will remove light skin debris and grease. A high-conductance gel reduces skin impedance. The skin between the stimulating and recording sites should be free of perspiration and gel to avoid short-circuiting the electrical current. Clean recording, stimulating, and ground electrodes are essential. Artifacts may also be reduced by ensuring that the wire cables for the stimulator, recording electrodes, and ground electrodes are not twisted on themselves or intertwined. Broken cable wires are a common cause of large stimulus artifacts. This cause is often overlooked because insulation of the wires prevents direct visual examination. Broken cable wires as a cause of excessive artifacts should always be considered when no other cause can be found.

If an artifact is above the baseline and is still decaying at the time of the peak of a sensory nerve action potential (SNAP), the latency-to-peak will shift to the left, and a smaller latency will be recorded.[28] If the stimulus artifact is below the baseline, and if the artifact is decaying at the time of the peak of the negative portion of the SNAP, the latency measured to the peak will be longer (Fig. 3-1).[28]

Motor Nerve Conduction Studies

The recording electrodes used are usually surface disc electrodes 1 cm in diameter. The active and reference electrodes may be either separate or mounted together as a bar electrode. The active electrode is placed over the middle of the muscle at the end-plate zone. The reference electrode is placed at a remote position, for example, the metacarpophalangeal joint when the abductor pollicis brevis or abductor digiti minimi is being recorded. The reference electrode records some volume-conducted activity, since a completely neutral point is not feasible. The position of the reference electrode must be standardized so that the parameters of the CMAP can be compared from one investigation to another. The position

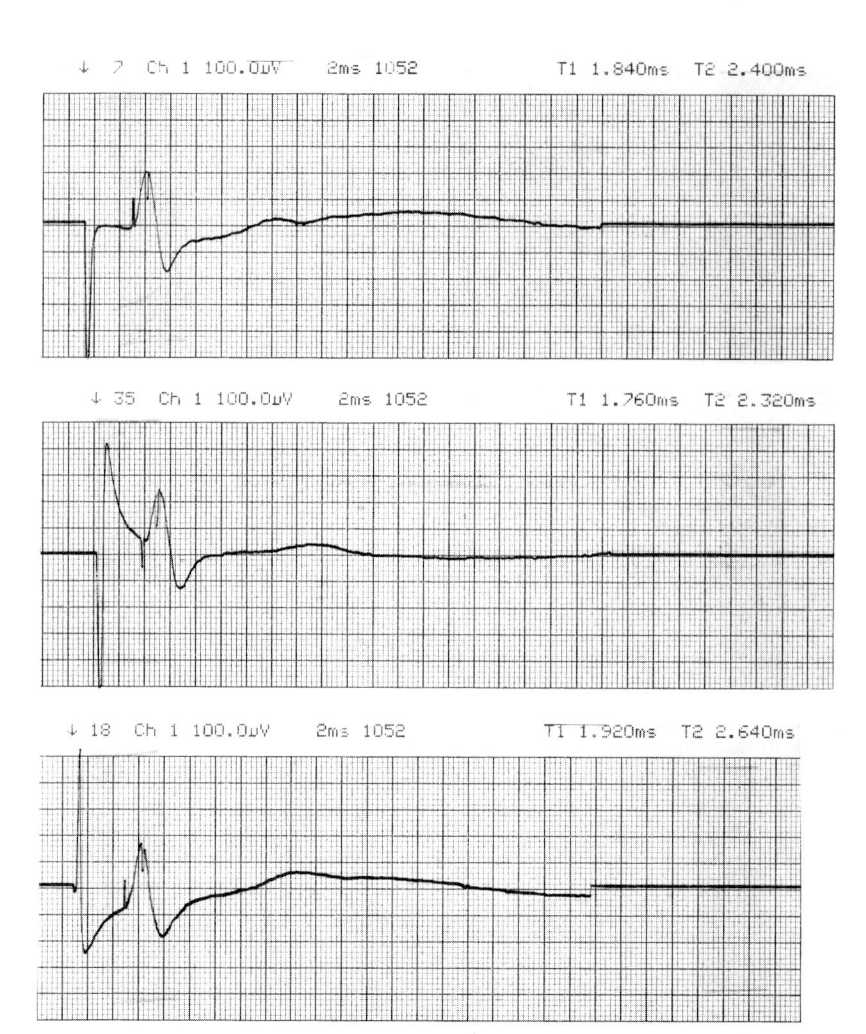

FIGURE 3-1 Effect of the stimulus artifact on the recording of the sensory potential: Sensory potentials were recorded from the base of the middle finger, and the median nerve was stimulated at the wrist. In the top trace the stimulus artifact completely returns to the baseline level. The onset latency of the sensory potential is 1.84 msec, and the peak latency is 2.40 msec. The middle trace shows a stimulus artifact above the baseline, which interferes with the recording of the sensory potential. The onset and peak latencies become shorter, measuring 1.76 msec and 2.32 msec, respectively. The bottom trace shows a stimulus artifact below the baseline, which has not decayed completely. The onset and peak latencies are falsely prolonged, measuring 1.92 msec and 2.64 msec, respectively.

of the recording electrode must be adjusted until it records from over the motor point. Recording over the motor point results in a biphasic CMAP with maximal amplitude and a sharp takeoff. A takeoff point that is not well defined causes errors in measuring the latency, and a longer latency is usually recorded (Fig. 3-2). If the recording electrode is either distal or proximal to the motor point, the CMAP will appear triphasic because a positive deflection precedes the main muscle response (Fig. 3-3, A). If the recording electrode is between two adjacent muscles, the shape of the CMAP is distorted and shows two peaks (Fig. 3-3, B). Errors in measurement of latency and amplitude can result from such recordings.

Surface electrodes are usually employed for recording, since they record over a larger area of

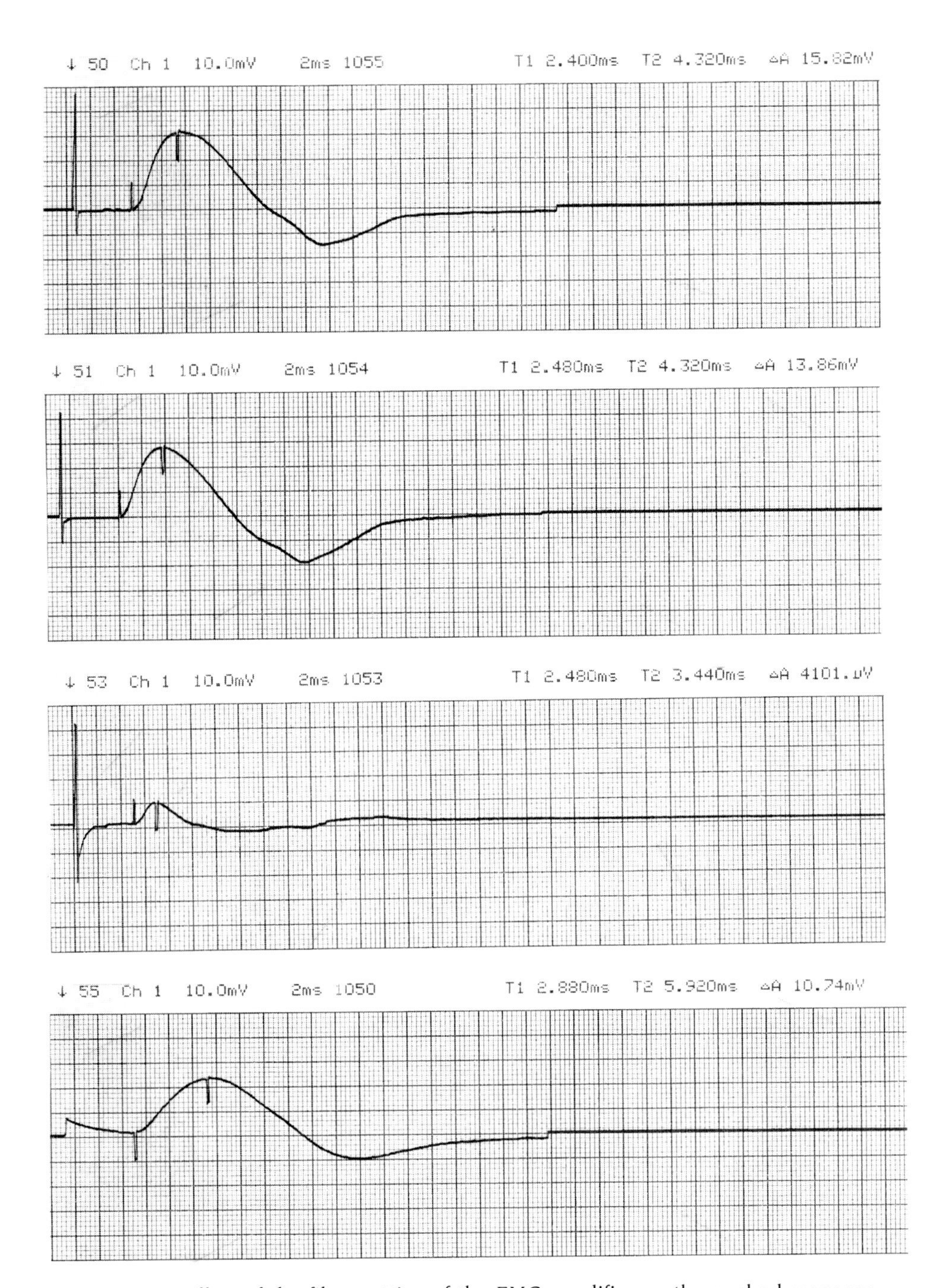

FIGURE 3-2 Effect of the filter setting of the EMG amplifier on the evoked response: Evoked motor responses were recorded from the abductor pollicis brevis by stimulating the median nerve at the wrist. The first trace was recorded with a 2 Hz–10 kHz filter; the amplitude of the CMAP measures 15.82 mV. The second and third traces were recorded with 20 Hz–10 kHz and 500 Hz–10 kHz filters, respectively, to show the effect of the exclusion of the low frequencies on the amplitude of the CMAP. The amplitudes of the CMAP measure 13.86 mV and 4.1 mV, respectively. An extra phase is seen in the CMAP recorded with the 500 Hz–10 kHz filter. The bottom trace was recorded with 2 Hz–200 Hz filter. Exclusion of frequencies above 200 Hz resulted in a CMAP of 10.74 mV. Note also that in the first three traces the onset of the CMAP is well defined, and the distal latencies measured were 2.40 msec, 2.48 msec, and 2.48 msec, respectively. In the bottom trace the onset of the CMAP is not as well defined, and the distal latency measured is longer (2.88 msec).

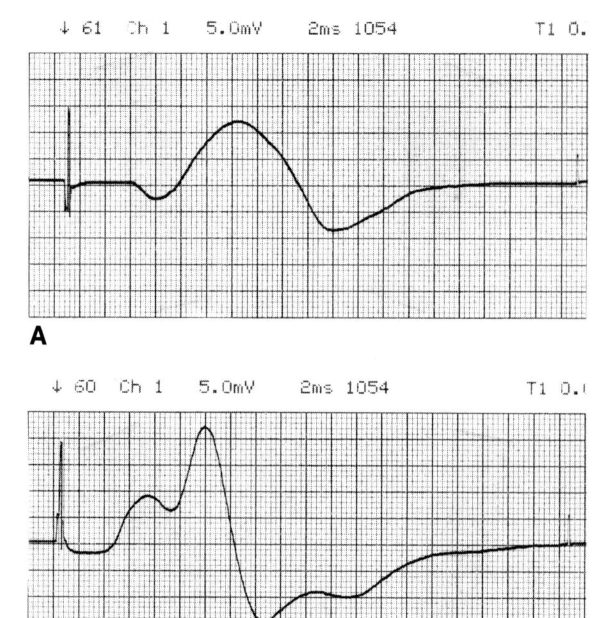

FIGURE 3-3 (A) CMAP obtained by recording at a point either distal or proximal to the motor point of the muscle under study. (B) CMAP obtained by recording between two adjacent muscles.

the muscle and thus record the activity of most of the muscle fibers from which a response is elicited. Recording with a needle electrode is done when an atrophic or deep muscle must be examined. In such situations, either a monopolar or a concentric needle can be used for recording. A monopolar needle is particularly useful because it records over a larger area than does the concentric needle. The CMAP therefore has a larger amplitude with this method. Some consider the CMAP to have a more constant shape with monopolar electrodes,[29] but opinions differ on this.[21] Recordings done with a needle electrode cannot be used to determine amplitude, since only those muscle fibers closest to the recording electrode are recorded. The CMAP recorded with a needle electrode is thus not representative of all of the muscle fibers from which a response has actually been elicited. The amplitude changes considerably when the electrode position is changed by a few millimeters.[29] The latency of the evoked potential recorded by the needle is longer than that recorded by the surface electrode, especially if the needle is placed in a superficial location in the muscle,[21] since the nerve fibers supplying the group of muscle fibers recorded by the needle may not be the fastest fibers.

In motor nerve studies the following parameters are usually measured:

Latency in milliseconds (msec), from onset of the stimulus to the time that the CMAP leaves the baseline. This measures the time it takes for the electrical impulse to elicit a response from the muscle fibers. The latency includes a delay of approximately 0.5 msec at the neuromuscular junction. It measures the conduction time along the fastest conducting nerve fibers.

Amplitude in millivolts (mV), measured from the baseline to the peak of the CMAP. This is an indication of the number of muscle fibers within the pickup area of the electrode.

Area, measured by taking the integral of the response curve within its duration. It is expressed as msec mV. Area and amplitude are directly correlated, but measurement of area is more reliable than measurement of amplitude, since the latter decreases the further away the active recording electrode is from the motor point. However, quantification of area commonly requires the assistance of a computer.

Shape of the CMAP, a valuable indication of

the degree of temporal dispersion of the elicited muscle fiber action potentials. It is well summated in the normal situation and in axonal lesions (Fig. 3-4, A and B). In demyelinating lesions; each nerve fiber is demyelinated to a different degree and hence is slowed to a different degree. This causes greater than normal variation in the conduction velocities between nerve fibers. The result is dispersion and prolonged duration of the CMAP (Fig. 3-4, C).

Conduction velocity, expressed in meters per second (m/sec), obtained by dividing the distance between two stimulus points by the difference in conduction times between these two points. Since the neuromuscular junction delay is common to both stimulus points, the difference in conduction time between these two points represents the time taken by the stimulus to travel between these points. Conduction velocity is a measure of the speed of the fastest conducting fibers.

The shape of the CMAP obtained with proximal and distal stimulation must be compared. In a normal patient the duration of the proximal CMAP is usually longer, and the amplitude is slightly smaller.[15] This is due to physiologic temporal dispersion from conduction at different rates along various sized myelinated fibers. The phenomenon is more pronounced when the distance between the stimulating and recording electrodes is increased. The occasional presence of an anomalous nerve connection, such as median–ulnar anastomosis in the forearm (Martin-Gruber anastomosis) and the accessory deep peroneal nerve in the leg, suggests the importance of comparing the shape of the CMAP obtained from proximal stimulation to that obtained from distal stimulation.[15] With the presence of an anomalous branch, the amplitude of the evoked CMAP on proximal stimulation is larger than that obtained with distal stimulation. The proximal CMAP is also preceded by an initial positive deflection (see Chap. 5 for further descriptions of anomalous nerve branches).

In motor nerve conduction studies with supramaximal stimulation, slowing the sweep speed (usually 5 msec/div. in the upper extremities and 10 msec/div. in the lower extremities) and using a sensitivity of 200 μV/div. demonstrates the presence of a small, late response called the F wave. This response occurs because antidromic stimulation of the fast-conducting nerve fibers causes a subsequent discharge of the anterior horn cells. The F wave can be recorded easily from the muscles of the hands and the feet. The H reflex is another late response. The H reflex is a monosynaptic reflex normally recorded from the soleus by stimulating the tibial nerve at the knee with a submaximal stimulus. In the presence of disorders of the peripheral nerves the F wave and the H reflex are usually abnormal earlier than are the results of routine conduction studies. (See Chap. 6 for detailed descriptions of the F wave and the H reflex.)

Sensory Nerve Conduction Studies

Sensory nerve conduction studies are performed by recording directly over the nerve. Stimulation can be done by antidromic or orthodromic techniques. Stimulation of a nerve in the direction opposite to the way it usually relays messages within the nervous system is called antidromic stimulation. Antidromic stimulation of a sensory nerve therefore entails stimulating the nerve at a proximal point and recording the evoked response at a distal site along the same nerve. Antidromic stimulation gives larger amplitudes of the sensory potential and is also less painful.[13] However, when a mixed nerve is stimulated antidromically, motor artifacts are commonly seen. Orthodromic conduction studies involve stimulating the nerve in the same direction that the nerve usually relays messages within the nervous system. In sensory conduction studies performed orthodromically the sensory nerve is stimulated peripherally, and the recording is done more proximally. In performing sensory nerve conduction studies the following parameters are usually measured:

Latency (msec), measured to the onset of the baseline deflection of the negative response (onset latency). This value divided into the distance between the stimulus point and the active recording electrode gives the conduction velocity, since no neuromuscular transmission is involved. The measurement to the peak of the negative potential (peak latency) is often used when a difference in latencies between two points is needed, because this measurement eliminates errors induced by the presence of stimulus artifacts. However, the peak latency is not representative of the fastest conducting fibers and therefore cannot be used for measuring conduction velocity.

Amplitude (μV), measured peak to peak, representing the number of nerve fibers that can be recorded by the electrode. However, there is no linear correlation between amplitude and number of axons. Amplitude decreases as the recording electrode moves away from the nerve and also if there is less than 4 cm between the active and reference electrodes.[7]

Shape changes, which are valuable for assessment of axonal or demyelinating neuropathies.

Averaging is a very useful technique that can be employed to improve the signal-to-noise ratio. It is particularly useful in the recording of evoked sensory responses. The signal, which is time-locked to the stimulus, is electronically summed and displayed as an evoked response, and the background noises that have no relationship to the stimulus disappear.

Factors Affecting Nerve Conduction Studies

Effects of Amplifier Settings

For motor nerve conduction studies the sensitivity setting is commonly 5 mV/div., for sensory nerve conduction studies the sensitivity is increased to 50 μV/div. The sensitivity is usually adjusted so that the amplifier is not overloaded

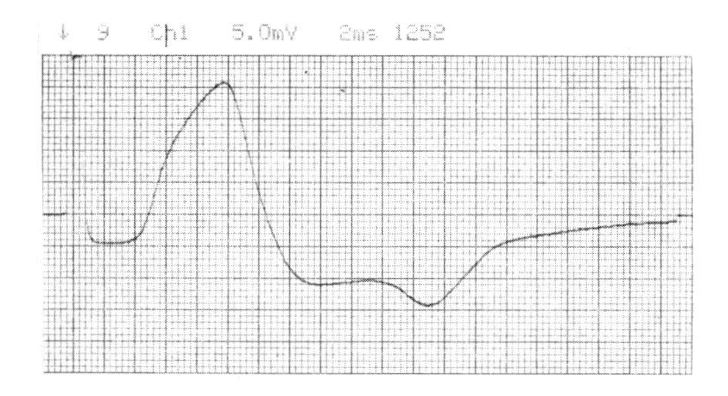

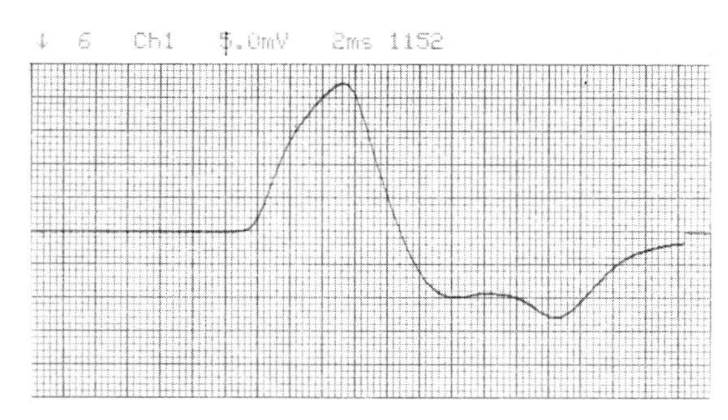

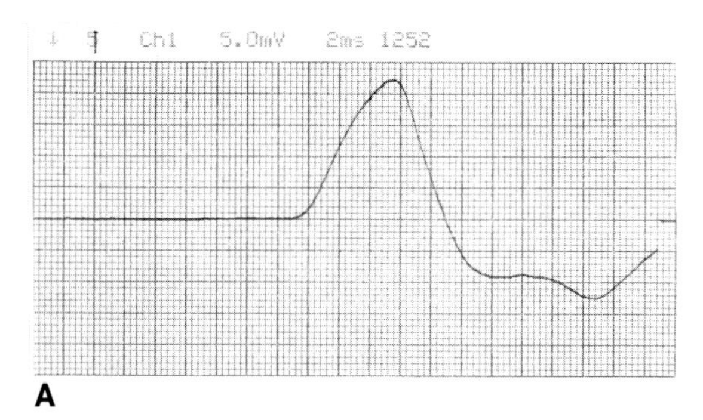

FIGURE 3-4 (A, *from top to bottom*) Normal CMAP from the abductor digiti minimi obtained from stimulation of the ulnar nerve at the wrist, below the elbow, and above the elbow. (B) CMAPs from the same muscle at the same stimulation sites in a patient with ulnar nerve entrapment at the elbow level, causing focal demyelination and axonal involvement. There is slowing of the conduction time across the elbow, and the amplitude of the CMAP drops significantly on stimulation above the elbow. (C) Tracings from a patient with Guillain-Barré syndrome. The CMAPs appear very small and dispersed because of the segmental demyelination that is present.
Note: A and B were recorded with 2 msec/div. sweep speed and 5.0 mV/div. sensitivity. C was recorded with 5 msec/div. sweep speed and a sensitivity of 2.0 mV/div.

and the amplitude of the total response can be observed. When the sensitivity is increased to a very sensitive amplification for motor nerve conduction studies, the latency measured may be shorter, since the first baseline deflection could be an intramuscular nerve action potential preceding the motor response.[7, 12, 14, 26] This potential would not be observed at low sensitivities. When the sensitivity is decreased, the latency measured tends to be longer, since the onset of the response is less well defined.

The sweep speed used for both motor and sensory nerve conduction studies is usually 2 msec/div. If the sweep speed is slowed, the latency tends to be shorter (Fig. 3-5). It is therefore essential that the same sensitivity and sweep speed be used for distal and proximal stimulations along the nerve to ensure the same degree of accuracy of measurement.

Filter settings employed by most laboratories for motor nerve conduction studies are the low-frequency (high-pass) filter at 2 Hz and the high-frequency (low-pass) filter at 10 kHz. The high-frequency filter should be as high as for the study of motor unit potentials because of the presence of low-amplitude multiphasic potentials in pathology.[27] For sensory studies the low-frequency filter is set at 32 Hz and the high-frequency filter at 3 kHz. If the high-frequency filter is decreased from 10 kHz to 2 kHz, the amplitude of the evoked response is depressed.[28] If the low-frequency filter is raised from 1.6 Hz to 16 Hz, the evoked response appears depressed and distorted owing to formation of an extra phase and an increase in the duration of the response.[28] See Figure 3-2 for examples of the effects of the filters on the CMAP.

The zero position of the strobe or time index

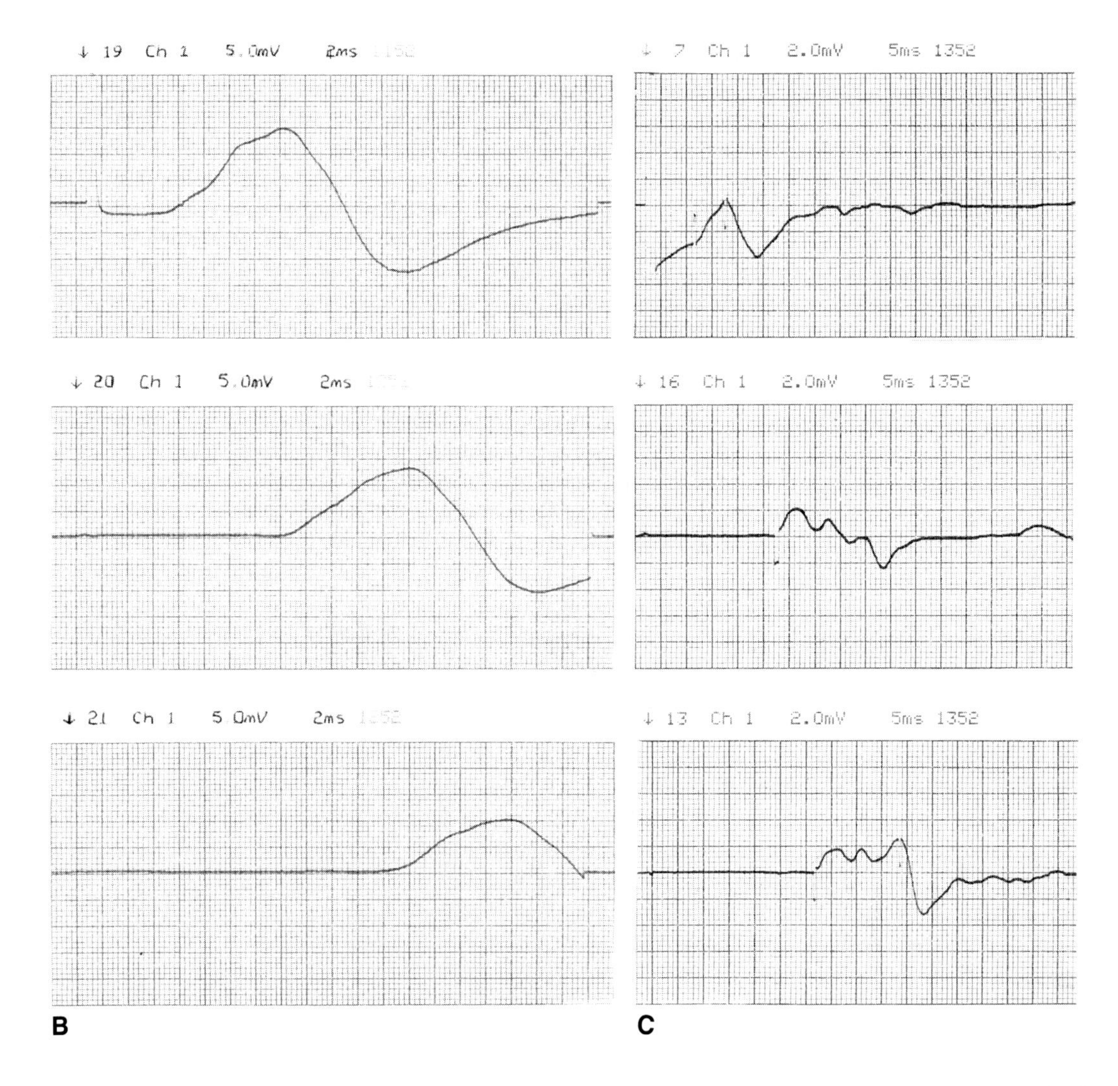

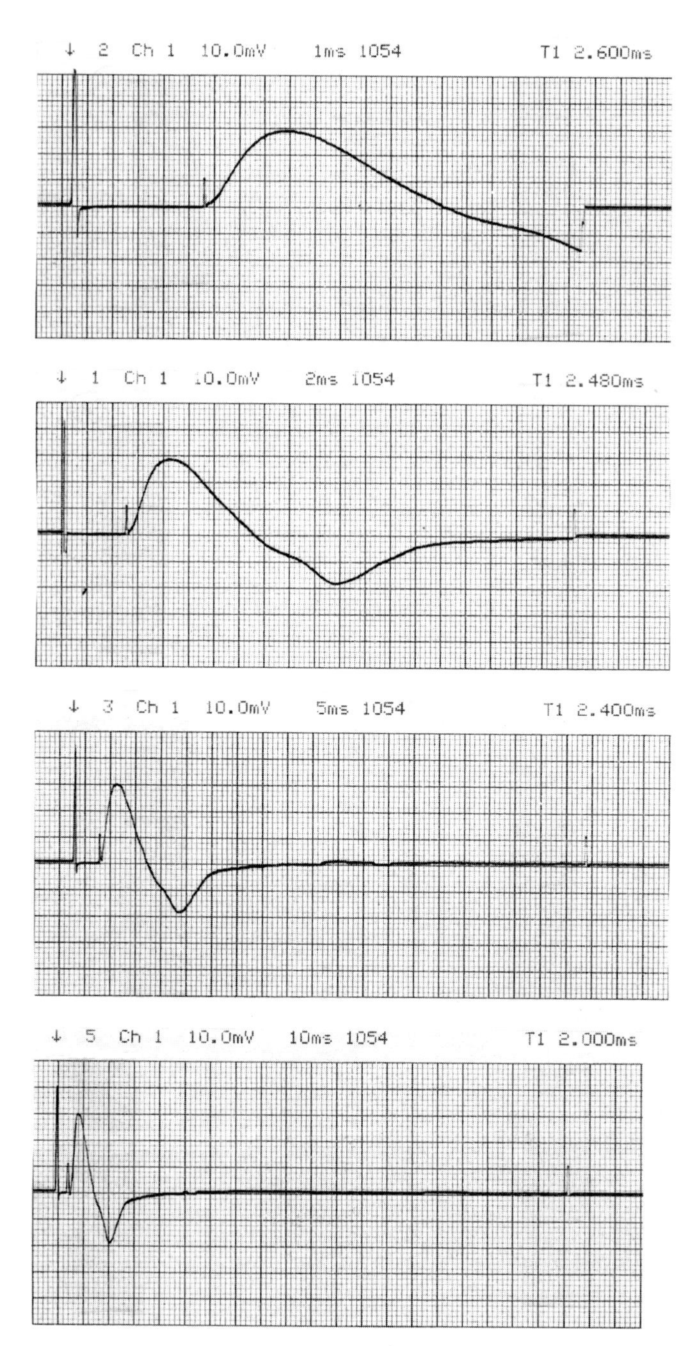

FIGURE 3-5 Effect of changing the sweep speed on the latency of the evoked response: Evoked motor responses have been recorded from the abductor pollicis brevis by stimulating the median nerve at the wrist. From the top down, the sweep speeds are 1 msec, 2 msec, 5 msec, and 10 msec/div. The sensitivity has been set at 10 mV/div. The distal motor latencies decrease progressively with the slowing of the sweep speed. The distal latencies are 2.60 msec (1 msec/div.), 2.48 msec (2 msec/div.), 2.40 msec (5 msec/div.), and 2.00 msec (10 msec/div.).

must be checked so that it coincides with the actual location of the stimulus artifact to avoid faulty latency measurements.

Each laboratory should set up its own normal values. If this is not possible and normal values from another laboratory are used, the methods used by that laboratory must be strictly employed. In particular, the same amplifier settings must be used.

Effects of Distance

The distal latencies depend on the distance between the stimulating and recording electrodes. Most laboratories perform distal latency measurements by stimulating at a fixed distance of 8 cm.[25] It is perhaps more convenient and faster to use anatomical landmarks than to stimulate at a fixed distance from the recording electrode.

However, with this method the standard deviation as a percentage of the mean value may be greater than with measured stimulation sites.[23]

The position in which the limb is held during stimulation should be maintained when you are measuring distances. This reduces the errors in distance measurements that would occur with repositioning of the limb.

Use of a metal tape is preferred for measuring distances. In certain situations in which the course of the nerve is not straight and surface contours interfere in the measurement of the length of the nerve (*e.g.*, for measuring the distance from Erb's point at the base of the neck to the axilla), obstetric calipers may be used. When a nerve is to be stimulated over a short segment, an interstimulus distance of not less than 10 cm should be chosen so as to reduce the percentage of error in measuring distances.

Effect of Temperature

The temperature of the limb to be studied for conduction velocity should be approximately 34° C to 35° C, in which case the intramuscular temperature may be assumed to be close to 37° C. The conduction velocity drops 2.4 m/sec for every degree Celsius drop in temperature. Both motor and sensory latencies can be falsely prolonged if the patient's hands or the feet are cold. However, there will be an increase in the amplitude and area of the SNAPs if the limb is cold.[9,10] In contrast, when slowing of the nerve is of neuropathic origin, a decrease in amplitude and area is common. Measuring the skin temperature and calculating the conduction velocity corrected for temperature is one way to compensate for temperature deviations.[16] Another way is to correct the temperature to a standard value by heating. The optimal way of measuring skin temperature is to use a thermoprobe. Using the dorsal aspect of your hand is a quick but inaccurate way of determining the skin temperature in a clinical setting. A hot pack can be placed for about 10 minutes on the segment of the limb to be examined. Running warm water over the patient's hands is a quick way of warming the limb.

Effect of Age

Conduction velocities in infants are approximately half those of adults.[11,30] Children do not achieve normal adult conduction velocity values until the age of 4 years. From 4 to 16 years the nerve conduction velocities are higher than the adult ranges. After age 16, nerve conduction velocity decreases with age.[6] After age 60 the mean nerve conduction velocity may be 10% slower than for adults less than 60 years of age.[18, 24]

Effect of Height

Conduction velocities tend to decrease with increasing height of the patient.[8]

Differences Between Various Nerves and Nerve Segments

The conduction velocities along the proximal nerve segments are faster than along distal segments.[12] This can be attributed to the temperature differential between the proximal and distal parts of the limb. The nerves of the lower extremities are generally slower than those of the upper extremities. This is probably due to a combination of the greater length and lower temperature of the nerves in the lower extremities.

Nerve Conduction Studies in Pathologic Situations

If no proximal response can be evoked but distal conduction studies appear normal in an examination performed 1 week or more after the onset of symptoms, complete neurapraxia may be the cause. There is total conduction block in complete neurapraxia, which is due to local demyelination. (The EMG in complete neurapraxia shows no spontaneous activity at rest and no motor unit potentials [MUPs] recruited on contraction.) In cases in which there is complete distal degeneration of the axons (neurotmesis), as seen with nerve transection, all conduction fails distal to the injury after the fourth day of injury.[22] (The EMG in neurotmesis shows spontaneous activity at rest at 10 to 21 days, depending on the proximity of the nerve lesion to the muscles of supply.)

When the CMAP on proximal stimulation is smaller than that obtained on distal stimulation and there is slowing of the conduction velocity between these two points, a partial conduction block due to restricted demyelination (partial neurapraxia) of the nerve segment between the two stimulus points should be considered as a possible cause. If the conduction velocity is very slow, there may be demyelination of most of the nerve fibers of this segment (segmental demyelination). If the conduction velocity is normal across a segment and the CMAP is similarly reduced for proximal and distal stimulation sites, a mild conduction block due to partial axonal involvement (axonotmesis) should be considered.

When peripheral neuropathy is suspected, sensory nerve conduction studies, including amplitude measurements, are essential, since sensory abnormalities are seen very early. Sural nerve conduction studies are particularly helpful, but other sensory nerves such as the median, ulnar, and radial should also be studied. If the sensory responses are poor, averaging can be performed. Studies of the H reflex and F response are also useful in evaluation for peripheral neuropathies.

Segmental demyelinating diseases of the peripheral nerves can cause the conduction velocities to be reduced to as low as 50% of normal values. The shape of the CMAP appears dispersed, especially with proximal stimulation. At times, slowing may be seen only at the most distal segments of the peripheral nerves, and hence only the distal latency may be prolonged. Acquired segmental demyelinating diseases (*e.g.*, Guillain-Barré syndrome) commonly involve the proximal nerves, including the facial nerves. In these diseases, multifocal conduction block causes the amplitude of the motor response to be much lower with proximal than with distal stimulation.

Mild axonal neuropathies cause little or no slowing of conduction velocities. They may cause depression of the amplitude and area of the CMAP, but the responses will not appear asynchronous or dispersed. However, when the involvement is severe, or when there is also degeneration of the overlying myelin sheath, the conduction velocity may drop to 30% below normal values. Axonal neuropathies affect the distal peripheral nerves more than the proximal peripheral nerves.

Stimulation of appropriate additional nerves must be done when the patient's clinical picture does not fit in the distribution of the peripheral nerves commonly studied, for example, stimulating the C8 nerve root or the proximal nerves of the brachial or lumbosacral plexus.

If routine conduction velocity determinations do not reveal abnormalities but the clinical symptoms suggest slowing along the slower motor nerve fibers, stimulation by the collision method can be done.[12,20] Measurement of conduction velocities of both the fastest fibers and the slowest fibers is possible with this technique. Two supramaximal shocks are given simultaneously at a proximal and a distal site. This results in a collision between the orthodromic and antidromic stimuli, and therefore no CMAP can be recorded with the proximal stimulus. The proximal stimulus is then given at a later interval, and a small CMAP is obtained from the recording site, since the fastest fibers now escape the collision. As the interstimulus interval is increased, the CMAP becomes progressively larger. The time interval at which the CMAP is the largest can be used to calculate the conduction velocity of the slowest fibers.

PRINCIPLES FOR EMG EXAMINATION AT REST

Instruct the patient to relax the muscle for this segment of the examination. Position the joint so that the muscle under examination is at a disadvantage for contraction (*e.g.*, bend the knee when examining the quadriceps). (Positions that work best for each muscle are described in Chap. 2).

Hold the needle as you would hold a pencil, and use a swift thrusting motion of the wrist to penetrate skin and muscle. The patient feels more discomfort if the needle is inserted slowly.

Examine rest-phase potentials with the sweep setting at 10 msec/div. and the sensitivity setting at 50 μV to 200 μV/div. Examine at least ten different sites in each muscle. One abnormal site out of 20 is not considered significant. The data are quantified by calculating the percentage of abnormal sites in each muscle. These data can be used for follow-up studies. When examining different sites within the muscle, withdraw the needle to the subcutaneous position and repenetrate the muscle fascia by holding the needle at a slight tangent. As soon as the fascia is penetrated, a "click" will be heard. Stop moving the needle as soon as this click is heard and watch the oscilloscope. Normal insertional activity stops as soon as needle movement stops. Repeat the same action at different depths of the muscle. The location with the best yield in abnormal spontaneous activity is close to or just under the fascia.

If end-plate potentials, previously known as 'nerve spikes,' are found or miniature end-plate potentials obtained, reposition the pin into another area (see later in this chapter). The patient will usually complain of pain when the pin is at the end plate. The positive waves found at the end plate are not significant for pathology. Insertional activity normally lasts less than 300 msec. It may be prolonged in association with increased muscle membrane irritability due to nerve or muscle disorders. It is reduced in muscle fibrosis.

Abnormal spontaneous findings include fibrillations, positive sharp waves, fasciculations, complex repetitive discharges, doublets, cramps, myotonic discharges, myokymia, and neuromyokymia. (These potentials are described individually later in this chapter.) If any of these potentials is found, you must investigate whether the findings occur in any specific anatomical distribution. Abnormal spontaneous activity may be found diffusely in disorders of the anterior horn cells, roots, plexi, peripheral nerves, and muscle. It may also be seen in diseases of the neuromuscular junction such as severe myasthenia gravis. Abnormal spontaneous activity may also be seen in metabolic disorders such as hyperkalemic periodic paralysis and acid maltase deficiency. Expand the investigation to include all four limbs and facial muscles if you suspect a generalized process.

Spontaneous activity has also been reported to be seen in upper motor neuron lesions such as those resulting from cerebrovascular accidents and spinal cord injury. It is more common in the upper than in the lower extremity and may be present without concomitant lower motor neuron involvement. It is believed to be due to neurophysiological aberration secondary to interruption of the descending pathways.[45]

Insertional Activity

Miniature End-Plate Potentials (Fig. 3-6)

GENERAL DESCRIPTION

Miniature end-plate potentials are nonpropagated subthreshold depolarizations of the end-plate region caused by spontaneous release of a single quantum of acetylcholine from the nerve terminal.[36]

SIGNIFICANCE

Miniature end-plate potentials are a normal finding in any muscle and are seen when the needle is in the end-plate region. When the needle is in this region the patient usually complains of a dull, aching pain that is relieved by moving the needle away from this region.

PARAMETERS

SHAPE Small, short negative spikes

DURATION 1 msec to 2 msec with concentric recordings. Off-line quantitative analyses of monopolar recordings of miniature end-plate potentials with the digitizer and Swedish Electrophysiologic Software (SES) range from 1 msec to 4.3 msec, with a mean of 2.3 ± 0.7 msec.

AMPLITUDE 10 μV to 50 μV with concentric recordings. Off-line quantitative analyses of monopolar recordings of miniature end-plate potentials with the digitizer and SES range from 16 μV to 100 μV, with a mean of 30.1 ± 10.8 μV.

RHYTHM Irregular

RATE 20 to 25/sec

SOUND Seashell murmur

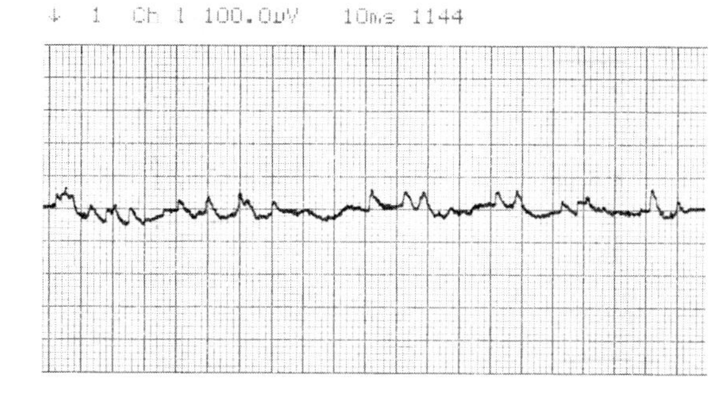

FIGURE 3-6 Miniature end-plate potentials. Calibrations: Sweep speed 10 msec/div., sensitivity 100 μV/div.

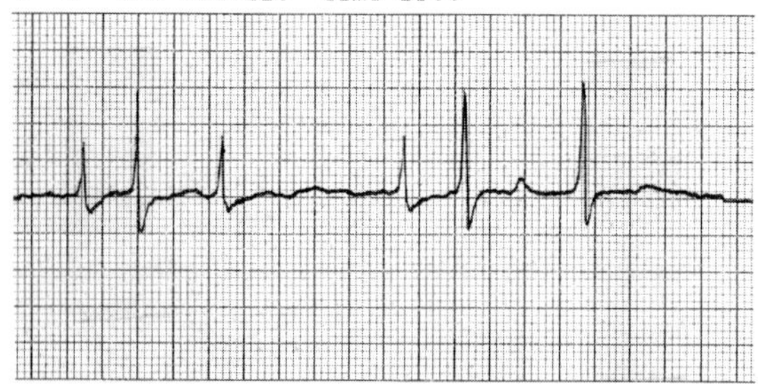

FIGURE 3-7 End-plate potentials. Calibrations: Sweep speed 10 msec/div., sensitivity 200 μV/div.

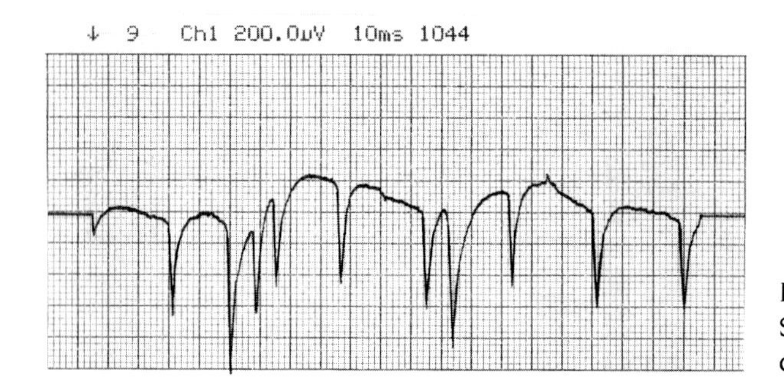

FIGURE 3-8 Positive sharp waves. Calibrations: Sweep speed 10 msec/div., sensitivity 200 μV/div.

End-Plate Potentials (Fig. 3-7)

GENERAL DESCRIPTION

End-plate potentials are discharges of single muscle fibers from irritation of intramuscular nerve terminals by needle movements.[32]

SIGNIFICANCE

End-plate potentials are a normal finding in any muscle.

PARAMETERS

SHAPE The initial phase is negative, followed by a positive phase.

DURATION 3 msec to 4 msec. Off-line quantitative analyses for monopolar needle recordings with the digitizer and SES range from 1.4 msec to 9.6 msec, with a mean of 4.1 ± 1.5 msec.

AMPLITUDE 100 μV to 200 μV. Off-line quantitative analyses for monopolar needle recordings with the digitizer and SES range from 107 μV to 1702.7 μV, with a mean of 629.5 ± 348.2 μV.

RHYTHM Irregular

RATE 5 to 50/sec

SOUND "Cracking" noise

Spontaneous Activity

Positive Sharp Waves (Fig. 3-8)

GENERAL DESCRIPTION

Positive sharp waves are a spontaneous discharge of single muscle fibers recorded when the tip of the recording electrode is positioned close to the damaged portion of the muscle membrane. They are monophasic in appearance, with a positive spike and a long negative tail. The negative portion is lower in amplitude and may continue up to 100 msec.[37]

SIGNIFICANCE

Positive sharp waves are similar to fibrillations but may appear earlier.[52]

PARAMETERS

DURATION 1 msec to 10 msec. Off-line quantitative analyses for monopolar needle recordings with the digitizer and SES range from 4.1 msec to 24.8 msec, with a mean of 11.9 ± 4.5 msec.

AMPLITUDE 50 μV to 1000 μV, with an average of 120 μV.[32] Off-line quantitative analyses for monopolar needle recordings with the digitizer and SES range from 44.3 μV to 2290.1 μV, with a mean of 392.2 ± 331.9 μV.

RHYTHM Regular

RATE 2 to 100/sec, with an average of 10/sec

SOUND Low thud

Fibrillations (Fig. 3-9)

GENERAL DESCRIPTION

Fibrillations are a spontaneous discharge of single muscle fibers. They are usually diphasic with initial positivity when recorded from outside the end-plate region. Fibrillations are occasionally triphasic. Take care to search for fibrillations outside the end-plate region, since fibrillations resemble end-plate activity if recorded in that region. Fibrillations are suppressed by cooling the muscle.

↓ 14 Ch1 200.0µV 10ms 1044

A

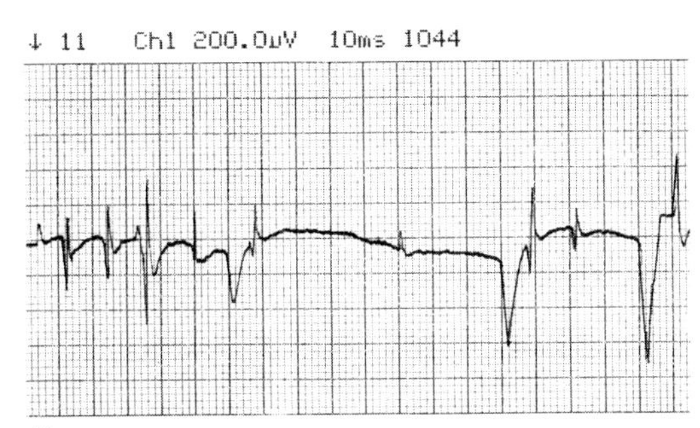

B

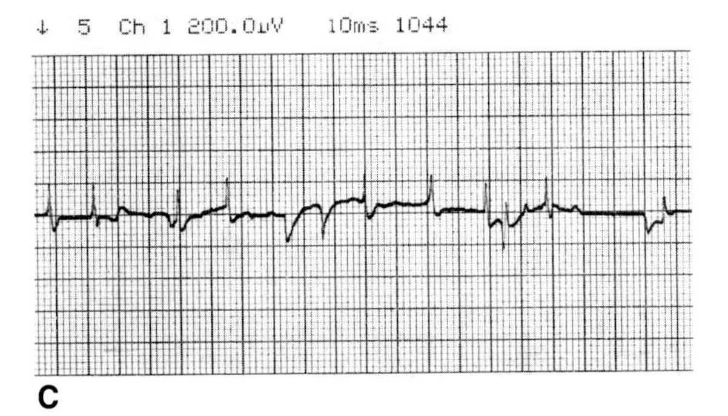

C

FIGURE 3-9 (A) Fibrillations. (B) Fibrillations and positive sharp waves. (C) End-plate potentials, positive sharp waves, and fibrillations. Calibrations: Sweep speed 10 msec/div., sensitivity 200 μV/div.

SIGNIFICANCE

Fibrillations are seen in association with lower motor neuron disorders but may also be seen in primary muscle disorders, severe neuromuscular junction disorders, and metabolic disorders such as hyperkalemic periodic paralysis. It is believed that fibrillations occur because the entire muscle fiber rather than just the end-plate region develops hypersensitivity to acetylcholine.[38]

PARAMETERS

DURATION 1 msec to 5 msec with concentric recordings.[46] Off-line quantitative analyses for monopolar needle recordings with the digitizer and SES range from 1.2 msec to 5.6 msec, with a mean of 2.9 ± 0.9 msec.

AMPLITUDE 20 μV to 200 μV. Off-line quantitative analyses for monopolar needle recordings with the digitizer and SES range from 37.3 μV to 2149.8 μV, with a mean of 355.1 ± 370.5 μV.

RHYTHM Usually regular. May also be irregular.

RATE 1 to 30/sec, with an average of 13/sec[32]

SOUND Clicking noises, similar to those of raindrops on a roof

Fasciculations (Fig. 3-10)

GENERAL DESCRIPTION

Fasciculations are a spontaneous discharge of a group of muscle fibers belonging to a single motor unit. They are usually accompanied by visible twitching of the skin and may be easier to recognize visually than by the needle electrode, since the needle electrode recording is focal. However, needle recordings may identify fasciculations in the deeper muscles.[41]

Fasciculations may originate from the anterior horn cells or along the peripheral nerve.[53] They may remain after peripheral nerve block. The exact site of origin of fasciculations is still not totally clear.

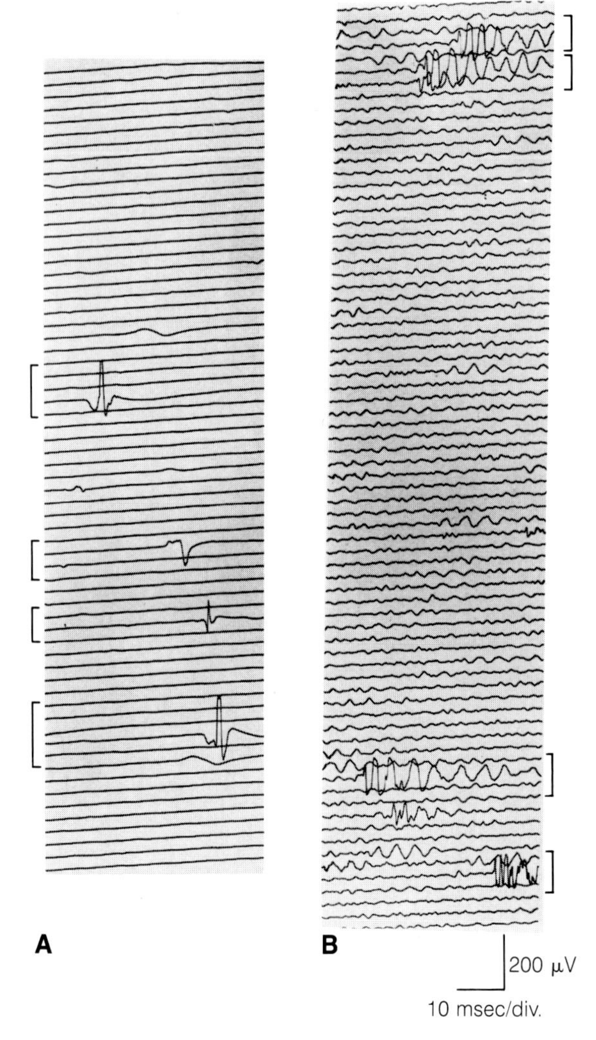

FIGURE 3-10 Fasciculations. (A) Benign. They are simple in shape and discharge at a faster rate than the fasciculations in B. (B) Malignant, as seen in amyotrophic lateral sclerosis. The fasciculations are larger in amplitude and longer in duration. They are also polyphasic in shape and appear very complex. Calibrations: Sweep speed 10 msec/div., sensitivity 200 μV/div.

SIGNIFICANCE

Fasciculations are usually seen in anterior horn cell disorders but may also be seen with chronic radiculopathies and chronic peripheral nerve diseases such as Guillain-Barré syndrome and Charcot-Marie-Tooth disease. They may also be seen in entrapment syndromes, tetany, thyrotoxicosis, and overdosage with anticholinesterase medications.[34] They are occasionally observed in normal muscles. Differentiation between benign and malignant fasciculations is difficult. Malignant fasciculations are best diagnosed by the concurrent presence of other signs of denervation such as various forms of spontaneous activity or changes in MUP parameters compatible with chronic or ongoing reinnervation.

PARAMETERS

SHAPE Diphasic, triphasic, or polyphasic. May change from discharge to discharge.

DURATION Similar to that of MUP: 5 msec to 15 msec

AMPLITUDE 300 μV to 5000 μV

RHYTHM Irregular

RATE 1 to 50/min. Benign fasciculations—one every 0.8 msec; malignant fasciculations—one every 3.5 msec[49]

SOUND Sudden-onset low popping noise

Complex Repetitive Discharges (Fig. 3-11)

GENERAL DESCRIPTION

Complex repetitive discharges represent a group of single muscle fibers (two to more than ten)

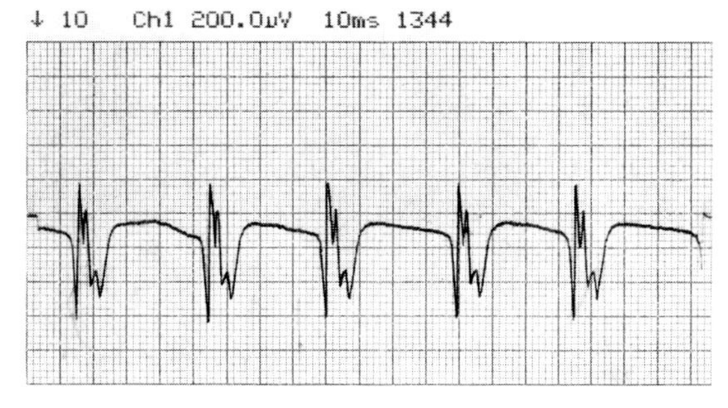

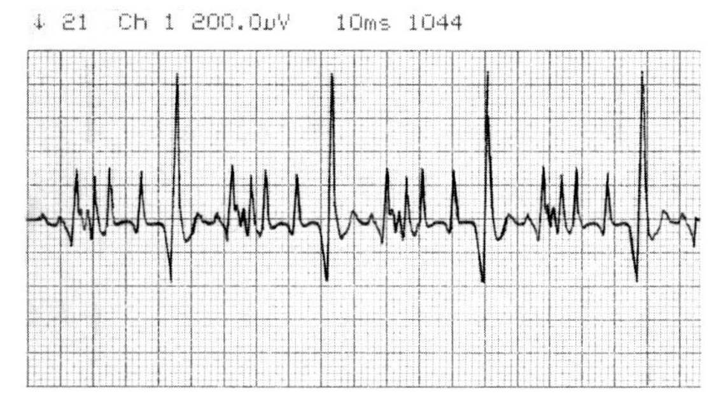

FIGURE 3-11 Complex repetitive discharges. Calibrations: Sweep speed 10 msec/div., sensitivity 200 μV/div.

firing in near synchrony and in the same order owing to the presence of a fibrillating single muscle fiber that acts as a pacemaker.[47] Ephaptic stimulation at low-threshold sites excites the adjacent muscle fibers. Complex repetitive discharges are seen in chronic slowly progressive denervation, dystrophic muscles with intact innervation, and normal sphincter muscles.

PARAMETERS

SHAPE Polyphasic, usually complex, very stable appearance at consecutive discharges

DURATION 50 msec to 100 msec

AMPLITUDE 50 μV to 1000 μV

RHYTHM Regular. May begin abruptly and end abruptly.

RATE 5 to 100/sec, with a mean of 40/sec. Usually maintains a certain rate for a short period.

SOUND Like that of a motorcycle engine or a dive bomber that does not dive

Doublets and Multiplets (Fig. 3-12)

GENERAL DESCRIPTION

Doublets and multiplets are almost identical MUPs firing two or more times at short intervals of 10 msec to 30 msec while the muscle is at rest. These MUPs can be voluntarily recruited.

SIGNIFICANCE

Doublets and multiplets can be increased with ischemia. They can also be seen with tetany and hyperventilation. They may infrequently be seen in motor neuron disease.[34]

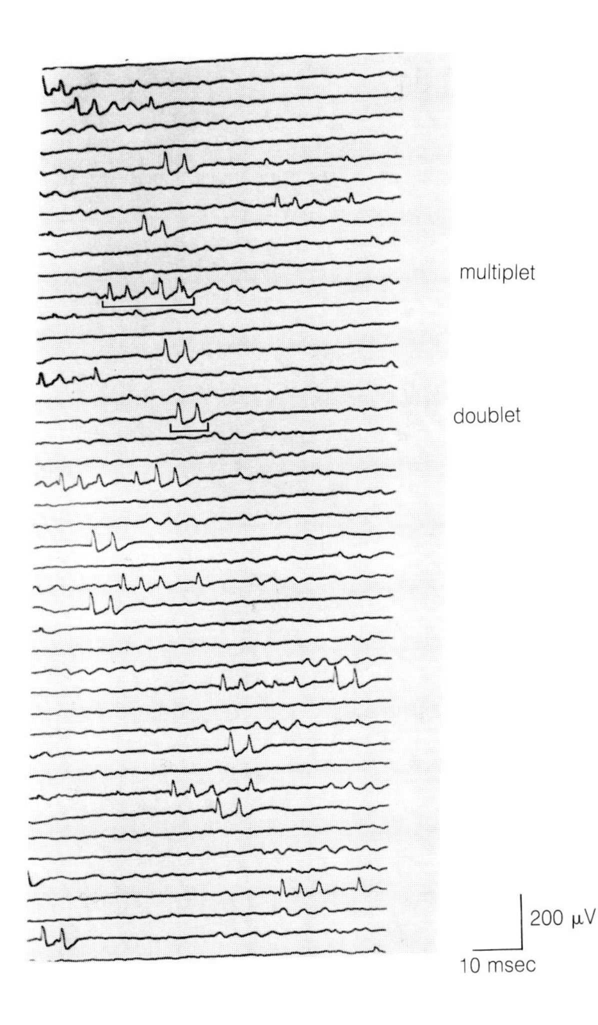

FIGURE 3-12 Doublets and multiplets. Calibrations: Sweep speed 10 msec/div., sensitivity 200 μV/div.

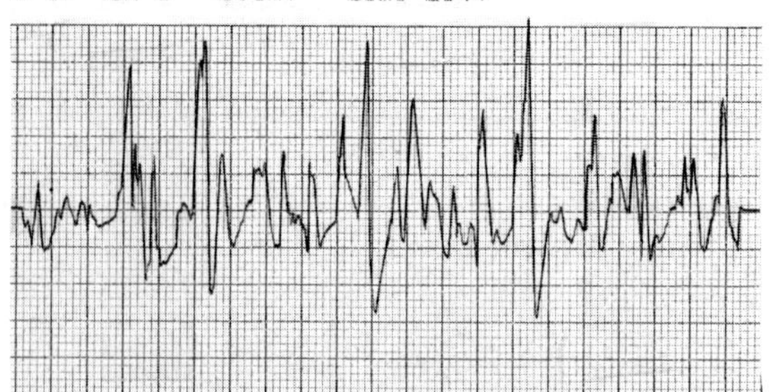

FIGURE 3-13 Cramps. Calibrations: Sweep speed 20 msec/div., sensitivity 5.0 mV/div.

Cramps (Fig. 3-13)

GENERAL DESCRIPTION

Cramps are high-frequency spontaneous discharges of motor units. The discharge usually starts abruptly when the muscle contracts strongly in a shortened position. It may end as abruptly as it begins.

SIGNIFICANCE

Cramps may be seen in association with salt depletion, chronic neurogenic atrophy, myxedema, pregnancy, and uremia. They may also occur as benign nocturnal cramps.

PARAMETERS

DURATION Similar to that of MUPs on maximal contraction

AMPLITUDE Similar to that of MUPs on maximal contraction

RHYTHM Irregular

RATE 40 to 60/sec, or up to 200 to 300/sec[44]

Myotonic Discharges (Fig. 3-14)

GENERAL DESCRIPTION

Myotonic discharges consist of single-fiber action potentials firing at high frequencies and usually declining to low frequencies. Discharges are usually triggered by a slight contraction, percussion, or the movement of a needle electrode.

SIGNIFICANCE

Myotonic discharges are seen in myotonia congenita, myotonia dystrophica, paramyotonia congenita, and hyperkalemic periodic paralysis.[31,43] They may be seen infrequently in polymyositis and acid maltase deficiency.[39] In myotonia congenita, there is low chloride conductance owing to abnormalities in the muscle membrane.[42] The cause of the myotonic discharges in the other forms of myotonic disorders has not yet been established.

PARAMETERS

SHAPE Similar to that of positive sharp waves or fibrillations

DURATION 1 msec to 10 msec (individual wave duration)

AMPLITUDE 10 μV to 1000 μV

RHYTHM Typically, the discharges wax and wane in frequency and amplitude, for example, from firing at 150/sec with amplitudes of 1000 μV to 20/sec at amplitudes of 10 μV.

RATE 20 to 150/sec

SOUND Similar to that of a dive bomber or of an accelerating and decelerating motorcycle engine[41]

Myokymia (Fig. 3-15)

GENERAL DESCRIPTION

Myokymia potentials resemble MUPs but fire at a fixed rate and rhythm while the muscle is at rest. They are usually accompanied by vermiform movements of the overlying skin.

SIGNIFICANCE

Myokymia is usually seen in association with multiple sclerosis,[40] brainstem glioma,[48] polyradiculoneuropathy,[35,51] facial palsy, radiation plexopathy,[33] and chronic nerve compression, such as carpal tunnel syndrome.[34]

PARAMETERS

DURATION Similar to that of MUPs

AMPLITUDE Similar to that of MUPs

RHYTHM Regular, recurring at intervals of 0.1 sec to 10 sec

RATE 2 Hz to 20 Hz, lasting 0.1 sec to 0.9 sec or continuous at 1 Hz to 5 Hz

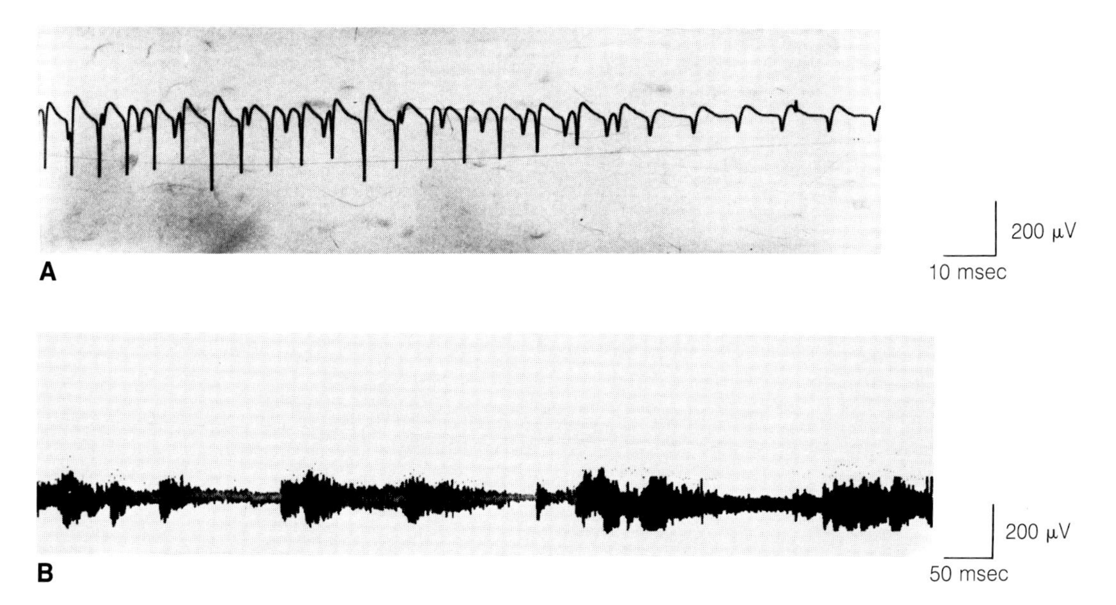

FIGURE 3-14 (A) Myotonic discharges in the form of a train of positive waves. These waves range in amplitude up to 500 μV at the left end of the trace, where the discharges are more rapid. At the right end of the trace the discharge frequency is lower, and the amplitude of the positive waves is smaller (100 μV). Calibrations: Sweep speed 10 msec/div., sensitivity 200 μV/div., fiberoptic paper speed 100 cm/sec. (B) Typical waxing and waning of myotonic discharges. Calibrations: Sweep speed 50 msec/div., sensitivity 200 μV/div. Fiberoptic paper speed 0.5 cm/sec.

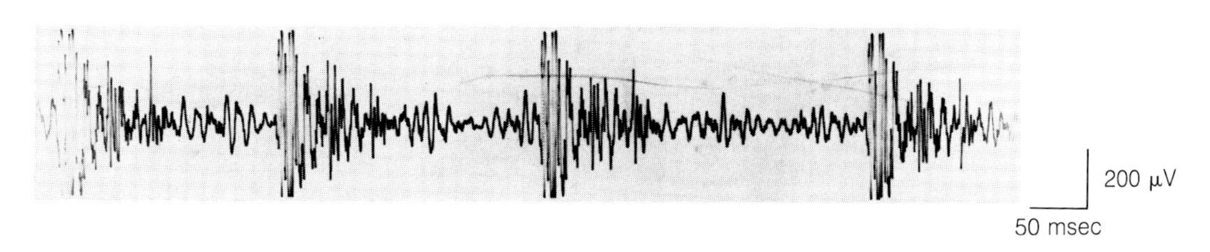

FIGURE 3-15 Myokymia. Calibrations: Sweep speed 50 msec/div., sensitivity 200 μV/div. Fiberoptic paper speed 100 cm/sec.

Neuromyotonia

Neuromyotonia is a rare form of spontaneous activity. The discharges continue even while the patient is asleep, under anesthesia, or under peripheral nerve block. Neuromyotonia may appear in the form of MUPs or fibrillations firing at rates of 100 Hz to 300 Hz. There is variation in amplitude as the spontaneous activity continues. It is seen in association with the syndrome of spontaneous fiber activity (Isaac's syndrome) and may also be seen with anticholinesterase poisoning, tetany, and chronic spinal muscular atrophies.[34, 50]

PRINCIPLES FOR EMG EXAMINATION ON MINIMAL CONTRACTION

The Motor Unit

The motor unit is the functional unit of the neuromuscular system. It consists of an anterior horn cell, its axon, and all of the muscle fibers supplied by the axon. Histochemically, different fiber types are present in muscle. Type I muscle fibers are rich in mitochondrial oxidative enzymes but poor in glycolytic enzymes such as adenosine triphosphatase (ATPase) and are therefore useful for aerobic metabolism. Type I motor units contract slowly, develop low tension,[124] and are resistant to fatigue. Type IIA muscle fibers are poor in mitochondrial oxidative enzymes and rich in ATPase enzymes. They are fatigue resistant, have a fast twitch contraction time, and develop moderate mechanical tension.[70,85] Type IIB fibers have a lower content of oxidative enzymes than do type IIA, are not resistant to fatigue, and develop high mechanical tension.[70,85] The alpha motor neurons supplying the type I muscle fibers are smaller than those supplying the type II muscle fibers. According to the principle of orderly recruitment, the smaller alpha motor neurons are activated before the larger ones.[90,101,120]

The muscle fibers of a motor unit are interspersed with the muscle fibers of other motor units.[79–81] It has been documented by fiber density determinations with single-fiber electromyography (SFEMG) that a mean of 1.5 muscle fibers of the same motor unit lie adjacent to each other.[118] Recent studies with SFEMG showed that each low-threshold motor unit in the biceps brachii may contain approximately 70 muscle fibers and that each low-threshold motor unit in the tibialis anterior may contain approximately 120 muscle fibers.[86] Generally, large limb muscles contain a few hundred muscle fibers per motor unit, whereas there may be only a few muscle fibers per unit in the laryngeal and ocular muscles.[84] The area over which the fibers of the same motor unit is distributed is called the motor unit territory. In the biceps brachii and the tibialis anterior this territory has been found to have a diameter of 5 mm to 10 mm.[64,113]

In most normal muscles each muscle fiber has a single motor end-plate. Exceptions to this are the extraocular muscles[78] and a small percentage of limb muscles,[74] including the biceps brachii.[100] The end-plates are located in the end-plate zone, which is usually in the middle of the muscle. However, the position and shape of the end-plate zone may vary from muscle to muscle. In the biceps brachii most of the end-plates are distributed within an irregular band 5 mm wide, spread longitudinally over an area of 40 mm.[66] In contrast, the end-plates in the deltoid muscle are arranged in an irregular sinusoid that crosses the middle of the muscle transversely.[74] In the sartorius the end-plates may be scattered over the length of the muscle.[74] In the tibialis anterior the end-plates are located in the periphery of the muscle.[55]

The Normal MUP

The MUP is the summated activity of the electrical fields of synchronously firing muscle fibers of a motor unit. The MUP is representative of the electrical activity of only a fraction of the fibers of a motor unit. The shape of the MUP is determined by the action potentials generated by individual muscle fibers, volume conduction within the muscle, orientation of the muscle fibers to the recording electrode, temporal dispersion of the action potentials, the recording equipment, and the type of electrode used.[76, 83, 111] The distant muscle fibers add the low frequencies to the initial and terminal portions of the MUP,[65] whereas the muscle fibers closest to the needle, usually five to ten fibers,[123] are responsible for the high-frequency major-spike portion of the MUP. The majority of MUPs are well summated. A well-summated MUP recorded from outside the end-plate region appears triphasic with an initial and terminal positive deflection and a central negative spike (Fig. 3-16). When one is recording over the end-plate region, the initial positive phase is not recorded, and the MUP is biphasic, consisting of an abrupt negative spike followed by a positive deflection (Fig. 3-17).[65] When the MUP recording is close to the tendon of the muscle fiber, there is often a positive deflection toward the end of the MUP (Fig. 3-18).[89] In our experience this phenomenon is common in certain muscles, such as the triceps and quadriceps, but can be seen in most muscles, especially with monopolar needle recordings. In concentric needle recordings this wave may not be seen because it is seen equally by both the core and the cannula and is thus cancelled.[83]

Generally, the onset of the MUP is better defined than its end. For visual estimation the duration of the MUP is measured from when the signal leaves the baseline until it returns. The duration reflects the number of muscle fibers in the pickup area of the electrode.[54] For a diagrammatic representation of the MUP and its parameters, see Figure 3-19.

The amplitude is measured peak to peak.[67] It represents the density and diameter of muscle fibers within the unit and the temporal summation of the various fibers.[64] Area is measured by taking the integral of the wave within the MUP duration. Area probably reflects the number of

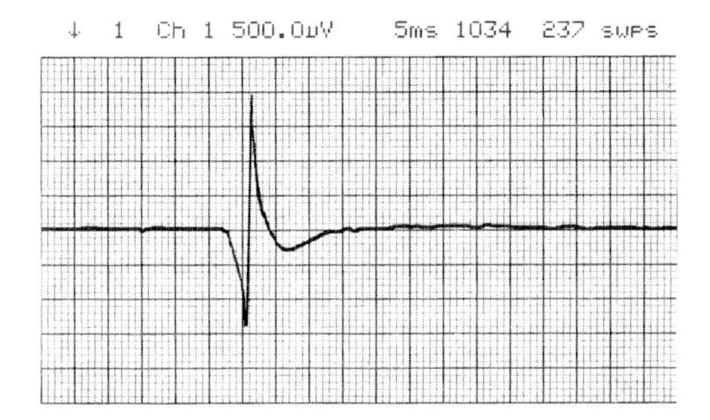

FIGURE 3-16 Averaged trace of a normal triphasic MUP. Calibrations: Sweep speed 5 msec/div., sensitivity 500 µV/div. Filter setting 20 Hz–10 kHz.

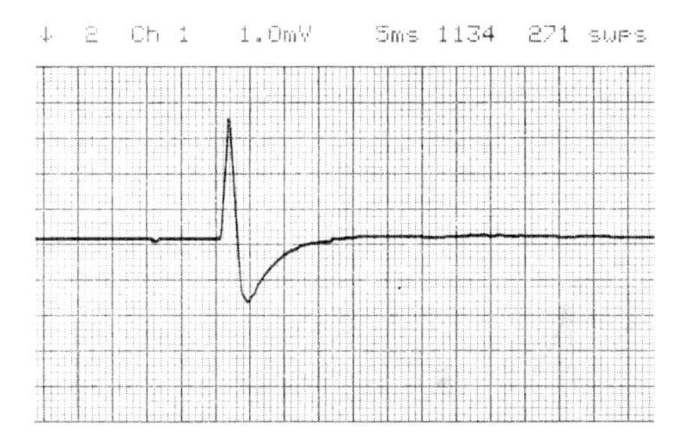

FIGURE 3-17 Averaged trace of a normal biphasic MUP recorded over the end-plate region of the muscle fibers. The initial deflection is negative, since the recording was done over the area of depolarization of the muscle fibers. Calibrations: Sweep speed 5 msec/div., sensitivity 1.0 mV/div. Filter setting 20 Hz–10 kHz.

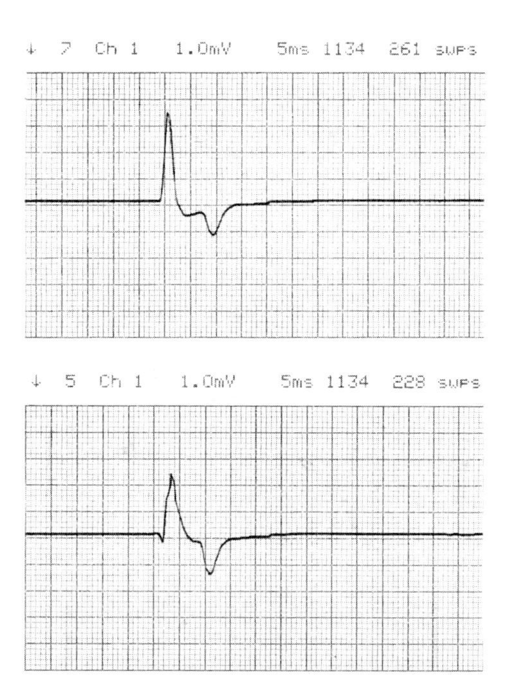

FIGURE 3-18 Averaged traces of MUPs showing positive deflections in the latter parts. These positive deflections occur when the recordings are done from the tendinous region of the muscle fibers. Calibrations: Sweep speed 5 msec/div., sensitivity 1.0 mV/div. Filter setting 20 Hz–10 kHz.

muscle fibers closest to the electrode but over a slightly larger territory than is reflected by amplitude measurements.[112] A phase is the section of the MUP that lies between two baseline crossings. The number of phases in an MUP is defined as the number of baseline crossings plus one. A turn is a polarity reversal with certain amplitude criteria between the previous turn and the next peak. For amplitude criteria, see Personal Experiences on Quantitative Analysis of the MUP on Minimal Contraction, later in this chapter. A certain percentage of the MUPs have more than four phases and are termed polyphasic MUPs. Those with more than four turns are known commonly as complex or serrated MUPs. Complex MUPs and polyphasic MUPs are caused by temporal dispersion. The ability to summate synchronously depends on the length of the nerve terminals, the rate of conduction along the nerve terminals and muscle fibers, the location of the end-plates on the muscle fibers, and the distance between the muscle fibers and the recording electrode. The spike duration (peak duration) is

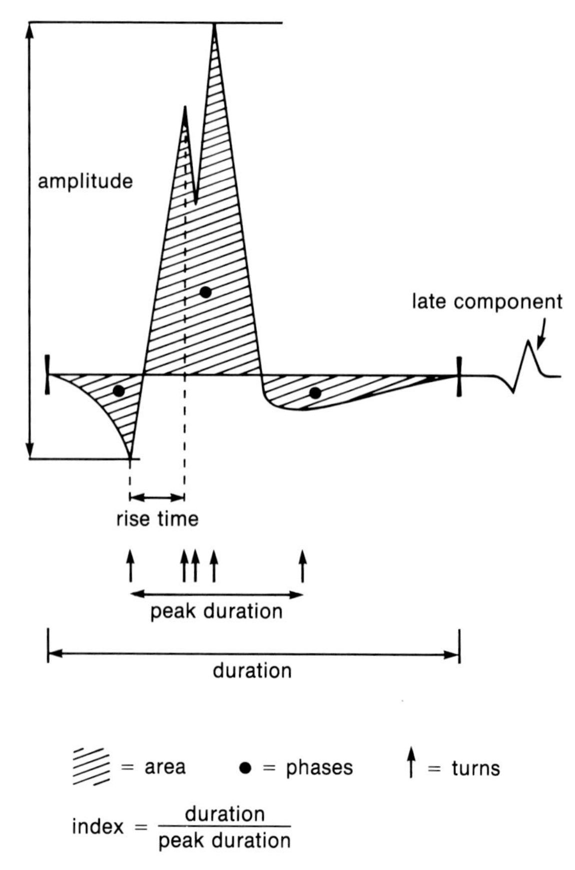

FIGURE 3-19 Diagrammatic representation of the MUP and its parameters.

the duration between the first and last turn and reflects the temporal dispersion of the muscle fibers closest to the electrode. Another important parameter for studying the MUP is variation in shape with consecutive discharges. This can be studied even with conventional EMG using a low-frequency filter of 500 Hz.[103,125] Normally the shape of the MUP is stable from one discharge to the next. It may vary in diseases such as myasthenia gravis and early reinnervation because of the increased jitter and blocking in the single-fiber action potentials that compose the MUP (Figs. 3-20 and 3-21).

Sometimes late components that are time locked to the spike segment may be seen at the end of the potential after the potential has returned to the baseline. Occasionally, it may be seen at the start of the potential. Although a definition of the term *late component* has not been completely formulated, any potential that is a part of an MUP and begins 2 msec or more after the spike segment of the MUP is generally considered a late component.[112] The late component usually represents the action potential of one muscle fiber.[69,77,98,119] It is formed because of depolarization from a newly regenerated nerve terminal that is conducting slowly because of poor myelination, or it may be due to the presence of ectopic end-plates or regenerating muscle fibers.[97] Usually, late components are rare, but in the biceps brachii, 5% of the MUPs may have a late component. Normally, it is very rare to see more than one late component to a single MUP (except, in our experience, in certain muscles such as the adductor longus). Since the late component is from only a single muscle fiber, the variability in neuromuscular transmission time (jitter) can easily be observed even while one is performing conventional electrodiagnosis, especially when the examination is performed with a 500-Hz–10-kHz filter (see Figs. 3-20 and 3-21).

It must be noted that the MUP parameters are different for different muscles[68] and may also vary with temperature,[65] age,[110] sex, and the degree of contraction. The MUP will increase in duration by approximately 10% per degree Celsius of temperature drop from 37° C to 30° C and by approximately 30% per degree Celsius from 30° C to 20° C.[65] The amplitude decreases 2% to 5% per degree Celsius fall in intramuscular temperature below 37° C. The percentage of polyphasic MUPs increases from 3% at 37° C to 10% to 15% at 30° C and 30% to 45% at 25° C.[65]

An increase in MUP duration with aging has been noted. The rate of increase is faster up to the age of 20 years than it is afterwards. The increase in duration has been attributed to the increase of the end-plate zone with growth of the muscles.[110] Amplitude and area are larger in males than in females owing to larger fiber diameter in males.[60] With increasing force of contraction, larger motor units are recruited. Therefore, MUP parameters obtained with low-threshold contraction are specific only for the same degree of contraction.

Technical Aspects of Recording the MUP

EMG Equipment

The filter settings suggested for accurate representation of the MUP are 2 Hz–10 kHz.[65] We have routinely used filter settings of 20 Hz–10 kHz and

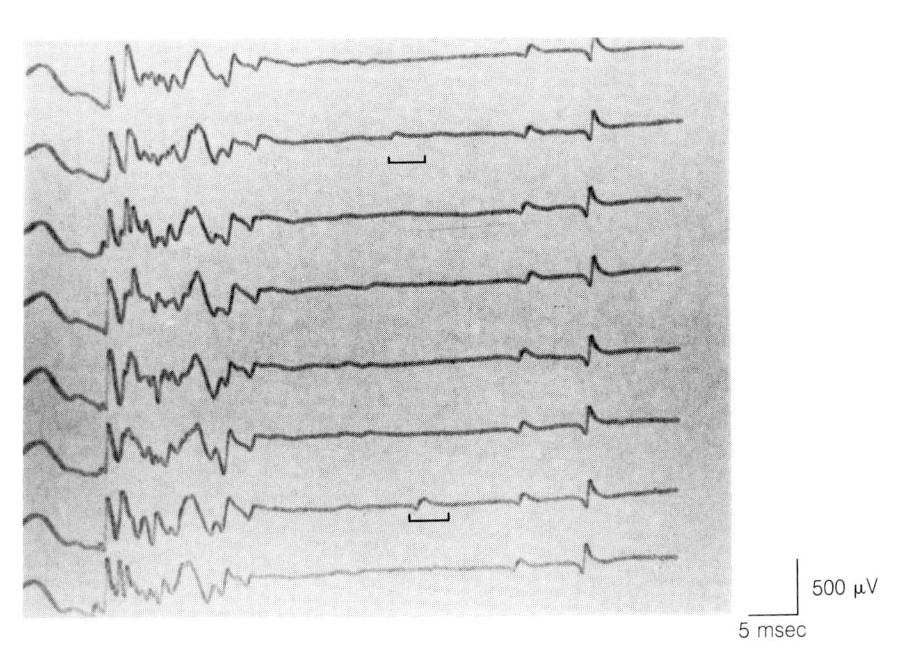

FIGURE 3-20 Serial discharges of a very complex polyphasic MUP seen in a patient with early reinnervation after a peripheral nerve injury. The recording is done with a monopolar needle. There is tremendous variation in shape of the main part of the complex polyphasic MUP. The small late components in the middle of the second trace from the top (*between brackets*) and the second trace from the bottom (*between brackets*) are often seen to block. The two late components at the far right of each show increased jitter. The jitter and variation in shape can be seen even with the monopolar needle when the low frequencies are restricted by using the filter setting of 500 Hz–10 kHz. Calibrations: Sweep speed 5 msec/div., sensitivity 500 μV/div. Filter setting: 500 Hz–10 kHz. Fiberoptic paper speed 5 cm/sec.

have found them to give MUP parameters comparable to those obtained with settings of 2 Hz–10 kHz, except for shorter durations.[73] If the low-frequency filter is set very low, excessive fluctuation of the baseline creates difficulty in recording the MUPs owing to intermittent blocking of the amplifiers. If the low-frequency filter is raised to 500 Hz, extra phases are induced.[115] With an increase of the high-limit filter, excessive noise from the electronic circuits interferes with the recordings.[115] When the high-frequency filter is reduced, depression of the spiky portion of the MUP occurs.

Use of a trigger circuit and delay line allows for detailed analysis of the MUP,[102,103] and the recording can be analyzed on line.

The suggested sweep speed setting for MUP analysis is 5 msec/div. The sensitivity is adjusted accordingly so that the peak-to-peak amplitude can be analyzed without overloading the amplifier. MUP parameters obtained from a given muscle with a given type of recording electrode are specific only to a given calibration of sweep speed and sensitivity.

The filter frequency used for sampling MUPs should be at least twice that of the highest frequency contained in the MUP to avoid aliasing.[57] Normal MUPs are adequately sampled at 5–10 kHz, while frequencies in the range of 10–20 kHz are desirable for sampling those with rise times of 100 μsec.[112]

The Recording Electrodes

Two commonly used needles in EMG are concentric and monopolar needles (Fig. 3-22). The concentric electrode records the potential differ-

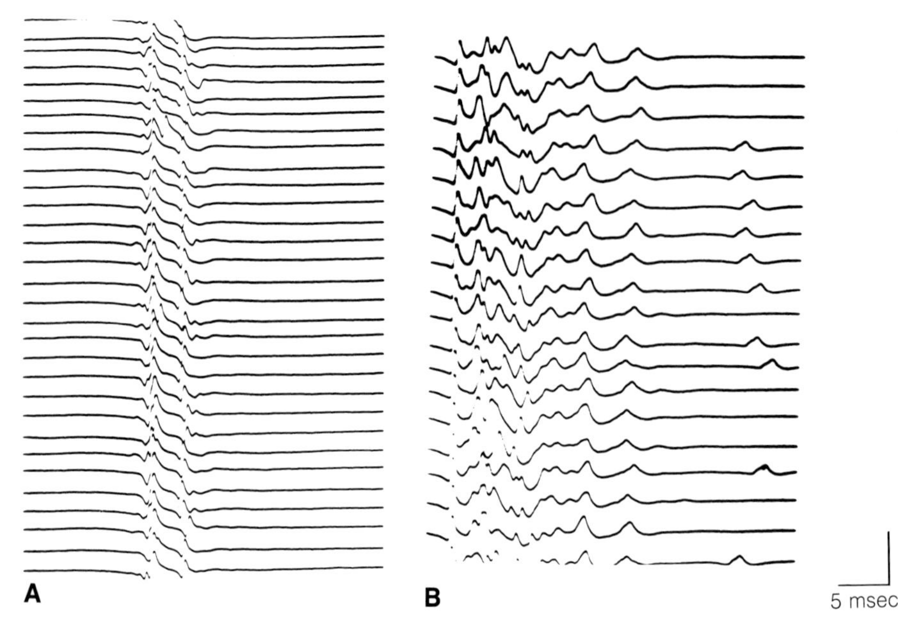

FIGURE 3-21 (A) Serial monopolar-needle recordings of a polyphasic MUP demonstrate shape variation at consecutive discharges. (B) A very complex polyphasic MUP with late components. The main portion of the MUP seen at the left end of the trace shows marked variation in shape with consecutive discharges. The late components at the far right are seen to have increased jitter and blocking. Calibrations: Sweep speed 5 msec/div., sensitivity 500 μV/div. Filter setting 500 Hz–10 kHz. Fiberoptic paper speed 5 cm/sec.

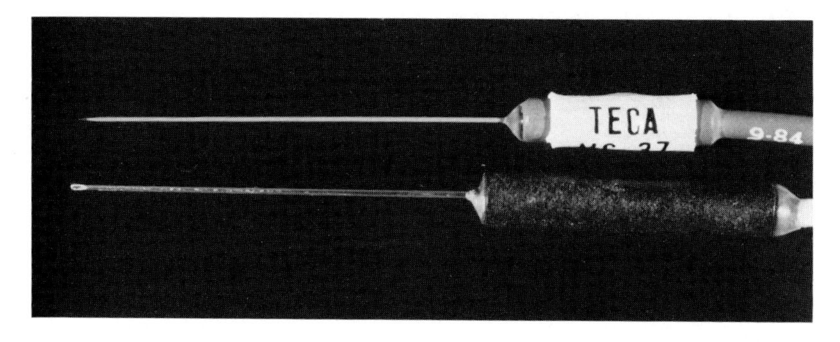

FIGURE 3-22 (*Top*) Monopolar needle with a recording area of 0.17 mm^2. (*Bottom*) Concentric needle with a recording area of 0.07 mm^2.

ence between the active core electrode and the cannula. Since tissue-to-core impedance is larger than tissue-to-cannula impedance, use of the concentric electrode reduces the common mode-rejection ratio of the amplifier. This necessitates use of a high-input impedance differential amplifier.[65] The recording area of the concentric needle is 0.07 mm^2. The recording surface, with dimensions of 580 μm × 150 μm, is asymmetrical with reference to the axis of the needle. Since the active and reference electrodes are in close proximity, the contributions of the electrical fields from the distant fibers are seen almost equally and are therefore not recorded. The recordings made with this needle are more selective than those of the monopolar electrode. However, the cannula may also record fibers close to it, and the activity of these fibers may be seen with inverse polarity before or after the main complex. The depth of recording may change the amplitude of the MUP, with higher amplitudes and longer durations seen at a deeper insertion, since the cannula then acts as a true reference electrode.[65,107,113] The angle with which the recording is done may also affect the amplitude of the MUP.[71]

The monopolar needle has a symmetrical recording area and has a larger area of exposed surface (0.17 mm^2). The reference electrode is usually placed on the skin. For these reasons the recordings obtained with the monopolar needle differ from those obtained with a concentric needle. Because the exposed area of the monopolar needle is larger, it has a lower impedance than that of the amplifier. Consequently, a fairly high common-mode rejection ratio can be obtained.[65] Because of its larger recording area, the MUP amplitudes and durations are larger than those recorded by the concentric needle.[88] In our experience the percentage of polyphasic MUPs is also higher than that recorded with the concentric needle. It must be noted that monopolar needles from different manufacturers may have different recording characteristics.

Methods for Studying MUP Parameters

The parameters of the MUP have been quantitated by Buchthal and colleagues using manual methods.[65] The MUPs were recorded on film, and an MUP was accepted for analysis if it appeared several times with similar shape. No attempts were made to achieve maximal amplitude with this method.[65]

It has been noted that the descriptive approach to MUP analysis is not sufficient for diagnosis of neuromuscular disease.[75,82] Recently, computerized analysis of the MUP has become possible.[58,59,91,95,96,100,108,114,121] One of the methods involves using the computer to choose an MUP from a series of MUPs. The selected MUP then serves as a template.[58,59,99,114,121] An MUP is analyzed when three to eight MUPs similar to the template are found. These MUPs may be averaged to improve the quality of the recordings. If no similar MUPs are found, a new template is chosen, and the previous template is discarded. A limitation of this method is that it fails to identify MUPs with shape variation at consecutive discharges.[112] The baseline is also noisier with the template method of MUP analysis.

MUP potential analysis may also be performed by the averaging method.[98] With this method an MUP is triggered for study. To analyze a specific MUP when several are firing simultaneously, a peak detector is used. This detector triggers the MUP from either the positive or negative peak within an adjustable window. The MUP that is triggered with either method is delayed and then averaged. A good signal-to-noise ratio is obtained after 16 to 512 runs.[112] If jitter and blocking are present, a given late component of an MUP may appear only intermittently or at varied intervals after the MUP. When that MUP is averaged, the effect is consequently to smooth out the MUP so that the presence of the late component is not apparent, or the late component may be distorted. Similarly, if there is instability in the muscle fibers giving rise to the turns in the spike portion of the MUP, averaging will result in loss of some turns, and the averaged trace appears smoother (Figs. 3-23 through 3-25). With the averaging method it is essential that only a single MUP be averaged. If more than one MUP is averaged, that trace must be discarded.

Practical Aspects of MUP Analysis on Minimal Contraction

Usually, before starting MUP analysis, we briefly explain the procedure to the patient so that he is able to give the proper amount of minimal contraction. To perform MUP analysis, instruct patient to listen to the firing rate of the MUP generated by a slight contraction. Ask him to keep the MUP firing constantly at a particular rate. If the patient relaxes too much, the MUP under study may be lost. Tell the patient immediately to contract again lightly, and if the needle has been held steady, the same MUP may sometimes be recruited if the effort of contraction is equivalent to the previous effort.

The positions for minimal contraction specifically described in Chapter 2 will facilitate the MUP analysis. Usually, a gravity-eliminating position is used so that the weak contraction required can be sustained for longer periods. This is important when the MUPs must be triggered and delayed to be studied in detail. It is easier to contract one MUP at a time without the influence of gravity.

Hold the needle in a manner similar to holding

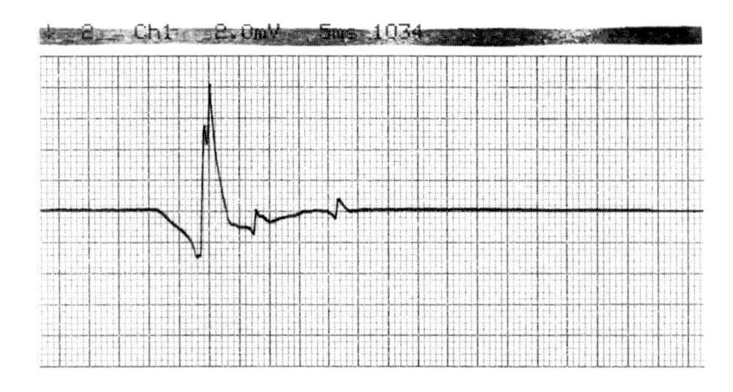

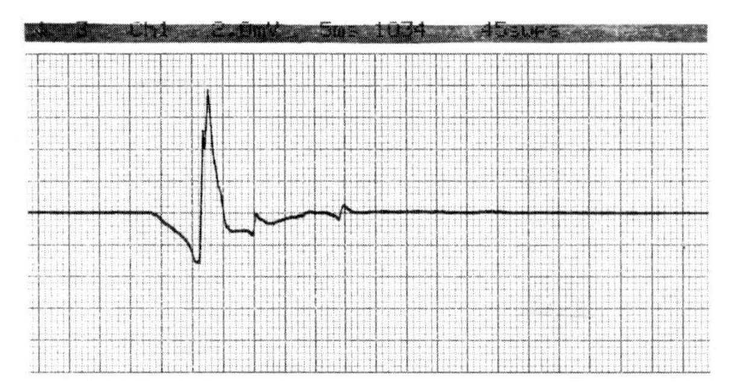

FIGURE 3-23 Influence of averaging on the MUP. (*Top*) A nonaveraged trace of an MUP. (*Bottom*) The same MUP after averaging. The two traces appear identical because the MUP components, including the late components, are stable. Calibrations: Sweep speed 5 msec/div., sensitivity 2.0 mV/div. Filter setting 20 Hz–10 kHz.

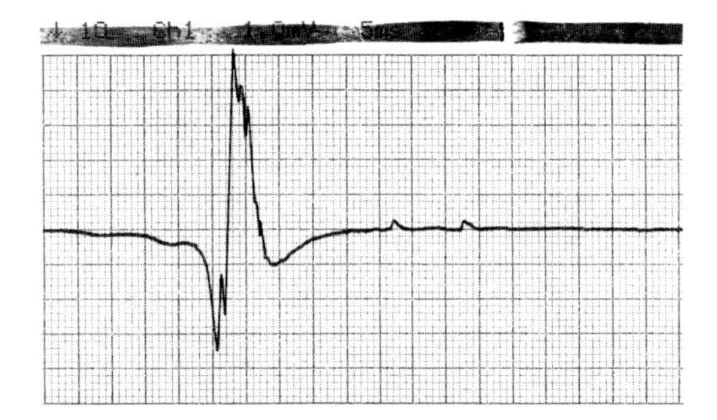

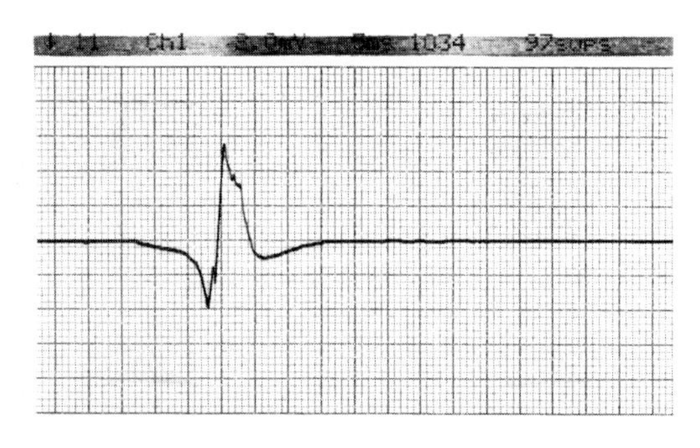

FIGURE 3-24 Influence of averaging on the MUP. (*Top*) Nonaveraged trace shows an MUP with two late components. Calibrations: Sweep speed 5 msec/div., sensitivity 1.0 mV/div. (*Bottom*) Same MUP after averaging. The presence of increased jitter and blocking in the late components led to the cancellation of the late components with averaging. This trace is displayed at a sensitivity of 2.0 mV/div. to show the peak-to-peak configuration of the MUP. Filter setting 20 Hz–10 kHz.

a pencil. Use your two medial fingers and wrist for support. Let the pulps of these two fingers rest lightly on or near the muscle under study. The needle is usually best held vertically or at a slight tangent, but the ultimate position depends on the direction of the muscle fibers.

The aim in positioning the electrode is to obtain a short rise time. The rise time is the time between the peak of the first positive deflection and the peak of the highest negative deflection. Rise time should be less than 500 μsec.[92] Manipulate the needle until the most spiky part of the potential has maximum negative polarity. This indicates that the needle is probably within 500 μm of the active fibers (Fig. 3-26). If the MUP has a prolonged rise time or a maximum amplitude in the positive direction, the needle is too far from the active muscle fibers. Such an MUP frequently has a falsely prolonged duration because there is a long negative deflection at the tail end of the potential (Fig. 3-27). This is more pronounced with monopolar than with concentric needle recordings. To get optimal recordings of the MUP the needle manipulation must be done with very fine coordinated movements. To improve the particular recording of an MUP, the needle is usually minimally rotated, moved slightly deeper, or retracted. As the needle approaches the area of the active muscle fibers, the MUP sounds also become crisper. The move-

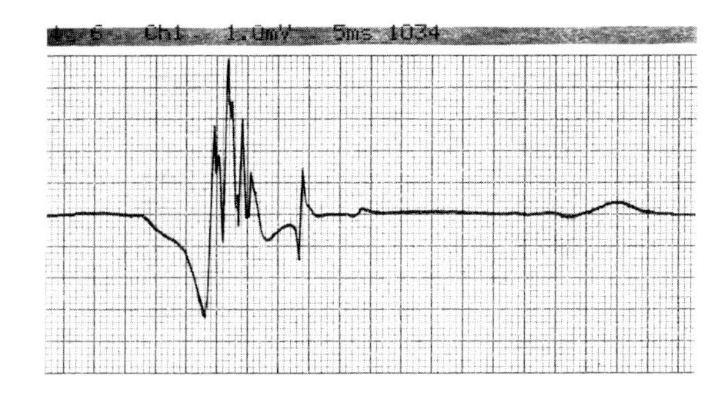

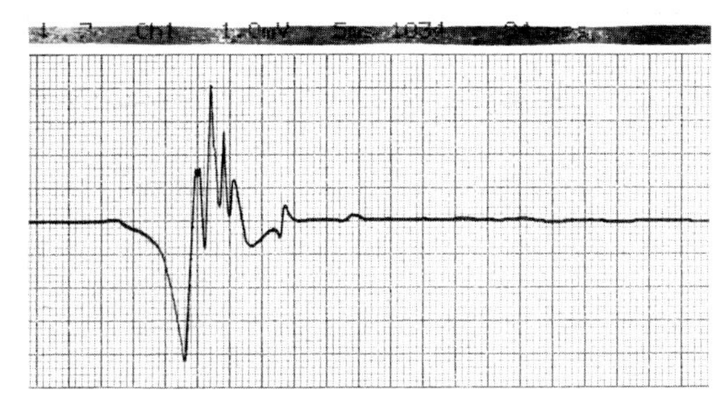

FIGURE 3-25 Influence of averaging on the MUP. (*Top*) A nonaveraged trace of a complex polyphasic MUP. (*Bottom*) The same MUP has been averaged, and the trace apppears smoother owing to the loss of some turns. This occurs when the MUP components are unstable owing to the presence of increased jitter. Calibrations: Sweep speed 5 msec/div., sensitivity 1.0 mV/div. Filter setting 20 Hz–10 kHz.

ments of the needle should be on the order of 0.1 mm to 0.3 mm. To ensure that different areas of the muscle are recorded, recording sites should be at least 3 mm apart.

The same MUP must be seen with the same amplitude and shape at least three to ten consecutive times to be superficially assessed. Many MUP parameters cannot be obtained with a free-running oscilloscope, thus limiting the information available with this method. A storage oscilloscope may be used to store the MUPs for more complete analysis. The disadvantage with this method is that two or more MUPs firing closely may be misinterpreted as a single polyphasic or complex MUP. In addition, MUP morphology cannot be seen in detail. The late components in particular may be missed. The optimal method for MUP analysis is to use a trigger circuit and delay line and, if necessary, to average the MUP as described previously so that the morphology can be assessed in detail. Averaging allows for the cancellation of artifacts or of MUPs that are not discharging synchronously with the triggered MUP.

MUP analysis should include measurement of the following parameters: amplitude, duration, area, number of phases and turns, and stability of the various components. Quantitation of the percentage of polyphasic MUPs is essential. The percentage of MUPs with one or more late components should also be noted.

Routinely, 20 MUPs are recorded in each muscle at multiple recording sites. The recording sites can be either within the same skin insertion point or at two to four different skin insertion sites. One abnormal MUP out of 20 is not considered significant for pathology. A 20% deviation from mean values may be useful for diagnosis of abnormality.[109] Using a range of values with defined upper and lower limits, as in macro EMG and jitter analysis,[116,118] may enable the electromyographer to detect abnormalities in an individual MUP even though the mean values of the parameters may still be normal. In our laboratory we consider a value three standard deviations above the mean to be abnormal. We use the lowest values found in our collection of normal data as the lower limit of normal. However, it may be necessary for each laboratory to set its own limits of normal.

When abnormalities are found, a thorough search must be done to see whether the abnormalities correlate with a specific lesion of a peripheral nerve, plexus, root, or anterior horn cell. Muscle cell diseases and neuromuscular junction transmission disorders must also be considered. The investigation should be extended to include all four extremities and the face, if needed.

MUPs in Nerve Disease—Neurogenic Reinnervation

In the early stages of reinnervation, MUPs are polyphasic, complex, of long duration, and of small amplitude. The newly incorporated muscle fibers may be seen as late components of the main MUP (Figs. 3-28 and 3-29, B and C). Unstable components show increased jitter and blocking (see Figs. 3-20 and 3-21). This phenomenon will remain as long as reinnervation continues and immature end-plates are present. Blocking has been noted to disappear 3 months

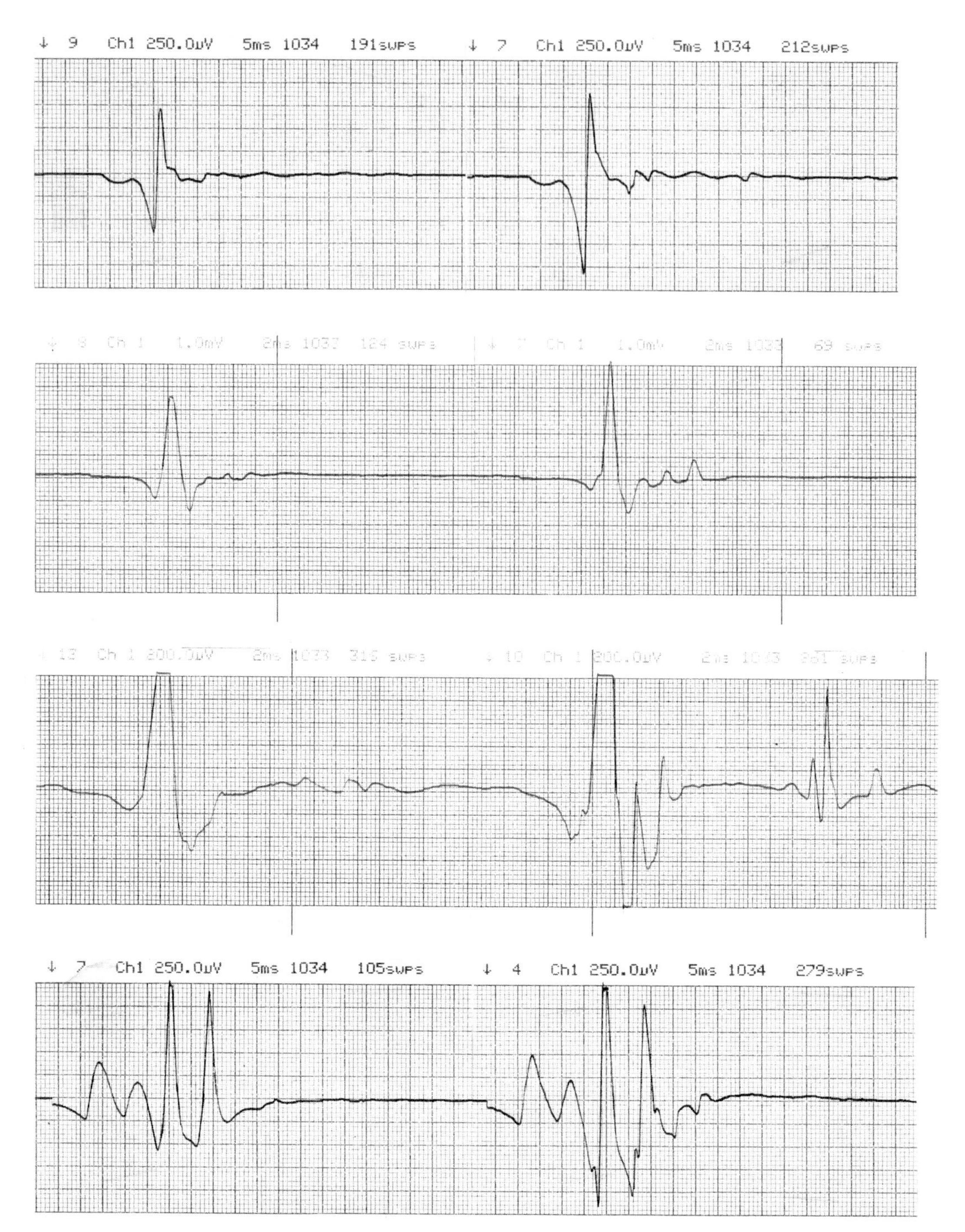

FIGURE 3-26 This series of tracings shows the influence of the position of the recording electrode on the MUP. The MUPs on the left were recorded with the needle at a position distant from the active muscle fibers. Those on the right are the same MUPs recorded by manipulating the needle so that the rise time is less than 500 μsec, indicating that the needle is within 0.3 mm of the active muscle fibers. Note that the MUPs on the right show more phases and turns, and the late components are well defined. Calibrations: All traces have been averaged and were recorded with sensitivity of 200 μV–250 μV/div., except for the second trace, which was recorded with sensitivity of 1.0 mV/div. The sweep speed for all traces is 5 msec/div. Filter setting 20 Hz–10 kHz.

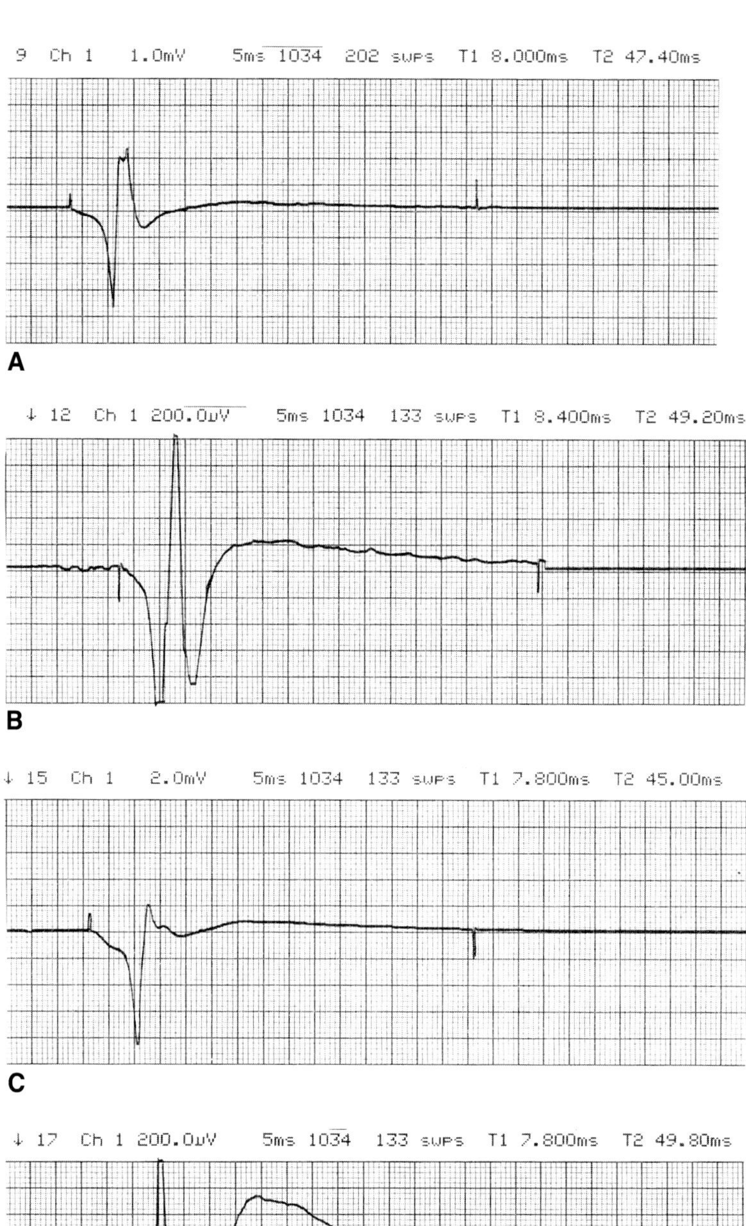

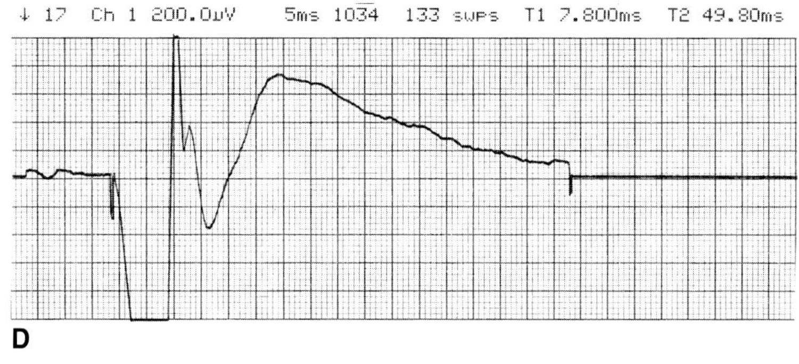

FIGURE 3-27 (A) An MUP in which the amplitude of the initial phase is more positive than the amplitude of the following negative phase. (B) The same MUP at an averager display gain of 200 μV/div. to illustrate falsely prolonged duration due to the formation of a negative deflection toward the end of the MUP. (C) Another MUP in which the amplitude of the initial positive phase is considerably larger than that of the following negative phase. (D) The same MUP seen in C at an averager display gain of 200 μV/div. The terminal negative deflection is seen to be more pronounced, which again falsely prolongs the duration. Calibrations: Sweep speed 5 msec/div., sensitivity 1.0 mV and 2.0 mV/div., respectively, for A and C. Sensitivity 200 μV/div. for B and D. Filter setting 20 Hz–10 kHz. *Note*: Vertical line indicators demarcate the duration in all traces. All traces have been averaged.

after reinnervation as the motor end plates mature.[118] Since conventional EMG records the summated activity of many muscle fibers, the detection of increased jitter and blocking may not be reliable. However, it can be suspected when variability of the amplitude and shape of the MUP is seen. When late components are present, the chance of detecting increased jitter and blocking on conventional EMG increases, since the late components usually represent the

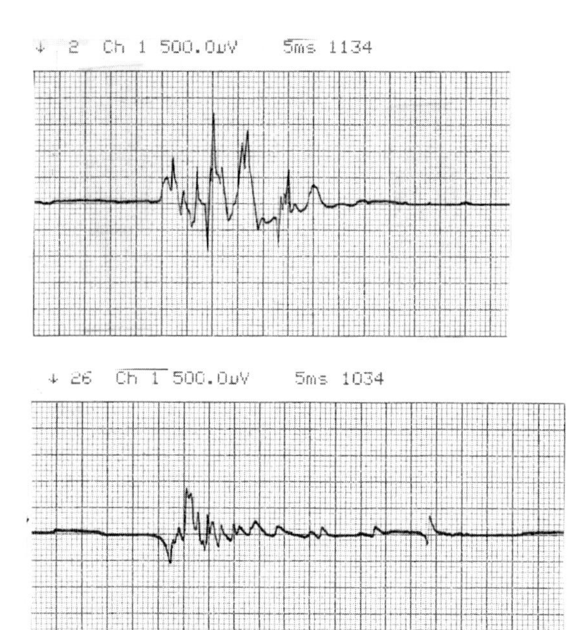

FIGURE 3-28 Very complex long-duration polyphasic MUPs. Calibrations: Sweep speed 5 msec/div., sensitivity 500 μV/div. Filter setting 20 Hz–10 kHz.

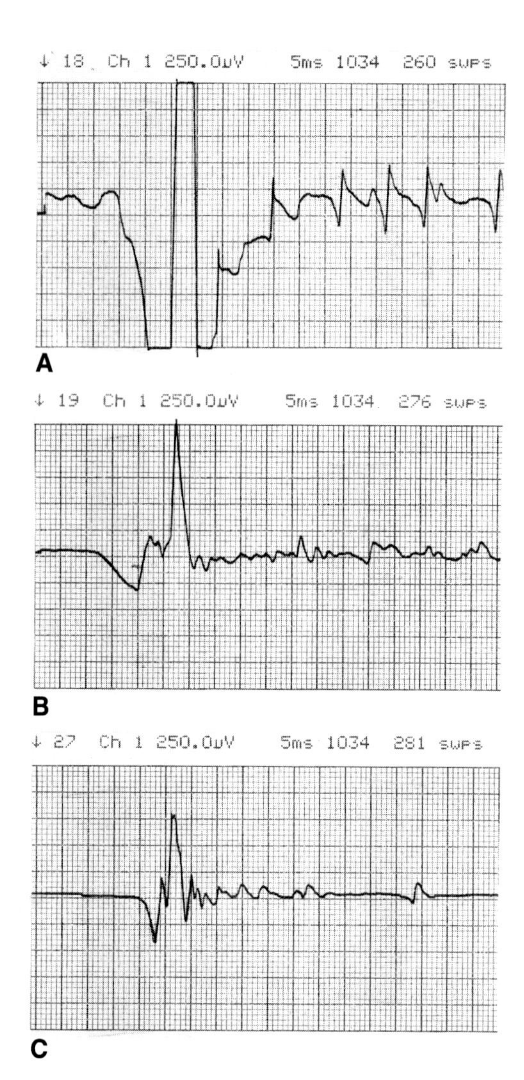

FIGURE 3-29 (A) An MUP that is of large amplitude and long duration because of chronic extensive re-innervation. However, there are multiple late components attached to the main MUP, indicating that the reinnervation is ongoing. (B and C) Very complex long-duration polyphasic MUPs. In both cases the main portion of the MUP is still of low amplitude, indicating that the reinnervation is more recent. Calibrations: Sweep speed 5 msec/div., sensitivity 250 μV/div. Filter setting 20 Hz–10 kHz.

action potentials of single muscle fibers. If doubt persists after conventional EMG, SFEMG may be performed in the muscle under suspicion for documentation of increased jitter or blocking. As the reinnervation process matures and becomes chronic, the MUPs appear very stable. They also become large in amplitude and long in duration and may become triphasic (Fig. 3-30) or noncomplex polyphasic in shape (Fig. 3-31). In anterior horn cell diseases, in which there is extensive collateral reinnervation over an extended period, amplitudes of the MUPs may be on the order of 10 mV or more (Fig. 3-32). If slow, ongoing denervation recurs, evidence of ongoing reinnervation can be observed as late components attached to the chronically enlarged triphasic or polyphasic MUP (Figs. 3-29, A, and 3-33).

MUPs *in Muscle Disease*

Generally, the MUPs in muscle disease are small in amplitude and short to normal in duration (Fig. 3-34).[62] There is a higher number of polyphasic MUPs. The reduced amplitude occurs because there is loss of muscle fibers and there are fewer muscle fibers per motor unit. This reduces the duration because the low-frequency contributions from the distant muscle fibers cannot be detected. The percentage of polyphasic MUPs in-

FIGURE 3-30 Averaged trace of a large-amplitude, long-duration triphasic MUP seen at calibrations of 200 μV/div. and sweep speed 5 msec/div. Filter setting 20 Hz–10 kHz.

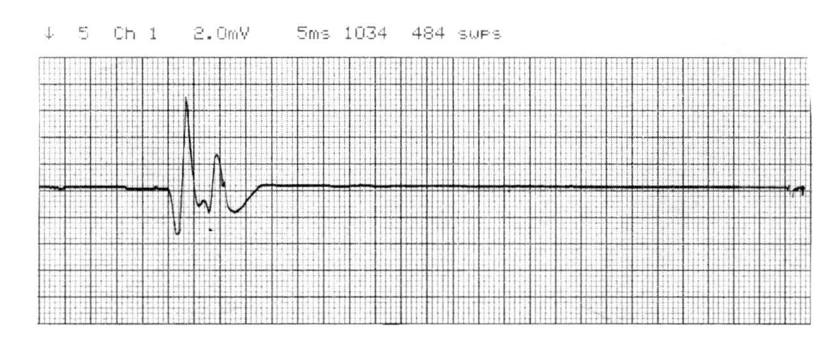

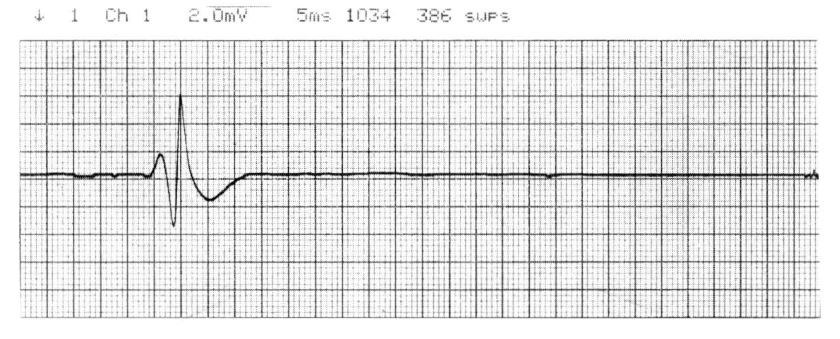

FIGURE 3-31 Averaged traces of large-amplitude, long-duration polyphasic MUPs indicating matured or completed extensive collateral reinnervation. Calibrations: Sweep speed 5 msec/div., sensitivity 2.0 mV/div. Filter setting 20 Hz–10 kHz.

creases because patchy loss of muscle fibers results in asynchronous summation and because of impaired propagation of impulses along the degenerating muscle membrane.[118] Splitting of the muscle fibers and muscle fiber budding increase the percentage of polyphasic MUPs. In addition, reinnervation of sequestered muscle fiber segments results in complex, long-duration, low-amplitude MUPs with multiple late components.

MUPs *in* Neuromuscular Transmission Defects

The MUPs in neuromuscular transmission defects may be normal in duration and amplitude at the beginning of the examination but may have varying amplitudes and shape as it progresses and fatigue sets in. If neuromuscular transmission defects are suspected, the patient must have repetitive stimulation studies; if these are nonconfirmatory, the patient should be referred to special EMG laboratories where SFEMG can be performed (Chap. 7). The presence of instability in the shape of the MUP due to increased jitter and blocking of its components is not indicative of myasthenia gravis but results from uncertain neuromuscular transmission. Routine conventional EMG must always be performed in cases of myasthenis gravis to detect or rule out concomitant disorders such as thyrotoxic myopathy, polymyositis, and steroid myopathy.[105]

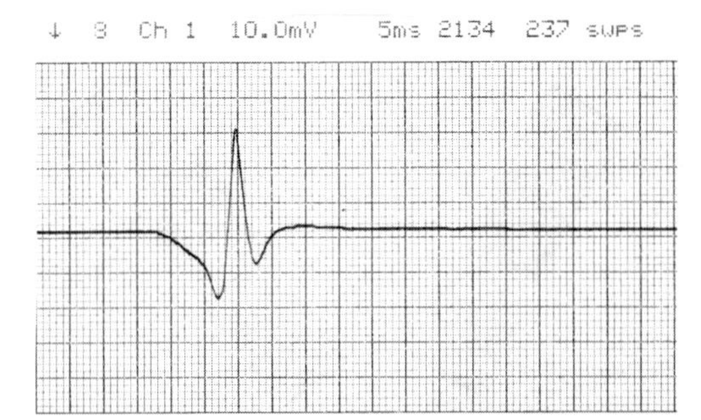

FIGURE 3-32 Averaged trace of a large-amplitude, long-duration triphasic MUP indicating matured or completed extensive collateral reinnervation. Calibrations: Sweep speed 5 msec/div., sensitivity 10.0 mV/div. Filter setting 20 Hz–10 kHz.

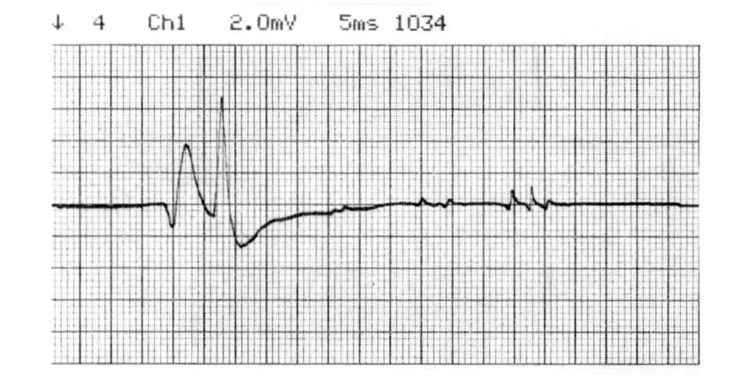

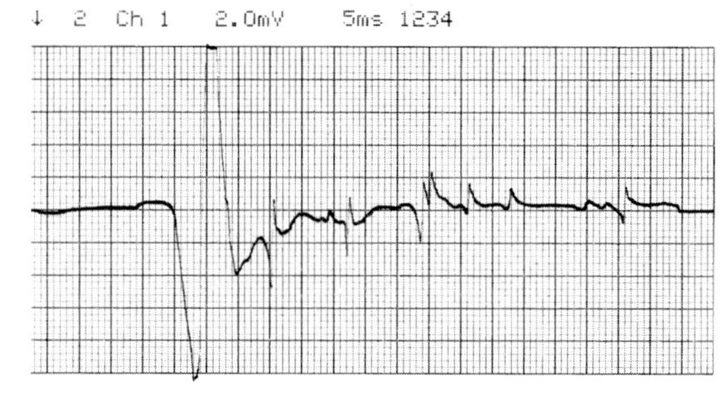

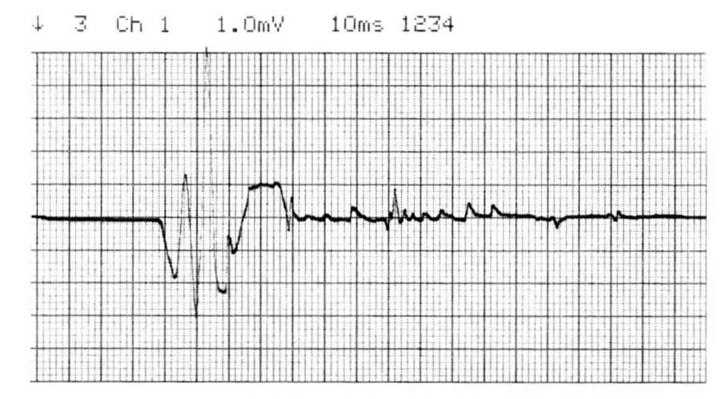

FIGURE 3-33 Large-amplitude, long-duration polyphasic MUPs with multiple late components. The main portion of these MUPs are of large amplitude owing to chronic extensive reinnervation. The presence of late components indicates that the reinnervation is ongoing. Calibrations: Sweep speed 5 msec/div., sensitivity 2.0 mV/div. for the top two traces and 1.0 mV/div. for the bottom trace. Filter setting 20 Hz–10 kHz.

MUPs *in Other* Diseases

In disuse atrophy there is an increased percentage of polyphasic MUPs but no change in MUP amplitude or duration.[69] In myotonic dystrophy the changes in MUPs are similar to those in muscle diseases. In addition, there is the characteristic presence of myotonic discharges. In myotonia congenita the MUP duration and amplitude have been reported to be normal.[63, 69]

Personal Experiences *on* Quantitative *Analysis of the* MUP *on* Minimal Contraction

Jennifer Chu-Andrews
Francis L. Bruyninckx
Rai-Chi Chan

The results described in this section are those obtained in our laboratory using the automatic MUP analysis program developed by Swedish Electrophysiologic Software (SES).[117] We studied the various MUP parameters in several different muscles to establish normal values for these muscles using the monopolar needle for recording. Normal values for MUP parameters with concentric recordings are available,[68,110] but until now there have been no standardized values for monopolar needle recordings from different muscles. The muscles studies were chosen to give a good representation of proximal and distal muscles that can be used in the identification of myopathic and neurogenic processes. The muscles studied were the biceps (long head, C5), deltoid (middle portion, C6), triceps (lateral head, C7), extensor digitorum (communis) (C7, C8), adductor longus (L3), vastus lateralis (L4), tibialis anterior (L5), and medial gastrocnemius (S1).

Subjects were screened, prior to inclusion in the study, for evidence of either systemic disease

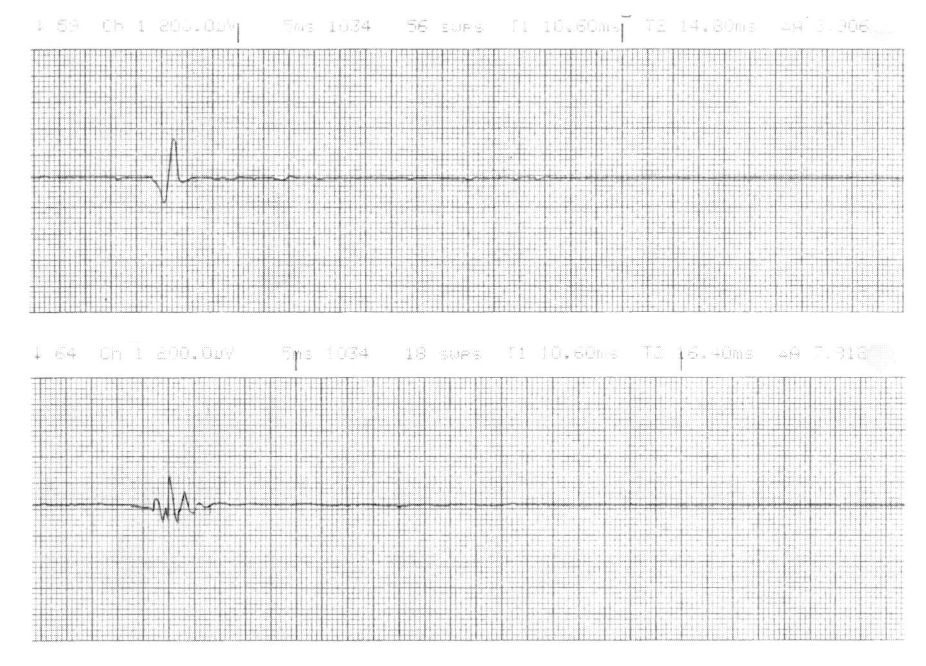

FIGURE 3-34 Averaged traces of small-amplitude, short-duration MUPs. The upper trace shows a triphasic MUP and the lower trace a polyphasic MUP. Calibrations: Sweep speed 5 msec/div., sensitivity 200 μV/div. Filter setting 20 Hz–10 kHz.

or peripheral problems in the muscles to be studied. Screening was on the basis of the history, clinical examination, and nerve conduction studies. To exclude the presence of peripheral neuropathy in these subjects, median and ulnar nerve conduction studies, including the F responses, and radial sensory nerve conductions were examined in the upper extremities. In the lower extremities the peroneal nerve (conduction studies, F responses), tibial nerve (conduction studies, F response from abductor hallucis and soleus and H reflex from soleus), and sural nerve were studied.

To establish normal values in the biceps, extensor digitorum (communis), and tibialis anterior, we studied ten normal subjects (five men and five women) from each decade between the ages of 20 and 76 years. Twenty MUPs were examined from each subject, for a total of 1000 MUPs. In each of the remaining muscles (deltoid, triceps, quadriceps, medial gastrocnemius) 400 MUPs were collected from 20 normal control subjects. Fifteen subjects were below and five subjects above age 60 years. Twenty subjects below the age of 40 years were also examined for MUP analysis in the adductor longus.

The EMG instrument used was the TECA* TD 20 interfaced with the Apple 2† minicomputer. All recordings were done with MG 37–type TECA monopolar needles with the surface reference electrode kept within 1 cm of the recording electrode. The MUPs accepted for analysis were those with rise times less than 500 μsec. The needle was manipulated to achieve this criterion. The MUPs were delayed, triggered, and averaged until the baseline on each side of the MUP was free from artifacts of 10-μV amplitude or more. This was usually achieved after 75 to 250 traces. The sweep speed used was 5 msec/div. The filter setting was 20 Hz–10 kHz. The analysis was done on line, and the data were stored on floppy diskette for further analysis.

The MUP analysis program from the SES was programmed to measure the following parameters:

Amplitude: Measured between the two highest peaks of the MUP

Duration: Measured from the time when the

* TECA Corporation, 3 Campus Drive, Pleasantville, NY 10570

† Apple 2 Computer, Inc., 10260 Bandley Drive, Cupertino, CA 95014

MUP left the baseline to the time of its return. Slope and amplitude criteria were used to pinpoint the exact time of departure and return of the signal to the baseline. The 50-μV levels of the MUP, as it first left and last returned to the baseline, were located. The starting point was found in the following way: from 10 msec before the first 50-μV point, a slope of 10 μV/msec (1-msec window) was identified, and then the 5-μV level is sought. The end point was found in the same way and defined by the 5-μV level.

Area: Measured as the integral of the rectified signal within its duration.

Phase: Any segment of the MUP that is between two consecutive baseline crossings, between the onset of the MUP and the first baseline crossing, or between the last baseline crossing and the return of the MUP to the baseline. The amplitude between the baseline crossings had to exceed 10 μV and the duration between the crossings more than 250 μsec for a phase to be counted.

Turn: A polarity reversal within the MUP. A turn was considered significant when there was at least 50 μV between the previous turn and the next polarity reversal under consideration.

Peak Duration: Measured as the time between the first and last significant turn of the MUP

Index: The ratio of MUP duration to peak duration

In addition to these parameters, the percentage of MUPs with at least five phases (polyphasic MUPs) and the percentage of MUPs with at least five turns (traditionally called complex or serrated MUPs and arbitrarily named polyturn MUPs) were analyzed. The MUP parameters are given in Tables 3-1 through 3-8.

The following major findings were seen on comparing the data from the different muscles:

Differences Among the Muscles

The MUPs of the biceps brachii were smallest in amplitude and area, had the shortest peak durations, and had the fewest phases and turns. These parameters indicate that the biceps brachii had smaller-sized MUPs that were also relatively simple in form. Like the biceps, the gactrocnemius and triceps also had MUPs that were relatively simple in form. MUPs in these muscles had fewer phases than did the other muscles. The gastrocnemius had the lowest percentage of MUPs with five or more turns. The triceps had

TABLE 3-1
MUP *Parameters in the Biceps* (Monopolar Needle Recordings)

Age (Years)	*Potentials* (No.)	*Amplitude* (mV)	*Duration* (msec)	*Peak Duration* (msec)	*Area* (msec mV)	*Phases* (No.)	*Turns* (No.)	*Index* (No.)	*Polyphasic* MUPs (%)	*Polyturn* MUPs (%)
20–29	200	0.6±0.3 (0.2–1.5)	15.1±4.1 (4.2–27.4)	2.2±1.6 (0.2–7.0)	0.9±0.5 (0.2–2.4)	3.2±0.8 (2.0–6.0)	2.9±1.1 (2.0–6.0)	12.4±11.6 (2.0–47.2)	10.0	10.0
30–39	200	0.6±0.3 (0.2–1.5)	14.0±3.2 (5.6–23.6)	2.0±1.4 (0.2–6.1)	0.8±0.4 (0.2–2.0)	3.3±0.8 (2.0–6.0)	2.9±1.1 (2.0–6.0)	13.9±13.5 (1.5–54.0)	15.0	10.0
40–49	200	0.7±0.3 (0.2–1.6)	14.7±4.2 (5.8–27.1)	2.3±2.2 (0.2–9.0)	0.9±0.5 (0.2–2.3)	3.4±0.9 (2.0–7.0)	3.1±1.2 (2.0–7.0)	11.9±10.4 (1.2–43.1)	10.0	20.0
50–59	200	0.8±0.4 (0.3–2.0)	14.7±3.6 (7.6–25.5)	2.4±1.8 (0.4–7.8)	1.0±0.5 (0.2–2.5)	3.3±1.2 (2.0–7.0)	3.3±1.1 (2.0–7.0)	11.8±10.3 (2.2–42.7)	15.0	15.0
Below 60	800	0.7±0.3 (0.2–1.6)	14.6±3.8 (4.2–26.0)	2.2±1.8 (0.2–7.6)	0.9±0.5 (0.2–2.4)	3.3±0.9 (2.0–6.0)	3.1±1.1 (2.0–6.0)	12.5±11.5 (1.2–47.0)	14.0±2.1 (5.0–20.0)	13.0±4.1 (5.0–25.0)
Above 60	200	0.9±0.4 (0.2–2.1)	16.2±4.5 (4.2–29.7)	2.9±2.1 (0.4–7.2)	1.3±0.6 (0.2–3.1)	3.4±1.0 (2.0–6.0)	3.3±1.4 (2.0–8.0)	9.4±8.8 (1.2–35.8)	15.0±4.0 (5.0–30.0)	17.0±2.1 (5.0–20.0)
All ages combined	1000	0.7±0.4 (0.2–1.9)	14.9±3.9 (4.2–26.6)	2.4±1.8 (0.2–7.8)	1.0±0.5 (0.2–2.5)	3.3±1.0 (2.0–6.0)	3.1±1.2 (2.0–7.0)	11.9±11.0 (1.2–44.9)	14.2±1.9 (5.0–20.0)	13.8±4.0 (5.0–25.0)

TABLE 3-2
MUP Parameters in the Deltoid (Middle Portion) (Monopolar Needle Recordings)

Age (Years)	Potentials (No.)	Amplitude (mV)	Duration (msec)	Peak Duration (msec)	Area (msec mV)	Phases (No.)	Turns (No.)	Index (No.)	Polyphasic MUPs (%)	Polyturn MUPs (%)
Below 60	300	0.9 ± 0.5 (0.2–2.4)	12.4 ± 1.9 (5.6–18.1)	2.7 ± 1.7 (0.2–7.8)	1.1 ± 0.6 (0.3–2.9)	3.4 ± 1.1 (2.0–7.0)	3.4 ± 1.3 (2.0–7.0)	8.3 ± 9.6 (1.4–37.1)	17.7 ± 9.0 (5.0–35.0)	20.0 ± 7.1 (5.0–40.0)
Above 60	100	0.9 ± 0.4 (0.2–2.1)	13.8 ± 1.9 (8.0–19.5)	3.0 ± 1.9 (0.2–8.7)	1.2 ± 0.6 (0.3–3.0)	3.6 ± 1.0 (2.0–7.0)	3.5 ± 1.3 (2.0–7.0)	10.5 ± 15.2 (1.6–56.1)	23.0 ± 4.5 (5.0–40.0)	24.0 ± 8.9 (5.0–50.0)
All ages combined	400	0.9 ± 0.5 (0.2–2.4)	12.7 ± 1.9 (5.6–18.4)	2.8 ± 1.7 (0.2–7.9)	1.1 ± 0.6 (0.3–3.0)	3.4 ± 1.4 (2.0–7.0)	3.4 ± 1.3 (2.0–7.0)	8.9 ± 11.3 (1.4–42.8)	19.0 ± 8.3 (5.0–40.0)	21.0 ± 8.7 (5.0–50.0)

TABLE 3-3
MUP Parameters in the Triceps (Lateral Head) (Monopolar Needle Recordings)

Age (Years)	Potentials (No.)	Amplitude (mV)	Duration (msec)	Peak Duration (msec)	Area (msec mV)	Phases (No.)	Turns (No.)	Index (No.)	Polyphasic MUPs (%)	Polyturn MUPs (%)
Below 60	300	1.4 ± 0.8 (0.3–3.8)	10.8 ± 2.2 (6.0–17.4)	3.1 ± 1.2 (0.4–6.7)	1.7 ± 0.8 (0.3–4.1)	3.1 ± 0.8 (2.0–6.0)	3.3 ± 1.1 (2.0–7.0)	4.2 ± 3.1 (1.5–13.5)	7.7 ± 5.5 (5.0–25.0)	16.1 ± 7.7 (5.0–40.0)
Above 60	100	1.4 ± 1.7 (0.5–3.5)	11.6 ± 1.8 (8.2–17.0)	3.3 ± 1.3 (0.4–7.2)	1.8 ± 0.8 (0.4–4.2)	3.3 ± 0.8 (2.0–6.0)	3.4 ± 1.0 (2.0–6.0)	4.3 ± 3.4 (1.6–14.5)	10.0 ± 3.5 (5.0–20.0)	14.0 ± 8.9 (5.0–40.0)
All ages combined	400	1.4 ± 0.7 (0.5–3.5)	11.0 ± 2.1 (6.0–17.3)	3.3 ± 1.2 (0.4–6.9)	1.7 ± 0.8 (0.3–4.9)	3.2 ± 0.8 (2.0–6.0)	3.4 ± 1.0 (2.0–6.0)	4.2 ± 3.1 (1.5–13.5)	8.3 ± 5.1 (5.0–20.0)	15.6 ± 7.8 (5.0–40.0)

TABLE 3-4
MUP Parameters in the Extensor Digitorum (Communis) (Monopolar Needle Recordings)

Age (Years)	Potentials (No.)	Amplitude (mV)	Duration (msec)	Peak Duration (msec)	Area (msec mV)	Phases (No.)	Turns (No.)	Index (No.)	Polyphasic MUPs (%)	Polyturn MUPs (%)
20–29	200	1.0 ± 0.5 (0.2–2.5)	14.5 ± 4.2 (4.8–27.1)	3.0 ± 1.7 (0.2–8.1)	1.3 ± 0.7 (0.2–3.4)	3.6 ± 1.1 (2.0–7.0)	3.5 ± 1.1 (2.0–7.0)	7.7 ± 7.2 (1.7–29.3)	20.0	20.0
30–39	200	1.0 ± 0.6 (0.2–2.8)	13.8 ± 2.6 (5.6–24.6)	3.3 ± 1.8 (0.4–8.5)	1.3 ± 0.7 (0.2–3.4)	3.6 ± 1.0 (2.0–7.0)	3.8 ± 1.4 (2.0–8.0)	6.3 ± 5.6 (1.5–23.1)	15.0	30.0
40–49	200	0.9 ± 0.6 (0.2–2.7)	13.8 ± 4.9 (7.0–28.5)	3.0 ± 1.8 (0.2–8.4)	1.1 ± 0.8 (0.2–3.5)	3.5 ± 1.1 (2.0–7.0)	3.5 ± 1.3 (2.0–7.0)	7.2 ± 6.9 (1.5–27.9)	15.0	20.0
50–59	200	1.0 ± 0.5 (0.3–2.5)	14.3 ± 4.9 (7.0–29.0)	2.9 ± 1.6 (0.4–6.1)	1.2 ± 0.7 (0.2–3.3)	3.7 ± 1.0 (2.0–7.0)	3.6 ± 1.3 (2.0–8.0)	7.4 ± 6.5 (1.5–26.9)	20.0	25.0
Below 60	800	0.9 ± 0.5 (0.2–2.4)	14.1 ± 4.4 (4.8–27.3)	3.0 ± 1.7 (0.2–8.1)	1.2 ± 0.7 (0.2–3.3)	3.8 ± 1.2 (2.0–7.0)	3.6 ± 1.3 (2.0–8.0)	7.1 ± 6.6 (1.5–26.9)	17.9 ± 2.4 (5.0–25.0)	24.6 ± 5.0 (5.0–40.0)
Above 60	200	1.1 ± 0.7 (0.2–3.1)	16.1 ± 6.5 (6.8–35.6)	3.2 ± 1.8 (0.2–8.6)	1.5 ± 0.9 (0.2–4.2)	3.6 ± 1.1 (2.0–7.0)	3.8 ± 1.4 (2.0–8.0)	8.0 ± 10.0 (1.5–38.0)	24.0 ± 5.5 (5.0–40.0)	31.5 ± 2.9 (5.0–40.0)
All ages combined	1000	1.0 ± 0.6 (0.2–2.8)	14.5 ± 4.9 (4.8–29.2)	3.1 ± 1.7 (0.2–8.2)	1.3 ± 0.8 (0.2–3.7)	3.6 ± 1.1 (2.0–7.0)	3.6 ± 1.3 (2.0–8.0)	7.3 ± 7.4 (1.5–29.5)	19.2 ± 3.6 (5.0–30.0)	26.0 ± 5.3 (5.0–40.0)

TABLE 3-5
MUP *Parameters in the Adductor Longus (Monopolar Needle Recordings)*

Age (Years)	*Potentials* (No.)	*Amplitude* (mV)	*Duration* (msec)	*Area* (msec mV)	*Phases* (No.)	*Turns* (No.)	*Polyphasic* MUPs (%)	*Polyturn* MUPs (%)
20–39	400	0.7±0.4 (0.2–1.9)	14.3±5.7 (3.8–31.4)	0.8±0.5 (0.2–2.3)	4.1±1.5 (2.0–7.0)	3.9±1.8 (2.0–10.0)	38.5	31.5

Note: MUPs with late components: 20.0%; MUPs with one late component: 17.5%; MUPs with two late components: 2.0%; MUPs with three/four late components: 0.5%.

TABLE 3-6
MUP *Parameters in the Vastus Lateralis (Monopolar Needle Recordings)*

Age (Years)	*Potentials* (No.)	*Amplitude* (mV)	*Duration* (msec)	*Peak Duration* (msec)	*Area* (msec mV)	*Phases* (No.)	*Turns* (No.)	*Index* (No.)	*Polyphasic* MUPs (%)	*Polyturn* MUPs (%)
Below 60	300	1.1±0.5 (0.3–2.6)	13.4±2.8 (6.2–21.8)	3.4±1.8 (0.4–8.8)	1.6±0.8 (0.4–4.0)	3.2±0.8 (2.0–6.0)	3.2±1.0 (2.0–6.0)	5.8±5.2 (1.5–21.4)	9.3±4.2 (5.0–20.0)	16.7±8.0 (5.0–40.0)
Above 60	100	1.4±0.8 (0.3–3.8)	14.5±3.4 (6.4–24.7)	4.2±2.2 (0.4–10.8)	2.1±1.0 (0.2–5.0)	3.4±1.1 (2.0–7.0)	3.8±1.4 (2.0–8.0)	5.5±6.2 (1.3–24.1)	15.0±7.9 (5.0–40.0)	29.0±9.9 (5.0–60.0)
All ages combined	400	1.2±0.6 (0.3–3.0)	13.7±2.9 (6.2–22.4)	3.6±1.9 (0.4–9.3)	1.7±0.9 (0.2–4.4)	3.2±0.9 (2.0–6.0)	3.4±1.1 (2.0–7.0)	5.7±5.5 (1.3–22.2)	10.8±5.2 (5.0–25.0)	19.8±9.3 (5.0–50.0)

the lowest percentage of MUPs with five or more phases. The tibialis anterior had MUPs with higher values for duration and area, indicating that this muscle has larger-sized MUPs. The adductor longus was unique among the muscles examined in that it had an unusually high number of MUPs with polyphases and polyturns.

Differences Between the Different Electrodes

MUPs recorded with the monopolar needle had higher mean values for amplitude, duration, and incidence of polyphases than MUPs recorded with the concentric needle. We found that the amplitude ranged from 0.2 mV to 3.8 mV, duration ranged 4.0 msec to 31.8 msec, and the percentage of polyphasic MUPs ranged from 5 to 40. Published values for amplitudes recorded with the concentric needle are in the ranges of 0.3 mV to 5.0 mV.[68] This range is larger than the one that we obtained with the monopolar recordings. The difference in the range of amplitudes may result from a difference in measurement techniques, since the present method of automatic analysis differs from the manual technique of the past. With concentric recordings, duration ranges from 3 msec to 16 msec, and the percentage of polyphasic MUPs ranges from 0.5 to 20.[68,122] The MUP parameters obtained by the two needles differ so greatly that normal values cannot be interchanged.

Sex Differences

Analysis of sex differences was done in the biceps, extensor digitorum (communis), and tibialis anterior. MUP potentials in men were significantly larger in amplitude and area in all three muscles ($P<0.01$). Duration was also longer in men ($P<0.01$), except in the biceps, where no significant differences were seen. The results for amplitude and area were in agreement with those found by Falck.[83] However, no differences in duration were found with different studies.[83, 94] No significant differences were seen between men and women in the number of phases or the index. No consistent differences were seen in the number of turns or the peak duration. These findings are in agreement with those of Falck.[83] Histolog-

TABLE 3-7
MUP *Parameters in the* Tibialis Anterior (*Monopolar* Needle *Recordings*)

Age (Years)	*Potentials* (*No.*)	*Amplitude* (*mV*)	*Duration* (*msec*)	*Peak Duration* (*msec*)	*Area* (*msec mV*)	*Phases* (*No.*)	*Turns* (*No.*)	*Index* (*No.*)	*Polyphasic* MUPs (%)	*Polyturn* MUPs (%)
20–29	200	1.0±0.6 (0.3–2.8)	15.5±4.8 (6.0–29.9)	2.9±1.6 (0.2–7.7)	1.3±0.7 (0.4–3.4)	3.6±1.0 (2.0–7.0)	3.6±1.4 (2.0–8.0)	8.3±8.7 (1.6–34.4)	20.0	25.0
30–39	200	1.0±0.5 (0.3–2.5)	15.1±3.7 (7.2–26.2)	3.5±2.3 (0.4–10.4)	1.4±0.8 (0.4–3.8)	3.6±1.1 (2.0–7.0)	3.6±1.5 (2.0–8.0)	7.1±6.5 (1.2–26.6)	20.0	20.0
40–49	200	1.3±0.7 (0.2–3.4)	16.1±5.6 (5.4–32.9)	3.6±1.8 (0.4–9.0)	1.9±1.1 (0.3–5.2)	3.6±1.0 (2.0–7.0)	3.9±1.4 (2.0–8.0)	6.2±4.1 (1.5–18.5)	15.0	30.0
50–59	200	1.2±0.6 (0.2–3.0)	16.4±5.2 (6.8–32.0)	3.7±2.1 (0.4–10.0)	1.9±1.0 (0.2–4.9)	3.5±1.0 (2.0–7.0)	3.7±1.2 (2.0–7.0)	6.0±4.4 (1.3–19.2)	15.0	30.0
Below 60	800	1.1±0.6 (0.2–2.9)	15.8±4.9 (5.4–30.5)	3.4±2.0 (0.2–6.4)	1.6±0.9 (0.2–4.3)	3.6±1.1 (2.0–7.0)	3.7±1.4 (2.0–8.0)	6.9±6.2 (1.2–25.5)	17.4±2.7 (5.0–25.0)	24.1±7.0 (5.0–45.0)
Above 60	200	1.4±0.9 (0.3–4.1)	18.1±6.3 (7.0–37.0)	3.6±2.1 (0.4–9.9)	1.9±1.2 (0.4–5.5)	3.9±1.4 (2.0–8.0)	4.0±1.5 (2.0–8.0)	7.2±6.0 (1.6–25.2)	23.5±4.9 (5.0–40.0)	35.5±3.3 (5.0–45.0)
All ages combined	1000	1.2±0.7 (0.2–3.3)	16.2±5.2 (5.4–31.8)	3.5±2.0 (2.0–9.5)	1.7±1.0 (0.2–4.7)	3.6±1.1 (2.0–7.0)	3.7±1.4 (2.0–8.0)	6.9±6.2 (1.2–25.5)	18.6±3.6 (5.0–30.0)	26.4±7.2 (5.0–45.0)

TABLE 3-8
MUP *Parameters in the* Medial Gastrocnemius (*Monopolar* Needle *Recordings*)

Age (Years)	*Potentials* (*No.*)	*Amplitude* (*mV*)	*Duration* (*msec*)	*Peak Duration* (*msec*)	*Area* (*msec mV*)	*Phases* (*No.*)	*Turns* (*No.*)	*Index* (*No.*)	*Polyphasic* MUPs (%)	*Polyturn* MUPs (%)
Below 60	300	1.3±0.6 (0.3–3.1)	10.2±1.9 (4.0–15.9)	2.7±1.1 (0.2–6.0)	1.5±0.7 (0.2–3.6)	3.3±1.0 (2.0–6.0)	3.1±1.0 (2.0–7.0)	4.9±4.2 (1.7–17.5)	9.0±3.9 (5.0–20.0)	10.8±6.8 (5.0–30.0)
Above 60	100	1.7±0.7 (0.3–3.8)	11.4±2.6 (7.0–19.2)	2.5±0.9 (0.4–5.5)	1.8±0.9 (0.4–4.5)	3.4±1.0 (2.0–6.0)	3.2±1.0 (2.0–6.0)	5.8±4.3 (2.4–18.7)	10.0±3.5 (5.0–20.0)	14.0±7.4 (5.0–35.0)
All ages combined	400	1.4±0.6 (3.0–3.2)	10.5±2.1 (4.0–13.8)	2.6±1.0 (0.2–5.6)	1.6±0.8 (0.2–4.0)	3.3±1.0 (2.0–6.0)	3.2±1.0 (2.0–6.0)	5.1±4.2 (1.7–17.7)	9.3±3.8 (5.0–20.0)	11.6±7.0 (5.0–30.0)

ically it has been demonstrated that the muscle fiber diameter of men is approximately 10% larger than that of women,[60] and this could account for the differences in amplitude, area, and duration.

Age Differences

Analysis of the effects of age in the muscles studied showed that the amplitude, duration, area, and percentage of polyphasic and polyturn MUPs were consistently greater in all muscles in subjects more than 60 years old ($P<0.01$). An increase in fiber density with increased age has been documented both by SFEMG[118] and by macro EMG.[116] The changes are most likely due to slow partial denervation and reinnervation.[61,72,93,118]

PRINCIPLES FOR EMG EXAMINATION ON MAXIMAL CONTRACTION

The Interference Pattern on Maximal Contraction

Interference patterns on maximal contraction are graded as "full," "reduced rich," "reduced poor," "discrete," and "single unit pattern" (Fig. 3-35).

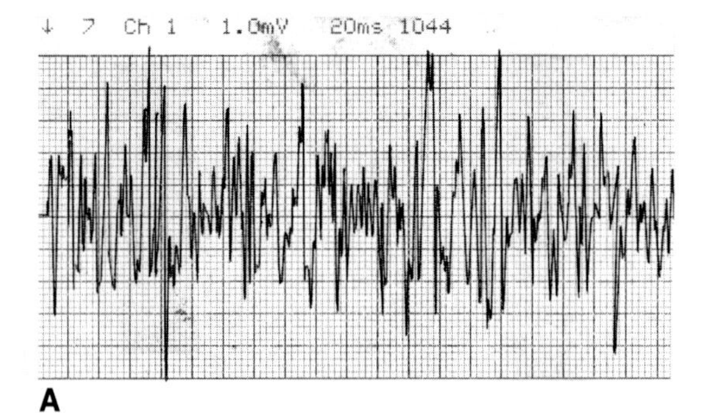

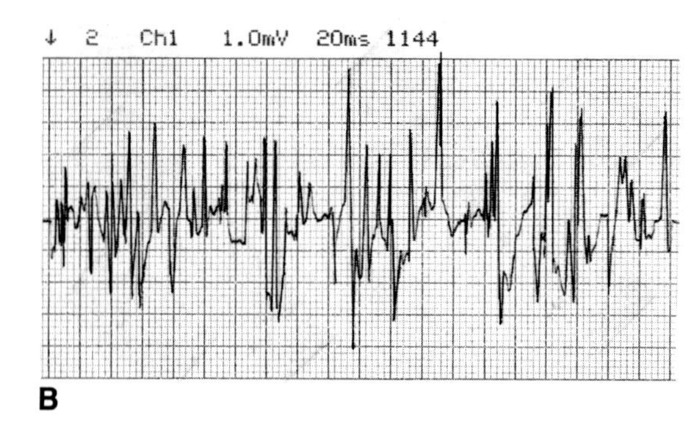

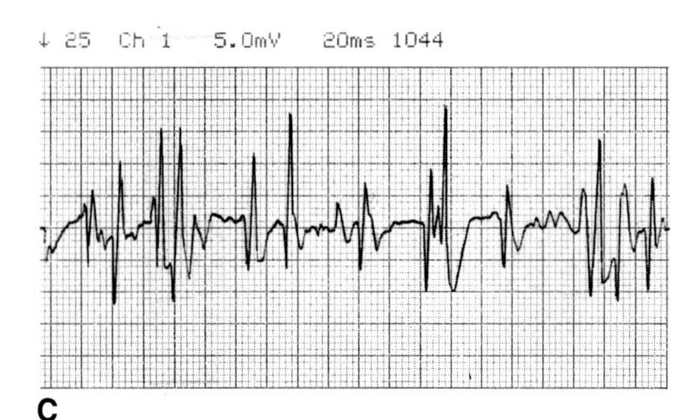

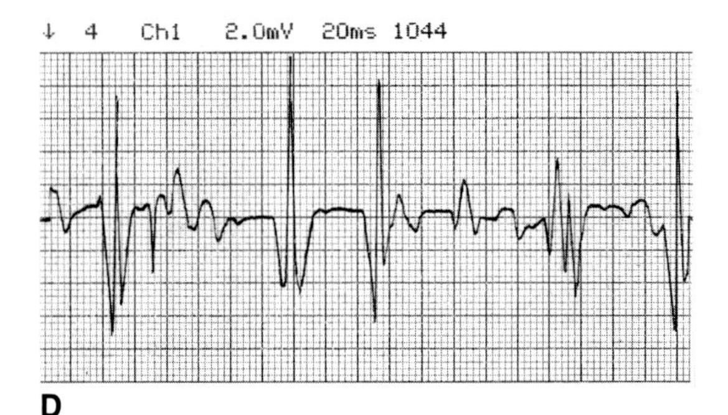

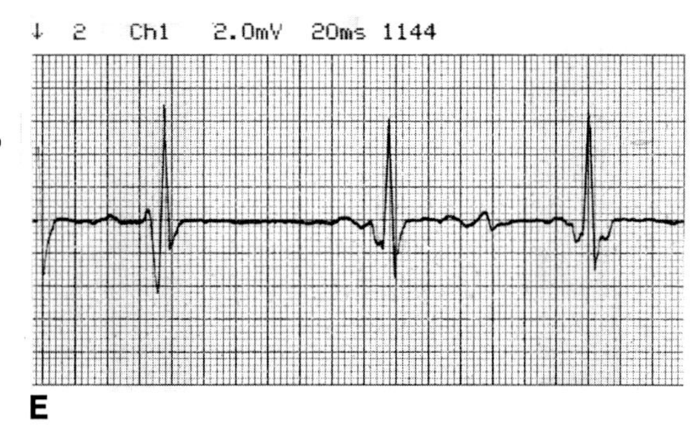

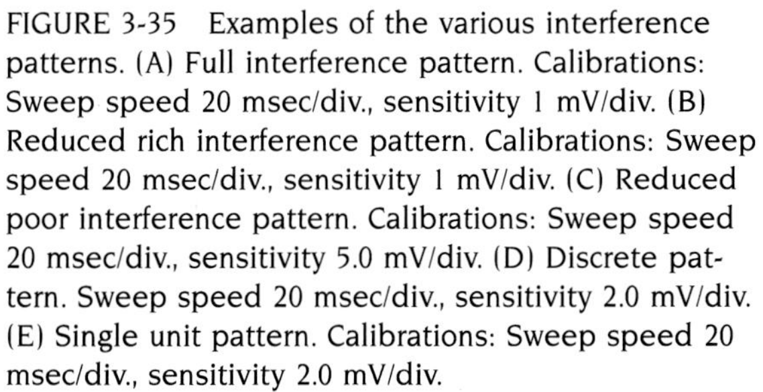

FIGURE 3-35 Examples of the various interference patterns. (A) Full interference pattern. Calibrations: Sweep speed 20 msec/div., sensitivity 1 mV/div. (B) Reduced rich interference pattern. Calibrations: Sweep speed 20 msec/div., sensitivity 1 mV/div. (C) Reduced poor interference pattern. Calibrations: Sweep speed 20 msec/div., sensitivity 5.0 mV/div. (D) Discrete pattern. Sweep speed 20 msec/div., sensitivity 2.0 mV/div. (E) Single unit pattern. Calibrations: Sweep speed 20 msec/div., sensitivity 2.0 mV/div.
Note: C through E were obtained from patients with chronic denervation and reinnervation.

The interference pattern is called "full" when the oscilloscope screen is filled with MUPs and the individual MUPs and the baseline cannot be identified.[135] It is "reduced" when the screen is not filled with MUPs. In this case, some MUPs can be identified individually, while others cannot be identified owing to overlapping from distant MUPs.[135] The interference pattern is called "reduced rich" when minor gaps are seen between the MUPs on full contraction. It is termed "reduced poor" if there are major gaps in the baseline but there are still enough MUPs that not all individual MUPs can be identified. The interference pattern is "discrete" when no interference is seen; in other words, each MUP can be identified individually. In a patient with the discrete interference pattern there will be only two or three MUPs on minimal contraction. A single unit pattern is seen when only one MUP is seen firing on maximal contraction.

Interference may be reduced for a number of reasons. Non-neurogenic causes for reduced interference include the following: The interference pattern may be reduced when the patient cannot produce full contraction because of pain, weakness, or upper motor neuron disease. If a muscle is very strong, the interference may not be full. Frequently, the patient may guard for fear of pain, or for functional reasons. If the patient voluntarily guards on full contraction because of functional problems, the resistance may give way in cogwheeling motion.

If the interference pattern is reduced for causes other than lower motor neuron involvement, there will not be a concomitant increase in the firing rate of the MUPs. Normally, MUPs fire at five to 15 per second on minimal contraction. On maximal contraction the firing rate increases to 25 to 50 per second. The index of recruitment is the ratio of the firing rate of one motor unit firing at a particular time to the total number of motor units firing at that time. This index is useful in distinguishing neurogenic from non-neurogenic causes of decreased recruitment. Normally, the recruitment index is less than 5.[127] In neurogenic situations there is a loss of MUPs and an increase in the firing rate of the remaining MUPs. The index of recruitment in this type of case may be on the order of 10 or higher.

Two other useful parameters to assess recruitment are the onset interval and the recruitment interval.[137] The onset interval is the interspike interval of the first recruited MUP when it begins to discharge. When a second MUP is recruited, the interspike interval of the first MUP is known as the recruitment interval. These intervals have been reported to be shortened in neurogenic and myogenic conditions.[136]

Normally, the amplitude of the MUPs on maximal contraction is between 2 mV and 5 mV in most muscles when recorded with concentric needles.[134] In our experience with monopolar needle recordings the amplitude of the interference pattern may range from 2 mV to 8 mV in most muscles. However, values up to 12 mV may be seen, particularly in hand muscles.[134]

Technical Aspects of Recording the Interference Pattern

The amplifier sweep speed is set at 20 msec/div. The sensitivity setting is at 1000 μV/div. when a monopolar needle is used. When a concentric needle is used, the sensitivity can be set at 500 μV/div. When the interference pattern is to be recorded qualitatively, the filter settings are the same as those suggested for MUP analysis: 2 Hz–10 kHz for concentric needles and 20 Hz–10 kHz for monopolar needles.

Practical Aspects of Recording the Interference Pattern

To examine the EMG on the prime mover, the joint on which the muscle acts is usually placed in its full range of motion. Certain antigravity muscles like the biceps brachii and the hamstrings give their strongest contraction in partial flexion, usually at about 60° of flexion.

Instruct the patient as follows: "Hold your joint in the position that I have placed it. Resist me when I push on you, and don't let me push you in any direction." The patient will give an isometric contraction of his muscle when you offer resistance.

It hurts the patient least if needle penetration is done while the muscle is fully contracted. The patient feels more pain if he contracts the muscle while the pin is deep inside the muscle. Should you need to examine the muscle for maximal contraction soon after minimal contraction, withdraw the needle first to a superficial location (*i.e.*, subcutaneous), get the muscle to contract fully, and then repenetrate the muscle for further examination.

The Interference Pattern in Pathology

NEUROGENIC INVOLVEMENT

The earliest sign of neurogenic involvement prior to the development of spontaneous activity is a reduced interference pattern. There will be poor recruitment of MUPs. The firing rate of the individual MUPs will be increased (Fig. 3-36).[144] The index of recruitment will be more than 5. If this ratio is greater than 10, it indicates loss of motor units.[127] The onset and recruitment intervals are also shorter.

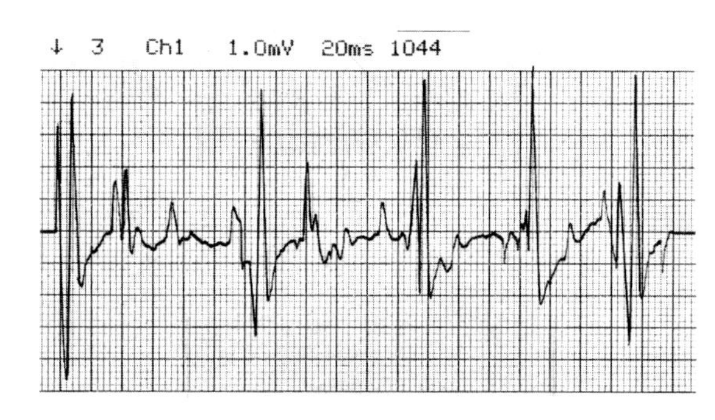

FIGURE 3-36 Discrete pattern on maximal contraction. The individual MUPs can be identified, and the rate of firing is rapid. This trace was from a patient with peripheral nerve injury. Calibrations: Sweep speed 20 msec/div., sensitivity 1.0 mV/div.

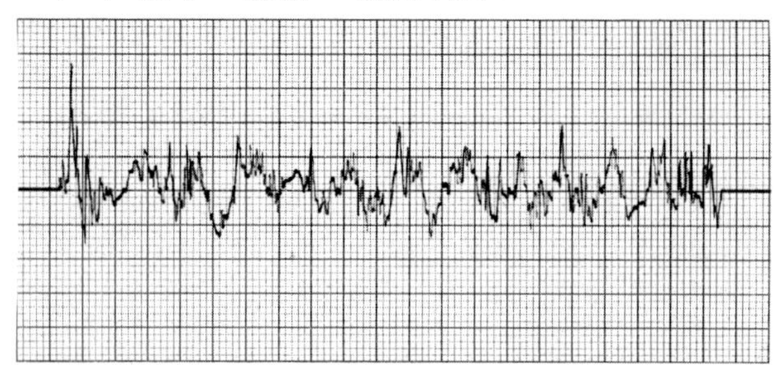

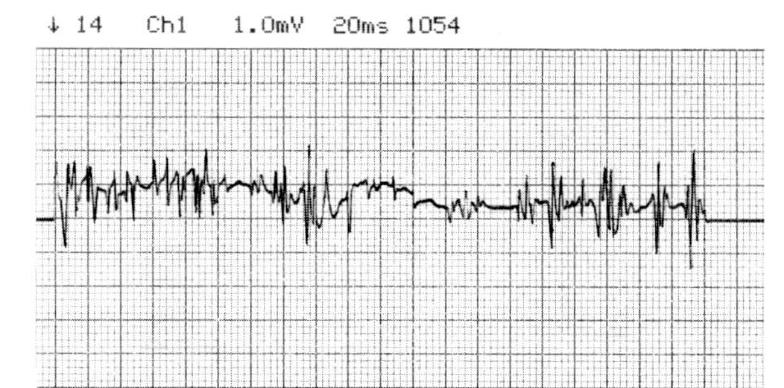

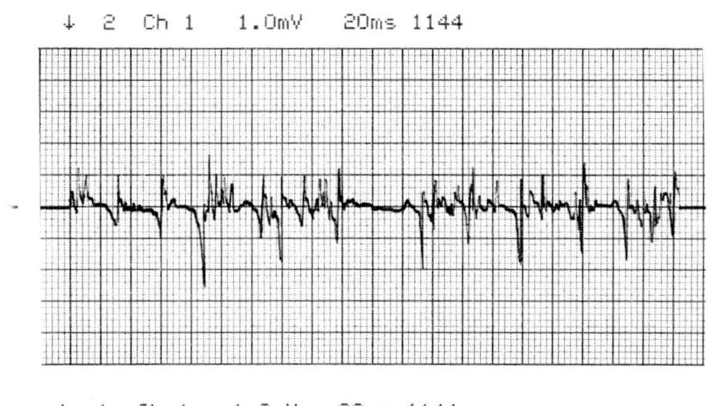

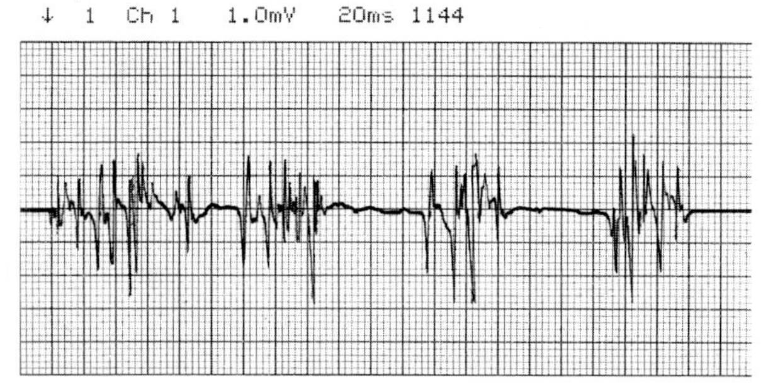

FIGURE 3-37 Examples of the various interference patterns that can be seen with myopathic involvement. The interference patterns in the top two traces were taken from myopathic muscles exerting a moderate degree of contraction. The interference in these two traces appears full even at moderate contraction, whereas the same effort on the part of a normal subject would generate less interference. The lower two traces were taken from patients with more severe myopathic involvement. Although the tracings were taken on maximal contraction, the interference pattern is less than in the two top tracings. This is because with more advanced disease, more muscle fibers are lost.

MYOPATHIC INVOLVEMENT

If the primary involvement is at the muscle cell level, the interference pattern may appear rich in relation to the degree of weakness exhibited by the muscle. The discharge frequency of the units is higher than normal.[128] An interference pattern can therefore be obtained at low forces of contraction. In severe cases or late cases in which most of the muscle fibers have been replaced by fat or fibrous tissue, the interference pattern is reduced proportional to the degree of weakness seen (Fig. 3-37).

Automatic Analysis of the Interference Pattern

Various methods have been developed to quantitate the interference pattern. The earliest methods involved frequency analysis[139] or correlating the mean electrical activity with the isometric strength.[133] Neither method has been widely used. These methods seemed to offer no advantage over the conventional method of visual analysis of the interference pattern.[134] The best known of the methods most recently developed for quantitating the interference pattern is that of Willison.[138,145] Two trains of pulses are analyzed. One train represents fixed voltage changes (amplitudes of 100 μV or more), and the other represents polarity reversals per second. The number of turns per second correlates with the frequency of the waveforms in the signal. Therefore, the number of turns per second can give information about the duration of the individual waveforms.[145] Thus, the turns-and-amplitudes method is able to differentiate between neurogenic involvement from nerve diseases and myopathic involvement. It is accurate in diagnosing myopathies, since the MUPs are short in duration and polyphasic. It is also useful for diagnosing neurogenic involvement when long-duration, large-amplitude MUPs are present. However, if there is reinnervation and if there are complex polyphasic MUPs, the results may be similar to those seen in myopathic involvement and therefore may be misleading. Although this method was very useful, it did not gain popularity because it is cumbersome and time consuming. Its main disadvantage is that a fixed load for a given muscle is needed, for example, 2 kg for the biceps brachii and triceps and 5 kg for the quadriceps.

Willison's method of analyzing turns and amplitudes was modified by others [129–131] Fuglsang–Fredriksen's modification entails applying a force that is relative to the maximum force for the individual subject.[129,130]

A ratio of the amplitude to the turns was analyzed by Smyth for a given force.[140,141] This method was also difficult to use, since the ratio varied with force. An index to express the relationship between turns and amplitudes has also been described for a given force.[126]

Stålberg and colleagues further modified the technique so that turns and amplitudes could be assessed without the force being kept constant.[142,143] A computer was used for analysis of a 300-msec epoch of contraction. Different forces of resistance were employed. The filter settings were 3.2 Hz–8 kHz. The sweep setting was 10 msec/div. The sensitivity was adjusted so that the amplitudes were not truncated. Sensitivity settings ranged between 200 μV and 1000 μV per division. The signals were digitized in a 12-bit A/D converter, with a sampling rate of 25 kHz. A turn was identified when the signal changed polarity and there was at least a 100-μV amplitude between the peaks. The amplitudes were expressed as mean amplitudes between the turns.

The subject was instructed to keep the contraction steady for 1 second. This was done with a wide range of forces, from minimal to strong contraction. The minimal contraction was required to produce more than a single motor unit pattern. Twenty data points were collected from each subject. A few seconds of rest were given between the recordings so that the frequency content of the EMG signal was not influenced by fatigue.[132]

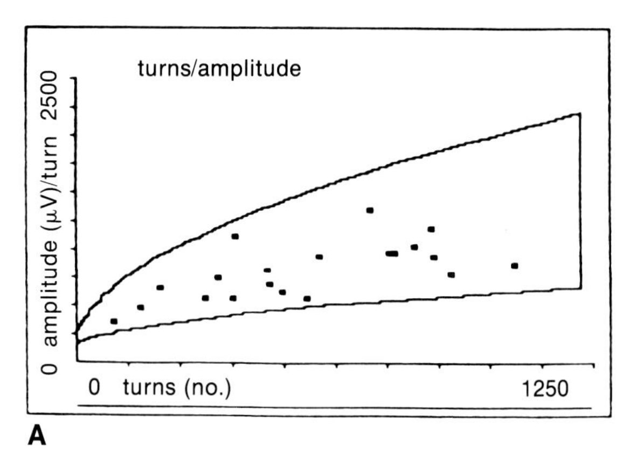

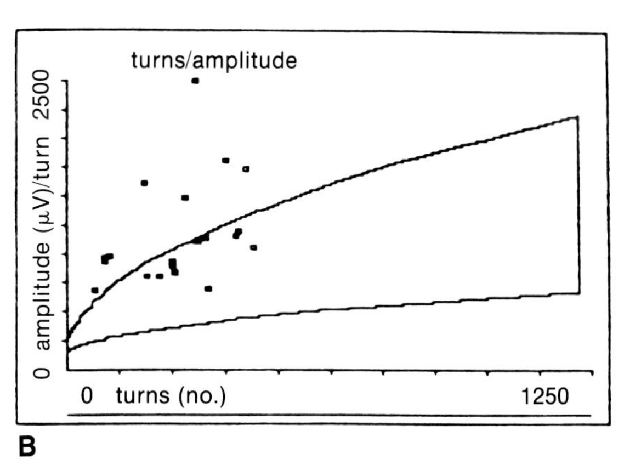

FIGURE 3-38 Automatic analysis of the interference pattern. (A) Normal pattern of data points collected within the boundaries of a normal cloud. (B) Recording from a patient with chronic reinnervation. Many data points appear in the upper left margin outside the upper limits of the cloud.

The relationship of turns to amplitudes was examined in each of several muscles, in men and women separately. Subjects below 60 and above 60 years of age were grouped separately. For each muscle, in each sex and age group, a "cloud" of normal values for amplitude as a function of turns was obtained. This cloud of normal values represents a region of approximately 95% confidence limits for amplitude values for a given turn value.[143] The normal clouds are available for the biceps brachii, extensor digitorum (communis), quadriceps (vastus lateralis), and tibialis anterior. See Figure 3-38, A, for an example of a normal cloud in the extensor digitorum (communis). The muscle is considered abnormal if two data points out of 20 are out of the limits of the cloud. The abnormal data points must be either above the upper limits of the cloud or below the lower limits of the cloud.

This method can distinguish myopathic from neurogenic involvement, particularly neurogenic involvement with chronic reinnervation. In myopathic cases the MUPs are of low amplitude and have a higher number of turns. Consequently, the abnormality is detected by the presence of data points that are below the lower border of the cloud (Fig. 3-39). In chronic reinnervation in which the amplitudes of the MUPs have increased and the number of turns has decreased, the abnormal data points are seen out of the cloud in the upper left quadrant (see Fig. 3-38, B).

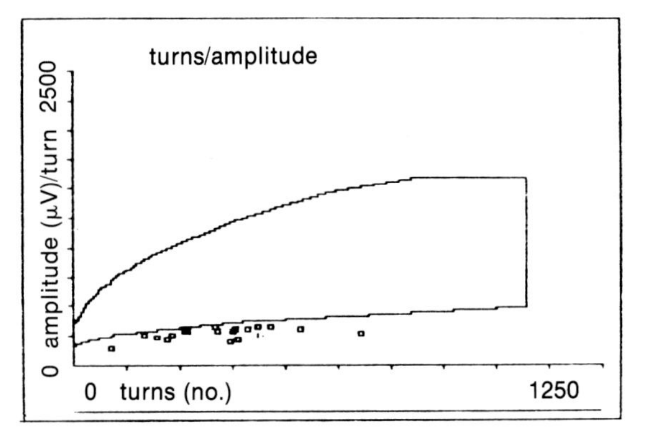

FIGURE 3-39 Automatic analysis of the interference pattern in myopathy. All of the data points appear in the lower part of the trace, below the lower margin of the cloud.

However, when there is active reinnervation with the presence of MUPs that are low in amplitude and polyphasic in shape, the findings with the turns-and-amplitude method may be similar to those seen with myopathic involvement. The turns-and-amplitude method of analysis of the interference pattern has been found to give the same diagnostic yield as the MUP analysis and the visual assessment of the interference pattern.[143] However, the method is very valuable for its ease of use, rapidity, and reproducibility.

REFERENCES

Introduction and General Principles

1. Alexander MA, Turk M: Pediatric considerations. In Johnson EW (ed) Practical Electromyography. Baltimore, Williams & Wilkins, 1980
2. Kimura J: Electrodiagnosis in Diseases of Nerve and Muscle: Principles and Practice. Philadelphia, FA Davis, 1983
3. Shahani BT: EMG in Central Nervous System Diseases. Woburn, MA, Butterworths, 1983
4. Skaggs H et al: Guidelines in EMG. Rochester, MN, Professional Standards Committee, American Association of Electromyography and Electrodiagnosis, 1979
5. Stolov WC: Instrumentation and measurement in electrodiagnosis. Minimonograph 16. Rochester, MN, American Association of Electromyography and Electrodiagnosis, 1981

Principles for Nerve Conduction Studies

6. Baer RD, Johnson EW: Motor nerve conduction velocities in normal children. Arch Phys Med Rehabil 46:698–704, 1965
7. Buchthal F, Rosenfalck A: Evoked action potentials and conduction velocity in human sensory nerves. Brain Res 3:1, 1966
8. Campbell WW, Ward LC, Swift TR: Nerve conduction velocity varies inversely with height. Muscle Nerve 3:436, 1980
9. Denys EH: The effect of temperature on the compound action potential in neuromuscular disease and normal controls. Electroencephalogr Clin Neurophysiol 43:598, 1977
10. Denys EH: The role of temperature in electromyography. Minimonograph 14. Rochester, MN, American Association of Electromyography and Electrodiagnosis, 1980
11. Gamstorp I: Normal conduction velocity of ulnar, median and peroneal nerves in infancy, childhood and adolescence. Acta Paediatr Scand (Suppl) 146:68–76, 1963

12. Gilliatt RW et al: Axonal velocities of motor units in the hand and foot muscles of the baboon. J Neurol Sci 29:249, 1976
13. Goodgold J, Eberstein A: Electrodiagnosis of Neuromuscular Diseases, 3rd ed. Baltimore, Williams & Wilkins, 1983
14. Gutmann L: The intramuscular nerve action potential. J Neurol Neurosurg Psychiatry 32:193, 1969
15. Gutmann L: Important anomalous innervations of the extremities. Rochester, MN, American Association of Electromyography and Electrodiagnosis, 1977
16. Halar EM, DeLisa JA, Brozovich FV: Nerve conduction velocity: Relationship of skin, subcutaneous and intramuscular temperatures. Arch Phys Med Rehabil 61:199, 1980
17. Henriksen JD: Conduction velocity of motor nerves in normal subjects and in patients with neuromuscular disorders. Master's Thesis, University of Minnesota, Minneapolis, 1956
18. Hodes R: Effects of age, consciousness, and other factors on human electrically induced reflexes (EIRs). Electroencephalogr Clin Neurophysiol (Suppl) 25:80, 1967
19. Hodes R, Larrabee MG, German W: The human electromyogram in response to nerve stimulation and the conduction velocity of motor axons. Arch Neurol Psychiatry 60:340, 1948
20. Hopf HC: Untersuchungen über die Unterschiede in der Leitgeschwindigkeit motorischer Nervenfasern beim Menschen. Dtsch Z Nervenheilkd 183:579, 1962
21. Horning MR, Kraft GH, Guy A: Latencies recorded by intramuscular needle electrodes in different portions of a muscle: Variation and comparison with surface electrodes. Arch Phys Med Rehabil 53:206–211, 1972
22. Kimura J: Electrodiagnosis in Diseases of Nerve and Muscle: Principles and Practice. Philadelphia, FA Davis, 1983
23. Kraft GH, Halvorson GA: Median nerve residual latency: Normal value and use in diagnosis of carpal tunnel syndrome. Arch Phys Med Rehabil 64:221–226, 1983
24. Mayer RF: Nerve conduction studies in man. Neurology (Minneap) 13:1021, 1963
25. Melvin JL, Harris DH, Johnson EW: Sensory and motor nerve conduction velocities in ulnar and median nerves. Arch Phys Med Rehabil 47:511–519, 1966
26. Simpson JA: Fact and fallacy in measurement of conduction velocity in motor nerves. J Neurol Neurosurg Psychiatry 27:381, 1964
27. Stolov WC: Requirements, safety feature and pitfalls. Recognition and correction of artifacts. In Techniques in Electromyography and Electrodiagnosis. First Annual Continuing Education Course. Rochester, MN, American Association of Electromyography and Electrodiagnosis, 1978
28. Stolov WC: Instrumentation and measurement in electrodiagnosis. Minimonograph 16. Rochester, MN, American Association of Electromyography and Electrodiagnosis, 1981
29. Thomander L, Stålberg E: Electroneurography in the prognostication of Bell's palsy. Acta Otolaryngol 92:221–237, 1981
30. Thomas PK, Lambert EH: Ulnar nerve conduction velocity and H–reflex in infants and children. J Appl Physiol 15:1, 1960

Principles for EMG Examination at Rest

31. Buchthal F, Engbaek L, Gamstorp I: Paresis and hyperexcitability in adynamia episodica hereditaria. Neurology (Minneap) 8:347, 1958
32. Buchthal F, Rosenfalck P: Spontaneous electrical activity of human muscle. Electroencephalogr Clin Neurophysiol 20:321, 1966
33. Daube JR: An electromyographer's review of plexopathy. In Neuromuscular Diseases as Seen by the Electromyographer. Second Annual Continuing Education Course. Rochester, MN, American Association of Electromyography and Electrodiagnosis, 1979
34. Daube JR: Needle examination in electromyography. Minimonograph 11. Rochester, MN, American Association of Electromyography and Electrodiagnosis, 1979
35. Daube JR, Kelly JJ Jr, Martin RA: Facial myokymia with polyradiculoneuropathy. Neurology (NY) 29:662, 1979
36. Fatt P, Katz B: Spontaneous subthreshold activity at motor nerve endings. J Physiol (Lond) 117:109, 1952
37. Goodgold J, Eberstein A: Electrodiagnosis of Neuromuscular Diseases, 3rd ed. Baltimore, Williams & Wilkins, 1983
38. Guth L: "Trophic" influences of nerve and muscle. Physiol Rev 48:645–687, 1968
39. Hudgson P et al: Adult myopathy from glycogen storage diseases due to acid maltase deficiency. Brain 91:435, 1968
40. Hjorth RJ, Willison RG: The electromyogram in facial myokymia and hemifacial spasm. J Neurol Sci 20:117, 1973
41. Kimura J: Electrodiagnosis in Diseases of Nerve and Muscle: Principles and Practice. Philadelphia, FA Davis, 1983
42. Lipicky RJ: Studies in human myotonic dystrophy. In Rowland LP (ed): Pathogenesis of Human Muscular Dystrophies. Proceedings of the Fifth International Scientific Conference of the Muscular Dystrophy Association. Amsterdam, Excerpta Medica, 1977
43. Morrison JB: The electromyographic changes in hyperkalaemic familial periodic paralysis. Ann Phys Med 5:153, 1960
44. Norris FH Jr, Gasteiger EL, Chatfield PO: An electromyographic study of induced and spontaneous muscle cramps. Electroencephalogr Clin Neurophysiol 9:139, 1957
45. Petty J Jr, Johnson EW: EMG in upper motor neuron conditions. In Johnson EW (ed) Practical Electromyography. Baltimore, Williams & Wilkins, 1980
46. Rosenfalck P, Buchthal F: Studies on fibrillation potentials of denervated human muscle. Electroencephalogr Clin Neurophysiol (Suppl) 22:130, 1962
47. Stålberg E, Trontelj JV: Single Fibre Electromyography. Old Woking, Surrey, Mirvalle Press, 1979
48. Tenser RB, Corbett JJ: Myokymia and facial contraction in brain stem glioma: An electromyographic study. Arch Neurol 30:425, 1974

49. Trojaborg W, Buchthal F: Malignant and benign fasciculations. Acta Neurol Scan (Suppl 13) 41:251, 1965
50. Warmolts JR, Mendell JR: Neurotonia: Impulse-induced repetitive discharges in motor nerves in peripheral neuropathy. Ann Neurol 7:245, 1980
51. Wasserstrom WR, Starr A: Facial myokymia in Guillain-Barré syndrome. Arch Neurol 34:576, 1977
52. Weichers DO: Mechanically provoked insertional activity before and after nerve section in rats. Arch Phys Med Rehabil 58:402, 1977
53. Wettstein A: The origin of fasciculations in motorneuron disease. Ann Neurol 5:295, 1979

Principles for EMG Examination on Minimal Contraction

54. Andreassen S, Jörgensen N: A model for the motor unit potential (abstr). Electroencephalogr Clin Neurophysiol 52:S116, 1981
55. Aquilonius SM, Arvidsson B, Askmark H, Gillberg P-G: Topographical localization of end-plates in cryosection of whole human biceps muscle. Muscle Nerve 5:418, 1982
56. Axelsson J, Thesleff S: A study of supersensitivity in denervated mammalian skeletal muscle. J Physiol 147:178, 1959
57. Bendat JS, Piersol AG: Random Data Analysis and Measurement Procedures. New York, John Wiley & Sons, 1971
58. Bergmans J: Computer assisted on line measurements of motor unit potential parameters in human electromyography. Electromyogr Clin Neurophysiol 11:161–181, 1971
59. Bergmans J: Computer assisted measurement of the parameters of single motor unit potentials in human electromyography. In Desmedt JE (ed) New Developments in Electromyography and Clinical Neurophysiology, Vol 2 pp 482–488. Basel, S Karger, 1973
60. Brooke MH, Engel WK: The histographic analysis of human muscle biopsies with regard to fiber types. 1. Adult male and female. Neurology (Minneapolis) 19:221–233, 1969
61. Brown WF: Functional compensation of human motor units in health and disease. J Neurol Sci 20:199–209, 1973
62. Buchthal F: Electrophysiological differences between myopathy and neuropathy. Excerpta Medica International Congress Series No. 147, pp 207–216. Amsterdam, Excerpta Medica, 1967
63. Buchthal F: An introduction to electromyography. Minimonograph 15. Rochester, MN, American Association of Electromyography and Electrodiagnosis, 1981
64. Buchthal F, Erminio F, Rosenfalck P: Motor unit territory in different human muscles. Acta Physiol Scand 45:72–87, 1959
65. Buchthal F, Guld C, Rosenfalck P: Action potential parameters in normal muscle and their dependence on physical variables. Acta Physiol Scand 32:200–215, 1954
66. Buchthal F, Guld C, Rosenfalck P: Innervation zone and propagation velocity in human muscle. Acta Physiol Scand 34:174–190, 1955
67. Buchthal F, Guld C, Rosenfalck P: Volume conduction of the spike of the motor unit potential investigated with a new type of multielectrode. Acta Physiol Scand 38:331–354, 1957
68. Buchthal F, Rosenfalck P: Action potential parameters in different human muscles. Acta Psychiatr Neurol Scand 30:125, 1955
69. Buchthal F, Rosenfalck P: On the structure of motor units. In Desmedt JE (ed): New Developments in Electromyography and Clinical Neurophysiology, Vol 1, pp 71–85. Basel, S Karger, 1973
70. Burke RE, Levine DN, Zajac FA: Mammalian motor units: Physiological–histochemical correlation in three types in cat gastrocnemius. Science 174:709–712, 1971
71. Butler BP, Ball RD, Albers JW: Effect of electrode type and position on motor unit potential configuration. Muscle Nerve 5:594–597, 1982
72. Campbell MJ, McComas AJ, Petito F: Physiological changes in aging muscles. J Neurol Neurosurg Psychiatry 36:174–182, 1973
73. Chu J, Chan RC: Changes in motor unit action potential parameters in monopolar recordings related to filter settings of the EMG amplifier. Arch Phys Med Rehabil 66:601–604, 1985
74. Cöers C, Woolf AL: The Innervation of Muscle: A Biopsy Study. Oxford, Blackwell Scientific Publications, 1959
75. Daube J: The description of motor unit potentials in electromyography. Neurology 28:623–625, 1978
76. Daube J: Needle examination in electromyography. Minimonograph 11. Rochester, MN, American Association of Electromyography and Electrodiagnosis, 1979
77. Desmedt JE, Borenstein S: Collateral reinnervation of muscle fibers by motor axons of dystrophic motor units. Nature 246:500–501, 1973
78. Dietert SE: The demonstration of different types of muscle fibers in human extraocular muscle by electron microscopy and cholinesterase staining. Invest Opthalmol 4:51–63, 1965
79. Dubowitz V, Brooke MH: Muscle biopsy: A modern approach. London, WB Saunders, 1973
80. Edström L, Kugelberg E: Histochemical composition, distributions of fibers and fatiguability of single motor units. J Neurol Neurosurg Psychiatry 31:424–433, 1968
81. Engel WK: The essentiality of histo- and cytochemical studies of skeletal muscle in the investigation of neuromuscular disease. Neurology 12:778, 1962
82. Engel WK: Brief, small, abundant motor unit action potentials: A further critique of electromyographic interpretation. Neurology 25:173–176, 1975
83. Falck B: Automatic analysis of individual motor unit potentials recorded with a special two channel electrode. Academic dissertation, Turku, Finland, 1983
84. Feinstein B, Lindegard B, Nyman E, Wohlfart G: Morphologic studies of motor units in normal human muscles. Acta Anat (Basel) 23:127–142, 1955
85. Garnett RAF, O'Donovan MJ, Stephens JA, Taylor A: Motor unit organizaiton of human medial gastrocnemius. J Physiol 287:33–43, 1979
86. Gath I, Stålberg E: In situ measurements of the innervation ratio of motor units in human muscles. Exp Brain Res 43:377–382, 1981

87. Goodgold J, Eberstein A: Electrodiagnosis of Neuromuscular Diseases 3rd ed. Baltimore, Williams & Wilkins, 1983
88. Guld C: On the Influence of the measuring electrodes on duration and amplitude of muscle action potentials. Acta Physiol Scand (Suppl) 89:30–32, 1951
89. Gydikov A: The potential of the motor unit. In Shachani M (ed): The Motor System: Neurophysiology and Muscle Mechanisms, pp 49–72. Amsterdam, Elsevier, 1976
90. Henneman E, Somjen G, Carpenter D: Functional significance of cell size in spinal motoneurons. J Neurophysiol 28:560–580, 1965
91. Hynninen P, Philipson L, Mandersson B, Elmqvist D: A computer based method for automatic motor unit potential analysis. Acta Neurol Scand 60 (Suppl 73):300, 1979
92. International Federation for Encephalography and Clinical Neurophysiology: Recommendations for the Practice of Clinical Neurophysiology. Amsterdam, Elsevier, 1983
93. Jennekens FGI, Tomlinson BE, Walton JN: Histochemical aspects of five limb muscles in old age: An autopsy study. J Neurol Sci 14:259–276, 1971
94. Kaiser E, Petersen I: Muscle action potentials studied by frequency analysis and duration measurements. Acta Neurol Scand 41 (Suppl 13):213–236, 1965
95. Kopec J, Hausmanowa-Petrusewisz I: On-line computer application in clinical quantitative electromyography. Electromyogr Clin Neurophysiol 16:49–64, 1976
96. Kunze K: Quantitative EMG analysis in myogenic and neurogenic muscle diseases. In Desmedt JE (ed): New Developments in Electromyography and Clinical Neurophysiology, Vol 2, pp 469–476. Basel, S Karger, 1973
97. Lang AH, Partanen VSJ: "Satellite potentials" and the duration of motor unit potentials in normal, neuropathic and myopathic muscles. J Neurol Sci 27:513–524, 1976
98. Lang AH, Vaahtoranta KM: The baseline, the time characteristics and the slow afterwaves of the motor unit potential. Electroencephalogr Clin Neurophysiol 35:387–394, 1973
99. Lee RG, White DG: Computer analysis of motor unit action potentials in routine clinical electromyography. In Desmedt JE (ed): New Developments in Electromyography and Clinical Neurophysiology, Vol 2, pp 454–461. Basel, S Karger, 1973
100. McComas AJ, Kereshi S, Manzano G: Multiple Innervation of human muscle fibers. J Neurol Sci 64:55–64, 1984
101. Milner-Brown HS, Stein RB, Yemm R: The orderly recruitment of human motor units during voluntary isometric contractions. J Physiol 230:359–370, 1973
102. Nissen-Petersen H, Guld C, Buchthal F: A delay line to record random action potentials. Electroencephalogr Clin Neurophysiol 26:100–106, 1969
103. Payan J: The blanket principle: A technical note. Muscle Nerve 1:423–426, 1978
104. Person RS, Kudina LP: Discharge frequency and discharge pattern of human motor units during voluntary contraction of muscle. Electroencephalogr Clin Neurophysiol 32:471–483, 1972
105. Petajan JH: Clinical electromyographic studies of the diseases of motor unit. Electroencephalogr Clin Neurophyiol 36:395, 1974
106. Petajan JH, Philip BA: Frequency control of motor unit action potentials. Electroencephalogr Clin Neurophysiol 27:66, 1969
107. Pollack V: The waveshape of action potentials recorded with different types of electromyographic needles. Med Biol Eng 9:657–664, 1971
108. Rathjen R, Simons DG, Peterson CR: Computer analysis of the duration of the motor unit potentials. Arch Phys Med Rehabil 49:524–527, 1968
109. Rosenfalck P, Rosenfalck A: Electromyography—Sensory and Motor Conduction: Findings in Normal Subjects, pp 1–49. Laboratory of Clinical Neurophysiology, Rigshospitalet, Copenhagen, 1975
110. Sacco G, Buchthal F, Rosenfalck P: Motor unit potentials at different ages. Arch Neurol 6:366–373, 1962
111. Stålberg E: Propagation velocity in human muscle fibers in situ. Acta Physiol Scand 70 (Suppl 287):1–112, 1966
112. Stålberg E, Andreassen S, Antoni L et al: Quantitative analysis of the motor unit potential—a proposition for standardized terminology and criteria for measurement. (In press)
113. Stålberg E, Antoni L: Electrophysiological cross section of the motor unit. J Neurol Neurosurg Psychiatry 43:469–474, 1980
114. Stålberg E, Antoni L: Microprocessors in the analysis of the motor unit and neuromuscular transmission. In Yamaguchi N, Fujisawa K (eds): Recent Advances in EEG and EMG Data Processing, pp 295–313. Amsterdam, Elsevier North-Holland, 1981
115. Stålberg E, Antoni L: Computer-aided EMG analysis. In Desmedt JE (ed): Progress in Clinical Neurophysiology, Vol 10, pp 186–234. Basel, S Karger, 1983
116. Stålberg E, Fawcett PRW: Macro EMG in healthy subjects of different ages. J Neurol Neurosurg Psychiatry 45:870–878, 1982
117. Stålberg S, Stålberg E: Swedish Electrophysiologic Software Program Manuals. Uppsala, Sweden, 1985
118. Stålberg E, Trontelj JV: Single Fibre Electromyography, p 67. Old Woking, Surrey, Mirvalle Press, 1979
119. Takahashi K: The coupling discharge in neurogenic muscular atrophy. Arch Neurol 14:617–623, 1966
120. Tanji J, Kato M: Firing rate of individual motor units in voluntary contraction of abductor digiti minimi muscle in man. Exp Neurol 40:771–783, 1973
121. Tanzi F, Taglietti V, Zucca G et al: Computerized EMG analysis. Electromyogr Clin Neurophysiol 19:495–503, 1979
122. Thage O, Trojaborg W, Buchthal F: Electromyographic findings in polyneuropathy. Neurology (Minneap) 13:273, 1963
123. Thiele B, Boehle A: Anzahl der Spike-Komponenten im Motor Unit Potential. EEG EMG 9:125–130, 1978
124. Warmolts JR, Engel WK: Open-biopsy electromyography. I. Correlation of motor unit behaviour with histochemical muscle fiber type in human limb muscle. Arch Neurol 27:512, 1972
125. Wiechers DO: Single fiber electromyography with a standard monopolar electrode. Arch Phys Med Rehabil 66:47–48, 1985

Principles for EMG Examination on Maximal Contraction

126. Cenkovich F, Hsu S-F, Gersten JW: A quantitative electromyographic index that is independent of the force of contraction. Electroencephalogr Clin Neurophysiol 54: 79–86, 1982
127. Daube JR: Needle examination in clinical electromyography. First Annual Continuing Education Course. Rochester, MN, American Association of Electromyography and Electrodiagnosis, 1978
128. Dietz V, Büdingen HJ et al: Discharge characteristics of single motor fibres of hand muscles in lower motoneurone diseases and myopathies. In Kunze K, Desmedt JE (ed): Studies on Neuromuscular Diseases, p. 122. Basel, S Karger, 1975
129. Fuglsang-Fredriksen A, Månsson A: Analysis of electrical activity of normal muscle in man at different degrees of voluntary effort. J Neurol Neurosurg Psychiatry 38:683–694, 1975
130. Fuglsang-Fredriksen A, Scheel U, Buchthal F: Diagnostic yield of analysis of the pattern of electrical activity and of individual motor unit potentials in myopathy. J Neurol Neurosurg Psychiatry 39:742–750, 1976
131. Hayward M: Automatic analysis of the electromyogram in healthy subjects of different ages. J Neurol Sci 33:397–413, 1977
132. Kadefors R, Kaiser E, Petersen I: Dynamic spectrum analysis of myo-potentials with special reference to muscle fatigue. Electromyogr Clin Neurophysiol 8: 39–74, 1968
133. Lenman JAR: Quantitative electromyographic changes associated with muscular weakness. J Neurol Neurosurg Psychiatry 22:306, 1959
134. Ludin HP: Electromyography in Practice. New York, Thieme Stratton, 1980
135. Nomenclature Committee: A glossary of terms used in clinical electromyography. Rochester, MN, American Association of Electromyography and Electrodiagnosis, 1980
136. Petajan JH: Clinical electromyographic studies of the diseases of the motor unit. Electroencephalogr Clin Neurophysiol 36:395, 1974
137. Petajan JH, Philip BA: Frequency control of motor unit action potentials. Electroencephalogr Clin Neurophysiol 27:66, 1969
138. Rose AL, Willison RG: Quantitative electromyography using automatic analysis: Studies in healthy subjects and patients with primary muscle disease. J Neurol Neurosurg Psychiatry 30:403–410, 1967
139. Richardson AT: The analysis of muscle action potentials in the differential diagnosis of neuromuscular disorders. Arch Phys Med Rehabil 32:199, 1951
140. Smyth DPL: Quantitative electromyography in babies and young children with primary muscle disease and neurogenic lesions. J Neurol Sci 56:199–207, 1982
141. Smyth DPL, Willison RG: Quantitative electromyography in babies and young children with no evidence of neuromuscular disease. J Neurol Sci 56:209–217, 1982
142. Stålberg E, Antoni L: Microprocessors in the analysis of the motor unit and the neuromuscular transmission. In Yamaguchi N, Fujisawa K (eds): Proceedings of the Conference on EEG and EMG, Data Processing, Kanazawa, Japan, pp 295–313. Amsterdam, Elsevier, 1981
143. Stålberg E, Chu J, Bril V et al: Automatic analysis of the EMG interference pattern. Electroencephalogr Clin Neurophysiol 56:672–681, 1982
144. Willison RG: Electrodiagnosis in motor neurone disease. Proc R Soc Med 55:1024, 1962
145. Willison RG: Analysis of electrical activity in healthy and dystrophic muscle in man. J Neurol Neurosurg Psychiatry 27:386–394, 1964

4

Notes on the Electrodiagnostic Features of Commonly Encountered Clinical Situations

Jennifer Chu-Andrews

ANTERIOR HORN CELL DISEASES

Nerve Conduction Studies

SENSORY

Results of sensory conduction studies are normal, since the lesion is proximal to the dorsal root ganglion.[6,8,11] Suspect coexistent entrapment neuropathies, pressure neuropathies, or end-stage disease if sensory abnormalities are noted.

Motor

Compound muscle action potential (CMAP) amplitude may be normal in the early stages but depressed in the later stages. The conduction velocity may be normal or slightly slowed when there is involvement of the large, fast-conducting nerve fibers.[6,7,11] Even if the large fibers are the effected fibers of a nerve, the conduction velocity will be at least 70% of normal because the smaller fibers will conduct normally. If there is involvement of the large fibers, the F responses may be delayed.[7]

REPETITIVE STIMULATION STUDIES

A decremental response (up to 20% decrement) may be seen on slow (2–3/sec) repetitive stimulation of nerves to atrophic muscles. Postexercise facilitation and exhaustion are also sometimes seen.[2,4,14]

EMG

GENERAL

The presence of abnormalities compatible with neurogenic involvement, if present in more than three roots in three separate extremities, so that the findings cannot be explained by a focal disease of the spinal cord, is evidence in favor of anterior horn cell disease.[11] If abnormalities are present in the muscles supplied by the cranial nerves, the head and neck may be counted as a separate extremity for the purpose of this criterion. Examination of the masseter and/ or genioglossus and the lateral muscles of the tongue is useful for documentation of involvement of the nuclei of the cranial nerves.

REST

Fibrillations, positive sharp waves, complex repetitive discharges, and fasciculations are usually present. Fasciculations may be complex, and their rate of discharge may be slow. The firing rate is typically one discharge every 3.5 msec.[20] Fasciculations are believed to result from spontaneous discharges from anterior horn cells or from axons of motor units that are still intact and therefore are not seen in muscles that have lost all innervation.[11,22] Similarly, the other forms of spontaneous activity disappear with end-stage denervation as the muscle fibers become fibrotic.

MINIMAL CONTRACTION

Because of collateral sprouting and incorporation of many muscle fibers into a motor unit, motor unit potentials (MUPs) are generally high in amplitude and long in duration.[23] A high incidence of polyphasia is usually observed.[4,9,11,12] Large-amplitude, long-duration noncomplex polyphasic and triphasic MUPs are seen when the reinnervation process is stable. In the presence of ongoing reinnervation the polyphasic MUPs are very complex in shape, with multiple late components. These MUPs vary in shape and form with consecutive discharges. Instability of the spike components of the main MUP and of the late components is due to increased jitter and blocking.[17,18] With use of fast sweep speeds (1 msec–0.5 msec) and a filter setting of 500 Hz–10 kHz, jitter and blocking can be observed even with conventional EMG.

MAXIMAL CONTRACTION

The interference pattern is reduced. In late stages the interference may be poor, discrete, or absent, depending on the degree of atrophy.

SFEMG

The presence of increased fiber density and stable potentials suggests that the disease process is slowly progressive. If the increased fiber density is seen in association with complex potentials that exhibit increased jitter and blocking, the disease process, while slow, is likely to be faster than if stable potentials are seen. Increased fiber density that is correlated with MUP morphology indicates the degree of reinnervation. Increase in fiber density is most pronounced if the neurogenic process is slow, since there is then enough time for axonal sprouting and reinnervation. Low fiber density together with stable potentials implies a slow neurogenic process with poor reinnervation. Low fiber density together with unstable potentials (*i.e.*, potentials with a high degree of jitter and blocking) implies a rapidly progressive neurogenic process.[17–19] SFEMG findings may be abnormal in muscles that are clinically unaffected.

Clinical Situations Associated With Anterior Horn Cell Diseases

Motor Neuron Disease

In amyotrophic lateral sclerosis, there is degeneration of the lower motor neurons in the spinal cord and brain stem. The 10th, 11th, and 12th cranial nerves are the most commonly affected cranial nerves. There is also degeneration of the motor cells in the cortex and degeneration of the corticospinal tracts. Death due to respiratory complications usually occurs within a few years. The electrodiagnostic features commonly seen in motor neuron disease include low-amplitude CMAPs, normal nerve conduction velocity studies, and a positive decrement with slow repetitive stimulation. On EMG there is widespread spontaneous activity at rest. There are large-amplitude, long-duration MUPs on minimal contraction. These MUPs appear stable if there is slow progression of the disease and unstable if there is rapid progression. There is poor recruitment on maximal contraction. Low CMAP amplitude, the presence of profuse fibrillations, varying shape of the MUPs, and a positive decrement have been found to be indicators of poor prognosis.[2,5,10]

Progressive Muscular Atrophy

The site of the lesion is primarily at the anterior horn cells. The disease is slower in progression than is amyotrophic lateral sclerosis.

Spinal Muscular Atrophy

The infantile type is known as Werdnig-Hoffmann disease. Spontaneous discharges of MUPs, which continue during sleep, are common. These potentials can be recruited voluntarily[3] and therefore differ from true fasciculations. The electrodiagnostic features are similar to those seen in amyotrophic lateral sclerosis. The prognostic indicators obtained from EMG are also similar.

The juvenile type is known as Kugelberg-Welander's disease and is more benign than the infantile type. Survival into adulthood is common. The nerve conduction studies are usually normal.[13,16,17] Spontaneous activity is sparse; if present, it is more prominent in the lower extremities, especially in the proximal muscles.[7] Myopathic changes of overwork in atrophic muscles may result in small-amplitude polyphasic MUPs.[1,10]

Poliomyelitis

Spontaneous activity is widespread and may be present for years if reinnervation is inadequate. The amplitudes of the spontaneous discharges become very small as time passes. With recent denervation the amplitudes of the fibrillations tend to be larger.[5] New onset of weakness in old poliomyelitis may be due to loss of residual MUPs with aging.[14,15] Progressive weakness may also result from neuromuscular transmission failure at the end-plates that were formed when reinnervation took place. This has been documented with SFEMG.[21]

Syringomyelia

Cavitation and gliosis are especially common in the cervical cord and medulla. Fibrillations and positive sharp waves are typically present in the upper extremities, especially in the intrinsic hand muscles. The lower extremities may show no involvement.

ROOT LESIONS

Nerve Conduction Studies

SENSORY

Studies are normal in amplitude and latency, since the involvement is proximal to the dorsal root ganglion. Suspect the presence of a coexistent entrapment syndrome, pressure neuropathy, or peripheral neuropathy if sensory abnormalities are noted.

MOTOR

Conduction velocities are normal. The evoked motor response may be depressed in amplitude owing to axonal loss. F-wave studies may be prolonged.[28,30] With involvement of the S1 root, the H reflex may be delayed or absent.[24,25,27,29,41] With cauda equina lesions the amplitude of the CMAP is frequently depressed asymmetrically.[36]

EMG

GENERAL

Abnormalities are localized to the distribution of a specific myotome, with involvement of the paraspinal muscles. The diagnosis of root involvement is best done by documentation of abnormal EMG findings in the paraspinal muscles and in at least three muscles supplied by three different peripheral nerves having a common root of origin. Since most muscles have innervation by more than one root, criteria for diagnosing involvement of a single root include normal findings in muscle groups supplied by adjacent nerve roots. For example, in pure L5 root involvement there may be abnormal findings not only in muscles with strong L5 root innervation, but also in muscles such as the medial gastrocnemius, which receives weak contributions from the L5 root. In such cases the soleus, which has little or no L5 root contribution, is normal.

When a root abnormality is found, bilateral examination is mandatory, even though there may be no symptoms in the contralateral extremity.[26] We have found the presence of fibrillations and positive sharp waves bilaterally in 1% of the patients with C6 root lesions, 0.5% of the patients with C7 root lesions, and 1% of the patients with C8 root lesions, even in the absence of symptoms in the other limb. Similarly, in the lower extremities, fibrillations and positive sharp waves were seen bilaterally in 0.5% of the patients with L2 and L3 root lesions, 1.0% of the patients with L4 root lesions, 7.5% of the patients with L5 root lesions, and 4.5% of the patients with S1 root lesions.

The findings in root lesions from spinal stenosis or degenerative diseases of the spine are frequently bilateral and at multiple root levels.[33,44] A unilateral herniated disc does not usually cause bilateral multiple root findings.[42] In our experience a central disc herniation often involves more than one root bilaterally. When involvement of multiple root levels is seen bilaterally, it is essential to rule out cauda equina or conus medullaris lesions. In cauda equina lesions the involvement may be from nerve roots L1 to S5. In conus medullaris lesions the sacral nerve roots, particularly the lower sacral roots, are commonly involved. Involvement of the lumbar nerve roots is uncommon.[36]

Because of overlapping of the nerve supply in the paraspinals, which are supplied by the posterior primary rami,[31] localization of the level of the nerve roots involved is best done by careful examination of multiple muscles of different myotomes supplied by the anterior primary rami.[34,35,46] Since the last level in the paraspinals is supplied by the S1 posterior primary ramus, involvement of the lower sacral myotomes is documented by involvement of the sphincter ani externus and the muscles of the perineum, such as the bulbospongiosus (bulbocavernosus).

The EMG examination detects electrophysiological changes and may be abnormal even though radiologic examinations, which detect structural changes, may show no abnormalities.[37] It must be emphasized that the role of EMG in radicular syndromes is in documentation of the root involved—not in localization of the level of the involved disc or vertebra.

REST

The earliest sign may be prolonged insertional activity. With acute and ongoing denervation, fibrillations and positive sharp waves are seen. The amplitudes of these discharges are high.[38] We have found them to range in amplitude from 600 μV to 2000 μV with monopolar needle recordings. The spontaneous activity should be seen in three or more muscles with different peripheral nerve supplies but with the same root contribution. With progressive denervation, complex repetitive discharges and even fasciculations can be seen. Residual damage from a previous root involvement may be noted as fibrillations with very small amplitude (10 μV–50 μV). Since the paraspinals are supplied by the posterior primary ramus, they may show the presence of spontaneous activity earlier than the limb muscles. This finding is related to the shorter distance between the paraspinals and the site of nerve root damage. The paraspinals usually show spontaneous activity within 7 to 10 days.[46] Fourteen to twenty-one days usually pass before the limb muscles show spontaneous activity. Similarly, reinnervation occurs earlier in the paraspinals than in the limb muscles. Consequently, spontaneous activity may be hard to detect in the paraspinals even if such activity is profuse in the limb muscles. On the other hand, if profuse spontaneous activity is noted at several paraspinal levels and this is in contrast to the findings in the limbs, metastases to the paraspinal muscles[39] or metabolic causes such as diabetes[40] should be considered.

Spontaneous activity may remain for a considerable period in the paraspinals after surgery of the spine. It has been suggested that spontaneous activity in the paraspinals is evidence of recurrent denervation when the muscles are examined approximately 3 cm lateral to the incision and to a depth of 3 cm to 5 cm.[34] However, a definite conclusion of recent pathology cannot be made even with this finding, since it may also be seen in the asymptomatic postlaminectomy patient.[43]

MINIMAL CONTRACTION

Increased polyphasia is seen within 4 to 7 days.[35,45] In our experience with quantitative MUP analysis using monopolar needle recordings, we have found that the polyphasic MUPs tend to be normal in duration in the early stages before reinnervation has begun. An increase in the percentage of normal-duration polyphasic MUPs above 30% to 35% in a myotomal distribution is suggestive of early root-level involvement.

In the presence of reinnervation the polyphasic MUPs have prolonged duration. When the reinnervation is very recent and active, the polyphasic MUPs are complex and may show variation in shape. Jitter and blocking in the late components may be observed. These findings are useful for detection of recent or recurrent radiculopathy. In particular, such findings are useful in a patient who has had surgery more than a year ago, since, as mentioned above, the presence of spontaneous activity in the paraspinals does not necessarily imply recurrent injury.

With very chronic and extensive reinnervation the amplitudes of the MUPs may reach 10 mV or more. If MUPs of these amplitudes are seen at several levels, involvement at the spinal cord level should be considered, especially if these amplitudes are seen bilaterally.

MUPs with chronic completed reinnervation are long in duration—30 msec or longer in our experience with quantitative MUP analysis using monopolar needle recordings. These MUPs are triphasic or noncomplex polyphasic. If there is continued reinnervation, such MUPs may be seen in association with the presence of single or multiple late components.

MAXIMAL CONTRACTION

The interference pattern is generally reduced. Depending on the degree of involvement, it may range from reduced rich to poor or discrete. The complete absence of MUPs is not common, since more than one root supplies the muscles. However, this pattern is sometimes seen in the peripheral muscles, especially if there is a concurrent peripheral nerve injury, for example, if a peroneal nerve injury coexists with an L5 root lesion.

The root supply of the muscles of the upper and lower extremities is given in Tables 4-1 and 4-2, respectively. The dominant root contributions are obtained through correlating EMG findings (indicated by the presence of fibrillations and positive sharp waves) with myelograms and actual surgical cases. Most of the data are from the 25 years of data collection from the EMG laboratory of the Department of Physical Medicine and Rehabilitation at the Hospital of the University of Pennsylvania. The reader is also referred to publications by Sharrard[45] and Hoppenfeld.[32]

PLEXUS LESIONS

Anatomy

See Appendix Figure 23 and Figures 1-16 through 1-20 for diagrams of the brachial plexus and its constituents.

Nerve Conduction Studies

SENSORY

The amplitudes are depressed, particularly on stimulation above the site of the lesion. The conduction velocities are slowed across the site of the lesion.[48,66] If the lesion is preganglionic, as in a root avulsion,[55] the sensory potentials will be normal, since the level of involvement is proximal to the dorsal root ganglion.

MOTOR

On the affected side, amplitudes are small, and the F responses are delayed, but the conduction velocities are usually normal. If the involvement is severe, with destruction of the largest, fastest nerve fibers, the conduction velocities will be slowed. Usually the conduction velocities are not slowed by more than 30% below normal, since the conduction velocity is maintained by the slower fibers. The distal latencies are also slowed. This slowing is seen in early reinnervation, when most of the nerve fibers are thin and poorly myelinated. In such instances there will be EMG evidence of reinnervation.

TABLE 4-1
Root Supply of the Upper Extremity

	Root(s)								
Muscle	C1	C2	C3	C4	C5	C6	C7	C8	T1
Sternocleidomastoid	·	●	·	·	·				
Levator scapulae			●	·	·				
Trapezius (upper portion)	·	·	●	·	·				
Trapezius (middle portion)			·	●					
Trapezius (lower portion)				●	·				
Rhomboideus major and minor					●				
Supraspinatus					●	·			
Infraspinatus					●	·			
Deltoid (anterior portion)					●	·			
Biceps (long head)					●	·			
Teres major					·	●			
Teres minor					·	●			
Deltoid (middle and posterior)					·	●			
Biceps (short head)					·	●			
Coracobrachialis					·	●			
Brachialis					·	●			
Brachioradialis					·	●			
Extensor carpi radialis longus					·	●			
Extensor carpi radialis brevis					·	●			
Supinator					·	●			
Pronator teres					·	●			
Serratus anterior					·	·	·		
Latissimus dorsi						·	·	·	
Pectoralis major (sternal portion)							·	·	·
Pectoralis major (clavicular portion)					·	·			

●, dominant supply; ·, additional supply

(continued)

TABLE 4-1 (*Continued*)
Root Supply of the Upper Extremity

Muscle	C1	C2	C3	C4	Root(s) C5	C6	C7	C8	T1
Triceps						·	●	·	
Anconeus							●	·	
Extensor digitorum (communis)							●	·	
Extensor digiti minimi							●	·	
Extensor carpi ulnaris							●	·	
Abductor pollicis longus							●	·	
Extensor pollicis brevis							●	·	
Extensor pollicis longus							●	·	
Extensor indicis							●	·	
Flexor carpi radialis						·	●		
Flexor digitorum superficialis							·	●	●
Flexor carpi ulnaris							·	●	
Flexor digitorum profundus							·	●	·
Flexor pollicis longus							·	●	·
Pronator quadratus								●	·
Abductor pollicis brevis								●	·
Flexor pollicis brevis								●	·
Opponens pollicis								●	·
Abductor digiti minimi								·	●
Adductor pollicis								·	●
Flexor digiti minimi brevis								·	●
Opponens digiti minimi								·	●
Palmar and dorsal interossei								·	●
Lumbricals								·	●

●, dominant supply; ·, additional supply

EMG

GENERAL

The abnormalities are seen in the distribution or more than two peripheral nerves. If a myotomal distribution is seen with no findings in the paraspinal muscles, the lesion may be due to involvement of the anterior primary ramus. With involvement of only the anterior primary ramus, the paraspinals are spared, since the spinal nerve and the ventral root itself are not involved. Careful mapping and quantitation of abnormal findings aid in localization of the plexus lesion, for example, whether the involvement of the brachial plexus is at the level of the cords, divisions, or trunks. Careful examination is needed to enable the examiner to document not only the level of involvement but also the extent of involvement so that a reasonable prognosis can be given. Examination of the contralateral extremity must be done to rule out bilateral involvement, which is not uncommon, especially in idiopathic brachial plexitis. Generally the EMG can provide more specific information on the extent and location of involvement of the plexus fibers than can the nerve conduction studies.[64]

REST

Fibrillations and positive sharp waves are seen in the distributions of the involved trunks, cords, or peripheral nerves.

TABLE 4-2
Root Supply of the Lower Extremity

Muscle	Roots L1	L2	L3	L4	L5	S1	S2	S3	S4
Psoas major	·	●	·						
Iliacus		●	·						
Gracilis		●	·						
Sartorius		●	·						
Adductor longus		·	●	·					
Adductor brevis		·	●						
Rectus femoris		·	●	·					
Vastus lateralis		·	·	●					
Vastus medialis		·	·	●					
Adductor magnus		·	·	●	·	·			
Tibialis anterior				·	●				
Extensor digitorum longus					●	·			
Extensor hallucis longus					●	·			
Peroneus tertius					●	·			
Extensor digitorum brevis					●	·			
Tibialis posterior				·	●	·			
Flexor digitorum longus					●	·	·		
Semitendinosus					●	·	·		
Semimembranosus					●	·	·		
Biceps femoris (short head)					●	·	·		
Tensor fasciae latae				·	●				
Gluteus medius				·	●	·			
Gluteus minimus				·	●	·			
Peroneus longus					·	●			
Peroneus brevis					·	●			
Medial gastrocnemius					·	●	·		
Lateral gastrocnemius					·	●	·		
Soleus						●	·		
Biceps femoris					·	●	·		
Gluteus maximus					·	●	·		
Piriformis					·	●	·		
Abductor hallucis						·	●		
Abductor digiti minimi (quinti)							●	·	
Interossei							●	·	
Sphincter ani externus							·	·	·
Bulbospongiosus (bulbocavernosus)							·	·	●

●, dominant supply; ·, additional supply

MINIMAL CONTRACTION

Increased polyphasia is seen. The polyphasic MUPs are normal in duration in early denervation. The MUPs are prolonged in duration with reinnervation. With early reinnervation the MUPs are highly polyphasic, of long duration, and of low amplitude. With chronic, progressive reinnervation the main MUP shows the presence of multiple late components, depending on the degree of reinnervation. If the reinnervation is recent, the individual components of the MUPs, especially the late components, show increased jitter and blocking. When the reinnervation process has matured, the MUPs are of high amplitude and long duration. They are triphasic or noncomplex polyphasic in shape with a stable configuration.

MAXIMAL CONTRACTION

The interference pattern is reduced, depending on the degree of motor units lost.

Injuries of the Brachial Plexus

Brachial plexus injuries can result from trauma (transections, missile injuries, or stretch injuries), complications of delivery (upper trunk lesions, known as Erb's palsy, and lower trunk injuries, known as Klumpke's paralysis), positioning in unusual postures as during surgery, malignancies of the nerves or surrounding tissues, metastases to the breast, and radiation plexopathies (myokymia may be seen at rest).[53,65]

Carrying a heavy rucksack on the shoulders and upper back may cause pressure on the upper trunk.[52] Injuries to the lower trunk or medial cord are common in true neurogenic thoracic outlet syndrome.[70] Such injuries are also seen with tumor infiltration from the upper lobe of the lung (Pancoast's tumor), in which case there may be associated Horner's syndome. A dislocation of the shoulder may injure the posterior cord,[53] but more likely the radial nerve. Isolated injuries of the middle trunk and lateral cord are rare.

In idiopathic brachial plexitis, also known as neuralgic amyotrophy,[61,63,68] the involvement may be limited to the distribution of a root, trunk, cord, or peripheral nerve.[53, 59, 69] The nerve conduction times of the proximal nerves such as the suprascapular, long thoracic, and axillary nerves may be delayed.[50,57,58,60] The accessory nerve, though not a derivative of the brachial plexus, is frequently involved, and the conduction time along this nerve may be delayed. The radial nerve is also often involved. The delay of conduction times is often seen after reinnervation has begun because conduction along newly myelinated, thin nerve fibers is slow. Not uncommonly, the anterior interosseous nerve may also be involved.[56,62] Involvement of the elements of the brachial plexus is patchy, and each peripheral nerve itself is involved in a patchy fashion. In addition, not all of the muscles supplied by a given nerve are necessarily involved or involved to the same degree.[57] The involvement is often more severe in muscles supplied by the upper trunk. The limb of the other side is sometimes also involved, but to a lesser extent and may therefore appear asymptomatic for some time.[67]

The innervation levels for the muscles supplied by the brachial plexus are provided in Table 4-3.

Injuries of the Lumbosacral Plexus

Injuries to the lumbosacral plexus may be caused by trauma (avulsion of lumbar nerve roots,[47,51] fractures of the pelvis), primary tumors or metastases to the pelvic viscera, and bleeding into the retroperitoneum, either from trauma or anticoagulant therapy.[49,54]

The innervation levels for muscles supplied by the lumbar plexus and sacral plexus are provided in Tables 4-4 and 4-5, respectively.

PERIPHERAL NEUROPATHIES

Electrodiagnostic studies help in determining whether the involvement of the peripheral nerves is primarily sensory, motor, or sensorimotor. These studies also aid in determining whether the involvement is predominantly demyelinative, axonal, or a combination of the two. Multiple peripheral nerves, including the facial nerves, may have to be examined bilaterally. In peripheral neuropathy the peripheral nerves of the lower extremities are most commonly affected. Hence, examination of the peripheral nerves of the lower extremities gives the highest diagnostic yield.

Demyelinative Neuropathies

Nerve Conduction Studies

SENSORY

Low-amplitude, asynchronous potentials with prolonged duration are seen. Distal latencies are very delayed.

MOTOR

Low-amplitude, asynchronous potentials are seen, especially on proximal stimulation. The de-

TABLE 4-3
Innervation Levels for Muscles Supplied by the Brachial Plexus

Muscle	*Anterior Primary Ramus(i) Trunk*	*Division(s)*	*Cord(s)*	*Peripheral Nerve(s)*
Rhomboideus major	Anterior primary ramus (C5)			Dorsal scapular
Rhomboideus minor	Anterior primary ramus (C5)			Dorsal scapular
Serratus anterior	Anterior primary rami (C5–C7)			Long thoracic
Supraspinatus	Upper trunk (C5, C6)			Suprascapular
Infraspinatus	Upper trunk (C5, C6)			Suprascapular
Deltoid	Upper trunk (C5, C6)	Posterior	Posterior	Axillary
Teres minor	Upper trunk (C5, C6)	Posterior	Posterior	Axillary
Teres major	Upper trunk (C5, C6)	Posterior	Posterior	Lower subscapular
Supinator	Upper trunk (C5, C6)	Posterior	Posterior	Radial
Extensor carpi radialis longus	Upper trunk (C5, C6)	Posterior	Posterior	Radial
Extensor carpi radialis brevis	Upper trunk (C5, C6)	Posterior	Posterior	Radial
Brachioradialis	Upper trunk (C5, C6)	Posterior	Posterior	Radial
Brachialis	Upper trunk (C5, C6)	Posterior	Lateral, posterior	Musculocutaneous, radial
Coracobrachialis	Upper trunk (C5, C6)	Anterior	Lateral	Musculocutaneous
Biceps brachii	Upper trunk (C5, C6)	Anterior	Lateral	Musculocutaneous
Pronator teres	Upper trunk (C5, C6)	Anterior	Lateral	Median (lateral head)
Triceps	Middle trunk (C7)	Posterior	Posterior	Radial
Extensor digitorum (communis)	Middle trunk (C7)	Posterior	Posterior	Radial
Extensor digiti minimi	Middle trunk (C7)	Posterior	Posterior	Radial
Extensor carpi ulnaris	Middle trunk (C7)	Posterior	Posterior	Radial
Abductor pollicis longus	Middle trunk (C7)	Posterior	Posterior	Radial
Extensor pollicis brevis	Middle trunk (C7)	Posterior	Radial	
Extensor pollicis longus	Middle trunk (C7)	Posterior	Posterior	Radial
Extensor indicis	Middle trunk (C7)	Posterior	Posterior	Radial
Latissimus dorsi	Middle trunk (C7)	Posterior	Posterior	Thoracodorsal
Flexor carpi radialis	Middle trunk (C7)	Ant/post	Lateral	Median (lateral head)
Pronator teres	Middle trunk (C7)	Ant/post	Lateral	Median (lateral head)
Flexor digitorum superficialis	Lower trunk (C8, T1)	Anterior	Medial	Median (medial head)
Flexor digitorum profundus (lateral half)	Lower trunk (C8, T1)	Anterior	Medial	Anterior interosseous
Flexor pollicis longus	Lower trunk (C8, T1)	Anterior	Medial	Anterior interosseous
Pronator quadratus	Lower trunk (C8, T1)	Anterior	Medial	Anterior interosseous
Abductor pollicis brevis	Lower trunk (C8, T1)	Anterior	Medial	Median
Opponens pollicis	Lower trunk (C8, T1)	Anterior	Medial	Median
Flexor pollicis brevis	Lower trunk (C8, T1)	Anterior	Medial	Median
Flexor carpi ulnaris	Lower trunk (C8, T1)	Anterior	Medial	Ulnar
Flexor digitorum profundus (medial half)	Lower trunk (C8, T1)	Anterior	Medial	Ulnar
Abductor digiti minimi	Lower trunk (C8, T1)	Anterior	Medial	Ulnar
Flexor digiti minimi	Lower trunk (C8, T1)	Anterior	Medial	Ulnar
Opponens digiti minimi	Lower trunk (C8, T1)	Anterior	Medial	Ulnar

pressed amplitude and asynchrony are due to the difference in the degree of involvement of different axons. The temporal dispersion becomes more noticeable when the distance from the recording electrode is increased. The distal conduction times and conduction velocities are markedly slowed. Determining the takeoff of the CMAP on proximal stimulation that corresponds to the takeoff on distal stimulation may be difficult because of the asynchrony of the response.

TABLE 4-4
Innervation Levels for Muscles Supplied by the Lumbar Plexus

Muscle	*Anterior Primary Ramus(i)*	*Division* (L2–L4)	*Branch*	*Peripheral Nerve*
Psoas major	L1–L3			
Adductor longus		Anterior	Anterior	Obturator
Adductor brevis		Anterior	Anterior	Obturator
Adductor magnus		Anterior	Anterior	Obturator
Gracilis		Anterior	Anterior	Obturator
Iliacus		Anterior	Posterior	Femoral
Pectineus		Anterior	Posterior	Femoral
Sartorius		Anterior	Posterior	Femoral
Vastus lateralis		Anterior	Posterior	Femoral
Vastus medialis		Anterior	Posterior	Femoral
Rectus femoris		Anterior	Posterior	Femoral

TABLE 4-5
Innervation Levels for Muscles Supplied by the Sacral Plexus

Muscle	*Anterior Primary Ramus(i)*	*Division*	*Peripheral Nerve*
Adductor magnus	L5,**S1**	Anterior	Tibial division of sciatic
Semitendinosus	**L5**, S1	Anterior	Tibial division of sciatic
Semimembranosus	**L5**, S1	Anterior	Tibial division of sciatic
Biceps femoris (long head)	L5, **S1**	Anterior	Tibial division of sciatic
Tibialis posterior	**L5**, S1	Anterior	Tibial
Flexor digitorum longus	**L5**, S1	Anterior	Tibial
Medial gastrocnemius	L5, **S1**, S2	Anterior	Tibial
Lateral gastrocnemius	L5, **S1**, S2	Anterior	Tibial
Soleus	L5, **S1**, S2	Anterior	Tibial
Abductor hallucis	S1, **S2**	Anterior	Medial plantar
Abductor digiti minimi (quinti)	S1, **S2**	Anterior	Lateral plantar
Sphincter ani externus	S2–S4	Anterior	Pudendal
Bulbospongiosus (bulbocavernosus)	S2–S4	Anterior	Pudendal
Tensor fasciae latae	L4, **L5**	Posterior	Superior gluteal
Gluteus medius	**L5**, S1	Posterior	Superior gluteal
Gluteus minimus	**L5**, S1	Posterior	Superior gluteal
Biceps femoris (short head)	**L5**, S1	Posterior	Common peroneal
Tibialis anterior	**L5**, S1	Posterior	Deep peroneal
Extensor digitorum longus	**L5**, S1	Posterior	Deep peroneal
Extensor hallucis longus	**L5**, S1	Posterior	Deep peroneal
Extensor digitorum Brevis	**L5**, S1	Posterior	Deep peroneal
Peroneus tertius	**L5**, S1	Posterior	Deep peroneal
Peroneus longus	L5, **S1**	Posterior	Superficial peroneal
Peroneus brevis	L5, **S1**	Posterior	Superficial peroneal
Gluteus maximus	L5, **S1**	Posterior	Inferior gluteal

In such situations recording with a needle pickup electrode may help, since the takeoff points are sharper with a needle recording.

Generally the conduction velocities are reduced to less than 50% of normal values because the lesion involves all nerve fibers homogeneously, large and small. If the conduction velocities are markedly slowed but the CMAPs do not show abnormal temporal dispersion, there may be uniform thinning of the myelin layers of the axons rather than multifocal involvement.

EMG

REST

In the early stages, when demyelinating neuropathy predominates, there may be silence at rest or a few positive sharp waves. Fibrillations are seldom seen.

MINIMAL CONTRACTION

A slight increase in polyphasia may be seen. The polyphasic MUPs are slightly longer or normal in duration and amplitude, since the polyphasia is caused by increased temporal dispersion rather than by reinnervation.

MAXIMAL CONTRACTION

The interference pattern is reduced in cases in which there is blocking of the impulse along the nerve.

Sensorimotor Neuropathies That Are Primarily Demyelinating

HEREDITARY DISEASES

Charcot–Marie–Tooth disease, type 1: autosomal dominant. Nerve studies show decreased motor conduction velocities, decreased amplitudes of sensory and motor responses, and prolonged distal latencies. The nerve conduction velocities average 25 m/sec.[80,84,91,97] There is little or no temporal dispersion because the myelin of the nerve fibers of a given nerve are homogeneously involved: the patient has more or less the same degree of involvement in all nerves. Blink reflexes are slower than normal.[88, 90]

Dejerine-Sottas disease—autosomal recessive, is the most severe form of sensorimotor peripheral neuropathy. Nerve conduction velocities are in the range of 3 m to 5 m/sec.[80]

Refsum's disease. Hypertrophic neuropathy, degeneration of the olivocerebellar tracts and anterior horn cells with defects in metabolism of phytanic acid

Cerebral lipidoses, which include metachromatic leukodystrophy and Krabbe's globoid leukodystrophy

ACQUIRED DISEASES

Guillain-Barré syndrome (postinfectious polyradiculopathy). It has been reported that the routine nerve conduction studies within the first 3 weeks are normal in Guillain-Barré syndrome.[82] Recently, it has been observed that the F responses and H reflexes may be absent or markedly delayed with the onset of the disease. Also seen at the time of onset of the symptoms are prolonged distal latencies and low-amplitude CMAPs. The CMAP amplitude often drops significantly from proximal to distal stimulation.[83] Reduced interference is often the only EMG abnormality in the initial stage. In the subacute stage, abnormalities in nerve conduction studies are more pronounced. The distal motor and sensory latencies are markedly delayed. The shape of the evoked responses is dispersed, especially with proximal stimulation. Facial nerve and blink reflex studies are also often abnormal.[88, 89] The conduction velocities are often slowed to 40% below normal.[76,87] Nerve conduction may continue to be slowed, even in the presence of clinical improvement. Prognosis is worst when the weakness is accompanied by axonotmesis with profuse fibrillations and positive sharp waves.

Chronic relapsing polyradiculopathy. When the inflammatory process in Guillain-Barré syndrome progresses beyond 6 weeks and continues intermittently, it is termed *chronic relapsing polyradiculopathy.*

Multiple myeloma affects the proximal and distal nerve segments about equally.[101]

Diphtheria. Segmental demyelination due to exotoxin of *Corynebacterium diphtheriae.* Clinical and electrophysiological features are similar to those of Guillain-Barré syndrome.

Leprosy. Conduction velocities have been reported to be extremely slowed,[95, 99] and conduction velocities of 2 m/sec have been reported.[85] Denervation may be seen in the muscles with atrophy.

Axonal Neuropathies

General

The nerves of the lower extremities are most commonly involved.

Nerve Conduction Studies

SENSORY

The amplitudes are depressed, but the shape is not asynchronous. The conduction times may be normal. In the later stages the sensory potentials may be absent. Sural nerve studies are particularly useful.

MOTOR

The amplitudes are depressed, but the configuration is smooth and not asynchronous. The conduction velocity is normal or mildly slowed. The conduction velocity, even if slow, will be at least 70% of normal, since the slowing is due to loss of the faster conducting fibers rather than to slowing along individual axons. If the distal motor responses are absent, the conduction velocity should be determined by using a proximal muscle. For example, record from the tibialis anterior and stimulate the peroneal nerve below and above the knee.

EMG

REST

Fibrillations and positive sharp waves are seen. These discharges are most prominent in the distal muscles, typically in the intrinsic muscles of the feet and hands. The involvement is usually symmetrical, and the lower extremities tend to be more involved than the upper extremities.

MINIMAL CONTRACTION

An increased percentage of polyphasic MUPs is seen. When the process of involvement is slow and the onset of denervation is recent, the polyphasic MUPs are of normal duration. If there is recent reinnervation, the polyphasic MUPs are very complex in shape, with jitter and blocking, especially in the late components. With very chronic reinnervation the MUPs are of long duration and high amplitude. They appear triphasic or noncomplex polyphasic in shape.

MAXIMAL CONTRACTION

The degree to which the interference is reduced depends on the amount of motor units lost.

Causes of Axonal Neuropathies

Axonal neuropathies are seen in association with the following:

Heavy-metal poisoning. Lead commonly causes radial neuropathy and involves the motor nerves of the upper extremities more than those of the lower extremities. Sensory involvement is not usually seen. Other heavy metals implicated include arsenic, mercury, thallium, and gold.

Drugs: Vincristine, phenytoin, isoniazid, dapsone, nitrofurantoin, and sodium cyanate

Organic compounds: Acrylamide, triorthocresylphosphate, methyl-N-butyl ketone, *n* hexane, and organophosphates. In toxic peripheral neuropathies due to acrylamide and triorthocresylphosphate poisoning, there is distal axonopathy of the large fibers, with retrograde involvement of the axons toward the cell body (dying-back neuropathy) and eventual involvement of the small fibers.[71, 72, 90] The distal latencies are delayed at the outset. Later, there is slowing of conduction velocities.

Uremia. Nerve conduction may deteriorate with increasing renal failure. Results of nerve conduction studies improve with dialysis or kidney transplant.[75, 96, 98]

Alcoholism. Results of sensory conduction studies may be more affected than those of motor conduction studies; usually the lower extremities are more involved than the upper extremities.[102] The degree of sensory nerve slowing is related to the degree of involvement of the sensory fibers.[92] The proximal and distal segments of the nerve may be equally involved.[81] Fiber density is increased on SFEMG.[100]

Carcinoma. Involvement may be predominantly sensory, or it may be a mixed sensorimotor involvement.[94]

Sarcoidosis. Distal sensorimotor peripheral neuropathy

Nutritional

Vitamin deficiencies (B_1, B_2, B_6, *and* B_{12})

Collagen vascular diseases: Periarteritis nodosa

Acute intermittent porphyria. Frequently affects motor nerves more than sensory nerves.

Neuronal Charcot-Marie-Tooth disease (hereditary motor sensory neuropathy, type 2). Results of peripheral nerve conduction velocity studies are normal. The amplitudes of the evoked motor and sensory responses may be depressed. With severe involvement there may be mild to moderate slowing of conduction velocities.[86] The EMG usually shows evidence of spontaneous activity at rest and very chronic extensive reinnervation and reduced interference on contraction.

Friedrich's ataxia. Commonly there is a normal to low-normal motor conduction velocity and CMAP amplitude. The sensory potentials are often small to absent.[81,93]

Mixed Demyelinative and Axonal Neuropathy

Nerve Conduction Studies

SENSORY

The distal latencies are prolonged, with small amplitudes.

MOTOR

The distal motor latencies are delayed. There is depression in amplitude and a dispersion of the CMAP. The conduction velocities are also mildly slowed, especially peripherally. This slowing is most pronounced in the lower extremity.

EMG

REST

The EMG shows either silence or fibrillations and positive sharp waves, depending on the degree of demyelination and axonal degeneration.

MINIMAL CONTRACTION

An increase in the incidence of polyphasic MUPs, either normal or slightly longer in duration, is seen when there is predominant demyelination. Evidence of chronic or active reinnervation is seen when the axonal lesions predominate.

MAXIMAL CONTRACTION

Interference is reduced proportional to the degree of demyelination or axonal involvement.

Diabetic Polyneuropathy

Diabetic polyneuropathy may present in several ways. Bilateral symmetrical peripheral neuropathy, starting with the peripheral nerves in the lower extremities, is due to a metabolic imbalance. Mononeuritis multiplex and mononeuritis are the results of vasculitis. Cranial neuropathy may be an initial presentation in diabetic neuropathy. Diabetic neuropathy sometimes predominantly involves large fibers.[73,78] If this is the case, the neuropathy is primarily from segmental demyelination.[81] Small fibers are sometimes predominantly involved, in which case damage is chiefly to the axons.[74, 81] When the involvement is both demyelinative and axonal, a mixture of large- and small-fiber involvement is common.

Also to be noted with diabetes is the occurrence of diabetic amyotrophy. In this situation there may be no evidence of peripheral neuropathy. There is pain in the thighs and lower paraspinal muscles, with rapid wasting of the thigh muscles owing to denervation. A good response to treatment for the underlying diabetes is usually seen.[77,79]

NEUROMUSCULAR JUNCTION DISEASES

Postjunctional Defects: Myasthenia Gravis

Myasthenia gravis is an autoimmune disease[131] in which antibodies destroy the postjunctional membrane. There is a frequent association with thymic disorders and thymoma.[114] Receptor antibodies that destroy the postsynaptic membrane are produced so that the membrane becomes

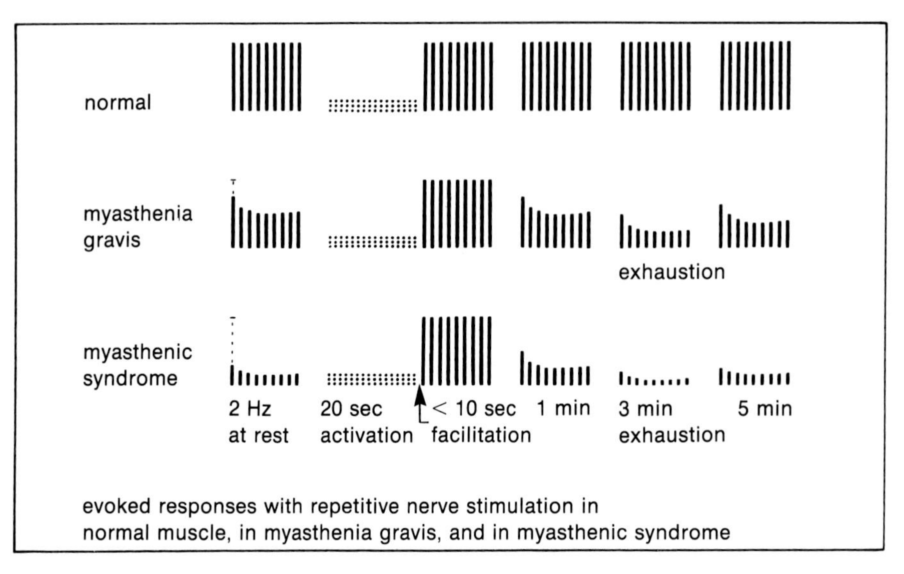

FIGURE 4-1 Schematic representation of the procedure and results of repetitive nerve stimulation in three different situations. (Stålberg E: Clinical neurophysiology tests of neuromuscular function. Didactic program, 29th Annual Meeting of the American Association of Electromyography and Electrodiagnosis, 1982)

very simplified and poorly formed.[103,113,123] The number of acetylcholine receptors is reduced.[115] The miniature end-plate potentials are of low amplitude but normal frequency. The amplitudes of the end-plate potentials are reduced.[110] The disease has a predilection for the extraocular muscles and the proximal musculature. Females are affected more often than males (2:1).

Nerve Conduction Studies

SENSORY

Results are normal.

MOTOR

Results of motor conduction studies are normal. The amplitude and area of the first CMAP evoked by a single shock can be either within normal limits or reduced, depending on the severity of the disease. The amplitude and area of the CMAP should therefore be measured.

REPETITIVE STIMULATION (FIG. 4-1)

Slow repetitive stimulation at a rate of two per second is used, since it is the most effective stimulation rate.[108, 109, 118, 126] Commonly, four stimuli are given. The amplitude and area of the first CMAP are compared to the amplitude and area of the fourth (or fifth) CMAP. If nine stimuli have been given, the responses to the first and ninth stimuli are compared. The amplitudes of the CMAPs usually decrease until the fourth or fifth stimulus.[107,120] (They often increase after the fifth.) A decrement of at least 10% by manual measurements or 5% by computer analysis is considered a positive result. The decrement is due to a progressive reduction in the amplitude of the end-plate potentials. Eventually the amplitude of the end-plate potentials is below threshold for firing.

The stimulation is repeated immediately after 20 seconds of isometric exercise for documentation of postexercise facilitation, a phenomenon that results from increased mobilization of acetylcholine immediately after exercise. Increased acetylcholine release causes the amplitudes of the end-plates to be larger.[108] This may cause the percentage of decrement seen on repetitive stimulation to be less immediately after the exercise than prior to the exercise. The first CMAP obtained after exercise may be larger in amplitude and area than the initial CMAP obtained at rest. This increase in amplitude and area is typically less than 100% of the amplitude and area of the initial CMAP. The maximal amplitude and area of the first CMAP obtained with postexercise facilitation may be an indication of the number of functioning endplates.[135]

The stimulation must then be repeated every minute for 5 to 10 minutes to detect postexercise exhaustion. Postexercise exhaustion results from depletion of the acetylcholine molecules that are immediately available for release at the nerve terminal.[108] This acetylcholine depletion may cause the percentage of the decrement seen on repetitive stimulation to be increased relative to the decrement obtained on repetitive stimulation of the muscle at rest. In severely myasthenic patients, if the exercise is prolonged for more than 20 seconds, the facilitation phase may be bypassed, and the exhaustion phase may be seen immediately after the exercise. With mild myasthenic involvement the postexercise exhaustion may not be seen after just 20 seconds of exercise, and the exercise may have to be prolonged for up to a minute.

In testing for myasthenia gravis it is essential to test the proximal muscles, such as the trapezius, biceps, and deltoid, and the facial muscles, since the test is more commonly positive in the proximal muscles and in muscles that are clinically weak. Patients who have never had repetitive stimulation studies but who are already taking anticholinesterase medications should have the medications withheld 12 hours prior to a test to be performed for initial diagnosis. This should, of course, be done only when it is clinically safe.[117,132] In follow-up studies the test should be performed at a constant interval after the last dose of medication. A rest period of 30 minutes prior to the test is essential. The limb to be tested should be warmed during this period to a skin temperature of 34°C or higher.

EMG

REST

Usually silent. Fibrillations and positive sharp waves may be seen in severely affected muscles and in the paraspinals in patients with severe myasthenia.

MINIMAL CONTRACTION

MUP parameters are usually normal. Commonly, there is variation in the shape of the MUP with consecutive discharges owing to increased jitter and blocking of the action potentials composing the MUP. In patients with chronic and severe disease the MUPs may resemble those seen in muscle diseases: depressed in amplitude and short in duration. In the case of a superimposed myopathy the MUPs are stable in configuration. The MUPs do not increase in amplitude after a rest period, as would be the case in myasthenia gravis alone.

MAXIMAL CONTRACTION

Interference is reduced proportional to the degree of neuromuscular junction delay and blockade. Some MUPs may fail to discharge completely. The amplitudes of successively recruited MUPs may decrease as the contraction continues.

SFEMG

Increased jitter and/or blocking can usually be seen in more than two pairs of potentials when 20 pairs of potentials are studied. Blocking on SFEMG can be expected if there is a decrement on repetitive studies. SFEMG is one of the most valuable tests for documentation of the disease, as well as for follow-up studies.[132,134–136]

Other Postjunctional Transmission Defects

Other postjunctional transmission defects are seen in association with drugs. These drugs include d-tubocurarine, decamethonium and suxamethonium, and the tetracyclines.[128,138] Penicillamine has also been noted to cause myasthenia.

In myotonia, muscle membrane refractoriness causes a decremental response to repetitive stimulation.

Prejunctional Defects: Myasthenic Syndrome

The myasthenic syndrome was first described by Eaton and Lambert.[122] It is seen in association with oat cell carcinoma of the lung[112] and has also been described in association with other malignancies. In the myasthenic syndrome a prejunctional defect causes impaired release of acetylcholine. The miniature end-plate potentials are of normal amplitude but low frequency.[110,111] Quantal content is low, but repetitive stimulation of the nerve terminal enhances this content.[120, 121] The muscles of the pelvic girdle are chiefly involved, the extraocular muscles rarely so. Peripheral neuropathy may be present, probably related to the presence of malignancy.

Nerve Conduction Studies

SENSORY

Results of conduction studies are normal unless there is an associated peripheral neuropathy.

MOTOR

The amplitude of the evoked motor response is very small, usually less than 2 mV. The conduction velocities are usually normal unless there is an associated peripheral neuropathy.

REPETITIVE STIMULATION (SEE FIG. 4-1)

Slow repetitive stimulation at a rate of two per second produces a decremental response in amplitude and/or area. A reduction in amplitude and/or area of more than 10% by manual estimates and 5% by computer estimates between the first and fourth responses (or between the first and ninth responses) is considered significant. When the stimulation is repeated immediately after 20 seconds of isometric exercise, a postexercise facilitation may be seen. This facilitation causes an increment in amplitude exceeding 100% of the response obtained at baseline, prior to the exercise. This effect lasts for approximately 20 seconds. To see this facilitation, repeat the test immediately after the exercise. Thereafter, the stimulation should be repeated at a rate of two per second every minute for 5 to 10 minutes. The amplitudes of the first evoked CMAP on each of these five to ten series of stimuli will be smaller than the amplitude of the response obtained at the onset of the test.

EMG

REST

Usually there is silence at rest unless there is denervation from associated peripheral neuropathy.

MINIMAL CONTRACTION

The MUP varies in shape at the beginning of the contraction. As the contraction continues, the individual components may increase in amplitude.[129]

MAXIMAL CONTRACTION

Interference appears more full as the contraction continues.

SFEMG

The increased jitter and blocking seen at the beginning of contraction decrease after exercise and increase with rest.[129] The fiber density is also increased.

Other Clinical Conditions Associated With Prejunctional Defects

Other clinical conditions associated with prejunctional blocking are *botulinum* intoxication,[105, 116, 127] hemicholinium poisoning,[104] and tick paralysis.[106, 125, 137]

Mixed Prejunctional and Postjunctional Transmission Defects

Prejunctional and postjunctional transmission defects are seen with kanamycin and neomycin toxicity,[104] as well as in association with extensive reinnervation, particularly in motor neuron disease,[124] poliomyelitis, syringomyelia, and axonal peripheral neuropathies. A decrement that is usually less then 20% is seen with reinnervation because of dysfunction in immature motor end-plates.

Practical Aspects of Repetitive Nerve Stimulation Studies

Any muscle can be used for repetitive nerve stimulation studies, but one should generally begin testing the muscle that is clinically most affected. The more proximal muscles usually give a higher yield of positive results, but they are more difficult to immobilize. However, since these muscles must be tested in the case of negative results on examination of the distal muscles, many examiners prefer to start the examination directly on the proximal muscles.

It is essential that the skin temperature of the limb be stabilized at 34°C. If the skin temperature is lower than 27°C, a false-negative result may be obtained because the decrement is abolished.[133]

Immobilization is essential so that movement artifacts do not interfere with the results. Hold the stimulator (usually a bar electrode) either steady or affix it to the limb so that variation in stimulus intensity due to movement of the stimulator does not occur. Needle stimulation can also be done.

Procedure

Allow the patient to rest for 30 minutes so that an uncontrolled decrement will not occur. This rest period is not needed if the test is being performed to document the diagnosis. However, it is essential if exact quantitative comparisons are to be made between successive examinations or if the effect of a drug is to be studied.[132, 133] Usually a series of nine stimuli is given. Compare the amplitude and area of the negative portion of the wave between the first CMAP to the amplitude and area of the fourth CMAP and to the amplitude and area of the ninth CMAP. Then ask the patient to contract the muscle under study isometrically for 20 seconds. Repeat the repetitive stimulation immediately, within 10 seconds, to document the presence of postexercise facilitation. You may miss this phase entirely in severely myasthenic patients if the exercise is longer than 20 seconds or if you do the test later after the exercise. Then repeat the test every minute for up to 5 minutes to document the presence of postexercise exhaustion. The following is a detailed guide to the examination of the most commonly examined muscles:

ABDUCTOR DIGITI MINIMI

Amplifier setting:
- Sweep speed: 2 msec/div.
- Sensitivity: Adjusted so as not to overload the amplifier (usually 5 mV/div.)
- Filter setting: 20 Hz–10 kHz
- Stimulus rate: 2/sec

Recording technique:
- Active electrode: At the middle of the muscle
- Reference electrode: On the base of the proximal phalanx of the fifth digit
- Ground electrode: On the ventral surface of the forearm

Stimulation technique: Place a bar electrode over the ulnar nerve at the patient's wrist so that a supramaximal response is achieved. When the positioning is satisfactory, immobilize the hand by strapping it and the forearm to an arm board.

BICEPS BRACHII

Amplifier setting:
- Sweep speed: 2 msec/div.
- Sensitivity: 5 mV/div.
- Filter setting: 2 Hz–10 kHz to allow for inclusion of the lower frequencies
- Stimulus rate: 2/sec

Recording technique:
- Patient position: Supine
- Active electrode: At the middle of the muscle
- Reference electrode: On the tendon of the biceps brachii
- Ground electrode: At the upper arm or on the wrist

Stimulation technique: Stimulate at Erb's point at a rate of one stimulus per second while trying to locate a good recording point and to ensure that the peak-to-peak amplitude can be visualized on the oscilloscope. When the recording point is satisfactory, the repetitive stimulation can be done. It is best to use a bar electrode for stimulation, since this electrode can be better stabilized than the stimulator with prongs. Immobilize the patient's arm by strapping it to an arm board. Since the entire brachial plexus tends to be stimulated, good immobilization is critical.

DELTOID

Amplifier setting:
- Sweep speed: 2 msec/div.
- Sensitivity: 5 mV/div.
- Filter setting: 2 Hz–10 kHz to allow for inclusion of the lower frequencies

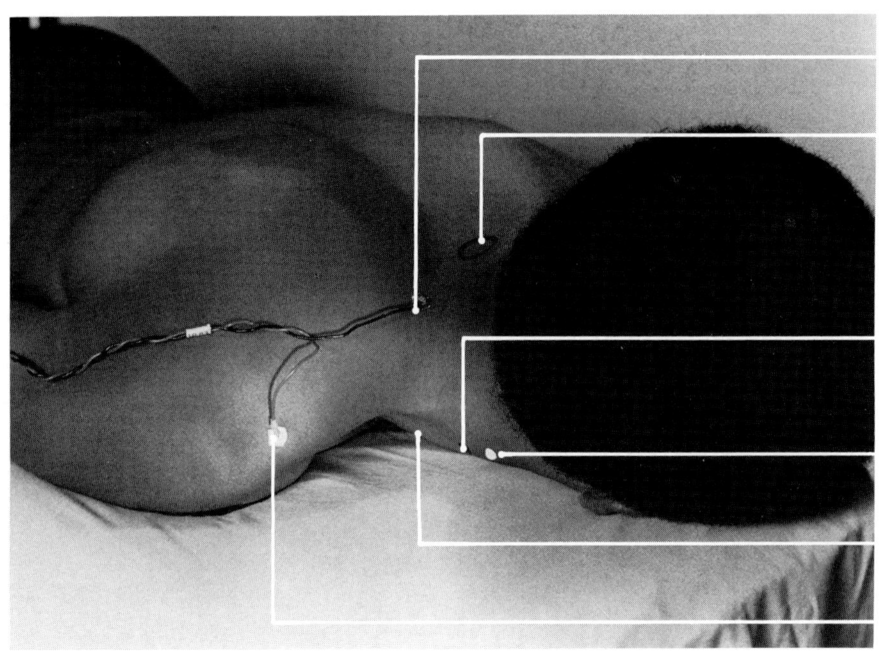

FIGURE 4-2 Repetitive stimulation study (accessory nerve stimulation).

Recording technique:
- Patient position: Supine
- Active electrode: On the most prominent portion of the deltoid
- Reference electrode: On the acromion
- Ground electrode: About the middle of the upper trapezius or on the wrist

Stimulation technique: Use supramaximal stimulation at a rate of one per second, as previously described, while trying to locate a good recording point. When the recording is satisfactory, the repetitive stimulation procedure can be started. A bar electrode is preferable to a stimulator with prongs, since the bar electrode can better be stabilized. The patient's arm can be immobilized by strapping it to the chest or having an assistant stabilize the arm against the chest. Arm immobilization can also be achieved by having the assistant stand at the angle between the patient's arm and chest and give downward pressure onto the patient's slightly abducted arm. Since the entire brachial plexus is stimulated, good immobilization is critical.

TRAPEZIUS (FIG. 4-2)

Amplifier setting:
- Sweep speed: 2 msec/div.
- Sensitivity: Usually 10 mV/div., but can be adjusted as needed
- Filter setting: 2 Hz–10 kHz

Recording technique:
- Patient position: Prone or semirecumbent
- Active electrode: Feel for the C7 spinous process and place the electrode 7 cm from this structure.
- Reference electrode: On the acromial process
- Ground electrode: On the arm

Stimulation technique: Stimulate at the midpoint of the posterior border of the clavicular head of the sternocleidomastoid. Use one stimulus per second to ensure that the recording is satisfactory before starting the repetitive stimulation procedure. For stimulation, a bar electrode is preferable to a stimulator with prongs, since the bar electrode can better be stabilized. Immobilize the arm to be examined by giving distal pressure at the tip of the shoulder to prevent shoulder elevation. Also give downward pressure over the scapula if the patient is prone. If the patient is semirecumbent or sitting, you can apply downward pressure over the upper arm and shoulder. This muscle is relatively easy to examine because only the accessory nerve is stimulated, and it is therefore easier to stabilize the limb.

FACIAL MUSCLES

Commonly examined are the orbicularis oculi and the nasalis.

- Amplifier setting:
  - Sweep setting: 2/sec
  - Sensitivity: 2 mV or 5 mV/div.
  - Filter setting: 20 Hz–10 kHz
- Recording technique for the nasalis:
  - Active electrode: On the wing of the ala nasi
  - Reference electrode: On the bridge of the nose or on the tip of the nose
- Recording technique for the orbicularis oculi:
  - Active electrode: On the inferior portion of the muscle
  - Reference electrode: On the zygomatic arch
- Stimulation technique: Stimulate at the anterior aspect of the ear at the level of the tragus.
- Test procedure: Allow the patient to rest for 30 minutes so that uncontrolled decrement will not occur. This period of rest is not needed if the test is being performed to document the diagnosis, but it is essential if exact quantitative comparisons are to be made between successive examinations or if the effect of a drug is to be studied.[133] Usually a series of nine stimuli is given. Compare the amplitude and area of the negative portion of the wave between the first CMAP to the amplitude and area of the fourth CMAP and to the amplitude and area of the ninth CMAP. Then ask the patient to contract the muscle under study isometrically for 20 seconds. Repeat the repetitive stimulation immediately, within 10 seconds, to document the presence of postexercise facilitation. You may miss this phase entirely if the exercise is longer than 20 seconds in patients with severe myasthenia or if you do the test later after the exercise. Repeat the test every minute for up to 5 minutes to document the presence of postexercise exhaustion.

MUSCLE DISEASES

Myopathic Disorders

Nerve Conduction Studies

SENSORY

Results are normal.

MOTOR

Conduction velocities are normal, but the amplitude of the CMAP is decreased proportional to the degree of atrophy.

EMG

GENERAL

It is essential to examine muscles that are clinically weak. The proximal muscles should be thoroughly examined.

REST

Fibrillations, positive sharp waves, and complex repetitive discharges are present. Fasciculations are never seen. Spontaneous activity disappears when muscle fibrosis occurs.

MINIMAL CONTRACTION

Owing to patchy loss of muscle fibers, there is poor temporal summation, and an increase in polyphasia results. The MUPs are generally small in amplitude and short in duration from loss of muscle fibers.[140] The shortened duration occurs because of the loss of distant muscle fibers that contribute to the low frequencies at the start and end of the MUP. Sometimes the duration may be prolonged, and late components may be present because of the reinnervation of muscle fibers that have regenerated by muscle fiber splitting or budding.[145] Innervation of myoblasts[147] or reinnervation of muscle fibers that were denervated by involvement of terminal nerve twigs or focal necrosis of muscle fibers also causes long-duration, complex polyphasic MUPs.

MAXIMAL CONTRACTION

Many MUPs are recruited relative to the force of contraction. This gives the interference pattern a full or slightly reduced pattern even when the muscle is clinically weak. The presence of high-frequency components from the many turns in the polyphasic MUPs may cause the interference pattern to sound high pitched and crackling. In late stages when there is substantial loss of muscle fibers, interference is reduced.

Myotonic Disorders

Nerve Conduction Studies

SENSORY

Amplitudes may be depressed owing to the presence of associated peripheral neuropathy (*e.g.*, in myotonic dystrophy).

MOTOR

Results are generally normal except in myotonic dystrophy, in which mild slowing is seen.[143,155] There may be a decremental response to repetitive stimulation, especially in myotonia congenita and paramyotonia congenita.[140,142] In paramyotonia there may be no CMAP on stimulation during the periods of weakness, owing to exposure to cold.

EMG

REST

Myotonic discharges characteristically wax and wane in amplitude and frequency. The myotonic discharges are usually in the form of fibrillations or positive sharp waves. The discharges may interfere with MUP analysis to such an extent that the muscle must be warmed to decrease the myotonic discharges. Cooling the muscle increases this type of discharge, except in paramyotonia, in which they disappear.[160] Myotonic discharges are initiated by a contraction, percussion over the muscle, or repetitive nerve stimulation.

MINIMAL CONTRACTION

An increase in polyphasia is seen. Low-amplitude, short-duration MUPs are seen in myotonic dystrophy, but the MUPs are normal in myotonia congenita.[140]

MAXIMAL CONTRACTION

The interference pattern is reduced when considerable loss of muscle bulk has occurred.

EMG *Characteristics of Specific Muscle Diseases*

I. Hereditary muscle diseases
   A. Muscular dystrophies
      1. Duchenne's muscular dystrophy, sex-linked recessive. Fibrillations, positive sharp waves, and complex repetitive discharges are commonly seen at rest.[144, 150, 156]
      2. Limb girdle dystrophy, autosomal recessive or sporadic. There is less spontaneous activity at rest than in Duchenne's muscular dystrophy.
      3. Fascioscapulohumeral dystrophy, autosomal dominant. The presence of fibrillations and positive sharp waves may vary in different muscles.[153]
   B. Myotonic diseases
      1. Myotonic dystrophy. There is predominant affectation of distal muscles. Clinical features of this disease include muscle weakness, cataracts, and dystrophic features in multiple organ systems. The myotonia disappears with exercise and increases with cold.
      2. Myotonia congenita. The myotonic involvement is diffuse. The patient's muscles also show hypertrophy. The myotonia disappears with exercise and increases with cold.
      3. Paramyotonia congenita. The myotonia increases with exercise and disappears with cooling, although the patient remains stiff. The muscles of the face and tongue are predominantly affected.[141]

C. Congenital myopathies. Examples of the congenital myopathies are central core disease, nemaline myopathy, congenital fiber-type disproportion, and myotubular myopathy. Spontaneous activity at rest is usually not seen with the first two diseases.[149,159] Occasionally, spontaneous activity is seen in congenital fiber-type disporportion.[149] It is usually seen in myotubular myopathy, and in this disease the spontaneous activity may include myotonic discharges at rest.[154,157]

D. Congenital metabolic myopathies
   1. Glycogen storage diseases
      (a) Pompe's disease (acid maltase deficiency). Fibrillations, positive sharp waves, and myotonic discharges may be seen at rest. There is no evidence of clinical myotonia.[146]
      (b) McArdle's disease (muscle phosphorylase deficiency). There is silence at rest on EMG during painful muscle cramps.[152]
      (c) Debrancher deficiency and muscle fructokinase deficiency. Profuse spontaneous activity is seen at rest.
   2. Disturbances in lipid metabolism. Examples include carnitine deficiency and carnitine palmityl transferase deficiency. Not infrequently, spontaneous activity is seen.
   3. Mitochondrial diseases (Kearns-Sayres disease). Mild myopathic changes are seen on EMG.
   4. Metabolic diseases
      (a) Hyperkalemic periodic paralysis. Insertional activity, fibrillations, positive sharp waves, and myotonic discharges are present at rest, and even more so during the paralytic period.[151] Responses to electrical stimulation may be absent during the paralytic phase.
      (b) Hypokalemic periodic paralysis. No evoked response or MUPs can be seen during the paralytic stage.[148]

II. Acquired muscle diseases
   A. Inflammatory muscle diseases
      1. Dermatomyositis and polymyositis. The spontaneous activity may be profuse.[139] The spontaneous activity diminishes as response to steroid therapy occurs. A decremental response may be seen in association with the presence of myasthenia gravis.[158]
      2. Other collagen vascular diseases with myopathic involvement: scleroderma, systemic lupus erythematosus, and rheumatoid arthritis
      3. Myositis may be seen with parasitic infections such as trichinosis and toxoplasmosis.
   B. Noninflammatory muscle diseases
      1. Endocrine disorders and disorders treated with corticosteroids
         (a) Hypothyroidism. Insertional activity is increased, and complex repetitive discharges may be seen at rest.
         (b) Hyperthyroidism. Myotonic discharges may be seen at rest.
         (c) Hypoparathyroidism. Doublets and multiplets may be seen at rest owing to increased muscle membrane instability associated with tetany.
         (d) Acromegaly
         (e) Steroid administration. No spontaneous activity is seen at rest. This finding is useful in differentiating the cause of weakness in patients with myositis treated with steroids.
      2. Myopathy may also be seen in chronic alcoholism and in malignancy.

REFERENCES

Anterior Horn Cell Diseases

1. Achari AN, Anderson MS: Myopathic changes in amyotrophic lateral sclerosis: Pathologic analysis of muscle biopsy changes in 111 cases. Neurology (NY) 24:477–481, 1974
2. Bernstein LP, Antel JP: Motor neuron disease: Decremental responses to repetitive nerve stimulation. Neurology (NY) 31:204–207, 1981

3. Buchthal F, Olsen PZ: Electromyography and muscle biopsy in infantile spinal muscular atrophy. Brain 93:15–30, 1970
4. Carleton AA, Brown WF: Changes in motor unit populations in motor neurone disease. J Neurol Neurosurg Psychiatry 42:42–51, 1979
5. Daube JR: EMG in motor neuron diseases. Minimonograph 18. Rochester, MN, American Association of Electromyography and Electrodiagnosis, 1982
6. Ertekin C: Sensory and motor conduction in motor neuron disease. Acta Neurol Scand 43:499–512, 1967
7. Hausmanova-Petrusevich I, Kopec J: Possible mechanism of motor conduction velocity changes in the anterior horn cell involvement. Electromyogr Clin Neurophysiol 13:357–365, 1973
8. Jusic A, Milic S: Nerve potentials and afferent conduction velocities in the differential diagnosis of amyotrophy of the hand. J Neurol Neurosurg Psychiatry 35:861–864, 1972
9. Kugelberg E, Taverner D: Comparison between the voluntary and electrical activation of motor units in anterior horn cell diseases. Electroencephalogr Clin Neurophysiol 2:125–132, 1950
10. Kuntz NL, Gomez MR, Daube JR: EMG in spinal muscular atrophy. Neurology (NY) 20:1002–1008, 1980
11. Lambert EH: Electromyography in amyotrophic lateral sclerosis. In Norris FH Jr, Kurland LT (eds): Motor Neuron Diseases, pp 135–153. New York, Grune & Stratton, 1969
12. Lambert EH, Mulder DW: Electromyographic studies in amyotrophic lateral sclerosis. Mayo Clin Proc 32:441–446, 1957
13. Moosa A, Dubowitz V: Motor nerve conduction velocity in spinal muscular atrophy of childhood. Arch Dis Child 51:974–977, 1976
14. Mulder DW, Lambert EH, Eaton LM: Myasthenic syndrome in patients with amyotrophic lateral sclerosis. Neurology (NY) 9:627–631, 1959
15. Mulder DW, Rosenbaum RA, Layton Jr DD: Late progression of poliomyelitis or forme fruste amyotrophic lateral sclerosis. Mayo Clin Proc 47:756–761, 1972
16. Ryniewicz B: Motor and sensory conduction velocity in spinal muscular atrophy: Follow-up study. Electromyogr Clin Neurophysiol 17:385–391, 1977
17. Schwartz MS, Moosa A: Sensory nerve conduction in the spinal muscular atrophies. Dev Med Child Neurol 19:50–53, 1977
18. Stålberg E, Schwartz MS, Trontelj JV: Single fibre electromyography in various processes affecting the anterior horn cells. J Neurol Sci 24:403, 1975
19. Stålberg E, Trontelj JV: Single Fibre Electromyography. Old Woking, Surrey, Mirvalle Press, 1979
20. Trojaborg W, Buchthal F: Malignant and benign fasciculations. Acta Neurol Scand 41 (Suppl 13):251–254, 1965
21. Weichers DO, Hubell SL: Late changes in the motor unit after acute poliomyelitis. Muscle Nerve 4:524, 1981
22. Wettstein A: Origin of fasciculations in motoneuron disease. Ann Neurol 5:295–300, 1979
23. Wohlfart G: Collateral regeneration from residual motor nerve fibers in amyotrophic lateral sclerosis. Neurology (Minneap) 7:124, 1957

Root Lesions

24. Aiello I, Rosati G, Serra G, Manca M: The diagnostic value of H index in S1 root compression. J Neurol Neurosurg Psychiatry 44:171–172, 1981
25. Braddom RL, Johnson EW: Standardization of "H" reflex and diagnostic use in S1 radiculopathy. Arch Phys Med Rehabil 55:161, 1974
26. Chu J: Lumbosacral radicular symptoms: Importance of bilateral electrodiagnostic studies (abstr.). Arch Phys Med Rehabil 62:522, 1981
27. Deschuytere J, Rossell N: Diagnostic use of monosynaptic reflexes in L5 and S1 root compression. In Desmedt JE (ed): New Developments in Electromyography and Clinical Neurophysiology, Vol 3, pp 360–366. Basel, S Karger, 1973
28. Eisen A, Schomer D, Melmed C: An electrophysiological method for examining lumbosacral root compression. Can J Neurol Sci 4:117–123, 1977
29. Fisher MA, Shivde AJ, Teixera C, Grainer LS: Clinical and electrophysiological appraisal of the significance of radicular injury in back pain. J Neurol Neurosurg Psychiatry 41:303–306, 1978
30. Fisher MA, Shivde AJ, Teixera C, Grainer LS: The F response—a clinically useful physiological parameter for the evaluation of radicular injury. Electromyogr Clin Neurophysiol 19:65–75, 1979
31. Gough JG, Koepke GH: Electromyographic determination of motor root levels in erector spinae muscles. Arch Phys Med Rehabil 47:9, 1966
32. Hoppenfeld S: Orthopaedic Neurology: A Diagnostic Guide to Neurologic Levels. Philadelphia, JB Lippincott, 1977
33. Jacobson RE: Lumbar stenosis—an electromyographic evaluation. Clin Orthop Rel Res 115:68–71, 1976
34. Johnson EW, Burkhart JA, Earl WC: Electromyography in postlaminectomy patients. Arch Phys Med Rehabil 53:407, 1972
35. Johnson EW, Melvin JL: Value of electromyography in lumbar radiculopathy. Arch Phys Med Rehabil 52:239, 1971
36. Kimura J: Electrodiagnosis in Diseases of Nerve and Muscle: Principles and Practice. Philadelphia, FA Davis, 1983
37. Knutsson B: Comparative value of electromyographic, myelographic and clinical–neurological examinations in disgnosis of lumbar root compression syndrome. Acta Orthop Scand [Suppl] 49:1, 1961
38. Kraft GH: Decay of fibrillation potential following nerve injury (Abstr). Muscle Nerve 7:565, 1984
39. La Ban MM, Grant AE: Occult spinal metastases—early electromyographic manifestations. Arch Phys Med Rehabil 52:223, 1971
40. Longstreth GF, Newcomer AD: Abdominal pain caused by diabetic radiculopathy. Ann Intern Med 86:166–168, 1977
41. Malcolm DS: A method of measuring reflex times applied in sciatica and other conditions due to nerve root compression. J Neurol Neurosurg Psychiatry 14:15, 1951
42. Op de Coul A, Lie T: A comparative electromyographic

study before and after operations for protruded lumbar disc. Electromyography 10:193–199, 1970
43. See DH, Kraft GH: Electromyography in paraspinal muscles following surgery for root compression. Arch Phys Med Rehabil 56:80, 1975
44. Seppalainen AM, Alaranta H, Soini J: Electromyography in the diagnosis of lumbar spinal stenosis. Electromyogr Clin Neurophysiol 21:55–66, 1981
45. Sharrard WJW: The segmental innervation of the lower limb muscles in man. Ann Col Surg 35:106, 1964
46. Weingarden HP, Mikolich LM, Johnson EW: Radiculopathies. In Johnson EW (ed): Practical Electromyography. Baltimore, Williams & Wilkins, 1980

Plexus Lesions

47. Barnett HG, Connolly ES: Lumbosacral nerve root avulsion: Report of a case and review of the literature. J Trauma 15:532, 1975
48. Bonney G, Gilliatt RW: Sensory nerve conduction after traction lesion of the brachial plexus. Proc R Soc Med 51:365, 1958
49. Chiu WS: The syndrome of retroperitoneal hemorrhage and lumbar plexus neuropathy during anticoagulant therapy. South Med J 69:595, 1976
50. Clein LJ: Suprascapular entrapment neuropathy. J Neurosurg 43:337, 1975
51. Coles CC, Miller KD Jr: Traumatic avulsion of the lumbar nerve roots. South Med J 71:334, 1978
52. Daube JR: Rucksack paralysis. JAMA 208:2447, 1969
53. Daube JR: An electromyographer's review of plexopathy. In Neuromuscular Diseases as seen by the Electromyographer. Second Annual Continuing Education Course. Rochester, MN, American Association of Electromyography and Electrodiagnosis, 1979
54. Emery S, Ochoa J: Lumbar plexus neuropathy resulting from retroperitoneal hemorrhage. Muscle Nerve 1:330, 1978
55. Jaeger R, Whiteley WH: Avulsion of the brachial plexus: Report of six cases. JAMA 153:633, 1953
56. Kiloh LG, Nevin S: Isolated neuritis of the anterior interosseous nerve. Br Med J 1:850, 1952
57. Kraft GH: Multiple distal neuritis of the shoulder girdle: An electromyographic clarification of "paralytic brachial neuritis." Electroencephalogr Clin Neurophysiol 27:722, 1969
58. Kraft GH: Axillary, musculocutaneous and suprascapular nerve latency studies. Arch Phys Med Rehabil 53:383, 1972
59. Martin WA, Kraft GH: Shoulder girdle neuritis: A clinical and electrophysiological evaluation. Milt Med 139:21, 1974
60. Olarte M, Adams D: Accessory nerve palsy. J Neurol Neurosurg Psychiatry 40:1113, 1977
61. Parsonage MJ, Turner JWA: Neuralgic amyotrophy: the shoulder-girdle syndrome. Lancet 1:973, 1948
62. Rennels GD, Ochoa J: Neuralgic amyotrophy manifesting as anterior interosseous nerve palsy. Muscle Nerve 3:160, 1980
63. Spillane JD: Localized neuritis of the shoulder girdle: A report of 46 cases in the MEF. Lancet 2:532, 1943
64. Stanwood JE, Kraft GH: Diagnosis and management of brachial plexus injuries. Arch Phys Med Rehabil 52:52, 1971
65. Thomas JE, Colby MY Jr: Radiation induced or metastatic brachial plexopathy? A diagnostic dilemma. JAMA: 222:1392, 1972
66. Trojaborg W: Electrophysiological findings in pressure palsy of the brachial plexus. J Neurol Neurosurg Psychiatry 40:1160, 1977
67. Tsairis P, Dyck PJ, Mulder DW: Natural history of brachial plexus neuropathy: Report on 99 patients. Arch Neurol 27:109, 1972
68. Turner JWA, Parsonage MJ: Neuralgic amyotrophy (paralytic brachial neuritis) with special reference to prognosis. Lancet 2:209, 1957
69. Weikers NJ, Mattson RH: Acute paralytic brachial neuritis: A clinical and electrodiagnostic study. Neurology (Minneap) 19:1153, 1969
70. Wilbourn AJ: True neurogenic thoracic outlet syndrome. Case Report 7. Rochester, MN, American Association of Electromyography and Electrodiagnosis, 1982

Peripheral Neuropathies

71. Aguayo AJ, Karpati G (eds): Current Topics in Nerve and Muscle Research. Amsterdam, Excerpta Medica, 1979
72. Asbury AK, Johnson PC: Pathology of Peripheral Nerve. Philadelphia, WB Saunders, 1978
73. Behse F, Buchthal F, Carlsen F: Nerve biopsy and conduction studies in diabetic neuropathy. J Neurol Neurosurg Psychiatry 40:1072, 1977
74. Brown MJ, Martin JR, Asbury AK: Painful diabetic neuropathy: A morphometric study. Arch Neurol 33:164, 1976
75. Cadilhac J et al: Follow-up study of motor conduction velocity in uraemic patients treated by hemodialysis. In Desmedt JE (ed): New Developments in Electromyography and Clinical Neurophysiology, Vol 2, pp 372–380. Basel, S Karger, 1973
76. Cerra D, Johnson EW: Motor nerve conduction velocity in "idiopathic" polyneuritis. Arch Phys Med Rehabil 42:159, 1961
77. Chokroverty S et al: The syndrome of diabetic amyotrophy. Ann Neurol 2:181, 1977
78. Chopra JS, Sawhney BB, Chakravorty RN: Pathology and time relationship of peripheral nerve changes in experimental diabetes. J Neurol Sci 32:53, 1977
79. Donovan WH, Sumi SM: Diabetic amyotrophy: A more diffuse process than clinically suspected. Arch Phys Med Rehabil 57:397, 1976
80. Dyck PJ, Lambert EH, Mulder DW: Charcot-Marie-Tooth disease: Nerve conduction and clinical studies of a large kinship. Neurology (Minneap) 13:1, 1963
81. Dyck PJ, Thomas PK, Lambert EH (eds): Peripheral Neuropathy. Philadelphia, WB Saunders, 1975
82. Eisen A, Humphreys P: The Guillain-Barré syndrome: A clinical and electrodiagnostic study of 25 cases. Arch Neurol 30:438, 1974

83. Flink R, Stålberg E, Ambler S, Rydin E: Early detection of Guillain-Barré syndrome. Presentation at the International Single Fiber EMG Symposium, Tromso, Norway, 1984
84. Gilliatt RW, Thomas PK: Extreme slowing of nerve conduction in peroneal muscular atrophy. Ann Phys Med 4:104, 1957
85. Goodgold J, Eberstein A: Electrodiagnosis of Neuromuscular Diseases. Baltimore, Williams & Wilkins, 1983
86. Harding AE, Thomas PK: The clinical features of hereditary motor and sensory neuropathy types I and II. Brain 103:259, 1980
87. Isch F et al: Measurement of conduction velocity of motor nerve fibres in polyneuritis and polyradiculoneuritis. Electroencephalogr Clin Neurophysiol 16:416, 1964
88. Kimura J: An evaluation of the facial and trigeminal nerves in polyneuropathy: electrodiagnostic study in Charcot-Marie-Tooth disease, Guillain-Barré syndrome, and diabetic neuropathy. Neurology (Minneap) 21:745, 1971
89. Kimura J: Conduction abnormalities of the facial and trigeminal nerves in polyneuropathy. Muscle Nerve 5:S142, 1982
90. Kimura J: Electrodiagnosis in Diseases of Nerve and Muscle: Principles and Practice. Philadelphia, FA Davis, 1983
91. Lambert EH: Electromyography and electric stimulation of peripheral nerves and muscles. In Depts. of Neurology, Physiology, and Biophysics, Mayo Clin and Mayo Foundation: Clinical Examinations in Neurology, 4th ed, pp 298–329. Philadelphia, WB Saunders, 1976
92. Mawdsley C, Mayer RF: Nerve conduction in alcoholic polyneuropathy. Brain 88:335, 1965
93. McLeod JG: An electrophysiological and pathological study of peripheral nerves in Friedreich's ataxia. J Neurol Sci 12:333, 1971
94. McLeod JG: Carcinomatous neuropathy. In Dyck PJ, Thomas PK, Lambert EH (ed): Peripheral Neuropathy, Vol 1, pp 1301–1313. Philadelphia, WB Saunders, 1975
95. McLeod JG et al: Nerve conduction studies in leprosy. Int J Lepr 43:21, 1975
96. Neilsen VK: The peripheral nerve function in chronic renal failure. IX. Recovery after renal transplantation: Electrophysiological aspects (sensory and motor nerve conduction). Acta Med Scand 195:171, 1974
97. Nielsen VK, Pilgaard S: On the pathogenesis of Charcot-Marie-Tooth disease: A study of the sensory and motor conduction velocity in the median nerve. Acta Orthop Scand 43:4, 1972
98. Oh SJ et al: Rapid improvement in nerve conduction velocity following renal transplantation. Ann Neurol 4:369, 1978
99. Swift TR et al: The peroneal and tibial nerves in lepromatous leprosy: Clinical and electrophysiologic observations. Int J Lepr 41:25, 1973
100. Thiele B, Stålberg E: Single fibre EMG findings in polyneuropathies of different aetiology. J Neurol Neurosurg Psychiatry 38:881, 1975
101. Walsh JC: The neuropathy of multiple myeloma: An electrophysiological and histological study. Arch Neurol 25:404, 1971
102. Walsh JC, McLeod JG: Alcoholic neuropathy: An electrophysiological and histological study. J Neurol Sci 10:457, 1970

Neuromuscular Junction Diseases

103. Appel SH, Almon RR, Levy N: Acetycholine receptor antibodies in myasthenia gravis. N Engl J Med 293:760, 1975
104. Argov Z, Mastalgia FL: Disorders of neuromuscular transmission caused by drugs. N Engl J Med 301:409, 1979
105. Cherington M: Botulism: Electrophysiologic and therapeutic observations. In Desmedt JE (ed): New Developments in Electromyography and Clinical Neurophysiology, Vol 1, pp 375–379. Basel, S Karger, 1973
106. Cherington M, Snyder RD: Tick paralysis: Neurophysiologic studies. N Engl J Med 278:95, 1968
107. Daube JR: Electrophysiologic testing for disorders of the neuromuscular junction. Minimonograph 8. Rochester, MN, American Association of Electromyography and Electrodiagnosis, 1978
108. Desmedt JE: The neuromuscular disorder in myasthenia gravis. 1. Electrical and mechanical response to nerve stimulation in hand muscles. In Desmedt JE (ed): New Developments in Electromyography and Clinical Neurophysiology, Vol 1, pp 241–304. Basel, S Karger, 1973
109. Desmedt JE, Borenstein S: Diagnosis of myasthenia gravis by nerve stimulation. Ann NY Acad Sci 274:174, 1976
110. Elmqvist D: Neuromuscular transmission defects. In Desmedt JE (ed): New Developments in Electromyography and Clinical Neurophysiology, Vol 1, pp 229–240. Basel, S Karger, 1973
111. Elmqvist D, Hoffman WW, Kugelberg J et al: An electrophysiological investigation of neuromuscular transmission in myasthenia gravis. J Physiol (Lond) 174:417, 1964
112. Elmqvist D, Lambert EH: Detailed analysis of neuromuscular transmission in a patient with myasthenic syndrome sometimes associated with bronchogenic carcinoma. Mayo Clin Proc 43:689, 1968
113. Engel AG, Santa T: Motor endplate fine structure. In Desmedt JE (ed): New Developments in Electromyography and Clinical Neurophysiology, Vol. 1, pp 196–228. Basel, S Karger, 1973
114. Engel WK et al: Myasthenia gravis. Ann Intern Med 81:225, 1974
115. Fambrough DM, Drachman DB, Satyamurti S: Neuromuscular junction in myasthenia gravis: Decreased acetylcholine receptors. Science 182:293, 1973
116. Gutmann L, Pratt L: Pathophysiologic aspects of human botulism. Arch Neurol 33:175–179, 1976
117. Jablecki C: Neuromuscular junction testing. Course A: Fundamentals of EMG. Fifth Annual Continuing Education Course. Rochester, MN, American Association of Electromyography and Electrodiagnosis, 1982
118. Johns RJ, Grob D, Harvey AM: Studies in neuromuscular

function. II. Effects of nerve stimulation in normal subjects and in patients with myasthenia gravis. Bull Johns Hopkins Hosp 99:125, 1956
119. Kao I, Drachman DB, Price DL: Botulinum toxin: Mechanism of presynaptic blockage. Science 193:1256, 1976
120. Lambert EH: Neurophysiological techniques useful in the study of neuromuscular disorders. Res Publ Assoc Res Nerv Ment Dis 38:247–273, 1960
121. Lambert EH, Elmqvist D: Quantal components of endplate potentials in the myasthenic syndrome. Ann NY Acad Sci 183:183, 1971
122. Lambert EH, Rooke ED, Eaton LM et al: Myasthenic syndrome occasionally associated with bronchial neoplasm: Neurophysiological studies. In Viets HR (ed): Myasthenia Gravis, pp 362–410. Springfield, IL, Charles C Thomas, 1961
123. Lefvert AK et al: Determination of acetylcholine receptor antibody in myasthenia gravis: Clinical usefulness and pathogenetic implications. J Neurol Neurosurg Psychiatry 41:394, 1978
124. Mulder DW, Lambert EH, Eaton LM: Myasthenic syndrome in patients with amyotrophic lateral sclerosis. Neurology (Minneap) 9:627, 1959
125. Murnaghan MF: Site and mechanism of tick paralysis. Science 131:418, 1960
126. Özdemir C, Young RR: Electrical testing in myasthenia gravis. Ann NY Acad Sci 183:287, 1971
127. Pickett JB, Berg B, Chaplin E et al: Syndrome of botulism in infancy: Clinical and electrophysiologic study. N Engl J Med 295:770, 1976
128. Pittinger CB, Eryasa Y, Adamson R: Antibiotic-induced paralysis. Anesth Analg (Cleve) 49:487–501, 1970
129. Schwartz MS, Stålberg E: Myasthenic syndrome studied with single fiber electromyography. Arch Neurol 32:815, 1975
130. Sears ML, Walsh FB, Teasdall RD: The electromyogram from ocular muscles in myasthenia gravis. Arch Ophthalmol 63:791, 1960
131. Simpson JA: Myasthenia gravis: A new hypothesis. Scott Med J 5:419, 1960
132. Stålberg E: Clinical electrophysiology in myasthenia gravis. J Neurol Neurosurg Psychiatry 43:622–633. 1980.
133. Stålberg E: Clinical neurophysiology tests of neuromuscular function. Didactic Program, 29th Annual meeting of the American Association of Electromyography and Electrodiagnosis, 1982
134. Stålberg E: Ekstedt J: Single fiber EMG and microphysiology of the motor unit in normal and diseased human muscle. In Desmedt JE (ed): New Developments in Electromyography and Clinical Neurophysiology, Vol 1, pp 113–129. Basel, S Karger, 1973
135. Stålberg E, Ekstedt J, Broman A: Neuromuscular transmission in myasthenia gravis studied with single fibre electromyography. J Neurol Neurosurg Psychiatry 37:540–547, 1974
136. Stålberg E, Trontelj JV, Schwartz MS: Single-muscle-fiber recording of the jitter phenomenon in patients with myasthenia gravis and in members of their families. Ann NY Acad Sci 274:189–202, 1976
137. Swift TR, Ignacio OJ: Tick paralysis: Electrophysiologic studies. Neurology (Minneap) 25:1130–1133, 1975
138. Wright EA, McQuillen MP: Antiobiotic-induced neuromuscular blockade. Ann NY Acad Sci 183:358, 1971

Muscle Diseases

139. Buchthal F, Pinelli P: Muscle action potentials in polymyositis. Neurology (Minneap) 3:424, 1953
140. Buchthal F: Diagnostic significance of the myopathic EMG. In Rowland LP (ed): Pathogenesis of Human Muscular Dystrophies. Proceedings of the Fifth International Conference of the Muscular Dystrophy Association. Amsterdam, Excerpta Medica, 1977
141. Burke D, Skuse NF, Lethlean AK: An analysis of myotonia in paramyotonia congenita. J Neurol Neurosurg Psychiatry 37:900, 1974
142. Burke D, Skuse NF, Lethlean AK: Contractile properties of the abductor digiti minimi muscle in paramyotonia congenita. J Neurol Neurosurg Psychiatry 37:894, 1974
143. Caccia MR, Negri S, Parvis VP: Myotonic dystrophy with neural involvement. J Neurol Sci 16:253, 1972
144. Desmedt JE, Borenstein S: Relationship of spontaneous fibrillation potentials to muscle fibre segmentation in human muscular dystrophy. Nature 258:531, 1975
145. Desmedt JE, Borenstein S: Regeneration in Duchenne muscular dystrophy: Electromyographic evidence. Arch Neurol 33:642, 1976
146. Engel AG et al: The spectrum and diagnosis of acid maltase deficiency. Neurology (Minneap) 23:95, 1973
147. Gardner-Medwin D: Studies of the carrier state in the Duchenne type of muscular dystrophy. 2. Quantitative electromyography as a method of carrier detection. J Neurol Neurosurg Psychiatry 31:124, 1968
148. Gordon AM, Green JR, Lagunoff D: Studies on a patient with hypokalemic familial periodic paralysis. Am J Med 48:185, 1970
149. Kimura J: Electrodiagnosis in Diseases of Nerve and Muscle: Principles and Practice. Philadelphia, FA Davis, 1983
150. Kugelberg E: Electromyography in muscular dystrophies. J Neurol Neurosurg Psychiatry 12:129, 1949
151. Layzer RB, Lovelace RE, Rowland LP: Hyperkalemic periodic paralysis. Arch Neurol 16:455, 1967
152. Layzer RB, Rowland LP: Cramps. N Engl J Med 285:31, 1971
153. Munsat TL, Piper D, Cancilla P, Mednick J: Inflammatory myopathy with fascioscapulohumeral distribution. Neurology (Minneap) 22:335, 1972
154. Munsat TL, Thompson LR, Coleman RF: Centronuclear ("myotubular") myopathy. Arch Neurol 20:120, 1969
155. Panayiotopoulos CP, Scarpalezos S: Dystrophia myotonica: Peripheral nerve involvement and pathogenic implications. J Neurol Sci 27:1, 1976
156. Pinelli P, Buchthal F: Muscle action potentials in myopathies with special regard to progressive muscular dystrophy. Neurology 3:347, 1952
157. Spiro AJ, Shy CM, Gonatas NK: Myotubular myopathy:

Persistence of fetal muscle in an adolescent boy. Arch Neurol 14:1, 1966
158. Vasilescu C et al: Myasthenia in patients with dermatomyositis: Clinical, electrophysiological and ultrastructural studies. J Neurol Sci 38:129, 1978
159. Warmolts JR, Wiechers DO: Myopathies. In Johnson EW (ed): Practical Electromyography. Baltimore, Williams & Wilkins, 1980
160. Wegmüller E, Ludin HP, Mumenthaler M: Paramyotonia congenita: A clinical, electrophysiological and histological study of 12 patients. J Neurol 220:251, 1979

5
Common Injuries and Entrapment Syndromes Involving the Peripheral Nerves*

Jennifer Chu-Andrews
Robert J. Johnson
Francis L. Bruyninckx

FACIAL AND TRIGEMINAL NERVES

Applied Anatomy

Facial Nerve (See Figs. 1-1 and 1-2)

The facial nerve (7th cranial nerve) is the nerve of the hyoid or second pharyngeal arch and supplies the muscles derived from the mesenchyme of that arch. These muscles are the facial muscles (called by some the "muscles of facial expression"), the stylohyoideus, the posterior belly of the digastricus, and the stapedius muscle within the middle ear. The facial nerve also carries some parasympathetic fibers, which are relayed through the pterygopalatine and submandibular (submaxillary) ganglia to then pass onward to innervate the lacrimal gland, the mucous glands of the nose, and the sublingual, submaxillary, and palatine salivary glands. Taste sensation from the anterior two thirds of the tongue travels over fibers that first run in the lingual nerve (a branch of the trigeminal), then leave the latter gathered together as the chorda tympani nerve, which enters the middle ear through the petrotympanic fissure. Within the middle ear cavity the chorda tympani travels posteriorward across the uppermost part of the tympanic membrane, between this membrane and the mucosa. It leaves the middle ear via the iter chordae posterius (the posterior canaliculus for the chorda tympani) and joins the facial nerve in the facial canal. The cell bodies of this sensory nerve are found in the geniculate ganglion of the facial nerve. The taste fibers just described and the parasympathetic fibers mentioned previously travel together in an independent, slender nerve that leaves the facial nerve as it exits from the petrous portion of the temporal bone to enter the internal auditory meatus. This combined group of afferent (taste) and visceral efferent (parasympathetic) fibers forms the nervus intermedius, which makes a second root of the facial nerve as it leaves the pontomedullary, or inferior pontine, sulcus of the brain stem. It stands between the main trunk of the facial nerve and the acoustic nerve; hence the name nervus intermedius.

As the facial nerve crosses the interval between the brain stem and the entrance into the internal auditory meatus, it is closely associated with the acoustic or vestibulocochlear nerve (8th cranial nerve). Both nerves crowd into the meatus, and both penetrate into small apertures in the bone at the fundus of the meatus. Acoustic neurinomata, which usually arise in the vestibular portion of the acoustic nerve, will, in time, not only damage and then destroy the nerve in which they arise, but such tumors also compress the cochlear and facial nerves. With continued expansion the tumor causes an erosion of the walls of the internal meatus and hence creates an asymmetric caliber of the right and left meatuses that is virtually diagnostic of the condition. The neurinoma mass, expanding toward the brain stem, grows into the angle between the pons and the medulla and hence the name cerebellopontine angle tumor. There are other types of tumor at this locus, however. The acoustic neurinoma cre-

* The applied anatomy portions of this chapter were written entirely by Robert J. Johnson, M.D.

ates what might be considered an entrapment syndrome within the internal acoustic meatus, but it is not traditionally identified as such.

When the facial nerve enters its foramen in the fundic end of the internal meatus, it begins its long and changing course within the substance of the petrous portion of the temporal bone.[72,120] The bony canal in which the nerve travels is called the facial canal. The canal, with its contained nerve, first runs laterally past the structures of the inner ear, and then, approaching the medial wall of the middle ear, or tympanic cavity, the facial canal makes a curved 90° flexure to run posteriorly. This flexure is referred to as the first external genu of the facial nerve. In its posteriorly running segment the canal bulges slightly into the middle ear along the medial wall of that cavity. After passing across the upper border of the fenestra vestibuli the facial canal makes another curved 90° flexure. This time it turns downward, and this flexure is called the second external genu of the facial nerve.

The nerve emerges from the stylomastoid foramen at the lower end of this vertical segment of the facial canal and is then external to the skull and immediately behind the base of the styloid process. After an anteroinferior course around the lateral side of the styloid process, the nerve divides into a temporofacial trunk and a cervicofacial trunk, each of which divides into several more branches, and these proceed forward in a cleft between the superficial and deep portions (lobes) of the parotid gland. A variable pattern of branches, which to some degree anastomose with one another, extends forward from the two major branches of the facial nerve.[139] From above downward, these branches are the temporal branches, the zygomatic branches, and the buccal branches, all from the temporofacial trunk. From the cervicofacial trunk there arise some lower buccal branches, a mandibular branch and sometimes a marginal mandibular branch, and the cervical branch, which supplies the platysma myoides muscle. All of the branches above the cervical branch pass to the regions of the face that their names suggest and, reaching the deep surface of the several facial muscles, penetrate and supply them.

Two small branches arise from the facial nerve while it runs within its canal in the temporal bone either at or very near the geniculate ganglion. The first of these is the greater petrosal nerve (formerly called the greater superficial petrosal nerve). This branch springs from the facial nerve at, or near, the geniculate ganglion and contains fibers of two types. One type is parasympathetic, and these fibers are relayed in the pterygopalatine ganglion, as mentioned earlier. The other type is special visceral afferent, or taste. These fibers arise in the palate and furnish a taste pathway other than through the lingual nerve and chorda tympani. By either route the cell bodies of the taste fibers are in the geniculate ganglion. Next, a very small twig leaves the facial nerve or the geniculate ganglion to join the tympanic plexus or the lesser petrosal nerve, which is the reassembled outflow from the tympanic plexus. The fibers in the lesser petrosal nerve are largely a continuation of the tympanic branch of the glossopharyngeal nerve and are preganglionic fibers to the otic ganglion. From the ganglion, postganglionic secretomotor fibers travel via the auriculotemporal branch of the trigeminal nerve to the parotid gland. In the more distal segment of the facial nerve, after the second external genu, as the nerve is descending vertically toward the stylomastoid foramen, a series of three branches arise. These are, in succession, the nerve to the stapedius muscle, the nerve to the chorda tympani and, finally, just above the stylomastoid foramen, a ramus communicans that joins the auricular branch of the vagus and thus assists in the supply of the skin of the external acoustic meatus and part of the skin of the tympanic membrane.

Just below the stylomastoid foramen the facial nerve gives off two branches before dividing into the two main trunks previously described. The first of these two branches in the neck, just below the base of the skull, is the digastric branch, which supplies the posterior belly of the digastric and stylohyoid muscles. The anterior belly of the digastric muscle is supplied by the mylohyoid branch of the mandibular division of the trigeminal nerve. The second branch of the facial nerve just below the base of the skull is the posterior auricular nerve. This slender twig runs posteriorly across the lateral aspect of the mastoid process and, ascending as it proceeds, finally reaches and supplies the occipitalis muscle. On its way, it also supplies the auricularis posterior muscle and gives very tiny twigs to each of the intrinsic auricular muscles. These muscles are rudimentary, and although there are six of them, they have no ability to modify the shape of the auricle. The auricularis anterior and superior are supplied by a small posteriorly directed twig from the highest temporal branch of the facial nerve as the latter heads for the frontalis and the upper part of the orbicularis oculi. The temporal and zygomatic branches supply, among other muscles, the palpebral portion of the orbicularis oculi in both the upper and lower lids. This palpebral portion is responsible for the very important motor side of the blink reflex.

Compression or entrapment neuropathy of the facial nerve while within the internal acoustic meatus has already been mentioned. Because of the anatomical relationships there, the two divisions of the acoustic nerve are involved along with the facial nerve in the presence of an expanding neurinoma. Thus, depending on the size of the tumor, the history may include vestibular abnormalities with vertigo and nausea, tinnitus progressing to deafness, and hemifacial spasm followed by facial palsy. As the tumor expands outside of the internal meatus, its expanding mass stretches and damages the nearby cranial nerves so that ultimately the trigeminal, the abducens, the glossopharyngeal, rootlets of the vagus, and even the hypoglossal nerves may be involved to some degree. The signs of this increasing involvement of the nerves are slowly added on as the tumor expands in the cerebellopontine angle. Loss of the corneal reflex because of trigeminal involvement is the only common sign, however, for the other nerves can be stretched to a surprising degree before they give rise to symptoms or signs.

The facial nerve may be damaged as it runs its course through the facial canal within the petrous portion of the temporal bone, which extends from the fundus of the internal acoustic meatus to the stylomastoid foramen.[13,40,177] Basal skull fractures, infections, and middle ear diseases may lead to lesions of the nerve within the facial canal. Bell's palsy is an idiopathic condition of unknown origin but of known pathology (in certain cases observed surgically), which usually occurs in the vertical segment beyond the second external genu, resulting in a facial muscle paralysis of varying degrees of severity and extent.[166] Tumors of the parotid gland, either in the deep part or lobe (deep to the facial nerve) or in the superficial part or lobe (superficial to the facial nerve), may by their expansion damage the facial nerve or some of its branches. Facial lacerations may also be the basis for disruption of branches of the facial nerve.

In the clinical identification of the locus of an intracranial or intratemporal lesion of the facial nerve, the sequence and location of the several branches and connections of the nerve become important. The branches of particular significance are the greater petrosal nerve, the nerve to the stapedius, the chorda tympani, and the posterior auricular nerve (which arises just below the stylomastoid foramen). Fractures of the petrous portion of the temporal bone may transect the nerve by virtue of the original shear along the fracture line or by hemorrhage at that site. Disruption of the facial nerve just before the origin of the greater petrosal nerve would include, in addition to the facial palsy, a loss of innervation to the lacrimal gland, the nasal glands, and the palatal glands. There would be some difficulty in identifying this loss and, especially, it must be remembered that the production of tears for the constant moistening of the cornea and conjunctiva is done by the accessory lacrimal glands, which lie in the superior and inferior fornices. These are the so-called basal secretors and are not under neural control. The lacrimal gland secretes on reflex stimulation from conjunctival irritation, nasal pain, certain emotional states, and so forth. Overflow lacrimation, on appropriate stimulus and on the opposite side only, might suggest the interruption of the innervation to the lacrimal gland, provided that there is not an occlusion of the nasolacrimal duct on that side.

Interruption of the facial nerve proximal to the origin of the nerve to the stapedius would cause a paralysis of the stapedius muscle, thereby eliminating the stapedius reflex with an attendant hyperacousia.[11] Interruption of the facial nerve proximal to the origin of the chorda tympani adds to the facial palsy a loss of the taste sensibility to the anterior two thirds of the tongue on the affected side. The loss of secretion of the sublingual and submaxillary salivary glands would not be detected except by special methods. Demonstration of normal function of the posterior auricular and occipitalis muscles in the presence of an otherwise complete facial palsy suggests that the damage to the facial nerve is in its parotid course, since the posterior auricular branch arises from the main nerve just below the stylomastoid foramen, but before becoming surrounded by the parotid gland.

Trigeminal Nerve (See Appendix Figs. 16 and 21)

The trigeminal nerve emerges from the lateral aspect of the midlevel of the pons as two roots. The much smaller motor root is superior but descends around the medial side of the larger sensory root and, passing inferior to the trigeminal ganglion, joins the mandibular division. These motor fibers are distributed to the muscles of mastication and to the tensor tympani, the tensor veli palatini, the mylohyoideus, and the anterior belly of the digastric. All of these muscles arise in the mesenchyme of the mandibular, or first, pharyngeal arch and are supplied by the nerve of that arch, which is the mandibular division of the trigeminal nerve.

The large sensory root expands abruptly into the trigeminal (or Gasserian) ganglion, in which lie the cell bodies of the great majority of the sensory fibers in the trigeminal nerve. The ganglion divides along its anterior margin into three great divisions, the ophthalmic or first, the maxillary or second, and the mandibular or third.

The ophthalmic division, passing through the superior orbital fissure, divides into three branches: the frontal, lacrimal, and nasociliary nerves. The frontal nerve passes forward against the very roof of the orbit, above the levator palpebrae superioris, dividing into the supratrochlear nerve and the supraorbital nerve. The former branch exits the orbit around the superomedial margin of the orbit to supply the medial end of the upper eyelid and the medial area of the forehead above the glabella. The supraorbital nerve divides into medial and lateral supraorbital branches, which leave the orbit through the supraorbital notch or foramen and supply the central portion of the upper eyelid and a broad area of the forehead extending back to the vertex.[104] The supraorbital notch is commonly identifiable on palpation with the fingertip or fingernail. If it has been converted to a foramen by ossification across the notch, its position may be obscure, but the emergent nerve branches can be located by virtue of their painfulness on compression against the bone. The lacrimal nerve passes forward through the orbit along the upper border of the rectus lateralis muscle and then, passing the lacrimal gland, gives a few fine twigs to the gland. The fibers in these branches to the gland were not originally in the lacrimal nerve, however. They have come, instead, from the pterygopalatine ganglion as postganglionic parasympathetic fibers that run first in the zygomatic branch of the maxillary nerve. These fibers next ascend, via an anastomotic loop in the lateral wall of the orbit, to join the lacrimal nerve some 10 mm proximal to the lacrimal gland. After that short course in the lacrimal nerve they finally gain the lacrimal gland for which they are secretomotor. The sensory fibers that make up the bulk of the lacrimal nerve pass onward, however, to be distributed into the skin of the lateral part of the upper eyelid. The nasociliary nerve enters the orbit through the superior orbital fissure and gives sensory supply to the bulbus oculi itself and, via the anterior ethmoidal nerve, to the medial and lateral parts of the anterior nasal mucosa. One small continuation of this nerve supplies the skin over the lower portion of the dorsum and sides of the external nose (external nasal branch).

The maxillary division of the trigeminal nerve leaves the middle cranial fossa via the foramen rotundum and appears in the uppermost part of the pterygopalatine fossa where the pterygopalatine (sphenopalatine) ganglion hangs suspended from it. Turning laterally, the maxillary nerve gives off the zygomatic branch, which enters the orbit to divide into the zygomaticofacial and zygomaticotemporal branches. Piercing bone, these two branches reach the skin of the malar eminence and the temple, respectively. The maxillary nerve then runs parallel to the inferior orbital fissure, which it enters when it reaches the level of the posterior end of the infraorbital sulcus. On entering the orbit the maxillary nerve becomes the infraorbital nerve as it runs forward, first in the sulcus and then in the canal, to emerge finally at the infraorbital foramen. Here its terminal branches supply the skin of the lower eyelid, the upper lip, the infraorbital skin intervening between eyelid and lip, and a variable portion of the ala nasi. The maxillary nerve also

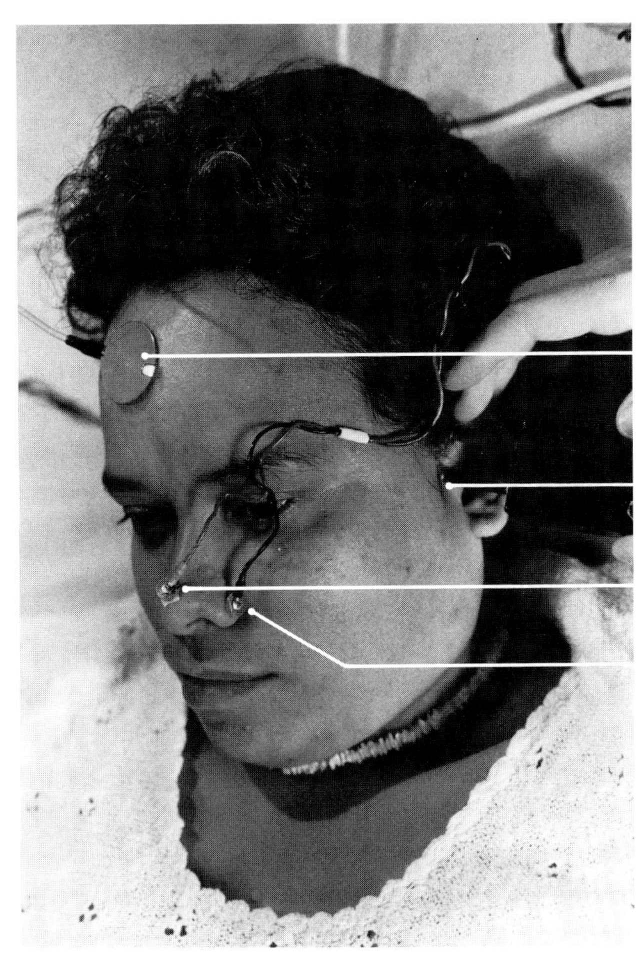

FIGURE 5-1 Facial nerve conduction study.

supplies the maxillary sinus, the upper teeth and gingiva, the posterior portions of both the medial (septal) and lateral walls of the nasal cavity, and the roof of the mouth, including the upper half of the vestibule of the mouth.

The mandibular division of the trigeminal gives origin to several muscular branches supplying the muscles of mastication plus the four addition muscles, previously cited, that also arise from the mesenchyme of the mandibular arch.[153] Its sensory branches are widely distributed to the mucosa and skin of the cheek (buccal nerve), the anterior two thirds of the tongue (lingual nerve), the lower teeth and gingiva and the lower lip and chin (mental branch of the inferior alveolar nerve), and the upper half of the external ear and a broad band of the skin of the side of the head from the level of the tragus to the level of the superior temporal line (auriculotemporal nerve).

Facial Nerve Conduction Study (Fig. 5-1)

Conduction Time

Amplifier setting:
  Sweep speed: 2 msec/div.
  Sensitivity: 2 mV/div.
  Filter setting: 20 Hz–10 kHz
Recording technique:
  Active electrode: On the nasalis
  Reference electrode: On the tip of the nose
    Note: Recording may also be done by placing the active electrode on the inferior

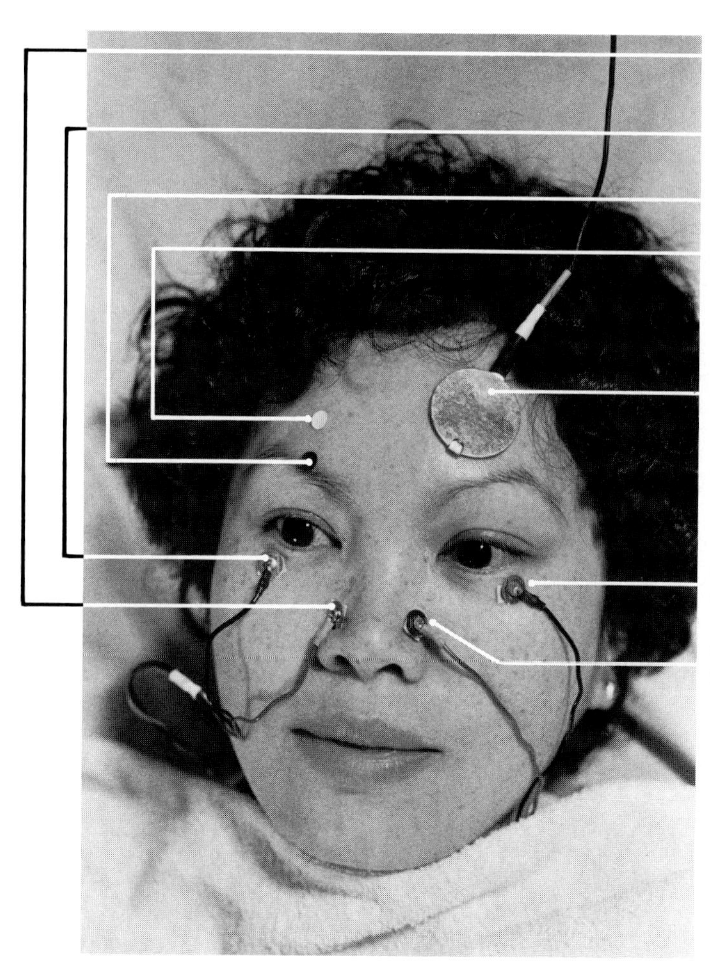

FIGURE 5-2 Blink reflex.
Note: The ground electrode may be placed on the chin, and the reference electrode may be placed on the temple.

and lateral portion of the orbicularis oculi approximately 1 cm below the inferior margin of the orbit and the reference electrode on the zygomatic process (see Fig. 5-2 for these electrode placements; they are identical to those described in the section on blink reflex).
Ground electrode: On the forehead or chin
Stimulation technique:
Use supramaximal current.
Stimulate with the cathode placed just anterior to the tragus of the ear.

Normal Values[101]

2.9 ± 0.4 msec. Conduction is considered delayed if longer than 4.1 msec (orbicularis oculi).

Blink Reflex Study (*Fig*. 5-2)

The blink reflex is obtained by stimulation of the supraorbital nerve and consists of two responses, R1 and R2. R1 is relayed through the pons[98] and is oligosynaptic; R2 is relayed through the pons and lateral medulla[103,167,231] and is multisynaptic. The R1 response is obtained by recording from the same side as the stimulation, whereas the R2 response is obtained bilaterally (Fig. 5-3, A). The R1 response is fairly reproducible, but the R2 response is variable. However, the R2 response is useful if there is a lesion along the facial nerve or trigeminal nerve.[101,103,167] In trigeminal nerve lesions the R2 response is delayed bilaterally. In facial nerve lesions it is delayed on the involved side with either ipsilateral or contralateral stimulation of the supraorbital nerve.

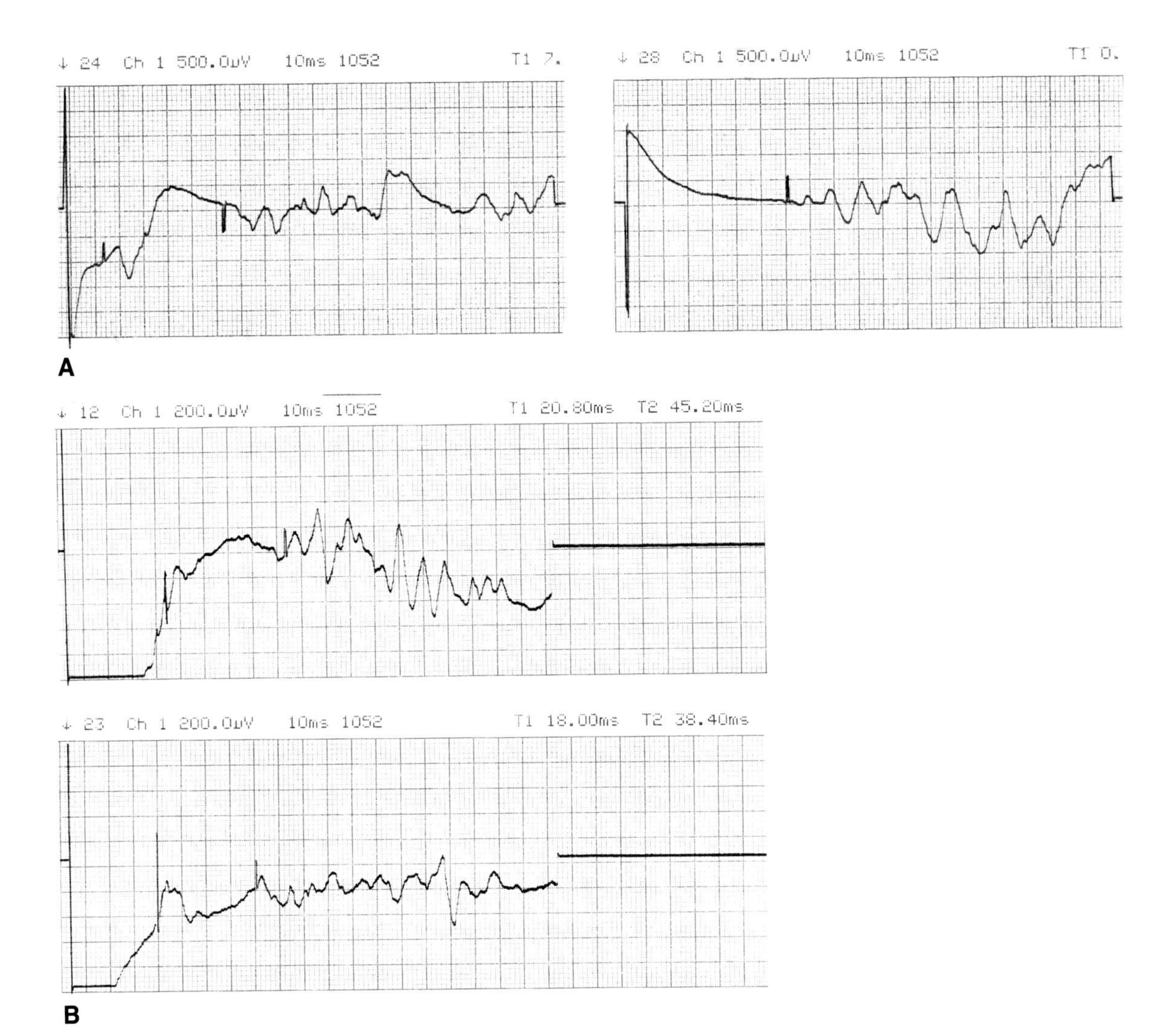

FIGURE 5-3 (A) Normal blink reflex recorded from the orbicularis oculi with supramaximal stimulation of the supraorbital nerve. The arrows on the left of each tracing indicate the position of the stimulus artifact. In the left trace the blink reflex was recorded from the orbicularis oculi ipsilateral to the side of stimulation. The first latency marker indicates the onset of the R1 response, and the second latency marker indicates the onset of the R2 response of the blink reflex. In the right trace the latency marker indicates the onset of the R2 response obtained simultaneously from the contralateral orbicularis oculi. (B) Abnormal blink reflexes from a patient with Guillain-Barré syndrome. The arrows on the left of each tracing indicate the position of the stimulus artifact. The first latency marker indicates the onset of the R1 response, and the second latency marker indicates the onset of the R2 response of the blink reflex. The blink reflexes were recorded from the side ipsilateral to the stimulus. The top trace was obtained with right supraorbital nerve stimulation, and the bottom trace was obtained with left supraorbital nerve stimulation. In both traces the R1 responses were delayed (20.80 msec and 18.00 msec, respectively), and the R2 response was delayed in the top trace (45.20 msec).

Conduction Time

Amplifier setting:
- Sweep speed: 10 msec/div.
- Sensitivity: 0.5 mV/div.
- Filter setting: 20 Hz–10 kHz

Recording technique:
- Active electrode: On the inferior portion of the orbicularis oculi at about the lateral third of the muscle
- Reference electrode: At the side of the nose or on the zygomatic arch
- Ground electrode: On the chin or forehead
- Stimulating electrode: Feel for the supraorbital groove. Stimulate at this point with the cathode over the supraorbital groove and the anode in the direction of the hairline.

Normal Values[101]

R1: 10.5 ± 0.8 msec (upper limit: 13.0 msec)
R2: 30.5 ± 3.4 msec (ipsilateral R2 upper limit: 40.0 msec)
R2: 30.5 ± 4.4 msec (contralateral R2 upper limit: 41.0 msec)

Comments

R1 responses between ipsilateral and contralateral stimulation should be less than 1.2 msec.[102] The ratio of the distal facial nerve latency and the R1 response should be in the range of 2.6 to 4.6.[102] The blink reflex has been found to be useful in the assessment of facial nerve palsies, acoustic neuroma, Guillain-Barré syndrome, diabetic polyneuropathy, Charcot-Marie-Tooth disease (type 1), and multiple sclerosis, and in the assessment of level of consciousness.[100,102]

Electrodiagnosis in Facial Nerve Lesions (Bell's Palsy)

Anatomy

See Figures 1-1 and 1-2 and Appendix Figure 22.

Nerve Conduction Studies

MOTOR

The facial nerve conduction time to the nasalis, orbicularis oculi, and orbicularis oris muscles and the amplitude and area of the respective compound muscle action potentials (CMAPs) are measured. If severe axonotmesis is present, there may be no evoked motor response. Absence of an evoked motor response within 7 days of the onset of symptoms is indicative of a poor prognosis.[166] The facial nerve conduction studies must be done bilaterally. The prognosis is best if the amplitude and area of the CMAPs are still normal more than 4 days after the onset of symptoms. The prognosis is good if the amplitude and area of the CMAP on the symptomatic side are above 30% of the amplitude and area on the asymptomatic side.[166] In this case an early clinical return can be expected, since the lesion is mainly a temporary conduction block (neurapraxia).[224] If the amplitude on the symptomatic side is less than 10% of the amplitude on the asymptomatic side, there will be a lag in improvement (sometimes more than 1 year) and incomplete recovery.[224]

BLINK REFLEX

On stimulation of the supraorbital nerve on the affected side, the R1 and R2 responses are delayed on the affected side, but the R2 response on the asymptomatic side is normal. On stimulation of the supraorbital nerve on the unaffected side, the R2 response on the affected side is delayed. Early return of the R1 or R2 response of the blink reflex after its absence signifies a good prognosis.[104]

EMG

GENERAL

In Bell's palsy the facial nerve is involved proximal to the stylomastoid foramen. The diagnosis can be confirmed by examination of these easily accessible facial muscles: frontalis, orbicularis oculi, nasalis, orbicularis oris, mentalis, and platysma.

REST

No spontaneous activity is seen if neurapraxia is the only lesion. If axonotmesis is present, fibrillations and positive sharp waves may be seen within 7 to 10 days of the onset of the lesion.

MINIMAL CONTRACTION

Evidence of even a few functioning motor unit potentials (MUPs) in each muscle usually signifies a good prognosis, provided that no further axonal degeneration occurs. Complex polyphasic MUPs with increased jitter and blocking in the individual components is seen with recent reinnervation.

MAXIMAL CONTRACTION

The interference pattern is reduced proportional to the degree of neurogenic involvement.

ACCESSORY NERVE

Applied Anatomy (See Figs. 1-1 *and* 1-2)

The origins of the fibers of the accessory nerve, which supplies the sternocleidomastoid and the trapezius, are from two quite different sources. The cranial (bulbar) part (or roots) arises from the caudal part of the nucleus ambiguus of the medulla, and these rootlets emerge caudal to, and in series with, the rootlets of the vagus nerve. Assembling together, these rootlets form a single trunk (the internal branch) that passes through the foramen jugulare in the same dural sleeve with the spinal part (or roots) of the accessory nerve. However, once through the foramen jugulare the cranial part of the accessory nerve leaves the dural sleeve, common to it and the spinal part, and passes over to join the vagus nerve. Thereafter the fibers of the cranial part are distributed in branches of the vagus nerve to the muscles of the larynx. The rostral and larger portion of the nucleus ambiguus sends its fibers out of the medulla in the rootlets of the vagus nerve to be distributed as branches of the vagus to the striated branchiomeric musculature of the pharynx and soft palate. Thus, the branchiomeric musculature of the pharynx, larynx, and soft palate is all supplied by the nucleus ambiguus but via two different pathways. The cranial part of the accessory nerve is really a special pathway for vagal nerve fibers.

The spinal part (or roots) of the accessory nerve arises in a totally different manner. The cell bodies of the fibers in the spinal roots are in the posterior part of the anterior grey column of the spinal cord through spinal segments C1 to C5. These fibers emerge from the spinal cord in rootlets that appear along the lateral side of the cord, approximately midway between the line of emergence of the ventral and dorsal roots of the spinal nerves. The rootlets of the spinal part of the accessory nerve ascend and unite in sequence to form a trunk that passes upward through the foramen magnum and then across the floor of the posterior cranial fossa to exit through the foramen jugulare in contiguity, but not continuity, with the cranial or bulbar part. This spinal part, so commonly referred to as the spinal accessory nerve, now descends below the base of the skull, passing posterolaterally to the internal jugular vein (70%) or between the internal jugular vein and the internal carotid artery (30%). The spinal accessory nerve descends across the tip of the transverse process of the atlas heading slightly posteriorly as it descends deep to the posterior belly of the digastricus and then deep to the upper end of the sternocleidomastoideus. For a very short interval the nerve appears in the upper lateral angle of the carotid triangle but is often concealed here by the lower pole of the parotid gland. Next the nerve penetrates to a variable extent into the substance of the deeper portion of the sternocleidomastoideus, giving innervation to the muscle as it passes through. The nerve reappears beyond the posterior border of the muscle somewhere between a point at the junction of the upper and middle thirds of the posterior border and a point at the midlevel of that border. The nerve now continues its course downward and posteriorly across the posterior triangle of the neck, where it lies immersed in the deep fascial covering of the posterior triangle. As it crosses the triangle, the nerve is parallel with and superficial to the levator scapulae. The nerve disappears under the cover of the anterior border of the trapezius some two to three fingers' breadth above the clavicle. Deep to the trapezius it contributes branches to the muscle and descends past the superior angle of the scapula, and then, medial to its vertebral border, it continues this vertical line of descent until it dwindles away. Its course across the posterior triangle of the neck may be roughly approximated by a line drawn from the tip of the transverse process of the atlas to the superior angle of the scapula.

Small branches from C3 and C4 of the cervical plexus lie parallel to and slightly below the spinal accessory nerve as it crosses the posterior triangle. These branches may blend with the spinal accessory or remain independent of it but, in any event, they send fibers into the muscle. Because of experiments in rhesus monkeys these branches from C3 and C4 have been claimed to be purely proprioceptive in man, as they are in the monkey.[27] Numerous clinical observations in man, however, seem to identify these twigs from C3 and C4 as an additional source of motor fibers to the trapezius. In a comparable manner, direct branches from C2 and C3 may aid in the motor innervation of the sternocleidomastoideus as well as supplying proprioceptive fibers.

Tumors adjacent to or in the foramen jugulare may compress the spinal accessory nerve either intracranially or extracranially. At either locus the tumor also is likely to damage the glossopharyngeal, vagus, and hypoglossal nerves to varying degrees. If the neoplasm is below the base of the skull, it may also damage the internal carotid nerve arising from the superior cervical sympathetic ganglion. This adds a partial Horner's syndrome (miosis and slight ptosis, but not the skin changes) to the paralysis of the last four cranial nerves (9th, 10th, 11th, and 12th). Lymph nodes occur along the course of the spinal accessory nerve just before and just after it passes deep to the sternocleidomastoid muscle. Metastases to these nodes from neoplasms of the nasopharynx may involve the spinal accessory nerve, and attempts to extirpate such nodes may lead to damage of the nerve during surgery.[142,158,245]

Destruction of the spinal accessory nerve proximal to the sternocleidomastoid muscle leads to the paralysis of most, if not all, of the fibers of that muscle and of at least half of the substance of the trapezius.[165] The upper half of the trapezius is usually the part that is noticeably atrophic and paralyzed. Nerve fibers from C3 and C4 via the cervical plexus may keep the lower part of the trapezius in some degree of functional competence. Paralysis of the upper trapezius allows the shoulder to droop, and the action of elevating the shoulder on command is weak. The unopposed actions of the levator scapulae and the rhomboids tend to rotate the scapula about an anteroposterior axis so that its inferior angle is medial to the superior angle and also tends to flare or wing backward so that it projects from the chest wall. The acromion is depressed, but the superior angle is not, since the superior angle is supported by the intact levator scapulae and the rhomboids. The action of forward flexion of the head is weakened on the side of the paralyzed sternocleidomastoid, with resulting slight rotation of the head toward the paralyzed side. The action of turning the head toward the side opposite the paralyzed muscle is also weakened.

Conduction Study

Technique

See Practical Aspects of Repetitive Nerve Stimulation Studies in Chapter 4 for a description of electrode placement and the site of stimulation. Normal conduction time to the upper trapezius (recorded 9 cm lateral to the C7 spinous process) is 2.3 ± 0.4 msec.[133]

Electrodiagnosis in Accessory Nerve Palsy

Nerve Conduction Study

The conduction time along the accessory nerve to the trapezius may be delayed. The amplitude of the evoked response may be reduced. It is important to compare the evoked motor responses bilaterally.

EMG

Evidence of denervation is seen in the trapezius and sternocleidomastoid. The upper trapezius is usually more involved.[245]

BRACHIAL PLEXUS AND SUPRASCAPULAR, MUSCULOCUTANEOUS, AND AXILLARY NERVES

Applied Anatomy

Brachial Plexus (See Figs. 1-16 Through 1-18 and Appendix Fig. 23)

The brachial plexus begins with the union of the anterior primary rami of spinal nerves C5 to T1 inclusive (called the roots of the brachial plexus). This is followed by separations and reunions of the nerve bundles until finally the five terminal branches are derived from the plexus. Although there are many minor and some major variations in the pattern of the plexus, only the most common form will be described.[95,203] The sequence is roots (5), trunks (3), divisions (6), cords (3), and terminal branches (5). (The number of each is indicated in parentheses.) In addition to the terminal branches there are a number of smaller collateral or side branches that arise chiefly from the cords but may also spring from the roots or trunks. With two exceptions all of the collateral branches are for the supply of muscles. The two exceptions are nerves that supply the skin of the medial side of the arm and forearm.

After passing laterally, beyond the sulcus for the spinal nerve on the superior surface of the transverse processes of the cervical vertebrae, the roots of the brachial plexus lie between the scalenus anterior and the scalenus medius muscles. These two muscles are close together above and separated below where they attach to the upper aspect of the first rib. Thus they form two sides of the tall, narrow interscalene triangle the base of which is the first rib. The five roots emerge into the posterior triangle of the neck in vertical sequence with a pronounced downward slant for the upper roots, but becoming more horizontal for C8, while the T1 root must ascend slightly to pass over the upper surface of the first rib. The T1 root is closely associated with the subclavian artery, which also escapes into the lower neck through the interscalene triangle. Both the artery and the T1 root rest on the first rib.

Roots C5 and C6 unite to form the upper trunk. Root C7 continues onward alone to form the middle trunk. Roots C8 and T1 unite to form the lower trunk. Each of the three trunks thus formed divides into an anterior and a posterior division. The anterior divisions of the upper trunk and the middle trunk then unite to form the lateral cord. The anterior division of the lower trunk continues alone to form the medial cord. The posterior divisions of each of the three trunks unite to form the posterior cord. The cords are named for their relationship to the axillary artery, which they surround, as it pierces very obliquely through the brachial plexus. The lateral cord divides into two terminal branches—the musculocutaneous nerve (C5, C6, C7) and the lateral root of the median nerve (C5, C6, C7). The medial cord divides into two terminal branches—the medial root of the median nerve (C8, T1) and the ulnar nerve (C8, T1). The posterior cord also divides into two terminal branches—the axillary nerve (C5, C6) and the radial nerve (C5–T1, inclusive). Thus, in the typical case, all roots of the brachial plexus send fibers into the median and radial nerves.

A glance at a brachial plexus shows that the musculocutaneous nerve could carry fibers from C5, C6, and C7, and it does, except that the contribution from C7 may be small or absent. The axilliary nerve could carry fibers from all root levels from C5 to T1, inclusive, but it does not, being limited to C5 and C6. The radial nerve could carry fibers from all root levels (C5–T1, inclusive), and it does. The median nerve, being formed by the union of medial and lateral roots, could receive fibers from all root levels (C5–T1, inclusive), and it does. The ulnar nerve, in the typical case, could receive fibers from C8 and T1, and it does. However, in some 10% to 20% of limbs the ulnar nerve carries a component of fibers from the C7 root. There are two ways that this may occur. One is that the middle trunk (C7) occasionally gives a direct branch to the medial cord, thus matching its usual branch to the lateral cord. Note that when this occurs there is an M-shaped pattern, which is the mirror image of the M-shaped pattern formed by the three terminal branches of the medial and lateral cords. The second way in which C7 fibers get into the ulnar nerve, and the more common of the two, is more devious than the path just cited. It involves C7 fibers in the lateral cord or in the lateral root of the median nerve leaving either of those bundles and, as a slender twig, piercing through the medial root of the median nerve to pass onward to join the ulnar nerve a centimeter or two beyond its origin. Sometimes this slender bundle of nerve fibers, instead of piercing the medial root of the median, doubles back in a recurrent fashion along the median nerve until these fibers reach the beginning of the ulnar nerve, which they then join. In this circumstance the arrangement is quite difficult to see and demonstrate during dissection.

Deviations in the size of the contributions from the roots into the trunks and from the trunks into the cords are mirrored in variations in the contributions to the individual terminal nerves or to the collateral branches of the brachial plexus. For the most part this is an expression of slight rostral or caudal displacement of the fibers of the roots of the plexus (prefixed and postfixed plexuses being a full segment shift upward or downward), thus incorporating more of C4 into the former and more of T2 into the latter. Although C4 contributes to the brachial plexus in some 50% of limbs, this contribution is minor and can be ignored for all practical purposes. In the prefixed plexus, however, the C4 contribution becomes considerably more important, while that of T1 dwindles.

As previously stated, the collateral branches of the cords of the plexus are chiefly to the muscles, as also are branches from the upper trunk and from the roots. Branches from the roots of the brachial plexus are numerous and include the long thoracic nerve (C5, C6, C7) to the serratus anterior, the dorsal scapular nerve (C5) to the rhomboideus major and minor and to part of the levator scapulae, a twig from C5 to join the phrenic nerve (in at least one third of cases), the nerve to the subclavius muscle (C5 and sometimes C6), and a number of small short twigs to the scaleni and longus colli. The long thoracic nerve descends along the medial wall of the axilla within the fascia covering the serratus anterior. The nerve gives twigs in sequence to each of the digitations of the serratus.

Collateral branches from the upper trunk include the suprascapular nerve (C5, C6) to the supraspinatus and infraspinatus muscles, and sometimes the dorsal scapular nerve and the nerve to the subclavius (when these two nerves fail to arise more proximally). Collateral branches from the lateral cord include the lateral pectoral nerve (C5, C6, C7) to pectoralis major (C5–T1, inclusive) and minor (C6, C7, C8) and sometimes the suprascapular nerve and the nerve to the subclavius muscle when they arise more distally than usual. Collateral branches from the medial cord include the medial pectoral nerve (C8, T1) to pectoralis major (C5–T1, inclusive) and minor (C6, C7, C8), the medial cutaneous nerve of the arm (C8, T1), and the medial cutaneous nerve of the forearm (C8, T1). These latter two branches are the only collateral branches of the brachial plexus that supply skin instead of muscles. Collateral branches from the posterior cord include the upper subscapular nerve (C5, C6) to the subscapularis muscle, the middle subscapular (thoracodorsal) nerve (C6, C7, C8) to the latissimus dorsi, and the lower subscapular nerve (C5, C6) to the teres major and the lateral part of the subscapularis muscle. Note that each of these three muscles of the posterior wall of the axilla is supplied by branches from the posterior cord of the plexus. The thoracodorsal nerve descends across the central area of the subscapularis muscle and then across the teres major to approach the deep surface of the latissimus dorsi near its anterior border. The several terminal branches penetrate into the muscle.

The clavicle crosses the brachial plexus at about the level of the division of the trunks into the anterior and posterior divisions. These divisions and the cords are in the axilla, while the trunks and roots are in the neck or above the clavicle. As the roots and trunks emerge between the scalenus anterior and scalenus medius and above the first rib (the three sides of the interscalene trigone), these plexus elements, plus certain of their collateral branches, are subject to impingement or compression from the adjacent structures as well as damage by external trauma. A strong downward thrust on the shoulder, especially when the head is bent to the opposite side, puts tension on the upper elements of the brachial plexus, since they are already slanting obliquely downward. Posterior displacement of the shoulder and rotation of the head and neck toward the opposite side further tense the brachial plexus around the scalenus medius.

The dorsal scapular nerve in its entirety and the upper two roots of the long thoracic nerve regularly pierce the substance of the scalenus medius as they pass to their destinations. The lower root of the long thoracic nerve, which arises from C7, usually passes across the anterior aspect of the scalenus medius to join with the upper two roots after they emerge from the substance of this muscle. Occasionally, however, the lowest root (from C7) of the long thoracic nerve is absent. Thus both the dorsal scapular nerve and the two roots of the long thoracic nerve have a relationship to this muscle such that they are potentially entrapped here by the pull of contracting muscle fasciculi during strong, prolonged, or repetitious contraction. These nerves may be stretched and perhaps angulated when the scalenus medius is hypertrophied from overactivity, or in spasm from cervical spondylosis or prolonged occupational postures. Strong downward pressure on the shoulder may so stretch the long thoracic nerve or, more likely, its rootlets from C5 and C6 as they pierce through the scalenus medius that a serratus anterior paresis ultimately results. Serratus anterior paralysis is manifested by winging of the scapula, particularly when the arm is held outstretched in front or when the patient pushes against a wall. Falls from a speeding motorcycle with one shoulder striking the curb or the tire of a parked car can give a powerful downward thrust to the shoulder. It should be remembered that a dorsal scapular nerve entrapment neuropathy, with weakness of the rhomboids and partial weakness of the levator scapulae, also results in a minor degree of winging of the scapula. The presence of an anomalous scalenus minimus muscle or a fibrous band representing it, as well as Sebileau's (vertebropleural) bands derived from the deep surface of the scalene fascia and from Sibson's fascia covering the pleural cupula, has at times been cited as the basis for nerve damage in this region. An anomalous cervical rib and the fibrous band that may complete its course have often been found to entrap or impinge on the lower trunk or other elements of the brachial plexus, as well as the subclavian artery itself. In the latter case there is a vascular element added to what might otherwise have been solely a nerve impingement. Variations in the anteroposterior spread of the tendinous lower ends of the scalenus anterior and medius may restrict the space available for the lower trunk of the brachial plexus or the T1 root, as well as the subclavian artery.[222] Thus, the base of the interscalene triangle formed by the first rib may be reduced to an acutely angled V by the encroachment of sharp tendinous adjacent boundaries of the two muscles. This, coupled with carrying a heavy weight such as a suitcase, on the affected side could lead to transitory nerve or artery impingement.

The term *thoracic outlet syndromes* is now commonly used to cover several neurovascular compression syndromes occurring in the root of the neck at the cervicobrachial junction zone, where neurovascular structures are passing between the apex of the axilla and the interscalene trigone or the superior thoracic aperture. The subclavian artery and vein emerge from the mediastinum through the superior thoracic aperture and are joined by the roots of the brachial plexus emerging through the interscalene trigone. The subclavian artery passes through the lower part of the interscalene triangle with the roots of the brachial plexus, but the subclavian vein passes over the first rib anterior to the scalenus anterior and therefore outside the triangle. Together, all of these structures pass over the first rib and descend through the truncated triangular apex of the axilla to enter the axillary fossa. This three-sided apical entry zone is bounded by the clavicle anteriorly, the lateral border of the first rib medially, and the superior border of the scapula posteriorly. There are several levels at which the emergent neurovascular structures may be compressed, but all may be loosely lumped together under the title *thoracic outlet syndromes*. These sites, predisposed to constrict or compress the great neurovascular structures of the upper limb, are as follows. (1) The interscalene triangle, where a cervical rib or variations in the manner of attachment of the scalene muscles to the first rib may compress the subclavian artery or elements of the brachial plexus. (2) The costoclavicular space, where the clavicle and the subclavius muscle make a very acute angle of variable degree with the first rib, which is narrowed still more as the shoulder is pushed backward and downward. This alone may produce neurovascular compression (costoclavicular syndrome). (3) More distally, the brachial plexus and the two great vessels and the coracoid process aided by the pectoralis minor, form an arch over the neurovascular structures. When the arm is hyperabducted, the brachial plexus and the great vessels are angulated and compressed as they pass under the coracoid process. The compression of the neurovascular structures is increased in hyperabduction by the downward projection of the head of the humerus, which becomes an added mass that the nerves and vessels must angulate around and therefore increases the tension on those structures. Compression of the neurovascular bundle against the coracoid process, with or without the added tension caused by the head of the humerus, is labeled the *hyperabduction syndrome*.

Variations in the precise anatomical arrangements in each of these syndromes produce variations in the clinical findings and symptoms. Some cases are purely vascular, some are more vascular than neural, and some are the reverse. Also, a purely vascular compression may result in neural symptoms owing to an ischemia of nerves. A cervical rib is one of the more common causes of nerve damage, yet it may occur without neural or vascular damage. A cervical rib may be present but cause no distress until, for reasons of descensus of the shoulder due to old age, weakness because of illness or lack of exercise, occupational activity, carrying a heavy bag, and so forth, a combination of factors precipitates the resultant syndome. Often there are subjective symptoms with only few, if any, objective findings. With thoracic outlet syndromes there is a great likelihood, because of the T1 involvement, for a simulation of an ulnar nerve lesion. On the other hand, when the median nerve seems to be implicated because of the distribution and type of findings, a cervical intervertebral disc degeneration is likely to be the cause. Brachial plexus injuries due to stretching, as in Erb's obstetric palsy or from falls on the shoulder with the head forced toward the opposite side, give rise to the so-called upper radicular syndrome involving fibers derived from C5 and C6 and sometimes C7. A lower radicular syndrome (of the Klumpke-Dejerine type) may result from the upper limb's being forcefully jerked upward, as in falls from scaffolding with the patient saving himself by grabbing a rope or other object so that his arm is stretched overhead. In this case, roots C8 and T1 may be damaged. This latter type of brachial plexus injury is much less common than is the Erb type. Horner's syndrome is often associated with the lower radicular syndrome because of damage to the preganglionic sympathetic fibers leaving the spinal cord over the T1 nerve.

It must not be forgotten that many persons have a cervical rib without ever experiencing any distress because of it. It is commonplace to find persons whose radial pulse disappears on hyperabduction, yet who have no complaint in relation to this. Some of these persons may at a later time and with appropriate circumstances develop some symptoms in relation to their heretofore silent aberration.

Suprascapular Nerve (See Figs. 1-13, B; 1-17; and 1-18 and Appendix Fig. 23)

The suprascapular nerve, which supplies the supraspinatus and infraspinatus muscles, receives its fibers from the C5 and C6 ventral divisions and usually arises from the upper trunk of the brachial plexus. In about half of body sides the suprascapular nerve also receives a contribution from C4. This contribution, when present, joins the C5 nerve and is usually quite small and relatively unimportant for practical purposes. However, in the prefixed type of plexus, it is large, with a corresponding reduction in the size of the contribution into the brachial plexus from the T1 root and hence a seeming upward shift or higher origin of the plexus. In keeping with the amount of muscle mass, or the total number of muscle fibers in the supraspinatus and infraspinatus muscles, the suprascapular nerve is rather large.

From its origin the suprascapular nerve parallels the posterior (inferior) belly of the omohyoideus muscle, which attaches to (arises from) the upper border of the scapula just medial to the suprascapular notch and partly also to the transverse scapular (suprascapular) ligament, which bridges the notch. Sometimes the ligament is ossified, converting the osseofibrous foramen into a purely bony foramen. As the nerve approaches the suprascapular notch, it is joined by the suprascapular (transverse scapular) artery and vein. Only the nerve, however, passes through the suprascapular notch, in which it is fixed in place by the transverse scapular ligament, which converts the notch into a foramen. This foramen is well filled by the nerve as it crosses over the upper border of the scapula. The suprascapular (transverse scapular) artery and vein cross the scapula above the transverse scapular ligament and therefore outside the osseofibrous foramen. Thereafter, the vessels closely follow the course of the nerve. Emerging from the foramen the suprascapular nerve lies deep to the supraspinatus muscle, sending twigs into the latter, and proceeds through the arch or notch formed by the spinous process with the acromion and the scapular neck, which supports the glenoid fossa. The arch, or notch, is called the greater scapular notch, which is to be clearly distinguished from the suprascapular notch. The nerve, with the accompanying vessels, passes through the great scapular notch and reaches the infraspinous fossa, where the nerve, lying deep to the infraspinatus, spreads branches into that muscle. The suprascapular nerve, its accompanying vessels, and the posterior belly of the omohyoideus are all under cover of the superior part of the trapezius as they approach the upper border of the scapula. Deep to the suprascapular nerve is the upper part of the serratus anterior.

In all movements of the scapula, up and down, forward and backward, and around, the lower end of the suprascapular nerve is fixed in the sharply edged, osseofibrous foramen formed by the suprascapular notch and its ligament. Various postures of the scapula may therefore produce tension on the suprascapular nerve.[228] The suprascapular nerve is put under tension when the shoulder is pushed forcibly downward, and is also tensed and stretched when the shoulder is rotated strongly forward, as in reaching widely to the left with the right hand while drawing the right arm across the front of the chest (hyperadduction). Stretching of the suprascapular nerve is inevitable with this motion, since the shoulder swings forward on a fixed radius represented by the clavicle, about a central axis, the sternoclavicular joint, which is several centimeters anterior to the point of origin of the suprascapular nerve from the upper trunk. Since the suprascapular nerve is held in the suprascapular notch by the transverse scapular ligament, and since the nerve well fills this foramen with its unyielding sides, it is evident that tension or stretching of the nerve may angulate and pinch the nerve here. Such prolonged or repetitious trauma to the nerve can lead to atrophy of the supraspinatus and infraspinatus muscles, as well as tenderness and pain along the course of the nerve.

Musculocutaneous Nerve (See Figs. 1-19 and 1-22)

The musculocutaneous nerve leaves the axilla and enters the arm by piercing the coracobrachialis. The nerve contributes a branch to the muscle, which arises prior to the level of penetration. Beyond the coracobrachialis the nerve lies between the biceps brachii and the brachialis and contributes muscular branches to both. Passing distally beyond these two muscles it continues as the lateral cutaneous nerve of the forearm.[159] While in the arm, the nerve is protected from external injury by the overlying biceps and from damage due to fracture of the humerus by the underlying brachialis. It might be expected that an entrapment neuropathy would occur where the nerve pierces the coracobrachialis, but this does not seem to be the case, for such reports are very rare.[16]

An anastomosis between the musculocutaneous and median nerves occurs deep to the biceps muscle in approximately one third of arms. This anastomosis allows fibers that should have left the lateral cord to travel into the median nerve but failed to do so to pass instead into the musculocutaneous. Such fibers leave the musculocutaneous nerve at this more distal level and then proceed into the median to finally reach their appropriate destination. The reverse arrangement is also possible, with fibers of the lateral cord that should have passed into the musculocutaneous nerve traveling instead into the lateral head of the median nerve and then at the more distal level switching back to the musculocutaneous, in which they finally reach their appropriate destination. The slant of the anastomotic trunk usually indicates the direction of travel of these fibers. The obvious significance of an anastomosis such as this, with the consequent aberrant course of the nerve fibers involved, is that nerve trauma and entrapment neuropathies could give unexpected muscle and sensory palsies or explain unexpected motor and sensory preservations.

Axillary Nerve (See Fig. 1-24)

After arising from the posterior cord of the brachial plexus the axillary nerve runs laterally and inferiorly (if the arm is pendant) across the anterior surface of the subscapularis to escape from the axilla by turning posteriorly, through the quadrilateral space. When the arm is adducted, the quadrilateral space is bounded by the anterior aspect by the subscapularis and the shoulder joint superiorly, the coracobrachialis and the surgical neck of the humerus laterally, the tendons of the latissimus dorsi and teres major inferiorly, and the long head of the triceps medially. The structures bounding the space differ somewhat when seen from behind, and of course, the four boundaries shift positions when the arm is abducted through 90°. The axillary nerve and the posterior humeral circumflex artery and vein pass through this space to reach the posterior aspect of the surgical neck of the humerus. The nerve, on appearing posteriorly, contributes a twig to the teres minor as this muscle forms the superior border of the quadrilateral space when seen from behind. Another twig, the upper lateral cutaneous nerve of the arm, passes around the posterior border of the deltoid to supply the skin overlying that muscle and the skin over the lateral head of the triceps. The main trunk of the axillary, curving around the surgical neck of the humerus, gives off several branches that penetrate into the deep surface of the deltoid, supplying it and sending a few small final branches through the deltoid and into the overlying skin.

A compression neuropathy of the axillary nerve, as it approaches the quadrilateral space, may occur with inferior dislocations of the head of the humerus.[12,148] The nerve is stretched and compressed about the downwardly protruding head of the humerus. The normal posterior angulation of the nerve through the quadrilateral space allows no slack or mobility of the nerve, and it becomes damaged either at once on occurrence of the dislocation or progressively as the dislocation continues unreduced. Of course, fractures of the surgical neck of the humerus pose a serious threat to the integrity of the axillary nerve and may even result in a compression neuropathy when the nerve is caught between fragments of the bone, but this is not the kind of intrinsic entrapment neuropathy that this chapter seeks to elucidate.

Determination of Conduction Across the Brachial Plexus (Cervical Nerve Root Stimulation Study) (Figs. 5-4 Through 5-6)

Conduction Time

Amplifier setting:
- Sweep speed: 2 msec/div.
- Sensitivity: 5 mV/div.
- Filter setting: 20 Hz–10 kHz

Recording technique:
- Patient position: Prone
- Recording electrode: On the biceps brachii, with the reference electrode on the tendon of the biceps. This gives information about the upper trunk and lateral cord.
- Recording electrode: On the triceps brachii, with the reference electrode on the tendon of the triceps. This gives information about the middle trunk and posterior cord.
- Recording electrode: On the abductor digiti minimi, with the reference electrode on the base of the proximal phalanx of the little finger. This gives information about the lower trunk and medial cord.

Stimulation technique*: Supramaximal current stimulation using a monopolar needle 50 mm in length with a surface reference electrode approximately 1 cm distal to the active electrode
- Upper trunk, lateral cord: Stimulate roots C5 and C6 together, with the needle 2 cm lateral to the C5 spinous process. Insert the needle until it touches the transverse process, then withdraw about 1 mm.
- Middle trunk, posterior cord: Stimulate roots C6, C7, and C8 with the needle inserted 2 cm lateral to the C6 spinous process. Insert the needle until it touches the transverse process, then withdraw about 1 mm.
- Lower trunk, medial cord: Stimulate nerve roots C8 and T1 with the needle inserted 2 cm lateral and slightly caudal to the C7 spinous process. Insert the needle until it reaches the transverse process of the C7 vertebra, then withdraw about 1 mm. Also stimulate the ulnar nerve at the axilla 25 cm from the sternal notch. The difference in latency between the cervical and the axillary values gives the plexus conduction time for the lower trunk or medial cord.

Normal Values[134]

Upper trunk, lateral cord: 5.3 ± 0.4 (4.8–6.2) msec.

Middle trunk, posterior cord: 5.4 ± 0.4 (4.4–6.1) msec.

Lower trunk, medial cord: 4.7 ± 0.5 (3.7–5.5) msec.

Contralateral latency difference: < 0.6 msec.

Comments

Cervical nerve root stimulation should be done bilaterally with similar distances between the recording and stimulating electrodes for comparison, since the latency difference between the two sides may be more reliable for detection of abnormality than is the absolute latency. C8 nerve root stimulation is more commonly performed

* Technique of MacLean[134]

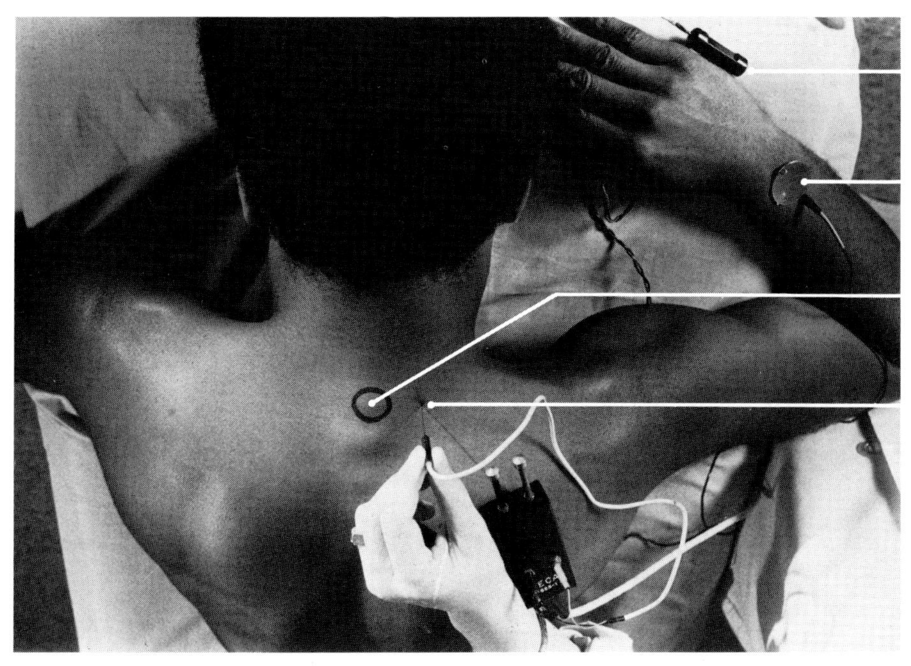

FIGURE 5-4 C8 nerve root stimulation study.

than stimulation of other roots. In particular, C8 root stimulation is done when thoracic outlet syndrome with entrapment of the C8 nerve root proximal to Erb's point is suspected. In such situations, stimulation at Erb's point produces normal values, since Erb's point is distal to the site of pathology.

Axillary, Musculocutaneous, and Suprascapular Nerve Conduction Studies (Fig. 5-7)

Conduction Time

Amplifier setting:
- Sweep speed: 2 msec/div.
- Sensitivity: 5 mV/div.
- Filter setting: 20 Hz–10 kHz

Recording electrode:
- Axillary nerve: The active electrode is on the most prominent portion of the deltoid, with the reference electrode on the acromion.
- Musculocutaneous nerve: The active electrode is on the most prominent portion of the biceps brachii and the reference electrode on the tendon of the biceps.
- Suprascapular nerve: Place the active electrode, a concentric or monopolar needle, in the supraspinatus or infraspinatus. Place the surface reference electrode 1 cm distal to the active electrode for recordings with a monopolar needle. (See Figs. 2-27 and 2-28 for identification of the supraspinatus and infraspinatus, respectively.) For the supraspinatus, insert the needle medial to and above the midpoint of the spine of the scapula. For the infraspinatus, insert the needle into the infrascapular fossa several centimeters medial to the lateral scapular border. The best location is between the trapezius (lower portion) and the teres major, where the infraspinatus is very superficial. For both the supraspinatus and infraspinatus the needle must be inserted until it gently touches the periosteum, then it is withdrawn 1 mm. This ensures that the needle is in the appropriate muscle and not in the overlying trapezius.

Stimulation technique:
- Use supramaximal stimulation.
- Stimulate at Erb's point. To locate this point, have the patient turn his chin away from

the side of examination so that you can palpate the clavicular head of the sternocleidomastoid at its origin from the clavicle. Stimulate immediately lateral to the clavicular head of the sternocleidomastoid where it attaches to the clavicle, with the cathode distal to the anode.

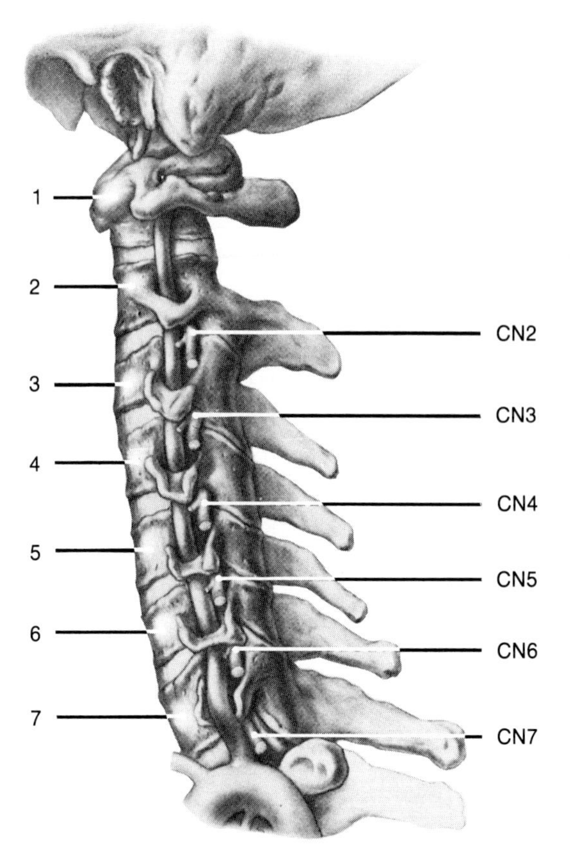

FIGURE 5-5 Side view of the cervical vertebrae, showing the proximity of the cervical nerves to the vertebral artery and to the transverse processes of the vertebrae. (Pitkin GP: Conduction Anesthesia, p 77. Southworth JL, Hingson RA [eds]: Philadelphia, JB Lippincott, 1946)

Normal Values[116]

Axillary nerve: 3.9 ± 0.5 (2.8–5.0) msec. Distance: 14.8–26.5 cm

Musculocutaneous nerve: 4.5 ± 0.6 (3.3–5.7) msec. Distance: 23.5–41.5 cm

Suprascapular nerve: See Figure 5-8 for abnormalities seen in nerve conduction studies in suprascapular nerve entrapment.

To supraspinatus: 2.7 ± 0.5 (1.7–3.7) msec. Distance: 7.4–13.8 cm

To infraspinatus: 3.3 ± 0.5 (2.4–4.2) msec. Distance: 10.6–19.5 cm

Comments

Bilateral examinations, with comparable distances used between the recording and stimulating electrodes, are usually performed. Differences greater than 0.5 msec to 0.6 msec on the symptomatic side may be considered significant for the presence of conduction delay.[116]

The sensory branch of the musculocutaneous nerve (lateral antebrachial cutaneous nerve) may be studied by stimulating at the lateral aspect of

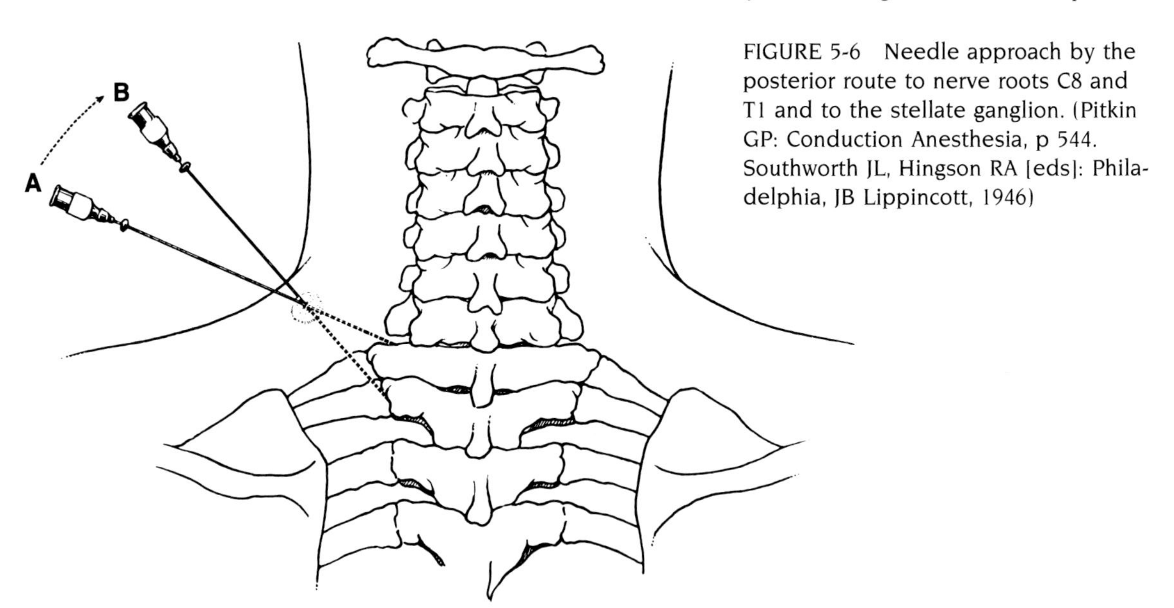

FIGURE 5-6 Needle approach by the posterior route to nerve roots C8 and T1 and to the stellate ganglion. (Pitkin GP: Conduction Anesthesia, p 544. Southworth JL, Hingson RA [eds]: Philadelphia, JB Lippincott, 1946)

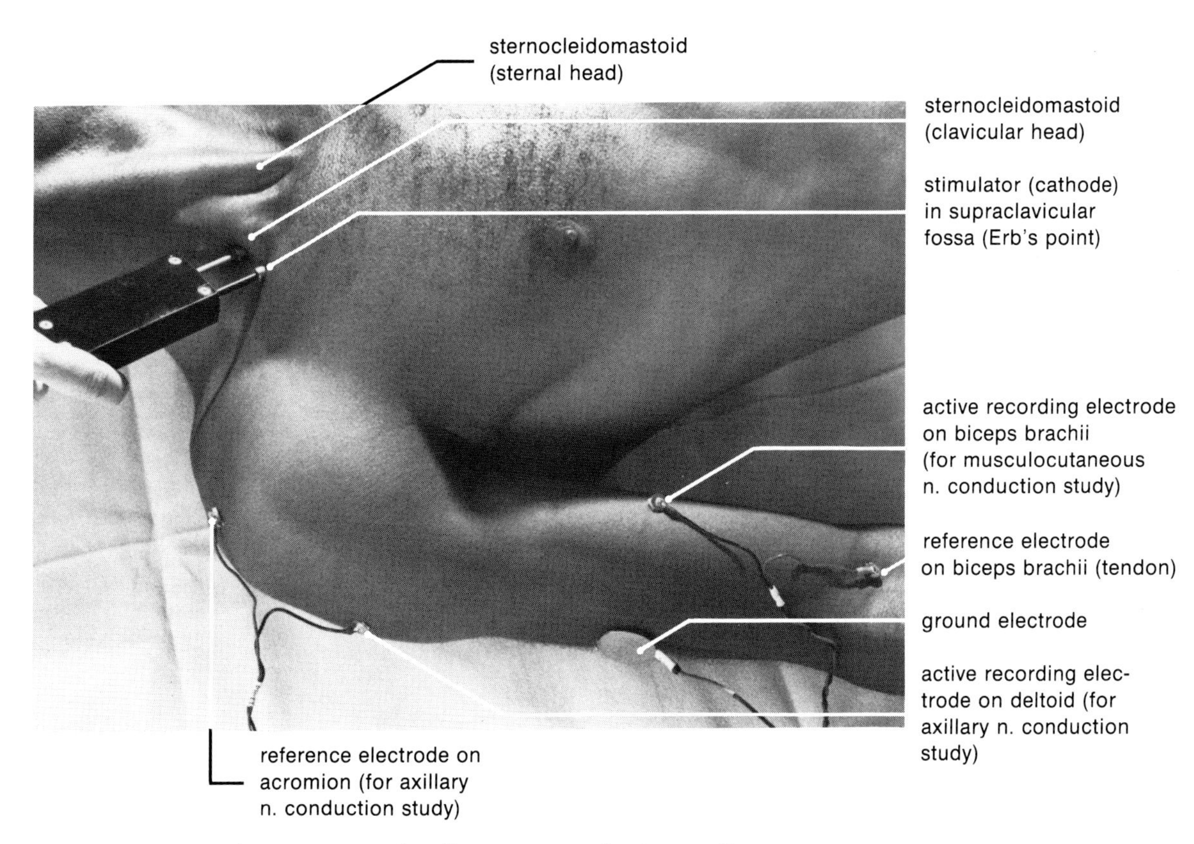

FIGURE 5-7 Musculocutaneous and axillary nerve conduction studies.

the biceps brachii tendon. The recording is done 12 cm distal to the stimulation site along a line joining the stimulus point to the radial artery.[133] The reference electrode is kept on the same line approximately 3 cm distal to the recording electrode. The normal parameters of this nerve in one study include onset latency 1.8 ± 0.1 msec, peak latency 2.3 ± 0.1 msec, conduction velocity 65 ± 3.6 m/sec, and amplitude 24 ± 7.2 μV.[207]

Electrodiagnosis in Thoracic Outlet Syndrome

Anatomy

See Figures 1-16 through 1-18 and Appendix Figure 23.

Nerve Conduction Studies

SENSORY

The amplitude of the ulnar nerve sensory potential recorded at the wrist may be smaller than that on the contralateral side,[61,128] since the involvement is distal to the dorsal root ganglion, that is, at the level of the plexus. The sensory potential may even be absent.[61] Decreased amplitude of the sensory potential of the median nerve has also been reported.[10] Abnormalities in the ulnar and median sensory nerve potentials should be seen in the absence of ulnar and median nerve distal lesions. If there are distal lesions along these nerves, they can be detected by the presence of focal slowing of these nerves at the wrist or elbow.

MOTOR

The amplitude of the evoked motor response from the abductor pollicis brevis on stimulation of the median nerve is smaller than normal.[242] Distal motor latencies and conduction velocities along the median and ulnar nerves are normal. The conduction velocity along the ulnar nerve from Erb's point to the axilla is slowed if the lesion is distal to the point of stimulation[19,233] but normal with more proximal lesions. However, it is difficult to obtain accurate conduction velocities along this segment because of volume conduction to adjacent nerves and errors in distance measurements.[30,38,63,240] C8 nerve root conduction time, if done bilaterally, may show a difference that is significant if it is more than 1 msec.[240] If thoracic outlet syndrome is present, F-wave conduction time may be prolonged[239,240] owing to loss of the largest myelinated fibers.

EMG

REST

Fibrillations and positive sharp waves may be seen in the muscles supplied by the C8 and T1 anterior primary rami, especially in the intrinsic hand muscles supplied by the median nerve.[242] The paraspinal muscles are not involved, since the lesion is at the level of the anterior primary rami.

MINIMAL CONTRACTION

Changes compatible with neurogenic reinnervation may be seen in the muscles supplied by the C8 and T1 anterior primary rami.

MAXIMAL CONTRACTION

The interference pattern is reduced proportional to the degree of neurogenic involvement.

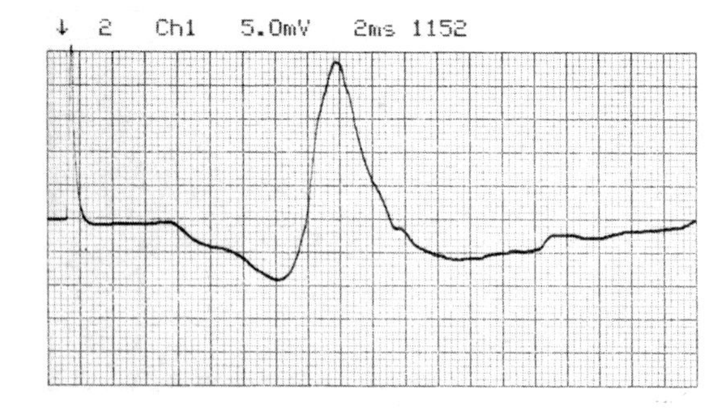

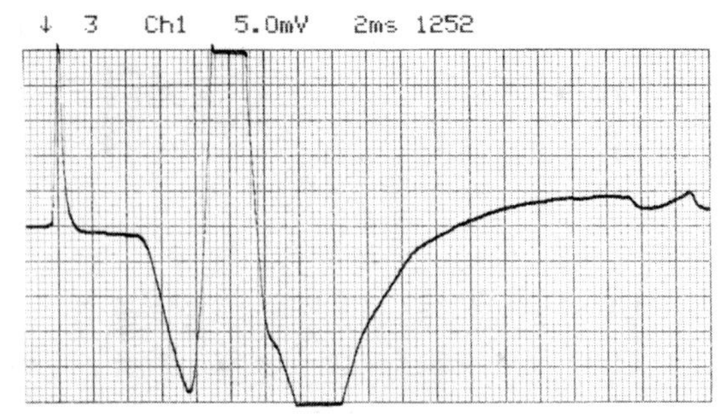

FIGURE 5-8 The top trace shows an evoked motor response from the left infraspinatus on stimulation of the left suprascapular nerve in a patient with suprascapular nerve injury. Compare with the recording obtained from the right infraspinatus with right suprascapular nerve stimulation (*bottom*). Sweep speed 2 msec/div., sensitivity 5.0 mV/div.

MEDIAN NERVE

Applied Anatomy (*See Appendix Fig.* 24)

Formed by the union of medial and lateral roots from the respective medial and lateral cords of the brachial plexus, the nerve trunk lies on the medial side of the arm in the groove between the biceps and brachialis muscles. In close relation to the brachial artery it descends lateral to the artery through the upper half of the arm, and at mid-arm level it crosses the brachial artery on its anterior aspect (but in approximately 5% of arms on the posterior side of the artery) to descend on the medial side of the artery, which in turn is medial to the strong cordlike tendon of insertion of the biceps. A variable, flat offshoot of the biceps tendon (the lacertus fibrosus or bicipital aponeurosis) spans the superficial surface of both the brachial artery and the median nerve to fuse into the antebrachial fascia covering the proximal muscle bellies of the forearm flexor muscles. Thus the artery and the nerve, descending through the cubital fossa, are covered partially by the bicipital aponeurosis, and both may be palpated here deep to that aponeurotic expansion.

In slightly fewer than 1% of humeri a bony process (the supracondylar process) is found approximately 5 cm above the medial epicondyle on the anteromedial surface of the humerus.[223] It is sometimes quite short but at other times 2 cm to 3 cm in length and arching anteromedially and downward. A fibrous band (the ligament of Struthers) continues from the tip of this process to the base of the medial epicondyle, thus forming a fibro-osseous foramen anterior to the medial intermuscular septum. The brachial (or ulnar) artery and the median nerve pass through this foramen in most cases. In most instances of this aberrant arrangement, there is no compression of the median nerve, and the patient is asymptomatic throughout life, but in a small percentage of persons who have the fibro-osseous foramen, symptoms may occur, often in adulthood. Thus, a median nerve entrapment neuropathy may occur at this level proximal to the origin of any of the muscular branches of the median nerve.[121,170]

Entering the forearm, the median nerve now gives off its first branch, which is to the pronator teres just before the main trunk passes between the superficial (humeral) head and the deep (ulnar) head of that muscle. The superficial head is much the larger and obscures the more slender, and often quite fibrous (tendinous), deep head. However, the relationship is variable, for the deep head may be missing, and at times, even when the deep head is present, the median nerve descends into the forearm beneath both heads of the pronator. Rarely, the nerve pierces through the substance of the superficial head. Tendinous fibers in either of the two heads may play against the median nerves or pinch it in a scissorlike grasp as the muscle contracts. Thus, in the appropriate limb and in the event of appropriate muscular action or overaction, the "pronator syndrome" may result.[111] It is possible that a well-developed bicipital aponeurosis may cause some degree of compression of the median nerve on strong (and repetitious) supination.[122] However, pain produced by forceful pronation, with some added tension created by elbow extension, is the usual confirmatory test of the pronator syndrome.[33] Branches to the forearm flexors arise in rapid sequence from the median nerve as it enters the interval between the heads of the pronator teres.

The anterior interosseous nerve is a branch of the median nerve that arises as the median nerve passes between the two heads of the pronator teres or at the inferior angle of the cubital fossa. The anterior interosseous branch descends in the interval between the flexor pollicis longus and the flexor digitorum profundus, lying directly on the interosseous membrane. This nerve supplies the flexor pollicis longus and the radial half of the flexor digitorum profundus (the portion that gives rise to the tendons for the index and middle fingers) and then descends on the deep or posterior side of the pronator quadratus, innervating that muscle. Sometimes the anterior interosseous nerve alone may be involved in a neuropathy, with inability to flex the distal phalanges of the thumb and index and middle fingers.[96,123,179,209,225] Loss of this action in the middle finger is variable because of ulnar nerve overlap (Martin-Gruber anastomoses).[210,243] A reduction in the power of pronation is another identifiable loss. The most characteristic sign of paralysis of this nerve, however, is inability to pinch the distal phalanges of the thumb and index finger strongly together because of paralysis of the flexor pollicis longus and the part of the flexor digitorum profundus that controls the distal phalanx of the index finger.[23,161,179] Injury of the main trunk of the median nerve with involvement of its several branches to the flexor muscles is more common than is an isolated lesion of the anterior interosseous nerve. Such an injury of the main trunk with its branches at the level of the pronator teres gives rise to the pronator syndrome, which will be discussed later.

Isolated paralysis of the anterior interosseous nerve without other median nerve damage occurs as a complication of supracondylar fractures of the humerus, particularly in children, but also in adults.[211,237] This is probably due to avulsion of the anterior interosseous nerve at its point of origin from the main trunk of the median nerve in the forearm, rather than to posterior compression against the median nerve at the level of the fracture.[24,141] The displacement of the distal fragment of bone, plus the hematoma mass, creates a traction force upward on the median nerve. The main trunk of the median nerve is loosely held in the forearm fascia, and it can be displaced and stretched upward. The anterior interosseous branch is more tightly bound in its groove between the deep muscles and against the interosseous membrane, and it is not displaceable; therefore, it cannot stretch upward sufficiently and becomes avulsed.

Several other anatomical variants and arrangements deep to the flexor digitorum superficialis may cause a compression of the anterior interosseous nerve. Among these variant structures are an accessory slip of origin of the flexor pollicis longus (Gantzer's muscle) and a tendinous band of origin of the flexor digitorum superficialis.[210] As with virtually all entrapment neuropathies, fractures and dislocations, as well as other types of extrinsic trauma, may play a role in causation.

Lying deep to the pronator teres, and at approximately the same vertical level as the pronator, is a fibrous arch formed by the upper border of the flexor digitorum superficialis between its origin from the medial epicondyle of the humerus and its origin from the oblique line of the radius. The median nerve passes under this fibrous arch to descend deep to the flexor digitorum superficialis. The entrapment neuropathy created by impingement of this fibrous arch against the median nerve is also labeled the "pronator syndrome," even though the pronator teres is not involved in causing the nerve injury.[147,200] Isolated contraction of the flexor digitorum superficialis becomes an identifying test for this variant of the pronator syndrome. Pain is produced by tension in the fibrous arch as the middle phalanx of the middle finger is flexed against resistance while the other fingers are held in passive extension.

The main trunk of the median nerve, after passing underneath the fibrous arch of the flexor digitorum superficialis, continues distally, held to the deep surface of the latter muscle by the investing fascia of the muscle. In the forearm some 5 cm above the distal flexion crease at the wrist the median nerve emerges from under the cover of the flexor digitorum superficialis by passing around the lateral border of that muscle to lie just medial to the tendon of the flexor carpi radialis. Here it is commonly covered, to a limited extent, by the tendon of the palmaris longus when the latter muscle is present. The nerve is, of course, also covered by the deep fascia of the forearm at this level. Beyond the distal flexion crease at the wrist the median nerve passes deep to the flexor retinaculum (the transverse carpal ligament) within the carpal tunnel.

The carpal tunnel is an osseofibrous canal at the level of the carpus. Its anterior wall is the flexor retinaculum. The posterior wall is formed by the carpal bones with their covering ligaments. The lateral wall is formed by the ridge of the trapezium and the tuberosity of the scaphoid bone, and the medial wall by the hamulus of the hamate and the pisiform. Thus the walls of the carpal tunnel are unyielding, and any encroachment on the enclosed space, such as by fracture or dislocation of a carpal bone, Colles' fracture, swelling of the ligaments, or osteoarthritic changes cause constriction of the contents.[110,174,175,220] Conversely, swelling of the contents due to local pathologic processes of systemic disease can also cause a constricting effect on the more yielding contents such as the median nerve.[217]

The contents of the carpal tunnel are the four tendons of the flexor digitorum profundus, the four tendons of the flexor digitorum superficialis plus the synovial sheath for these tendons (the common flexor sheath or ulnar bursa), the tendon of the flexor pollicis longus with its synovial sheath (the radial bursa), and the tendon of the flexor carpi radialis (which, in a sense, lies in the lateral wall of the tunnel, for it is in its own ligamentous tube formed by the lateral end of the flexor retinaculum). Thus there are ten tendons within the carpal tunnel. The median nerve is an important eleventh structure passing through at a most superficial position immediately against the deep surface of the retinaculum. Occasional additional variant structures within the canal are a persistent arteria mediana (which may rarely be large enough to cause median nerve compression), anomalous small muscles, and unusually distal extensions of the muscle bellies of elements of the two long flexor muscles.[14,33,210,228]

Entrapment neuropathy in the carpal tunnel is manifested by thenar muscle weakness and atrophy and diminished sensibility or paresthesias over the cutaneous distribution of the median nerve beyond the flexor retinaculum. Bear in mind that only the common and proper palmar digital branches of the median nerve can be involved; the palmar cutaneous branch escapes injury.

Near the inferior border of the flexor retinaculum the median nerve typically divides into three common palmar digital nerves: one to the thumb, one to the interspace between the second and third metacarpals, and one to the interspace between the third and fourth metacarpals. Each of these subsequently divides into two proper palmar digital nerves plus one proper palmar digital nerve that arises directly from the median nerve and then passes to the radial side of the index finger. The precise manner of division of these several common digital nerves is, however, quite variable. In addition to the cutaneous distribution of these common palmar branches, they also supply the two radial lumbricales. One additional branch—the muscular branch to the thenar muscles, often called the recurrent branch because, after clearing the retinaculum, it curves laterally and slightly upward to supply the abductor pollicis brevis, the opponens pollicis, and the flexor pollicis brevis (superficial head)—arises from the median nerve at the lower border of the retinaculum. This recurrent muscular branch occasionally pierces the lower border of the flexor retinaculum and thus can be individually entrapped, giving rise to a purely motor palsy limited to the three thenar muscles and without any sensory component.

The palmar cutaneous branch arises some 5 cm above the distal flexion crease at the wrist and descends into the palm superficial to the flexor retinaculum. In carpal tunnel syndrome this nerve is spared, and its area of distribution in the palmar skin shows normal sensation. Obviously, this can be used in determining the level of a median nerve lesion.

Distally in the palm, the common palmar digital nerves divide into the proper palmar digital nerves, which pass distally anterior to the deep transverse ligaments of the palm, accompanied by the corresponding vessels and the lumbricales muscles. In the distal part of each intermetacarpal space are two of these proper digital nerves, each passing to its respective side of the adjacent fingers. Anterior to this grouping of nerves, vessels and lumbrical muscles, which lie within each space between the long flexor tendons, lies the superficial transverse ligament of the palm. This ligament is more distal in the palm than is the deep ligament and extends into the interdigital web of skin. From the medial and lateral sides of each digital extension of the palmar aponeurosis there pass septumlike sheets of connective tissue fibers that reach and blend with the tissue of the deep transverse metacarpal ligament. Thus these septumlike sheets from the palmar aponeurosis complete tunnels for the four sets of long flexor tendons. At the same time they form the medial and lateral walls of the three intermetacarpal tunnels, cited above as the passageways for the digital nerves and vessels and the lumbrical muscles as they extend into the webspace tissue distal to the distal transverse palmar crease.

The proper digital nerves passing distally through these fibrous-walled intermetacarpal tunnels have little free space available to them for shifting or for accommodating the swelling of tissue. Hence, swelling of the adjacent tendons or their digital synovial sheaths causes compression on the enclosed proper palmar digital nerves. Tumors arising in this locality may also be a rare basis for compression. The most common mechanism of nerve compression here is a single severe trauma or multiple, repetitious trauma of lesser degree. Severe blows to the palm or crushing injuries of the hand, with or without fracture, may be the basis of an entrapment neuropathy in the palm. Excessive or forceful hyperextension at the metacarpophalangeal joint is another cause of entrapment neuropathy. In this circumstance the proper palmar digital nerve is drawn taut across the unyielding distal edge of the deep transverse metacarpal ligament. Occupational uses of the hand or habitual postures of the fingers may also be causal factors. If there is strong radial or ulnar deviation of the fingers as hyperextension of the metacarpophalangeal joint occurs, there will be even greater tautness of the proper palmar digital nerves.

Since there are two proper digital nerves in each intermetacarpal tunnel, it is evident that the area of pain and sensory loss or paresthesia is projected to the adjacent sides of two fingers; if only one of the two nerves is damaged, only the corresponding half of one finger will be involved.

Digital nerve neuropathy can obviously occur from repetitious external compression, such as occurs in some occupations and recreational activities involving the frequent use of certain tools or implements, notably scissors, staple guns, hand saws, and bowling balls. The nerve may be palpably thickened and very tender at the site of the compressive neuropathy.

Anastomoses Between Nerves in the Forearm and Hand

There are several levels of anastomoses between the median nerve and the ulnar nerve in the forearm and hand.[209,210,215] The median and ulnar nerves are linked to each other by one or two grossly recognizable trunks that may be in the proximal or distal parts of the forearm in the plane between the deep and superficial long flexors. These are referred to as the Martin-Gruber anastomoses. Sometimes the anastomosing bundles are quite small and are in the substance of the flexor digitorum profundus. The anterior interosseous nerve may convey the median nerve fibers to the anastomotic trunks or filaments. The nerve fibers may travel either way in the anastomotic nerves. Herein lies the explanation for the all-ulnar-nerve hand, the all-median-nerve hand, and the various lesser degrees of anastomosis.

An anastomosis may occur more distally between median and ulnar nerves as they descend into the hand. This occurs in the thenar eminence and in the palm and is apparently an anastomosis of purely motor nerve fibers, again accounting for variation in the innervation of the intrinsic muscles of the hand. When this anastomosis occurs in the hand, it is referred to as the Riche-Cannieu anastomosis. Such anastomoses do not alter the spinal cord or spinal nerve level of origin of the fibers, but they do modify the course of the fibers to their final destination. In essence, all of these variably present distal anastomoses between peripheral nerves may be thought of as continuations of the interchange of fibers seen proximally in the brachial plexus. Therefore, lesions of the nerves at different levels can give paralyses of muscles or sensory loss of unexpected and varying nature. This fact, in addition to the varying degrees of nerve damage, explains the variety of findings in different cases of the same entrapment neuropathy.

In the forearm the anterior interosseous branch of the median nerve occasionally gives small twigs that pierce the interosseous membrane at various levels or pass around its lower end to anastomose with the posterior interosseous nerve from the radial nerve (Rauber's anastomosis). These fibers are then carried down the forearm and possibly onto the dorsum of the hand when the posterior interosseous nerve extends that far. An anastomosis sometimes occurs between the posterior interosseous nerve and the deep branch of the ulnar nerve. This anastomosis is largely buried in the substance of the first and second dorsal interosseous muscles and is referred to as the Froment-Rauber anastomosis. An alternate path is for twigs from the posterior interosseous nerve to innervate the first and second dorsal interosseous muscles directly. In this case the fibers enter the radial nerve at the brachial plexus level instead of passing into the ulnar nerve. Thus, some fibers from the T1 spinal nerve and spinal cord segment that pass through the brachial plexus and that *should* travel into the ulnar nerve pass into the radial nerve directly or pass first into the median nerve and then through the interosseous membrane into the posterior interosseous nerve (Rauber's anastomosis). They then anastomose with the deep branch of the ulnar nerve between or in the substance of the first and second dorsal interosseous muscles (Froment-Rauber's anastomosis). As elsewhere, the occurrence of such variable and circuitous routes of nerve fibers to specific muscles explains the variability of signs and symptoms in the various entrapment syndromes.

Median Nerve Motor Conduction Study (Fig. 5-9)

Conduction Velocity

Amplifier setting:
- Sweep speed: 2 msec/div.
- Sensitivity: 5 mV/div.
- Filter setting: 20 Hz–10 kHz

Recording technique:
- Active electrode: Place the recording portion of the bar electrode on the midpoint of the abductor pollicis brevis. (Separate disc electrodes may be preferable, however, since they tend to record higher amplitudes of the CMAPs. In this case the reference electrode can be better positioned to be a true reference electrode than is possible with the fixed spacing necessary with the bar electrode.) When you are using separate discs, the distance between the active and reference electrodes must be standardized. The amplitudes recorded with bar electrodes and those recorded with separate electrodes are not interchangeable.
- Reference electrode: In the region of the base of the proximal phalanx of the thumb
- Ground electrode: On the dorsum of the hand between the active recording electrode and the stimulation site at the wrist

Stimulation technique:
- Use supramaximal current.

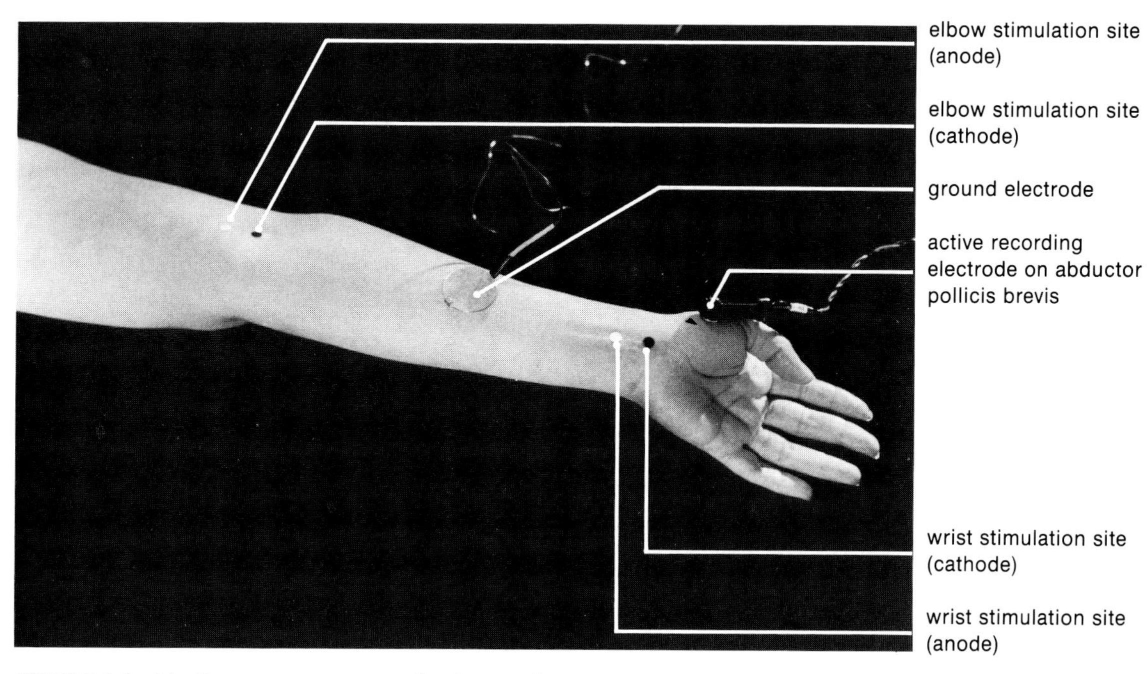

FIGURE 5-9 Median nerve motor conduction study.
Note: The wrist stimulation site is at the distal wrist crease between the tendons of the flexor carpi radialis and the palmaris longus. The proximal stimulation site is at the distal elbow crease, medial to the biceps brachii tendon. The ground electrode is placed on the flexor surface of the forearm for photographic purposes, but its ideal location is on the dorsum of the hand between the wrist stimulation site and the active recording electrode.

Wrist: Stimulate at the level of the most distal wrist crease between the tendons of the flexor carpi radialis and palmaris longus. (Stimulus duration is usually 0.1 msec, stimulus strength usually 150–300 V.)

Elbow: Stimulate at the bend of the elbow, medial to the tendon of the biceps brachii. In obese patients the nerve is made more accessible to stimulation by bending the elbow. (Stimulus duration is usually 0.1–0.5 msec, stimulus strength usually 150–300 V.)

F Wave

Amplifier setting:
- Sweep speed: 5 msec/div.
- Sensitivity: 200 μV/div.
- Filter setting: 20 Hz–10 kHz

Method: Stimulate with supramaximal current at the wrist 10 to 20 times and measure the F wave with the shortest latency. Keep the cathode distal. (Stimulus duration is usually 0.1 msec, stimulus strength 150–300 V.)

Normal Values

See Table 5-1.

Median–Ulnar Nerve Anastomosis in the Forearm (Martin-Gruber Anastomosis)

The presence of a Martin-Gruber anastomosis may be suspected when the shape and the amplitude of the CMAP obtained with proximal stimulation of the median nerve is different from that obtained with distal stimulation. The presence of this anastomosis is confirmed by obtaining an evoked motor response from the first dorsal interosseous or hypothenar muscles by stimulating the median nerve at the elbow.

Generally, when the parent nerve of an anom-

TABLE 5-1
Normal Values for Median Nerve Motor Conduction Studies

Age (Years)	Data (No.)	Amplitude (mV)	Distal Latency (msec)	Conduction Velocity (m/sec)	F Latency Minus Distal Latency (msec)
20–29	100	12.6 ± 2.6 (7.4–17.8)	3.1 ± 0.4 (2.3–3.9)	56.4 ± 3.3 (49.8–63.0)	23.8 ± 1.9 (20.0–27.6)
30–39	100	12.6 ± 2.9 (6.8–18.7)	3.1 ± 0.3 (2.5–3.9)	56.7 ± 3.7 (49.3–64.1)	23.7 ± 1.7 (20.3–27.1)
40–49	100	12.0 ± 2.5 (7.0–17.0)	3.2 ± 0.3 (2.2–3.8)	55.1 ± 3.2 (48.7–61.5)	23.8 ± 1.7 (20.4–27.2)
50–59	100	10.9 ± 2.1 (6.7–15.1)	3.2 ± 0.4 (2.8–4.0)	54.1 ± 3.8 (46.4–61.7)	24.8 ± 2.2 (20.4–29.2)
Below 60	400	12.0 ± 2.5 (7.0–17.0)	3.2 ± 0.4 (2.8–4.0)	55.6 ± 3.5 (48.6–62.6)	24.0 ± 1.9 (20.2–27.8)
Above 60	50	9.9 ± 2.5 (4.9–14.9)	3.4 ± 0.4 (2.6–4.2)	51.9 ± 4.1 (43.7–60.1)	25.4 ± 2.2 (21.0–29.8)
All ages combined	450	11.6 ± 2.5 (6.6–16.6)	3.2 ± 0.4 (2.8–4.0)	54.8 ± 3.6 (47.6–62.0)	24.3 ± 2.0 (20.3–28.3)

alous nerve is stimulated, the following findings are usually seen (Fig. 5-10): A potential recorded over a muscle innervated by the parent nerve contains an initial positive deflection on proximal stimulation. This positive deflection is not seen on distal stimulation. The initial positive deflection is the result of a volume-conducted response from stimulation of adjacent muscles supplied by the anastomotic nerve. The amplitude of the proximal CMAP is larger than that of the distal response, since both the parent nerve and the anomalous nerve fibers are stimulated. Hence, the CMAP obtained is the recording of muscle fibers elicited by stimulation of the nerve of interest as well as neighboring muscle fibers supplied by the anomalous nerve.

With anomalous innervations the calculated conduction velocity is erroneously fast if the proximal latency is measured to the onset of the initial positive deflection rather than to the onset of the first negative deflection. This falsely shortens the proximal latency, and a spuriously fast conduction velocity results. This effect is accentuated in the presence of carpal tunnel syndrome[74] because the median nerve entrapment at the wrist prolongs the distal latency but does not affect the conduction time across the anastomotic nerve.

Comments

Traditionally, median nerve motor conduction studies are performed by applying the distal stimulation 8 cm from the recording electrode.[144,145] This is believed to give a smaller standard deviation about the mean value than when one uses a fixed anatomical point such as the distal wrist crease as the landmark for distal stimulation.[118] In our laboratory, however, we have used the most distal wrist crease because it is at the proximal edge of the flexor retinaculum and is therefore closer to the carpal tunnel. Stimulation at this point is not influenced by contributions from the segment of the median nerve at the lower forearm. Technically, it is also faster and more convenient, since no measurements are involved. It is essential that our normal values be used only when our method, as described above, is employed.

Median Nerve Sensory Conduction Study (Fig. 5-11)

Conduction Time

Amplifier setting:
- Sweep speed: 2 msec/div.
- Sensitivity: 20–50 μV/div.

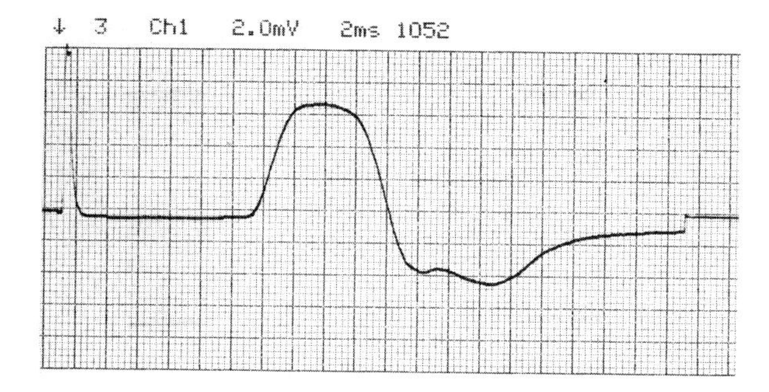

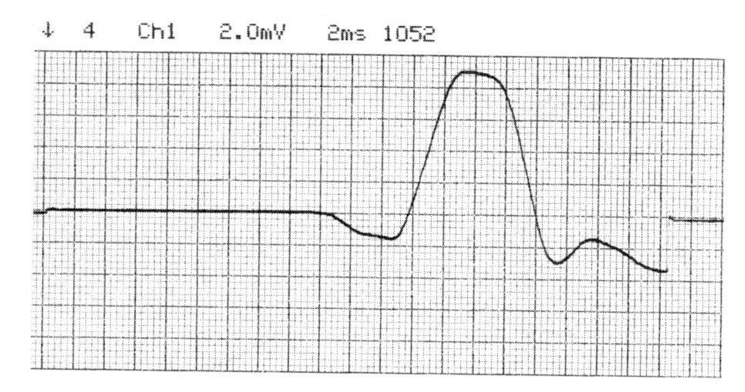

FIGURE 5-10 Martin-Gruber anastomosis. The top tracing shows the CMAP from the abductor pollicis brevis on stimulation of the median nerve at the wrist. The distal motor latency is prolonged owing to the presence of carpal tunnel syndrome. The bottom tracing shows the proximal CMAP obtained from stimulation of the median nerve at the elbow. The proximal response is larger in amplitude than the distal response, and a positive deflection precedes the CMAP.

Filter setting: 20 Hz–2 kHz

Recording technique (antidromic):

Midpalm: Place the active recording portion of the bar electrode 5 cm distal to the stimulating electrode in the axis of the third digit.

Third digit: Place the active recording portion of the bar electrode at the base of the proximal phalanx of the third digit.

Fourth digit: Place the active recording portion of the bar electrode on the lateral portion of the base of the proximal phalanx of the fourth digit.

Reference electrode: If you are using separated reference and active electrodes, the reference electrode should be no more than 4 cm away from the active electrode.

Ground electrode: On the dorsum of the hand between the stimulus site at the wrist and the recording site at midpalm

Stimulation technique:

Use supramaximal current.

Wrist: Stimulate at the level of the most distal wrist crease, between the tendons of the flexor carpi radialis and palmaris longus. (Stimulus duration is usually 0.05 msec, stimulus strength 150–300 V.)

Normal Values

See Table 5-2.

Comments

Artifacts occurring during recording can be reduced by spreading the patient's fingers apart and lifting the hand off the examination bed or arm board. Traditionally, stimulation of the median nerve is done 14 cm proximally from the active recording electrode, which is placed at the base of the third digit.[87] This level is also used for performing median nerve motor conduction studies. We stimulate the median nerve at the level of the most distal wrist crease because the stimulator is then just above the proximal edge of the carpal tunnel. We have found this method of stimulation, coupled with midpalmar recordings, to be sensitive in the detection of mild sensory abnormalities from early entrapment of the median nerve at the wrist. Our procedure must be followed if our normal values are to be used.

The median nerve sensory potential may also be recorded from the third digit, and antidromic stimulation can be done at 1-cm increments from midpalm to the distal forearm. If the stimulus is

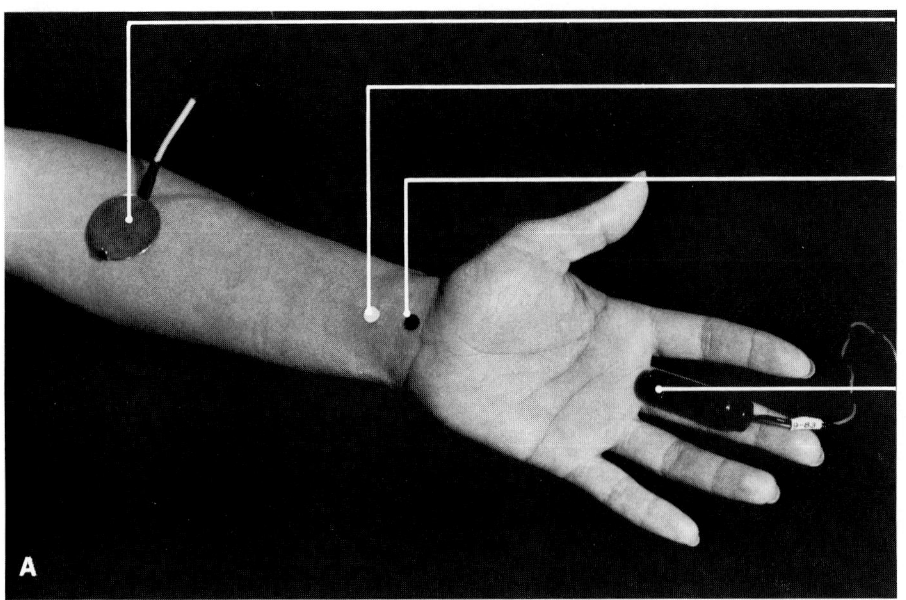

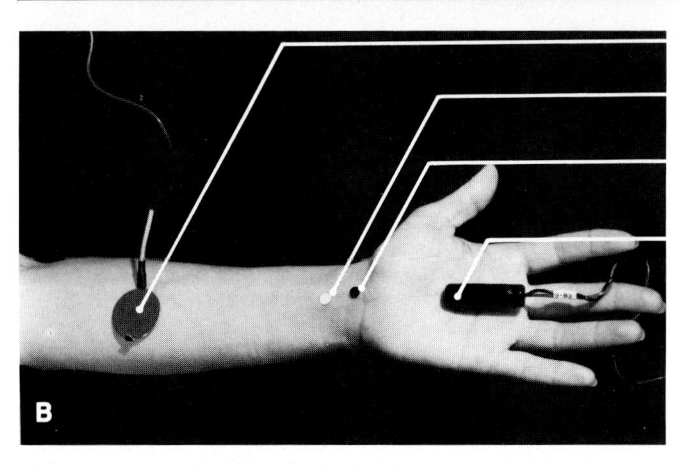

FIGURE 5-11 (A) Median nerve sensory conduction study. (B) Median nerve midpalmar sensory conduction study.
Note: The ground electrode is placed on the flexor surface of the forearm for photographic purposes, but its ideal location is on the dorsum of the hand between the wrist stimulation site and the active recording electrode.

moved proximally from the midpalm, a latency change of 0.16 msec to 0.2 msec/cm is normally observed.[99] A sudden increase beyond this range indicates involvement of the median sensory fibers at a specific site. This increase is most commonly found 2 cm to 4 cm distal to the origin of the flexor retinaculum; the origin of the flexor retinaculum is at the same level as the distal wrist crease. This method is useful in differentiating distal sensory neuropathy from local entrapment of the median nerve, such as is seen in carpal tunnel syndrome.[99]

Electrodiagnosis in Carpal Tunnel Syndrome

Anatomy

See Figures 1-27 through 1-29 and Appendix Figure 24.

Nerve Conduction Studies

SENSORY

Distal sensory latency is prolonged earlier than distal motor latency.[18,145,202,227,241] Sensory poten-

TABLE 5-2
Normal Values for Median Nerve Sensory Conduction Studies (Antidromic)

Age (Years)	*Data (No.)*	*Midpalm Amplitude (μV)*	*Midpalm Peak Latency (msec)*	*Digit 3 Amplitude (μV)*	*Digit 3 Peak Latency (msec)*	*Digit 4 Amplitude (μV)*	*Digit 4 Peak Latency (msec)*
20–29	70	113.9 ± 40.8 (31.4–195.5)	1.6 ± 0.1 (1.4–1.8)	76.5 ± 31.9 (12.7–140.3)	2.7 ± 0.2 (2.3–3.1)	46.5 ± 19.6 (12.0–105.7)	2.7 ± 0.3 (2.1–3.3)
30–39	80	106.4 ± 41.3 (23.8–189.0)	1.6 ± 0.1 (1.4–1.8)	71.9 ± 28.4 (15.1–128.7)	2.8 ± 0.2 (2.4–3.2)	43.5 ± 17.5 (12.0–78.5)	2.7 ± 0.3 (2.1–3.3)
40–49	65	98.5 ± 36.8 (24.9–172.1)	1.7 ± 0.1 (1.5–1.9)	67.5 ± 24.6 (18.3–116.7)	2.8 ± 0.2 (2.4–3.2)	41.5 ± 19.1 (12.0–79.7)	2.8 ± 0.2 (2.4–3.2)
50–59	50	94.7 ± 36.1 (22.5–166.9)	1.8 ± 0.1 (1.6–2.0)	56.7 ± 25.4 (15.0–107.5)	2.8 ± 0.2 (2.4–3.2)	33.8 ± 14.8 (12.0–63.4)	2.8 ± 0.2 (2.4–3.2)
Below 60	265	103.4 ± 38.8 (25.8–181.0)	1.7 ± 0.1 (1.5–1.9)	68.2 ± 27.7 (12.3–123.6)	2.8 ± 0.2 (2.4–3.2)	41.3 ± 17.8 (12.0–76.9)	2.8 ± 0.3 (2.2–3.4)
Above 60	30	72.3 ± 34.9 (15.0–142.1)	1.7 ± 0.2 (1.3–2.1)	50.7 ± 18.3 (14.1–87.3)	2.9 ± 0.2 (2.5–3.3)	25.9 ± 9.2 (8.0–44.3)	2.8 ± 0.3 (2.2–3.4)
All ages combined	295	97.2 ± 38.1 (21.0–173.4)	1.7 ± 0.1 (1.5–1.9)	64.7 ± 26.1 (12.5–116.9)	2.8 ± 0.2 (2.4–3.2)	38.2 ± 16.5 (8.0–71.2)	2.8 ± 0.3 (2.2–3.4)

tial amplitudes are also depressed. Comparison of the median and ulnar sensory conduction latencies to the ring finger also aids in the diagnosis.[86] Prolongation of the sensory latencies across the wrist with midpalmar stimulation is usually the earliest finding.[17,31] Measurement of the sensory latency with midpalmar stimulation helps to differentiate distal sensory delay due to carpal tunnel syndrome from that due to distal neuropathy. To improve the sensitivity of the recordings, Kimura[99] has described stimulation from the midpalm to the distal forearm in 1-cm increments.

MOTOR

Distal motor latency is delayed, and the amplitude may be depressed. Because the recording is done distal to the site of entrapment, a depressed amplitude may not reflect axonal degeneration but may instead be due to partial neurapraxia or a mixture of the two.[102] This is best differentiated by EMG or by comparing the CMAP obtained from the abductor pollicis brevis on stimulation just proximal and just distal to the carpal tunnel. The CMAP obtained with stimulation just distal to the carpal tunnel is bigger than that obtained on stimulation proximal to the carpal tunnel if the pathology is neurapraxia.

A very useful method for detection of early carpal tunnel–type involvement is to calculate the residual latency. The residual latency is the difference between the distal motor latency and the quotient obtained when the distance between the cathode at the distal stimulation point and the active recording electrode is divided by the conduction velocity. The mean value, as reported by Kraft and Halvorson,[118] ranges from 1.4 msec to 2.5 msec (mean value 1.97 ± 0.27 msec). To obtain this mean the distal motor latency was measured with sensitivity at 200 μV/div. and sweep speed at 2 msec to 5 msec/div. The residual latency is useful in helping one to decide whether there is a concomitant carpal tunnel syndrome in a patient with peripheral neuropathy or whether the slowed distal latency is attributable solely to peripheral neuropathy.

Another useful method when there is a question of carpal tunnel syndrome in a patient with peripheral neuropathy is to determine the terminal latency index (TLI).[199] This index is the ratio of the conduction velocity in the distal segment of a nerve to the proximal velocity. (Of course, the calculation of distal conduction velocity includes the delay at the neuromuscular junction.) It is calculated by using the formula

$$\frac{\text{terminal distance (mm)}}{\text{conduction velocity (m/sec)} \times \text{terminal latency (msec)}}$$

The mean TLI for the median nerve in normal subjects was 0.433 ± 0.045 (0.356–0.550).[199]

Although the F response from the abductor pollicis brevis may be delayed, the F-minus-M latency is normal in the absence of coexisting proximal nerve disease (see Table 5-1 for our normal values on F − M).

A median-to-ulnar-nerve anastomosis in the forearm may be concomitant with carpal tunnel syndrome.

It is essential that electrodiagnostic studies be performed bilaterally in cases of carpal tunnel syndrome, since the incidence of bilaterality is high.[6] Ulnar nerve motor and sensory conduction studies and radial nerve sensory conduction studies should routinely be performed in these cases. If these are abnormal, sural nerve studies must be performed to rule out the presence of generalized peripheral neuropathy.

EMG

GENERAL

Neuropathic changes are seen in the abductor pollicis brevis and opponens pollicis. EMG of other limb muscles must be done to rule out proximal lesions such as coexisting cervical radiculopathy, especially along nerve roots C6 and C7.[249]

Electrodiagnosis in Pronator Teres Syndrome

Anatomy

See Figures 1-25 and 1-26 and Appendix Figure 26.

Nerve Conduction Studies

SENSORY

The amplitudes of the sensory potentials in the digits supplied by the median nerve may be depressed, and the durations may be prolonged with stimulation of the median nerve at the wrist and elbow. The distal latencies may be normal.[150]

MOTOR

The distal latency to the thenar muscles may not be delayed.[150] The conduction velocity along the forearm segment may be mildly slowed.

EMG

Since the entrapment occurs distal to the origin of the branch that supplies the pronator teres, this muscle is spared, but the signs of denervation are observed in all other distal muscles supplied by the median and anterior interosseous nerves.

Electrodiagnosis in Anterior Interosseous Nerve Syndrome

Anatomy

See Figure 1-28 and Appendix Figure 24.

Nerve Conduction Studies

SENSORY

Amplitude and latency are normal in the digits supplied by the median nerve on stimulation of this nerve at the wrist or elbow. (The anterior interosseous nerve has no sensory supply to the digits.)

MOTOR

Results of routine conduction studies of the median nerve are normal.[161] Latencies to the flexor pollicis longus or pronator quadratus may be delayed when compared to the contralateral side, and the duration of the evoked motor response may be prolonged.[161]

EMG

Evidence of denervation is seen in the muscles supplied by the anterior interosseous nerve, namely the flexor pollicis longus, flexor digitorum profundus (lateral half), and pronator quadratus. The involvement may be bilateral.[156]

The EMG examination should not be limited to the distribution of this nerve, since anterior interosseous nerve palsy may be associated with idiopathic brachial plexitis.[184]

ULNAR NERVE

Applied Anatomy (*See Appendix Fig.* 25)

Arising from the medial cord of the brachial plexus, at about the level of the lower border of the pectoralis minor, the ulnar nerve enters the arm by crossing the tendons of the latissimus dorsi and teres major muscles. At first it lies close to the brachial artery, but at about mid-arm level it inclines posteriorly and parts company with the artery, then pierces the medial intermuscular septum to descend posterior to that septum thereafter. The septum becomes increasingly well defined as it travels downward to the medial epicondyle. In the lower half of the arm the ulnar nerve is in intimate relationship with the medial head of the triceps. The ulnar nerve descends behind the medial epicondyle of the humerus, which is here variably grooved for the nerve. Sometimes shallow and sometimes deeper, the groove does not trap or anchor the nerve even when the elbow is flexed. In fact, subluxation of the nerve may be freer in flexion than in extension. Injury may occur at this level by direct trauma or by the irritation of recurring subluxation of the nerve with elbow flexion and extension.

Below the medial epicondyle the nerve enters the forearm by passing across the elbow joint against the ulnar collateral ligament and under cover of the aponeurotic arch of connective tissue that bridges the humeral (epicondylar) and ulnar (olecranon) heads of the flexor carpi ulnaris (the cubital tunnel). Here the nerve is rather snugly held, and encroachments from any source or side are likely to compress the nerve within this osseofibrous tunnel. The distance between the tip of the medial epicondyle and the medial border of the tip of the olecranon is greater in full flexion of the elbow than it is in extension. Accordingly, the aponeurotic arch of bridging fibers between the humeral and ulnar heads of the flexor carpi ulnaris is drawn tight in full flexion. This reduces the space between the fibrous arch and the floor of the tunnel. In some, prolonged full flexion sufficiently compresses the ulnar nerve in the cubital tunnel to cause annoying but transient paresthesia and even muscular weakness in the hand. Additional reduction of the caliber of the cubital tunnel may occur in arthritis of the elbow joint, especially with bony lipping and thickening of the ligaments, with new or old fractures of the area that distort the cubital tunnel by callus or poor reduction.[94] If the fracture is in a child, the growth plates may be damaged, and years later the unequal growth may lead to an increase in the carrying angle (cubitus valgus), with consequent increased tension on the nerve, especially with elbow flexion. Such delayed onset of the symptoms and findings is referred to as tardy ulnar palsy.[48] The greater carrying angle usually to be seen in women may account in part for the greater frequency of occurrence of cubital tunnel syndrome in women. However, carpal tunnel syndrome also occurs more often in women than in men, so other factors may be responsible for the sex difference. Space-occupying lesions such as tumors may precipitate the development of cubital tunnel syndrome, and occasionally an aberrant muscle slip from the medial head of the triceps may cross the nerve at the upper margin of the cubital tunnel and may cause the syndrome. Naturally, external forces such as prolonged or repetitious compression of the ulnar nerve in the cubital tunnel, or behind the medial epicondyle, caused by resting the elbow and proximal forearm against the firm arm of a chair or the edge of a bed, desk, or table may cause damage to the nerve. As the nerve lies behind the epicondyle and in the cubital tunnel it is supplied by the superior and inferior ulnar collateral arteries and the posterior ulnar recurrent artery, which anastomose as they run in close relationship to the nerve.[163] There are occasional cases of postoperative ulnar palsy in which, apparently, no external compressive force occurred. It is possible that these cases can be explained by a fall in blood pressure during the surgery, thereby causing a critical period of ischemia in an already abnormal nerve in the cubital tunnel.

In some cases of anterior translocation of the ulnar nerve in the treatment of cubital tunnel syndrome, a postsurgical iatrogenic entrapment neuropathy occurs a little below mid-arm level. This is due to the relative fixation of the nerve as it passes through or underneath the arcade of Struthers.[210] With anterior displacement of the nerve, it becomes angulated and stressed at this level. Without translocation this passage of the nerve under the arcade is not known to cause a neuropathy. To prevent this postsurgical entrapment, it has been advocated that the nerve be freed by sectioning the arcade of Struthers and resecting the medial intermuscular septum at the time of translocation. It must be understood that the arcade of Struthers is a separate entity from the ligament of Struthers, which I cite in my discussion of the median nerve neuropathy that occasionally occurs in the presence of a supracondylar process. The arcade of Struthers is a commonly identifiable fascial and aponeurotic arch that straps the ulnar nerve in place against the medial head of the triceps, some 6 cm to 10 cm above the medial epicondyle. It is formed by the combination of the medial intermuscular septum, the deep fascia of the triceps, and the aponeurotic origin of a thin sheet of triceps muscle fibers arising from the septum.

The ulnar nerve descends through the forearm, lying on the flexor digitorum profundus and deep to the overlapping anterior border of the flexor carpi ulnaris and the other superficial forearm flexors. High in the forearm, it sends a branch to each of the two heads of origin of the flexor carpi ulnaris, as well as a twig to the flexor digitorum profundus. Usually, the latter twig supplies the portion sending tendons to the little and ring fingers, but it occasionally supplies the part serving the middle finger as well. The nerve or nerves that supply the two heads of the flexor carpi ulnaris may arise above the arching aponeurosis that extends between the two heads, and these branches may therefore be spared in the compression of the ulnar nerve that gives rise to cubital tunnel syndrome.

At approximately the junction of the middle and distal thirds of the forearm the ulnar nerve gives off the dorsal cutaneous branch to the hand. Thereafter, the ulnar nerve gradually becomes more superficial between the tendon of the flexor carpi ulnaris and the medialmost tendon of the flexor digitorum superficialis. In this place it commonly gives off a small palmar cutaneous branch that supplies the proximal portion of the palm on the ulnar side.

Entering the hand, the ulnar nerve, in company with the ulnar artery, lies deep to the palmaris brevis muscle and is lodged in a groove created by the pisiform bone and the hamate with its prominent palmar process, the hamulus.[71,107] This bony groove is covered over by an expansion from the tendon of the flexor carpi ulnaris, fibers of the flexor retinaculum, and fibers of origin of the abductor digiti minimi and the flexor digiti minimi brevis. The deep fascia of the forearm extends across the level of the wrist joint to end as a superficial lamina of the flexor retinaculum, and this aids in covering the aforementioned groove. Thus, the groove housing the ulnar nerve and vessels is converted into an osseofibrous canal known as Guyon's canal or tunnel (also called the distal ulnar tunnel). Within this 4-cm-long canal the ulnar nerve divides into its superficial and deep terminal branches. The superficial branch is sensory except for fibers to the palmaris brevis.[79,176] Extending distally, the superficial branch crosses superficial to the fibers of origin of the abductor digiti minimi and the flexor digiti minimi brevis to divide into a proper digital branch to the ulnar side of the little finger and a common palmar digital branch. This latter nerve then contributes a branch to the radial side of the little finger and a branch to the ulnar side of the ring finger. Usually there is also a communicating or anastomotic branch that joins the closest common palmar digital branch of the median nerve. The deep branch of the ulnar nerve is purely motor and passes deeply between the abductor digiti minimi and the flexor digiti minimi brevis proximally or at their origins. This deep branch gives twigs to the three hypothenar muscles and continues distally deep to the flexor digiti brevis to curve radialward around the hamulus of the hamate ultimately to supply all of the interossei (both palmar and dorsal), the two medial lumbricals, the adductor pollicis, and the deep head of the flexor pollicis brevis. Compression neuropathy in Guyon's canal may give rise to a motor loss (deep branch), a sensory loss (superficial branch), or a mixed motor and sensory neuropathy.[43] In spite of the subcutaneous fat, the palmaris brevis, and the dense fascial fibers overlying the contents of the canal of Guyon, both the ulnar nerve and the ulnar artery are subject to trauma here. Pushing and pounding with this proximal part of the hand can lead to thrombosis of the ulnar artery and neuropathy of the ulnar nerve. In the latter circumstance the palmar cutaneous branch and the dorsal branch of the ulnar nerve are intact, and only the digital branches of the superficial terminal branch of the ulnar nerve in the hand show the altered sensibility. Neuropathy of the deep branch, which supplies the hypothenar muscles, the two medial lumbricals, the interossei, the adductor pollicis, and the deep head of the flexor pollicis brevis, leads to atrophy and paralysis of those muscles. The superficial branch is purely sensory except for supplying the palmaris brevis when this branch has not arisen from the main trunk. To simplify the statement of the motor distribution of the ulnar nerve in the hand, it may be said that it supplies all of the intrinsic hand muscles except the two lateral lumbricals and two and one half thumb muscles that are supplied by the median nerve.

Total destruction of the ulnar nerve at the wrist or of its deep branch in the distal ulnar tunnel gives rise to the "ulnar claw hand." In this condition the unopposed action of the extensor digitorum tendons to the little and ring fingers (radial nerve) results in hyperextension at the metacarpophalangeal joints of these digits, since the interossei and lumbricals that would flex these joints are paralyzed. Flexion of the interphalangeal joints of these fingers by the long flexors, particularly the profundus, occurs because the ulnar nerve damage is distal to the profundus innervation, and the interossei and the lumbricals for these two fingers do not exert their usual extensor action on the interphalangeal joints. Atrophy of the hypothenar muscles and of the interossei is apparent. The little finger is likely to be slightly abducted owing to the unopposed action of the extensor digiti minimi (supplied by the radial nerve). When the median nerve alone is destroyed at the wrist level, the thumb tends to be adducted, extended, and in the plane of the palm because of the loss of the abductor pollicis brevis, flexor pollicis brevis (superficial head), and opponens pollicis. The thumb is incapable of true opposition to the fingers. The loss of the two radial lumbricals diminishes the extensor action on the interphalangeal joints of the index and middle fingers and also the flexor power at the metacarpophalangeal joints of those two digits; hence, the index and middle fingers are somewhat extended at the metacarpophalangeal joints and somewhat flexed at the interphalangeal joints. When both median and ulnar nerves are destroyed at the wrist, the loss of action of the interossei for flexion of the metacarpophalangeal joints and for extension of the interphalangeal joints of the index and middle fingers allows the unopposed action of the long flexors and the extensor digitorum to pull the index and middle fingers into the same posture of clawing described for the lesion of the ulnar nerve at the wrist. This combined lesion is a true (or total) claw hand, or *main en griffe*. The isolated median nerve lesion at the wrist does not give a "median claw hand," as sometimes erroneously stated, but instead a simian hand (*main en singe*). Destruction of the median nerve above the elbow causes paralysis of the flexor pollicis longus and flexor digitorum profundus to the index and middle fingers (typically), as well as paralysis of the flexor digitorum superficialis. This leaves unopposed action of the thumb extensors and the extensor digitorum to the index and middle fingers. Accordingly, these digits tend to remain extended while the ring and little fingers flex. This is a posture called the "hand of benediction" by some clinicians.

Other causes of ulnar entrapment neuropathy at Guyon's canal include occupational trauma, anomalous muscle arrangements, carpal bone fractures, ganglia (protruding from carpal joints), and ulnar artery thrombosis.[194] Ganglia are the most common causes, according to published reports.[185,197,221]

Variations in the muscular distribution of the ulnar nerve become more understandable with consideration of the distal anastomoses between nerves, as previously described. Such variations in innervation of the intrinsic hand muscles explain the variations in the observed paralyses in cases of ulnar (or median) nerve compression neuropathies.[34,51,76,77,191]

Motor Conduction Study (*Fig.* 5-12)

Conduction Velocity

Amplifier setting:
- Sweep speed: 2 msec/div.
- Sensitivity: 5 mV/div.
- Filter setting: 20 Hz–10 kHz

Recording technique:
- Active electrode: Place the recording portion of the bar electrode on the midpoint of the abductor digiti minimi. Separate electrodes may give higher CMAP amplitude, since the reference electrode can be better positioned to be more of a true reference

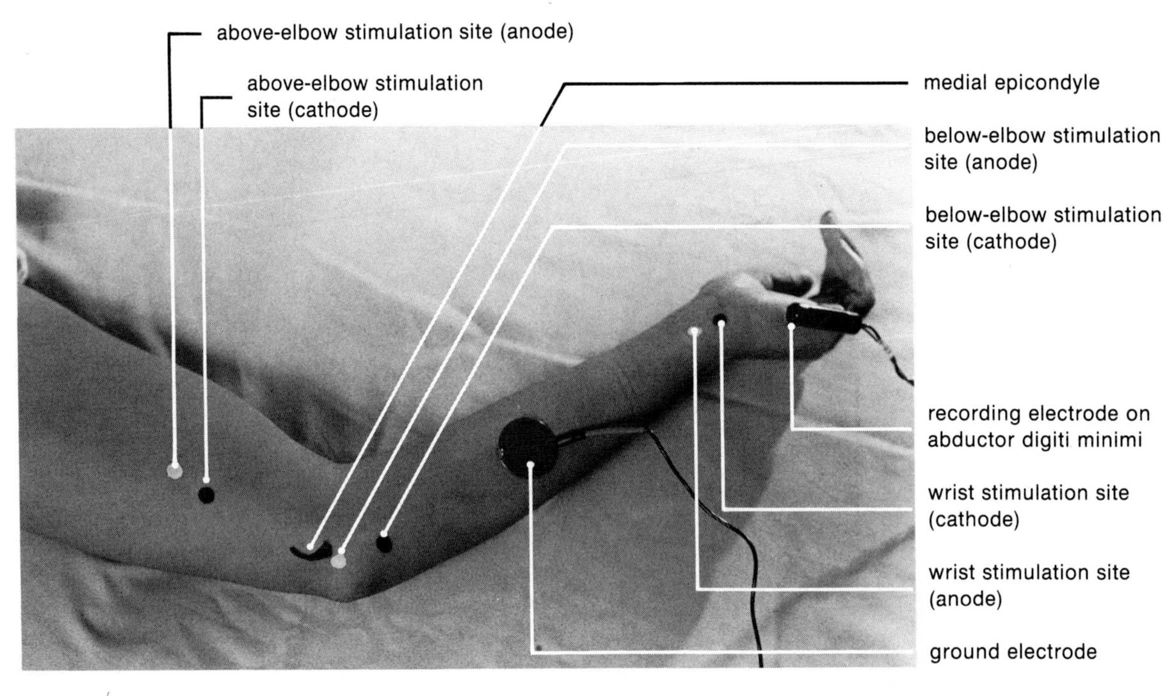

FIGURE 5-12 Ulnar nerve motor conduction study.
Note: The wrist stimulation site is at the distal wrist crease, lateral to the flexor carpi ulnaris tendon. The below-elbow stimulation site is located by placing the stimulator anode on the lower border of the medial epicondyle. The above-elbow stimulation site is 10 cm proximal to the below-elbow stimulation site with elbow bent 45°. The ground electrode is placed on the flexor surface of the forearm for photographic purposes, but its ideal location is on the dorsum of the hand between the wrist stimulation site and the active recording electrode.

electrode than the fixed spacing necessary with a bar electrode. However, it is essential that the placement of the reference electrode be standardized; the amplitudes obtained with the bar electrode and the separate electrodes are not interchangeable.

Reference electrode: In the region of the medial aspect of the base of the proximal phalanx of the fifth digit

Ground electrode: On the dorsum of the hand between the active recording electrode and the stimulation site at the wrist

Stimulation technique:

Use supramaximal stimulation.

Wrist: Stimulate at the level of the most distal wrist crease, just lateral to the tendon of the flexor carpi ulnaris.

Below elbow: Feel for the lower edge of the medial epicondyle and place the anode of the stimulator at this level so that the cathode stimulates below the elbow.

Above elbow: Bend the elbow 45° and measure a distance of 10 cm proximally from the below-elbow stimulation point. Use a metal tape and measure carefully, with the tape measure closely applied to the skin surface. You should be able to palpate the nerve at this level. Remeasure the distance after stimulation, since the stimulation is over a short segment, and errors in measurement affect the results significantly. Usually, the difference in conduction velocity values between the below-elbow and across-elbow segments is less than 10 m/sec.

Note: The ulnar nerve can also be stimulated at the axilla, medial to the coracobrachialis. It can be stimulated at the supraclavicular fossa at Erb's point, which is

TABLE 5-3
Normal Values for Ulnar Nerve Motor Conduction Studies

Age (Years)	*Data (No.)*	*Amplitude (mV)*	*Distal Latency (msec)*	*Across-Elbow Conduction Velocity (m/sec)*	*Below-Elbow Conduction Velocity (m/sec)*	*F Latency Minus Distal Latency (msec)*
20–29	100	8.7 ± 2.0 (4.7–12.7)	2.5 ± 0.3 (1.5–3.1)	55.8 ± 4.6 (46.6–65.0)	59.1 ± 3.4 (52.3–65.9)	24.2 ± 1.9 (20.4–28.0)
30–39	100	8.7 ± 1.5 (5.7–11.7)	2.5 ± 0.3 (1.5–3.1)	55.2 ± 4.9 (45.4–65.0)	58.1 ± 4.1 (49.9–66.3)	24.4 ± 1.9 (20.6–28.2)
40–49	100	8.6 ± 1.7 (5.2–12.0)	2.5 ± 0.3 (1.9–3.1)	54.3 ± 4.8 (44.7–63.9)	57.6 ± 3.8 (50.0–65.2)	24.6 ± 2.1 (20.4–28.8)
50–59	85	8.4 ± 1.7 (5.0–11.8)	2.5 ± 0.3 (1.9–3.1)	52.8 ± 3.7 (45.4–60.2)	56.4 ± 3.7 (49.0–63.8)	25.1 ± 2.0 (21.0–29.0)
Below 60	385	8.6 ± 1.7 (5.2–12.0)	2.5 ± 0.3 (1.9–3.1)	54.5 ± 4.5 (45.5–63.5)	57.8 ± 3.8 (50.2–65.4)	24.6 ± 2.0 (20.6–28.6)
Above 60	50	7.8 ± 1.9 (4.0–11.6)	2.5 ± 0.3 (1.9–3.1)	49.9 ± 3.7 (42.5–57.3)	54.2 ± 3.3 (47.6–60.8)	26.0 ± 2.0 (22.0–30.0)
All ages combined	435	8.4 ± 1.8 (4.8–12.0)	2.5 ± 0.3 (1.9–3.1)	53.6 ± 4.4 (44.8–62.4)	57.1 ± 3.7 (49.7–64.5)	24.8 ± 2.0 (20.8–28.8)

at about the junction of the clavicular head of the sternocleidomastoid and the medial end of the clavicle. This point is at the level of the C6 vertebra. Traditionally, the distal stimulation site at the wrist is 8 cm from the recording electrode.[144] Our normal values should be used only when the recording methods described in this section are employed. The elbow position must be standardized, since this affects the conduction velocity across the elbow.[22]

F Wave

Amplifier setting:
- Sweep speed: 5 msec/div.
- Sensitivity: 200 μV/div.
- Filter setting: 20 Hz–10 kHz

Method: Stimulate 10 to 20 times with supramaximal current at the wrist and measure the F wave with the shortest latency. (Stimulus duration is usually 0.1 msec, stimulus strength usually 100–300 V.)

Normal Values

See Table 5-3.

Sensory Conduction Study (Fig. 5-13)

Conduction Time

Amplifier setting:
- Sweep speed: 2 msec/div.
- Sensitivity: 20–50 μV/div.
- Filter setting: 20 Hz–2 kHz

Recording technique (antidromic):
- Midpalm: Place the recording portion of the bar electrode at the midpalmar level in line with the fifth digit 5 cm distal to the distal wrist crease.
- Fifth digit: Place the active recording portion of the bar electrode at the base of the fifth digit.
- Reference electrode: If you are using separate electrodes for recording and reference, place the reference electrode at least 4 cm from the active electrode.
- Ground electrode: Over the dorsum of the hand between the stimulus site at the wrist and the recording site at the midpalm

Stimulation site:
- Wrist: Stimulate at the most distal wrist crease, on or just lateral to the tendon of the flexor carpi ulnaris.

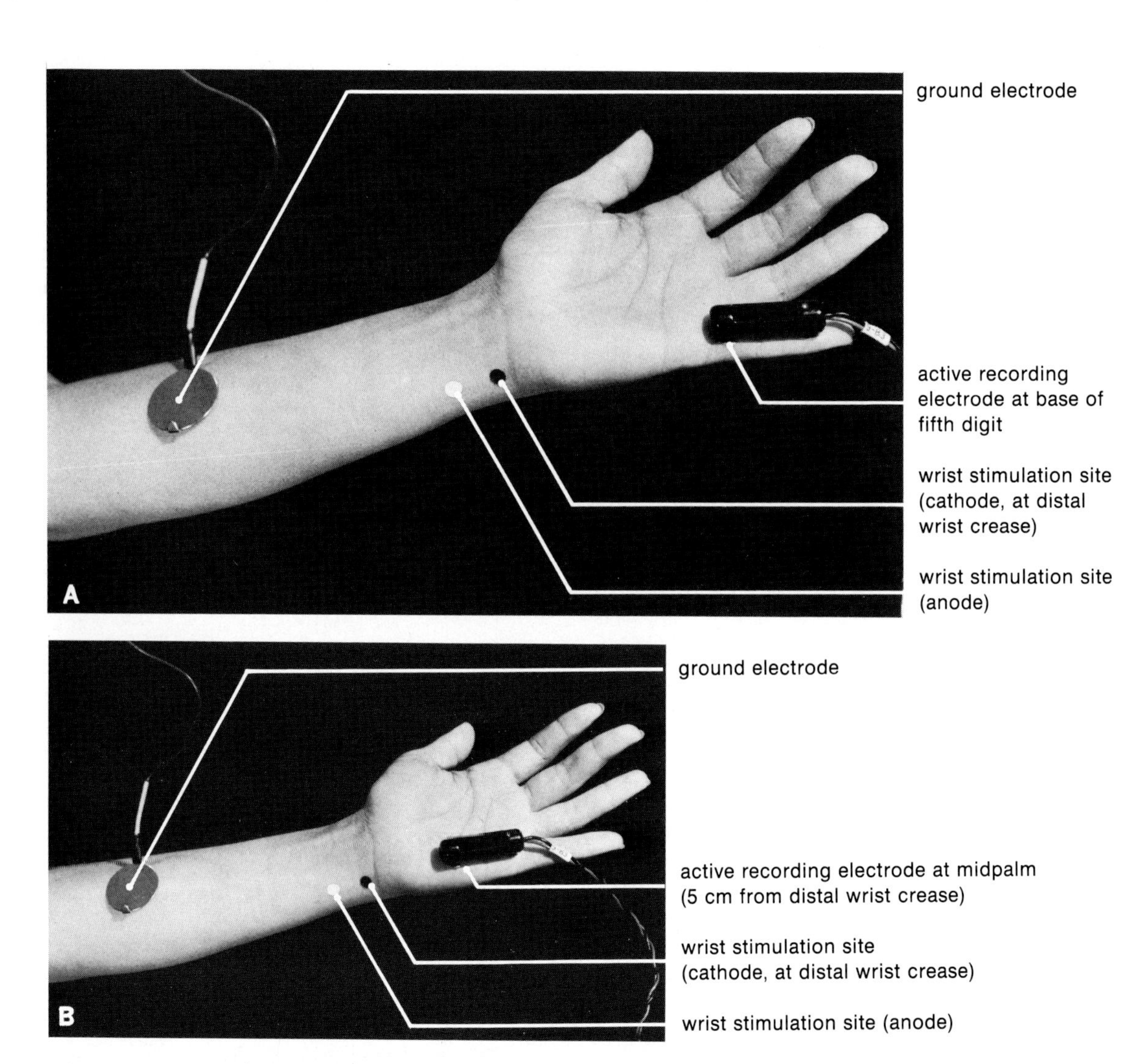

FIGURE 5-13 (A) Ulnar nerve sensory conduction study. (B) Ulnar nerve midpalmar sensory conduction study.

Normal Values

See Tables 5-4 and 5-5.

Comments

Artifacts occurring during recording can be reduced by spreading the patient's fingers and lifting the hand off the examination bed or arm board. Traditionally, stimulation of the ulnar nerve at the wrist is done 14 cm proximal to the recording electrode. The recording electrode itself is placed at the base of the fifth digit.[87] Because normal values vary with different procedures, our values should be used only in conjunction with the method of stimulation described above.

The dorsal cutaneous branch of the ulnar nerve can be studied by placing the recording electrode at the intermetacarpal space between the fourth and fifth digits on the dorsum of the hand. The reference electrode is placed 4 cm distally. The site of stimulation is 8 cm proximal to the recording electrode, with the stimulator between the tendon of the flexor carpi ulnaris and the ulna. One study reports the normal conduction velocity to be 60.0 ± 4.0 m/sec and amplitude to be 20.0 ± 6.0 μV.[81]

TABLE 5-4
Normal Values for Ulnar Nerve Sensory Conduction Studies (Fifth Digit, Antidromic)

Age (Years)	*Data (No.)*	*Amplitude (μV)*	*Peak Latency (msec)*
20–29	100	60.8 ± 27.2 (20.0–115.0)	2.5 ± 0.2 (2.1–2.9)
30–39	100	57.7 ± 27.1 (20.0–111.9)	2.6 ± 0.2 (2.2–3.0)
40–49	100	52.0 ± 25.9 (10–103.8)	2.6 ± 0.2 (2.2–3.0)
50–59	100	42.0 ± 18.6 (10.0–79.2)	2.6 ± 0.2 (2.2–3.0)
Below 60	400	53.1 ± 25.0 (10.0–103.1)	2.6 ± 0.2 (2.2–3.0)
Above 60	80	35.5 ± 18.6 (9.0–72.7)	2.7 ± 0.3 (2.1–3.3)
All ages combined	480	49.6 ± 23.8 (9.0–97.2)	2.6 ± 0.2 (2.2–3.0)

Electrodiagnosis in Ulnar Nerve Entrapment at the Elbow

Anatomy

See Figures 1-23, 1-26, 1-28, and 1-38 and Appendix Figure 25.

Nerve Conduction Studies

SENSORY

When you are stimulating the ulnar nerve antidromically at the wrist and recording from the fifth digit, the sensory nerve action potential (SNAP) may be either normal or depressed in amplitude, depending on the degree of axonal involvement. With severe or very chronic lesions, the SNAP obtained at the fifth digit on stimulation above the elbow is depressed compared to that obtained on stimulation below the elbow. If the SNAP is recorded at the axilla by orthodromic stimulation of the ulnar nerve distally, the amplitude appears normal with above-elbow stimulation but depressed with below-elbow stimulation.[60] The amplitude of the sensory potential along the dorsal cutaneous nerve of the forearm (branch of ulnar nerve) is depressed, or it may not be obtainable.

TABLE 5-5
Normal Values for Midpalmar Nerve Studies (Fifth Digit, Antidromic)

Age (Years)	*Data (No.)*	*Amplitude (μV)*	*Peak Latency (msec)*
20–70	100	34.6 ± 22.9 (10.0–80.4)	1.5 ± 0.1 (1.3–1.7)

MOTOR

With focal demyelination, conduction velocity is slowed across the elbow by more than 10 m/sec[45] compared to the velocity in the forearm or axillary segments. The amplitude of the CMAP is depressed, and the shape is dispersed on stimulation above the site of the lesion. The exact site of involvement can be determined by stimulating the nerve in 1-cm serial increments along the elbow segment.[146] This is best performed with a needle. The site of the lesion is that site where the amplitude drops significantly or the shape of the potential becomes more dispersed. There may be no significant drop in amplitude across the elbow level with mild axonal involvement. With more severe involvement the proximal amplitude is depressed, although the conduction velocity across the elbow may not be notably slowed. With very severe or chronic involvement, there is considerable loss in CMAP amplitude. In addition, there is slowing of conduction velocity across the elbow and distal to it.[60] There may be only slight slowing in the upper arm.

EMG

Signs of denervation are seen in the forearm muscles as well as in the intrinsic muscles of the hand supplied by the ulnar nerve. When the injury to the ulnar nerve is an external compressive lesion (*e.g.*, from leaning on the elbows or from tight plaster casts), the EMG changes may be more evident in the medial portion of the flexor digitorum profundus and flexor carpi ulnaris than in the intrinsic muscles of the hand. This is due to the relative distribution of the various fascicles in the ulnar nerve at the level of the medial epicondyle.[215,218] However, the flexor carpi ulnaris can be spared, since this muscle may be supplied by the ulnar nerve from above the level of the elbow. Other muscles must also be examined to exclude the presence of proximal pathology such as coexisting cervical radiculopathy, especially along the C8 and T1 nerve roots, or much more rarely, thoracic outlet syndrome or lower trunk plexopathy.

Electrodiagnosis in Ulnar Nerve Entrapment at the Wrist

Anatomy

See Figures 1-26 and 1-27 and Appendix Figure 25.

Nerve Conduction Studies

SENSORY

Responses recorded from the fifth digit or midpalm on stimulation of the ulnar nerve at the wrist may be depressed in amplitude when the involvement of the ulnar nerve is proximal to or within Guyon's canal.[33] With entrapments proximal to or within the canal, both the deep motor and the superficial sensory branches are involved. With more distal lesions the superficial sensory nerve is not involved,[201] and the sensory potential recorded from the fifth digit is normal. In entrapments of the ulnar nerve at the wrist level the sensory potential along the dorsal cutaneous nerve of the forearm (branch of the ulnar nerve) is normal, since this branch arises from the ulnar nerve 6 cm to 8 cm above the wrist.[81,97]

MOTOR

The motor conduction time along the ulnar nerve to the first dorsal interosseous muscle is delayed if the deep branch of the ulnar nerve is involved after the hypothenar muscles have been supplied.[9,42,201] If the branch to the hypothenar muscles is also involved, the motor conduction time to this muscle group is also delayed. The amplitude of the CMAP obtained from the first dorsal interosseous muscle and/or the hypothenar muscles is depressed.

EMG

REST

Fibrillations and positive sharp waves can be seen in the intrinsic muscles supplied by the deep branch of the ulnar nerve (*i.e.*, the hypothenar muscles, interossei, medial two lumbricals, and adductor pollicis). The hypothenar muscles may be less involved, especially in lesions at or distal to Guyon's canal, since they are also supplied by the ulnar nerve proper. The muscles supplied by the ulnar nerve in the forearm are essentially normal.

MINIMAL CONTRACTION

An increase in polyphasia and other signs of reinnervation may be seen. Chronic reinnervation can be seen as high-amplitude, long-duration MUPs, whereas ongoing reinnervation is seen as complex polyphasic MUPs that may also have late components exhibiting increased jitter and blocking.

MAXIMAL CONTRACTION

Interference is reduced proportional to the degree of neurogenic involvement.

RADIAL NERVE

Applied Anatomy (See Appendix Fig. 26)

The radial nerve arises as a branch of the posterior cord of the brachial plexus and descends across the anterior surface of the subscapularis muscle and the tendons of the latissimus dorsi and teres major to leave the axilla and enter the arm. While the nerve is still within the axilla, a sensory and a muscular branch usually arise. The sensory branch is the posterior cutaneous nerve of the arm. The muscular branch is the nerve to the long head of the triceps. Sometimes a branch to the medial head of the triceps (the ulnar collateral branch) also arises from the main trunk within the axilla.

Passing into the arm, the radial nerve runs between the long head of the triceps and the medial aspect of the humerus, thereafter winding onto the posterior aspect of the humerus and descending in the radial (musculospiral) sulcus of that bone. Here it is overlaid by the lateral head of the triceps, and inferior to the latter is the origin of the medial head of the triceps. Thus the nerve lies close against the bone while in the radial sulcus between the areas of origin of the lateral and medial heads of the triceps. During this part of its course it gives off branches to both the lateral and medial heads of the triceps, the anconeus, and the posterior cutaneous nerve of the forearm. The branch to the anconeus descends through the substance of the medial head of the triceps and across the elbow joint to reach the deep surface of the anconeus.[5,64,181]

At about the junction of the middle and lower thirds of the humerus, the radial nerve winds around the lateral aspect of the arm at the upper limit of the lateral supracondylar ridge and pierces the lateral intermuscular septum to come to lie between the brachioradialis and brachialis. Thus, the nerve briefly passes across a lateral crest of bone with no muscle covering it. Next it descends across the elbow anterior to the lateral epicondyle, still nestled in the deep crevice between the brachioradialis and the brachialis. After giving twigs to the brachioradialis, the extensor carpi radialis longus, and a small inferolateral portion of the brachialis, the radial nerve divides into the superficial branch and the deep branch, or posterior interosseous nerve.

Still concealed beneath the cover of the brachioradialis, the superficial branch descends on the anterior aspect of the forearm to about the junction of the middle and lower thirds of the forearm, where it turns posteriorly around the radial side of the forearm to emerge from under cover of the tendon of the brachioradialis along its posterior border. The nerve pierces the deep fascia and ramifies to be distributed as branches to the posterior aspect of the radial half of the hand and finally as dorsal digital branches to the proximal phalanges of the first three digits. This superficial branch of the radial nerve has been reported to be damaged by such things as handcuffs, tight wristwatch bands, and casts as it crosses the dorsum of the lower end of the radius and over the wrist.

The deep branch, or posterior interosseous nerve, first descends anterior to the neck of the radius and then winds laterally to reach the upper border of the supinator. There it slips between the superficial and deep laminae of the supinator. Descending through the substance of the supinator it reappears at, or near, the lower border of that muscle. Prior to entering the supinator, the deep branch of the radial gives one branch to the extensor carpi radialis brevis (although commonly this branch arises from the beginning of the superficial branch of the radial nerve) and one to the supinator muscle itself. Emerging from the substance of the supinator this posterior interosseous nerve quickly gives three rather short branches to the extensor digitorum, the extensor digiti minimi, and the extensor carpi ulnaris, all of which are superficial muscles. Two longer branches of the posterior interosseous nerve descend until each divides into two terminal twigs. The more lateral of these longer branches supplies the abductor pollicis longus and extensor pollicis brevis, while the more medial nerve supplies the extensor pollicis longus and the extensor indicis (proprius). Thus the four deep extensor muscles of the forearm are supplied by these two longer branches. The branch to the extensor pollicis longus is prolonged beyond its supply to that muscle and insinuates itself between it and the extensor pollicis brevis to gain the level of the interosseous membrane. At this deep position it continues its course distally to end as fine filaments to the wrist joints and carpal joints.

The passage of the posterior interosseous nerve between the laminae of the supinator is particularly noteworthy because of the possibility of entrapment here. The superior fibers of the superficial lamina of the supinator are often aponeurotic or fibrous (in 30% of limbs of adults) throughout the middle area of the length of this upper border.[208] This fibrous border overlying the posterior interosseous nerve is commonly strongly curved, almost like an inverted arch. It is generally referred to as the arcade of Frohse but sometimes called the "radial tunnel" or "supinator slit." Since these superior fibers of the muscle are usually aponeurotic at their superior end (in 70% of cases), the variable extension of the aponeurotic nature of these upper fibers further inferiorward until they cross the penetrating nerve is what constitutes the fibrous arcade. Even as purely muscular fibers, their taut contraction in strong supination may be able to compress the posterior interosseous nerve to a damaging degree. Clearly, however, from cases seen at surgical exploration, it is the fibrous arcade that is more likely to damage the nerve with strong repetitious supinator effort.

Neuropathy of the posterior interosseous nerve may be caused by compression from the arcade of Frohse, by tumors or ganglia encroaching on the space beneath the arcade, or by extrinsic trauma.[14,20,67,186] It is apparent that with a nerve lesion at this site, the brachioradialis, the extensor carpi radialis longus, the extensor carpi radialis brevis, and the supinator itself will still be functional, while the extensor digitorum, the extensor digiti minimi, and the extensor carpi ulnaris would be paretic. The four extensor muscles of the deep layer (abductor pollicis longus, extensor pollicis brevis, extensor pollicis longus, and extensor indicis) would also be weakened or fully paralyzed. The palsy of the extensor carpi ulnaris with preservation of the two radial extensors would result in weakness of wrist extension and a definite tendency to radial deviation on extension because of the unopposed or unbalanced action of the extensor carpi radialis longus, which inserts into the base of the second metacarpal. Extensor carpi radialis brevis is more central in its insertion and hence is more nearly a pure extensor. Inability to extend the metacarpophalangeal joints of the fingers and weakness of extension and abduction of the thumb would also be evident. The symptoms are likely to be exacerbated on forceful resisted supination of the forearm. This should be performed with the forearm in 90° of flexion to reduce the action of the biceps in supination. Tenderness over the nerve as it passes under the arcade of Frohse and Tinel's sign elicited by tapping at that site are likely to be found.[149,162]

Certain other radial nerve compression neuropathies are of some importance but cannot be called entrapment neuropathies. They are, instead, neuropathies due to extrinsic trauma. Such compression neuropathies may occur in the axilla or at its posterior border as the radial nerve crosses the tendons of the latissimus dorsi and teres major and extends into the arm in relation to the long head of the triceps. In crutch palsy, in which excessive weight is born on the axillary plate of the crutch instead of on the handpiece, the pressure on the radial nerve presses and stretches it against the above-mentioned muscles. These muscles all tend to be in contraction during the crutch use, thus providing a firm background for damage to the nerve rather than a soft protective substrate. In some circumstances, particularly when excessive padding that broadens the axillary plate of the crutch is used and when the arm is held adducted, the radial nerve may be compressed laterally and forced against the humerus and the tense long head of the triceps. The shoulder straps of a backpack may compress the radial nerve as the straps pass across the medial side of the arm at the base of the axilla, especially if the straps are made of a wide, firm material.[29] The median and ulnar nerves may also be compressed by the shoulder straps of a pack, particularly when the wearer is riding a bicycle. Rifle slings, when worn about the proximal portion of the arm to steady the rifle while one is on the firing range, have been the cause of nerve trunk compression against the humerus. Prolonged pressure against the radial nerve as it winds about the lateral side of the humerus, where it pierces the lateral intermuscular septum, as may occur when the abducted and externally rotated arm is hanging over the resistant side board of a bed, can cause a radial nerve palsy in a sleeping drunk (Saturday night palsy). This somewhat descriptive name also designates the occurrence of radial palsy in the patient who sleeps long and soundly in a chair with a straight wooden back with his arm thrown over the resistant upper margin of the chair. Although the circumstances are different, the mechanism here is very much like crutch palsy. Even prolonged compression of the radial nerve in the radial sulcus can cause neuropathy, in spite of the protection of the overlying lateral head of the triceps. Compression against a firm object or edge adds to the likelihood of this occurrence during prolonged sleep in a narcotized or anesthetized patient. The prolonged sleep or coma of emaciated or debilitated persons (those with small flaccid muscles) on a hard but flat surface may result in compression neuropathies, especially if the subject's own body weight is over a limb pressed to the floor or ground.

With compression neuropathy occurring in the radial nerve as it pierces the lateral intermuscular septum, the three heads of the triceps and the anconeus are spared. It is likely that the lower lateral cutaneous nerve of the arm and the posterior cutaneous nerve of the forearm will also be spared. However, the tendency for these cutaneous nerves to be spared clinically is not necessarily due to a more protected anatomical position but may be due more to the fact that the areas of distribution of both nerves are subject to much overlap from nerves not arising from the radial. Furthermore, there is some evidence that

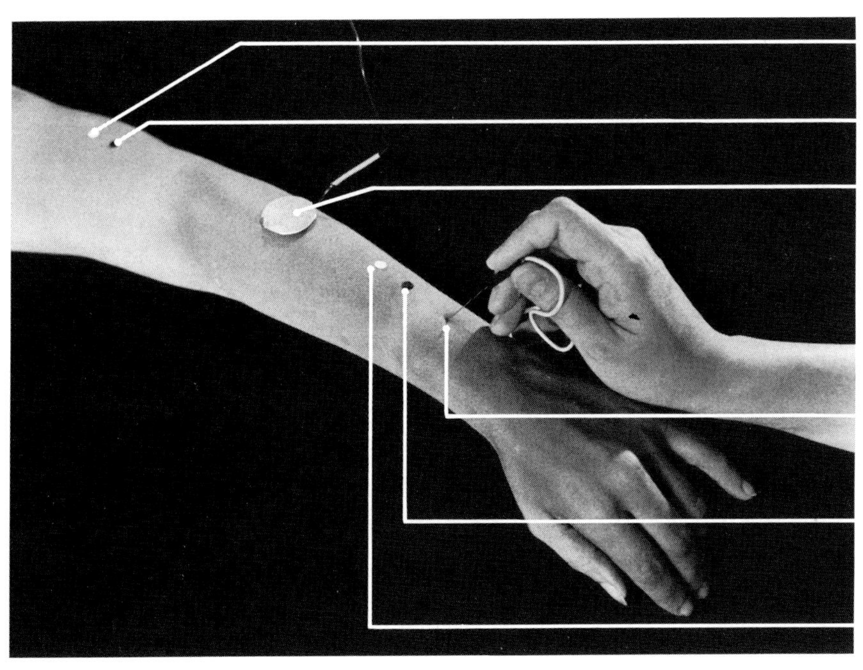

FIGURE 5-14 Radial nerve motor conduction study.

sensory fibers are less susceptible to damage from pressure than are motor fibers.

Motor Conduction Study (*Fig.* 5-14)

Conduction Velocity

Amplifier setting:
- Sweep speed: 5 msec/div.
- Sensitivity: 1 mV/div.
- Filter setting: 20 Hz–10 kHz

Recording technique:
- Active electrode: Place the concentric needle in the extensor indicis. Surface electrodes may also be used for recording, in which case the active electrode is placed on the extensor indicis and the reference electrode is placed on top of the ulnar styloid process.
- Ground electrode: Over the extensor surface of the forearm between the active recording electrode and the stimulating electrode

Stimulation technique:
- Use supramaximal current.
- Lower forearm: Stimulate in the line of the lateral aspect of the head of the ulna approximately 3 cm to 4 cm proximal to the recording needle. (Stimulus duration is usually 0.1–0.2 msec, stimulus strength usually 150–300 V.)
- Lower arm (above elbow): Stimulate approximately 5 cm to 6 cm proximal to the lateral epicondyle between the brachialis and the brachioradialis muscles. Abduct the arm 10°, keep the forearm pronated, and bend the elbow 10° to 15°. (Stimulus duration is usually 0.1–0.2 msec, stimulus strength 200–300 V.)
- Radial sulcus: Stimulate at the midpoint of an imaginary line joining the acromion and lateral epicondyle.
- Neck: Stimulate at Erb's point. (Stimulus duration is usually 0.1–0.2 msec, stimulus strength usually 200–300 V.)

Normal Values[84]

Proximal segment (neck to lower arm) mean velocity: 72.0 ± 6.3 m/sec (range: 56–93 m/sec).

Distal segment (lower arm or above elbow to lower forearm) mean velocity: 61.6 ± 5.9 m/sec (range: 48–75 m/sec).

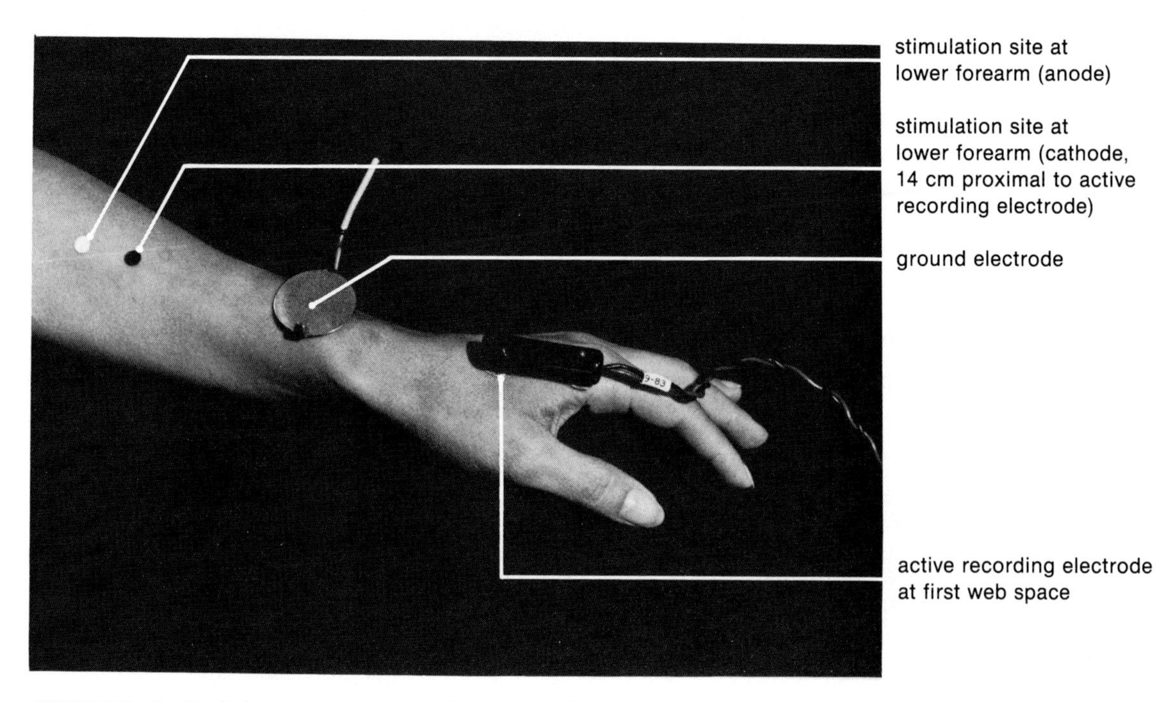

FIGURE 5-15. Radial nerve sensory conduction study.

Comments

This nerve conduction study is sometimes difficult to perform because of the deep location of the nerve. Errors in distance measurements are common, since using a tape measure includes the bulk of the muscles under or between which the radial nerve lies. Therefore, the measured length far exceeds the true length of the nerve. Obstetric calipers are useful for obtaining more accurate distance measurements.

Sensory Conduction Study (*Fig. 5-15*)

Conduction Time

Amplifier setting:
- Sweep speed: 2 msec/div.
- Sensitivity: 20–50 μV/div.
- Filter setting: 20 Hz–2 kHz

Recording technique:
- Active electrode: Place the recording portion of the bar electrode in the first web space, just above the junction of the base of the first and second metacarpals.
- Reference electrode: In the region of the head of the second metacarpal bone. If you are using separate electrodes, place the reference electrode preferably no more than 4 cm distal to the active electrode.
- Ground electrode: Over the extensor aspect of the lower forearm between the recording and stimulating electrodes

Stimulation technique:
- Use supramaximal current.
- Lower forearm: 14 cm proximal to the recording site, over the lateral margin of the radius

Normal Values

See Table 5-6.

Electrodiagnosis in Radial Nerve Lesions at the Radial Sulcus

Anatomy

See Figures 1-22 through 1-26 and Appendix Figure 26.

Nerve Conduction Studies

SENSORY

The amplitude may be depressed and the conduction velocity slowed. If the entrapment is severe, the sensory potential may be absent.

TABLE 5-6
Normal Values for Radial Nerve Sensory Conduction Studies (Antidromic)

Age (Years)	*Data (No.)*	*Amplitude (μV)*	*Onset Latency (msec)*	*Conduction Velocity (m/sec)*
20–29	100	26.0 ± 14.7 (10.0–55.4)	2.4 ± 0.2 (2.0–2.8)	60.0 ± 4.3 (51.4–68.6)
30–39	100	26.3 ± 9.6 (10.0–45.5)	2.4 ± 0.2 (2.0–2.8)	58.5 ± 4.3 (49.9–67.1)
40–49	100	25.0 ± 9.9 (10.0–44.8)	2.4 ± 0.2 (2.0–2.8)	58.7 ± 5.1 (48.5–68.9)
50–59	100	23.4 ± 9.0 (10.0–41.4)	2.4 ± 0.2 (2.0–2.8)	58.2 ± 4.5 (49.2–67.2)
Below 60	400	25.2 ± 11.0 (10.0–47.2)	2.4 ± 0.2 (2.0–2.8)	58.9 ± 4.6 (49.7–68.1)
Above 60	75	21.0 ± 8.4 (8.0–37.4)	2.5 ± 0.2 (2.1–2.9)	56.7 ± 5.5 (45.7–67.7)
All ages combined	475	24.3 ± 10.6 (8.0–45.5)	2.4 ± 0.2 (2.0–2.8)	58.4 ± 4.8 (48.8–68.0)

MOTOR

Conduction velocity along the segment of the radial nerve from Erb's point to the middle of the radial sulcus is slowed if the lesion involves the segment above the middle of the sulcus. If the lesion is below the middle of the radial sulcus, the conduction velocity is slowed along the segment from the middle of the sulcus to the lower arm. The CMAP is absent on distal stimulation in severe axonotmesis but present in neurapraxia or partial axonotmesis. An evoked response distal to the site of the lesion obtained more than 4 days after the onset of symptoms signifies a good prognosis.[56]

EMG

Evidence of denervation may be seen in all muscles supplied by the radial nerve except the long head of the triceps.[229] Absence of denervation in the anconeus aids in localizing the lesion to be below the middle of the radial sulcus, since this muscle receives its innervation from the radial nerve at the level of the middle of the radial sulcus.

Electrodiagnosis in Posterior Interosseous Nerve Syndrome

Anatomy

See Figures 1-34 and 1-35 and Appendix Figure 26.

Nerve Conduction Studies

SENSORY

The posterior interosseous nerve has no sensory supply. The distal sensory latency and the amplitude of the superficial radial nerve are normal.

MOTOR

The amplitude of the evoked motor response may be depressed, and the motor conduction time to the extensor indicis may be delayed.

EMG

The usual level of entrapment is under the arcade of Frohse,[157] a fibrotendinous arch under which the radial nerve passes to enter the supinator. With this type of entrapment the supinator may or may not be involved, since some or all of its motor supply may accompany the posterior interosseous nerve through the arcade of Frohse.[21] The extensor carpi radialis brevis, which receives its supply from the posterior interosseous nerve above the supinator, is spared in this type of lesion. The brachioradialis and extensor carpi radialis longus are supplied by the radial nerve proper and may therefore not be involved either. All muscles supplied by the posterior interosseous nerve distal to the supinator are involved. These are the extensor digitorum (communis), extensor digiti minimi, extensor carpi ulnaris, abductor pollicis longus, extensor pollicis longus and brevis, and extensor indicis. Involvement of the posterior interosseous nerve above the level of the supinator involves this muscle. In this situation the extensor carpi radialis brevis is also involved, as sometimes is the extensor carpi radialis longus when this muscle receives innervation from the posterior interosseous nerve.[210]

LUMBOSACRAL PLEXUS AND ILIOHYPOGASTRIC, ILIOINGUINAL, GENITOFEMORAL, LATERAL CUTANEOUS, OBTURATOR, SUPERIOR GLUTEAL, INFERIOR GLUTEAL, POSTERIOR FEMORAL CUTANEOUS, AND PUDENDAL NERVES

Applied Anatomy

Lumbosacral Plexus (See Appendix Fig. 27)

The roots of the lumbosacral plexus are the anterior primary rami of spinal nerves L1 to S5, inclusive. It is usual to include the first coccygeal primary ramus (Co 1) as well. After a short course these anterior primary rami divide into ventral and dorsal divisions, which can be compared to the anterior and posterior divisions of the upper, middle, and lower trunks of the brachial plexus. The ventral divisions, as in the upper limb, finally send their fibers to the morphologically ventral (flexor) muscles, while the dorsal divisions, again, as in the upper limb, send their fibers to the morphologically dorsal (extensor) muscles. However, it must be borne in mind that there is a 90° rotation of the lower limb, which places the morphologically ventral muscles in medial and posterior position and the morphologically dorsal muscles in an anterior and lateral position. Thus, if an adult assumes a position with the right and left palms and the right and left soles of the feet brought into apposition, the flexor and extensor surfaces of the upper and lower limbs will correspond with each other, as they do in the fetus. The preaxial and postaxial borders of the upper and lower limbs will also correspond.

The nerves formed from the ventral divisions are the iliohypogastric and ilioinguinal, the genitofemoral, the obturator, the tibial portion of the sciatic plus the nerves to the hamstring muscles, the nerve to obturator internus and gemellus superior, the nerve to the quadratus femoris and gemellus inferior, half of the posterior femoral cutaneous (with a more medial distribution), and the pudendal. The nerves formed from the dorsal divisions are the lateral femoral cutaneous, the femoral, the superior and inferior gluteal, the common peroneal portion of the sciatic, half of the posterior femoral cutaneous (with a more lateral distribution), the perforating cutaneous branch of S2 and S3 (when it exists as a separate entity), and the perineal branch of S4. Thus the ventral divisions of the anterior primary rami of these spinal nerves contribute to the innervation of the morphologically ventral (flexor) muscles and their overlying skin, while the dorsal divisions of the anterior primary rami of these spinal nerves contribute to the innervation of the morphologically dorsal (extensor) muscles and their overlying skin. The anterior primary rami of lumbar nerves L1 through L4 pass behind the psoas major muscle, contributing twigs to it, and thereafter pass obliquely laterally and caudally across the anterior surface of the quadratus lumborum, contributing twigs to it.

Iliohypogastric and Ilioinguinal Nerves (See Appendix Fig. 27)

The iliohypogastric and ilioinguinal branches of L1 pass beyond the lateral border of the quadratus lumborum to penetrate either the aponeurosis or the muscular part of the transversus abdominis. These two nerves thereafter run in the fascial interval (the neurovascular plane) between the latter muscle and the internal oblique. They then (sometimes still as one) proceed in this interval around the flank, immediately above the iliac crest, until they reach the anterior part of the abdominal wall approximately 2 cm to 3 cm medial to the anterior superior spine of the ilium and, commonly, a like amount inferior to the level of the spine. At this point the two nerves usually perforate the substance of the internal oblique to come to lie in the areolar interval between the internal oblique and the aponeurosis of the external oblique.

The iliohypogastric nerve pierces the aponeurosis of the external oblique some 2 cm to 3 cm superior to the superficial inguinal ring and then supplies the skin superior to the symphysis pubis. On its way along the crest of the ilium the nerve contributes a twig downward across the crest to supply the skin over the lateral hip region, descending toward the level of the greater trochanter.

Like the iliohypogastric nerve, the ilioinguinal nerve gains the same fascial interval between the internal oblique and the aponeurosis of the external oblique, but it penetrates the latter by passing through the superficial inguinal ring and thereafter supplies the skin of the anterior aspect of the scrotum (or the anterior part of labium majus), the root of the penis, and a small area of the thigh below the inguinal ligament. Entrapment neuropathy may occur just medial to the anterior superior spine of the ilium as the ilioinguinal nerve makes its abrupt penetration through the substance of the internal oblique.[114] The damage to the nerve may result from traction on the nerve as it changes course in penetrating the muscle. At this pentration site the nerve is relatively fixed to the muscle, and strong contraction of the internal oblique could overextend the nerve. Since ilioinguinal nerve entrapment sometimes follows herniorrhaphies and appendectomies, it would appear that the slowly contracting scar tissue at the incision site can entrap the nerve.

Because the ilioinguinal nerve is the source of innervation to the internal oblique and transversus abdominis in the inguinal area, these muscles may become weakened and allow localized bulging of the abdominal wall below the level of the nerve entrapment and thus suggest the development of a hernia. The muscles of the lower abdominal wall are stretched, and perhaps the nerve itself is tensed when the thigh is extended fully, as in walking. There may be a tendency for some patients to offset that tension by assuming a slightly bent-over posture. The sensory distribution of the ilioinguinal nerve is to the anterior aspect of the scrotum (or the anterior part of labium majus) and to the skin just above and just below the inguinal ligament. The sensory manifestations of entrapment of the ilioinguinal nerve may be paresthesia (often burning pain) or hypesthesia in the cutaneous area mentioned. Pressure in the area where the nerve pierces the internal oblique may reproduce the characteristic burning pain, and Tinel's sign may be elicited by tapping here.

Genitofemoral Nerve (See Appendix Fig. 27)

The genitofemoral nerve arises from two roots, L1 and L2. These roots pass ventrally into the psoas major, wherein they unite to emerge on its anterior surface as a single trunk. The nerve descends, piercing the psoas fascia and thereby escaping from within the psoas sheath, then continues downward, centered over the prominence of the psoas. As it nears the level of the inguinal ligament, it divides into two branches, the genital branch and the femoral branch. The genital branch passes via the deep inguinal ring into the inguinal canal to emerge at the superficial inguinal ring. It then supplies the cremaster muscle and the skin of the scrotum or labium majus and the immediately adjacent skin of the thigh. The femoral branch descends into the thigh deep to the inguinal ligament, as does the psoas muscle itself, on the anterior aspect of which the branch rests. The nerve passes through the saphenous opening to supply the skin over the femoral trigone (Scarpa's triangle).

Like the roots of the femoral and obturator nerves, the genitofemoral nerve may be compressed and irritated by retroperitoneal and retrorenal tumors, hematomata, and abscesses.[66,132,135,160] Surgical observations in some right-sided cases of genitofemoral neuropathy suggest that the cause was by entrapment of the nerve in scar tissues or fibrosis occurring posterior to the cecum and appendix as they related to the distal portion of the nerve where it lies on the anterior surface of the psoas. Onset of causalgic symptoms has followed appendectomy. Neurolysis of the nerve at this site has given relief of symptoms. The burning pain (causalgia) felt over its cutaneous distribution may be difficult to distinguish from that of ilioinguinal nerve neuropathy. The absence of a trigger point at the anterior abdominal wall or entrapment site near the anterior superior iliac spine aids in the differential diagnosis. Tension in the lower abdominal wall by the contraction of muscles and by forceful hyperextension of the thigh does not influence genitofemoral neuropathy as it does ilioinguinal nerve lesions.

Lateral Femoral Cutaneous Nerve (See Appendix Fig. 27)

The lateral femoral cutaneous nerve from L2 and L3 is formed behind the psoas major and then appears along the lateral border of that muscle at about the level of the iliac crest posteriorly. Thereafter, it runs forward on the surface of the iliacus muscle, but deep to the iliacus fascia, until it reaches the region of the anterior superior spine of the ilium. Here the nerve exits the abdominal cavity into the thigh by passing through the narrow angle between the lateralmost end of the inguinal ligament and the anterior border of the iliacus muscle and the anterior superior spine. Sometimes it pierces the inguinal ligament, but more commonly it passes out of the false pelvis still deep to the iliacus fascia, which it then pierces just inferior to the anterior superior spine. Still descending, it next passes on either the superficial or deep side of the upper end of the sartorius to lie immediately deep to the fascia lata. At a variable point, some 3 cm to 8 cm inferior and slightly medial to the anterior superior spine of the ilium, the nerve pierces the fascia lata and divides into anterior and posterior branches, which descend supplying the anterolateral skin of the thigh as far down as the knee.

An entrapment syndrome of the lateral femoral cutaneous nerve, commonly called meralgia paresthetica, was one of the first to be recognized (since 1895).[50,59,85,140,151,172,195,213] There are two sites to be considered: first, as the nerve passes posterior to or through the lateral end of the inguinal ligament approximately 1 cm medial to the anterior superior spine. At this site, it is also escaping from beneath the iliacus fascia, and the latter may contribute to its degree of fixity at this point. Furthermore, the nerve here passes either medial or lateral to the origin of the sartorius from the anterior superior spine. Sometimes it penetrates the sartorius. Either of these relationships to the muscle adds a definite tethering effect.

The second site of interest is where the nerve pierces the fascia lata. As previously stated, this is quite a variable point, but commonly no more than 8 cm below the anterior superior spine. Often the nerve has already divided into its anterior and posterior branches, and thus there are two sites of penetration. Because this latter point (or points) of penetration is almost vertically below the anterior superior spine of the ilium, it is evident that wide abduction or strong extension of the thigh (or the correlated lateral bending or backward leaning of the torso) increases the distance between the first and second points of penetration. The upper point is where the nerve is quite fixed by surrounding connective-tissue structures; the lower one is ordinarily a round or slitlike aperture that does not so much tether the nerve as dictate the descending axis. An early paresthesia of a tingling or burning nature within the skin area of the lateral femoral cutaneous nerve is later followed by a slow subsidence of the paresthesia, until only a much smaller area of hypesthesia remains as a residuum of the syndrome. It is possible for the nerve to be damaged by direct trauma to the thigh. Penetrating wounds that sever the nerve tend to cause a more distressing syndrome, with severe and persistent paresthesias. Tight belts or trousers and the low-lying waistband of tight shorts have all been incriminated at one time or another as the cause of a compressive neuropathy of the nerve.

Femoral nerve neuropathy, which gives a more anterior area of paresthesia, must be differentiated, as well as radiculopathy involving L2 and L3 due to a herniated disc or paraspinal tumor. In either of these conditions there is motor loss, particularly in the quadriceps femoris, as well as sensory loss, whereas the lateral femoral cutaneous nerve is purely sensory. Rarely, retroperitoneal tumors may compress roots of origin of the lateral femoral cutaneous nerve, but such masses are also likely to damage the roots of origin of the femoral and obturator nerves.

Obturator Nerve (See Fig. 1-40 and Appendix Fig. 27)

The obturator nerve arises from the ventral divisions of the anterior primary rami of spinal nerves L2, L3, and L4. The branches of origin unite in and behind the psoas major, and the nerve thereafter descends to emerge around the medial border of the psoas major at the level of the upper aspect of the lateral mass of the sacrum. It then descends across the sacroiliac joint to enter the true (lesser) pelvic cavity, where it lies in close proximity to the descending branch of L4, which joins with L5 to form the lumbosacral trunk.

Briefly, the obturator nerve follows the medial border of the psoas, but then the psoas follows the brim of the pelvis (linea terminalis), and the obturator nerve descends into the lesser pelvis to lie on the fascial covering of the obturator internus as the nerve continues its oblique descent toward the obturator canal. Entering the canal in company with the obturator artery and vein, the nerve divides into anterior and posterior branches as the parent trunk descends across the superior border of the obturator internus.

Passing out of the obturator canal into the thigh, the posterior branch of the obturator nerve pierces the anterior portion of the obturator externus muscle, supplying it and continuing on to descend between the adductor brevis and the adductor magnus and contributing twigs to both. This posterior branch penetrates into the upper part of adductor magnus and, passing obliquely downward through the muscle, it appears posterior to the adductor magnus and enters the upper end of the popliteal fossa to pierce the oblique popliteal ligament (the posterior aspect of the knee joint capsule) and give sensory innervation to the cruciate ligaments and the covering synovial membrane.

The anterior branch of the obturator nerve descends anterior to the obturator externus and adductor brevis muscles, but posterior or deep to the pectineus and adductor longus. Occasionally it aids in the supply of the former, and it regularly supplies the latter. At this level it contributes a sensory branch to the hip joint. As it descends between the adductor longus and adductor brevis, it sends twigs into each and becomes subcutaneous at mid-thigh level by passing medially between the adductor longus and the gracilis. Its terminal branch supplies a hand-sized area of skin on the medial side of the thigh.

It was previously pointed out that the beginnings of this nerve from the lumbar plexus may be involved by retroperitoneal masses or hematomata, that compression neuropathy of the obturator nerve may thus occur, and that this is often found in association with femoral neuropathy produced by the same compressing mass. In this circumstance the motor loss in the thigh musculature is very extensive and severe. Clinical evidence of an obturator palsy consists of both sensory and motor changes. The motor deficit is some degree of weakness of the adductor muscles of the thigh. The weakness of the adductor longus and brevis and the superior part of the adductor magnus (the inferior portion is supplied by the tibial part of the sciatic nerve), plus weakness of the gracilis and obturator externus, causes noticeable instability of the hip joint during walking. The patient assumes a wide-based gait because of the abduction of the affected limb. On testing, a clear reduction in adduction strength and a minimal reduction in the power of external rotation of the thigh (loss of the obturator externus) are found. On the sensory side, the painfulness, paresthesias, and sensory deficit involve the medial aspect of the thigh above the knee level, and in some patients there is pain in the knee joint itself. Occasionally, this latter symptom may lead to an initial suspicion that the patient's problem is a purely orthopaedic one. Hyperextension or strong abduction of the thigh may increase the pain sensations in the thigh and knee because of increased tension in the obturator nerve in these postures.

As the nerve descends across the brim of the pelvis at the sacroiliac joint, it may be damaged by compression from metastatic tumor in the internal iliac nodes or by severe osteophytic changes in the joint. It is when the nerve passes through the rigid-walled obturator canal, which is bounded by the superior pubic ramus and the obturator membrane, that it is subject to a classic but uncommon entrapment syndrome. Fracture of the superior pubic ramus or more extensive pelvic fractures elsewhere that allow a shift of the position of the segment of the pelvis concerned may cause entrapment or a compression neuropathy. Entrapment of the nerve within the obturator canal may occur by herniation of a variety of structures crowding into the 3-cm-long canal and compressing the nerve. The contents of the hernia may be a short loop or knuckle of small intestine, a Richter's hernia of bowel wall, a portion of bladder wall, the end of the uterine tube, the vermiform appendix, or even Meckel's diverticulum. The obturator neuropathy thus caused may produce no more than pain in the knee and on the medial side of the thigh (the Romberg-Howship sign), with the patient being unaware of any muscular weakness, although appropriate testing may reveal some adductor weakness. The mass of the hernia may not be recognized in Scarpa's triangle on physical examination, and the signs and symptoms of strangulation may not have developed. This hernia is much more common in women than in men, and vaginal examination may reveal the laterally placed intrapelvic tender mass anchored at the entrance to the obturator canal. Such a hernia usually occurs after age 60 years, particularly in women who have borne several children. Wasting of body fat seems to predispose to the development of the hernia, and chronic cough may add to the likelihood.

Superior Gluteal Nerve (See Appendix Fig. 29)

Formed by the union of branches from the dorsal divisions of the anterior primary rami of spinal nerves L4, L5, and S1, the superior gluteal nerve, like its counterpart, the inferior gluteal nerve, arises from the dorsal surface of the lumbosacral plexus and accordingly supplies the posterior muscles of the proximal part of the lower limb. In company with the superior gluteal artery and veins, the nerve exits the pelvic cavity by passing through the slitlike aperture between the upper margin of the greater sciatic foramen and the upper margin of the piriformis muscle as the latter muscle exits from the pelvic cavity. This slitlike aperture is called the foramen suprapiriforme, and only the structures cited above leave the lesser pelvis and pass through this slit to enter the gluteal area. Accompanied by the counterpart vessels, the nerve divides into a superior branch and an inferior branch as it runs forward in the fascial plane between the gluteus minimus and the overlying gluteus medius. The superior branch is distributed primarily to the gluteus medius but occasionally sends some twigs into the underlying gluteus minimus. The inferior branch contributes twigs into both muscles as it passes forward between them horizontally. At the anterior border of these two gluteal muscles the nerve escapes between them from the fascial interval and then gives its final twigs into the deep surface of the overlying tensor fasciae latae muscle.

Because the superior gluteal nerve arises from some of the same ventral divisions as does the common peroneal portion of the sciatic nerve, one of the anomalies that befalls the common peroneal may also occur with the superior gluteal nerve, either in conjunction with the anomaly of the common peroneal or, quite rarely, independently. In about 10% of the body sides there is a high or plexus level of separation of the common peroneal and tibial nerve portions of the sciatic, with the common peroneal nerve piercing the piriformis as it exits from the pelvis, rather than going through the foramen infrapiriforme in conjunction with the tibial nerve. This foramen is the slitlike interval between the lower margin of the piriformis and the lower part of the greater sciatic foramen (here primarily formed by the sacrotuberous ligament and the coextensive coccygeus muscle). Thus, in such cases the superior gluteal nerve may occasionally run with the common peroneal nerve as it pierces the piriformis, or, rarely, the superior gluteal nerve may take this aberrant pathway into the gluteal area all by itself. In this circumstance an entrapment neuropathy may occur in the superior gluteal nerve.[180] However, just as with this aberrant course of the common peroneal nerve, there is far more likelihood that the variant course of the nerve is innocent and will not produce any recognizable disturbances in the life of the patient. Additional factors of anatomy, function, or pathology are necessary for this variation to be harmful.

Clinical signs of superior gluteal nerve palsy, from whatever cause, include loss or reduction of abductor strength at the hip joint and reduction of the strength of medial rotation of the thigh, both due to weakness of the gluteus medius and minimus. If the patient is supine, it is likely that the affected side will show a toeing-out owing to the incompetence of the medial rotation action of the anterior portion of the gluteus minimus, in particular. The loss of abductor competence that is tested for in the supine position is also manifested in the patient's posture and gait. During the swing phase of walking, the unsupported side of the pelvis (the side with the foot off the ground) drops because the paralyzed gluteus medius and minimus (of the side with the foot on the ground) cannot hold the ilium of this paralyzed side at the proper distance from the greater trochanter against the weight of the torso projected downward in the midline of the pelvis (the line of the center of gravity). The patient tries to compensate for this effect by listing toward the paralyzed side, thus seeking to keep his center of gravity over the head of the femur on the affected side. This repetitious series of events in walking gives rise to the expression "the gluteus medius gait."

Inferior Gluteal Nerve (See Appendix Fig. 29)

The inferior gluteal nerve arises from the dorsal divisions of the anterior primary rami of L5, S1, and S2 and leaves the lesser pelvic cavity through the foramen infrapiriforme to lie posterior to the broad, flattened sciatic nerve as it too descends through the foramen. Both nerves lie deep to the gluteus maximus, and close beside them on their medial side is the posterior femoral cutaneous nerve, which has also entered the gluteal region through the foramen infrapiriforme. Because of the close relationship of the sciatic nerve, the inferior gluteal nerve, and the posterior femoral cutaneous nerve in the gluteal area, one lesion, such as a sciatic hernia, a gunshot wound, or an injection of noxious chemicals, may damage all three nerves. The inferior gluteal nerve divides into several branches that penetrate the deep aspect of the gluteus maximus.

Destruction or neuropathy of the inferior gluteal nerve greatly weakens extension of the hip joint, causing difficulty in climbing stairs and standing up from a seated position. When the patient is bent forward at the hip, while standing, the gluteus maximus is important in straightening up the torso. The gluteus maximus is an external rotator of the thigh, and this function should be compared with that of the opposite side in muscle testing. Owing to atrophy of the muscle, the prominence of the buttock diminishes, and this causes the hollow or depressed area between the belly of the gluteus maximus and the prominence of the greater trochanter to be less noticeable than on the normal side. Furthermore, the horizontally disposed gluteal (infragluteal) fold tends to sag and is shallower than normal. The gluteal fold is not created by the lower border of the gluteus maximus but, in fact, obliquely crosses the latter. The fold is created by adherence of the superficial fascia and skin to the underlying deep fascia covering the gluteus maximus. A strengthening band of fibers in the fascia, to which the overlying tissues are adherent, determines the level and configuration of the gluteal fold. Atrophy of the muscle allows this band to sag and thus alters the gluteal fold. The fold might be thought of as an extension crease for the hip joint.

Posterior Femoral Cutaneous Nerve

The posterior femoral cutaneous nerve arises from both the ventral and dorsal divisions of the anterior primary rami of S1, S2, and S3, and when the two parts of the sciatic nerve are separated by part of the piriformis muscle, the posterior femoral cutaneous nerve is also in two parts. These are then separated as a dorsal part with a lateral skin distribution and a ventral part with a medial skin distribution. The area of skin supplied by the posterior femoral cutaneous nerve includes the lower region of the skin of the buttock (the inferior cluneal branches), the posterior aspect of the skin of the thigh, the popliteal fossa, and the upper area of the calf. Its lower limit varies somewhat, and branches occasionally extend below the calf, overlapping with branches of the sural nerve. Regularly a branch arises proximally and passes medially across the ischiopubic ramus to make a limited contribution to the innervation of the skin of the perineum, overlapping with the pudendal nerve. The posterior femoral cutaneous nerve at first lies on the posterior aspect of the sciatic nerve deep to the gluteus maximus. It then descends into the thigh just deep to the fascia lata. Near the level of the knee joint it pierces the fascia lata as two or three slender branches that supply the overlying skin. No specific entrapment syndromes have been described for this nerve. Presacral retroperitoneal hemorrhage or tumor involving levels S1, S2, and S3 would equally afflict the roots of the posterior femoral cutaneous nerve and the lower roots of the sciatic nerve. Therefore, in lesions of the sciatic nerve in which there is no evidence as to whether the lesion is in the pelvis or thigh, it might be of some diagnostic help during the physical examination to discover that the cutaneous distribution of the posterior femoral cutaneous also shows sensory loss, for this would indicate that the lesion is probably intrapelvic.

Pudendal Nerve

The pudendal nerve arises from anterior primary rami S2, S3, and S4 and represents the ventral divisions of these roots. Accordingly, it travels anteriorly in the perineum, where it becomes the major source of cutaneous innervation and the sole source of muscular innervation. The counterpart contributions of S2, S3, and S4 to the dorsal divisions are the perforating cutaneous nerve from S2 and S3 and the perineal branch of S4. The perforating cutaneous nerve is so named because it perforates the sacrotuberous ligament and ends by being distributed to a small area of skin over the lower medial part of the buttock. It is, however, often absent because its fibers have used the posterior femoral cutaneous nerve or the pudendal nerve to reach their expected destination. The perineal branch of S4 supplies the coccygeus muscle and sends a small twig onto the superior surface of the levator ani, contributing to the innervation of that muscle. The other part of this nerve pierces the coccygeus and, crossing the posteriormost part of the ischiorectal fossa, sends fibers into the posterior portion of the sphincter ani externus. The major innervation of the latter muscle, however, is from the inferior rectal branch of the pudendal nerve.

The pudendal nerve itself, after forming in the pelvic cavity, exits almost at once through the slit between the lower border of the piriformis muscle and the upper borders of the fused sacrospinous ligament and the coccygeus muscle. This slit is the foramen infrapiriforme, and after passing through it, the nerve is present briefly in the gluteal area. The pudendal nerve descends behind the sacrospinous ligament and the spine of the ischium, to which the ligament attaches, and then curves forward into the ischiorectal fossa in a fascial canal (the pudendal canal of Alcock). The course of the nerve is immediately above the curving falciform margin of the sacrotuberous ligament as it reaches the tuberosity of the ischium.

While in the pudendal canal the pudendal nerve gives off an inferior rectal (hemorrhoidal) branch that is the primary source of innervation to the sphincter ani externus and the overlying skin. The main trunk of the pudendal nerve escapes from the pudendal canal just before it reaches the coronal plane of the posterior edge of the urogenital diaphragm. It then divides into the perineal nerve and the dorsal nerve of the penis or clitoris. The perineal nerve in turn divides into three branches: the posterior scrotal (or labial), the superficial (entering the superficial perineal compartment), and the deep (entering the deep perineal compartment). The superficial branch supplies the transversus perinei superficialis, ischiocavernosus, and bulbospongiosus. The deep branch enters the deep perineal compartment (the space between the superior and inferior fascial layers of the urogenital diaphragm) and supplies the transversus perinei profundus and the specialized portion of this muscle referred to as the sphincter urethrae membranaceae (the external urinary sphincter or voluntary sphincter). The dorsal nerve of the penis (or clitoris) traverses the deep perineal compartment and exits from its anterior edge to run along the dorsal aspect of the penis (or clitoris), supplying the skin of the penis, including the glans. No specific entrapment syndrome has been reported for the pudendal nerve.

Determination of Conduction Across the Lumbar Plexus (Lumbar Nerve Root Stimulation Study) (Fig. 5-16)

Conduction Time

Amplifier setting:
- Sweep speed: 5 msec/div.
- Sensitivity: 5 mV/div.
- Filter setting: 20 Hz–10 kHz

Recording technique:
- Patient position: Supine for femoral nerve stimulation and prone for lumbar nerve root stimulation
- Active electrode: Surface electrode on the vastus medialis
- Reference electrode: On the quadriceps tendon
- Ground electrode: On the ventral aspect of the thigh

Stimulation technique (needle stimulation):
- Use supramaximal current.
- Proximal stimulation: Feel for the L4 spinous process. Stimulate the L2–L4 nerve roots with a 50-mm monopolar needle inserted approximately 2 cm to 3 cm lateral and proximal to the spinous process of the L4 vertebra until the needle touches the transverse process of the vertebral body, then withdraw approximately 1 mm.

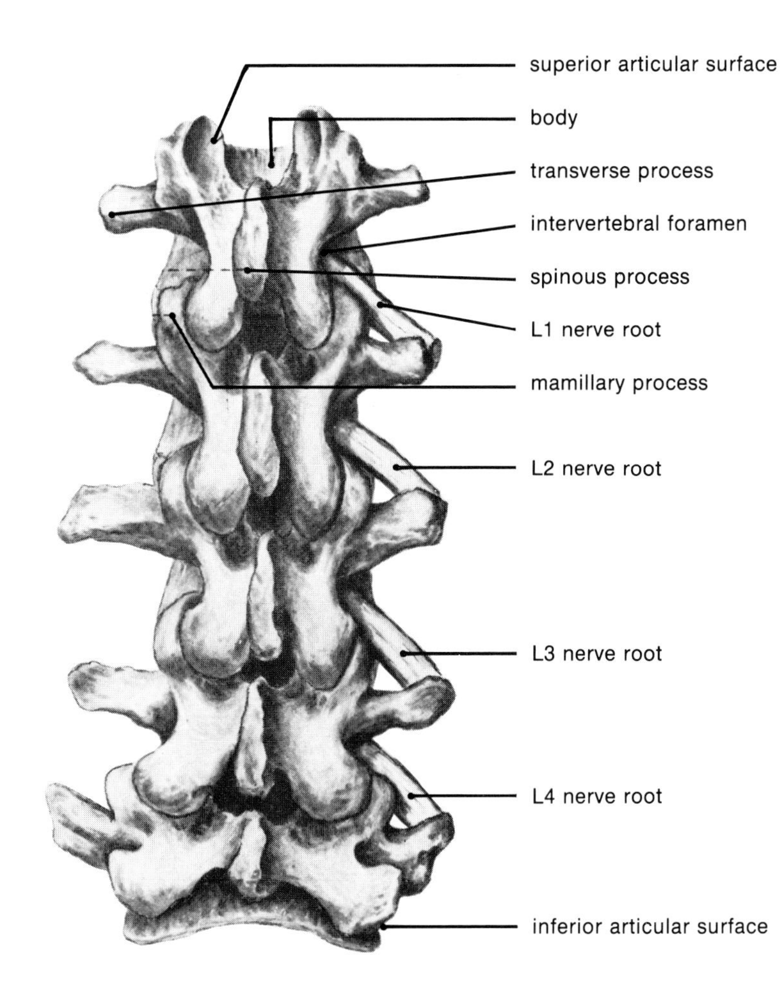

FIGURE 5-16 Posterior view of the lumbar vertebrae, showing the relationship of the lumbar nerve roots to the transverse processes of the vertebrae (for lumbar nerve root stimulation study),
Note: The L4 nerve root can be stimulated electrically by inserting the needle approximately 3 cm lateral to the spinous process to reach the transverse process of the L4 vertebra. (Pitkin GP: Conduction Anesthesia, p 535. Southworth JL, Hingson RA [eds]: Philadelphia, JB Lippincott, 1946)

Distal stimulation: Stimulate the femoral nerve below the inguinal ligament. Surface stimulators are usually used.

Normal Values[134]

Lumbar plexus latency (difference between proximal and distal latencies): 3.4 ± 0.6 msec (range 2.0–4.4 msec)
Contralateral latency difference: <0.7 msec

Determination of Conduction Across the Sacral Plexus (First Sacral Nerve Root Stimulation Study) (Figs. 5-17 and 5-18)

Conduction Time

Amplifier setting:
Sweep speed: 2 msec/div.
Sensitivity: 5 mV/div.
Filter setting: 20 Hz–10 kHz
Recording technique:
Patient position: Prone
Active electrode: On the motor point of the abductor hallucis
Reference electrode: At the base of the proximal phalanx of the great toe
Stimulation technique (needle stimulation):
Proximal stimulation: Feel for the posterior superior iliac spine and stimulate with a 50-mm monopolar needle electrode. Insert the needle until it touches the bone, then withdraw slightly.
Distal stimulation: 1 cm medial to the midpoint of the imaginary line joining the greater trochanter and the ischial tuberosity

Normal Values[134]

Sacral plexus latency (difference between proximal and distal latencies): 3.9 ± 0.7 msec (range: 2.5–4.9 msec)
Contralateral latency difference: < 0.9 msec

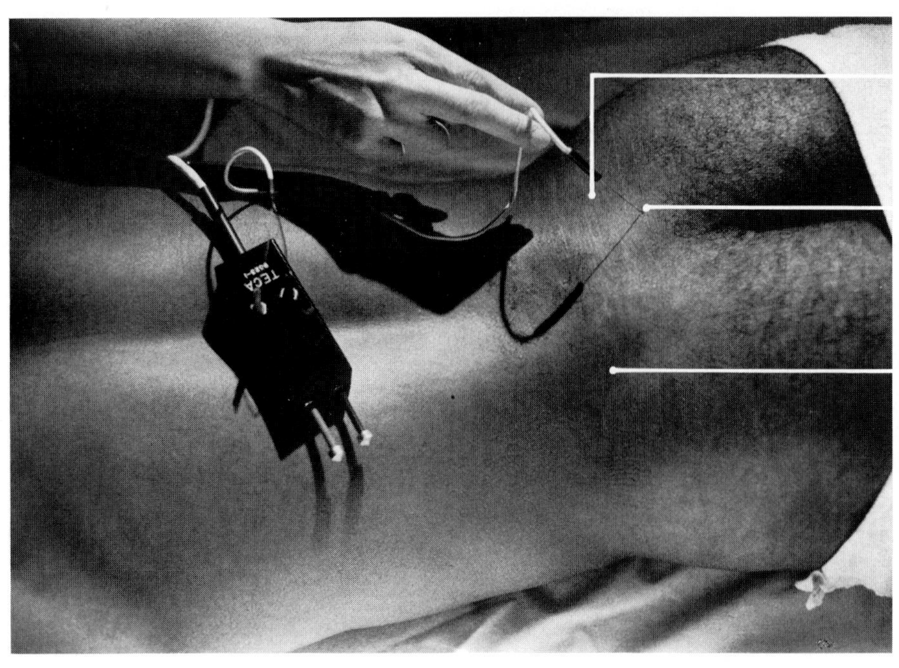

FIGURE 5-17 First sacral nerve root stimulation study.

Electrodiagnosis in Lateral Femoral Cutaneous Nerve Entrapment (Meralgia Paresthetica)

Nerve Conduction Studies

SENSORY

The sensory potential along the lateral femoral cutaneous nerve may be delayed and the amplitude depressed relative to that seen along the contralateral side. It may even be absent. This nerve should be studied bilaterally, since nerve conduction studies at this location are technically difficult to perform. Bilateral studies are essential if the response on the symptomatic side is absent. The SNAP is often obscured by the motor response from the quadriceps owing to inadvertent stimulation of the femoral nerve. The lateral femoral cutaneous nerve can be studied antidromically or orthodromically. With the antidromic method, stimulation is performed 1 cm medial to the anterior superior iliac spine, and the recording is made along the line of the anterior superior iliac spine at a distance of 12 cm to 16 cm. One study reports a normal conduction velocity of 57.5 ± 8.6 m/sec (range: 45.0–68.2 m/sec), with amplitudes of 2 μV to 10 μV.[195]

EMG

EMG should be performed to rule out pathology of the L2 and L3 nerve roots, as well as of the femoral nerve.

Femoral Nerve

Applied Anatomy (See Appendix Fig. 28)

The anterior primary rami of nerves L2, L3, and L4 each contributes to the formation of the femoral and obturator nerves. The femoral nerve is formed by the union of the posterior divisions and the obturator nerve by the anterior divisions of the anterior primary rami in question. Thus the femoral nerve supplies the morphologically dorsal part of the limb, and the obturator nerve innervates the morphologically ventral part. The femoral nerve is formed by the union of the three nerve trunks while they are still concealed behind the psoas major. The femoral nerve descends obliquely downward and appears at the lateral border of the psoas in the deep troughlike angle or groove between this muscle and the iliacus. In this groove it descends through the false pelvis and exits by passing posterior to the inguinal

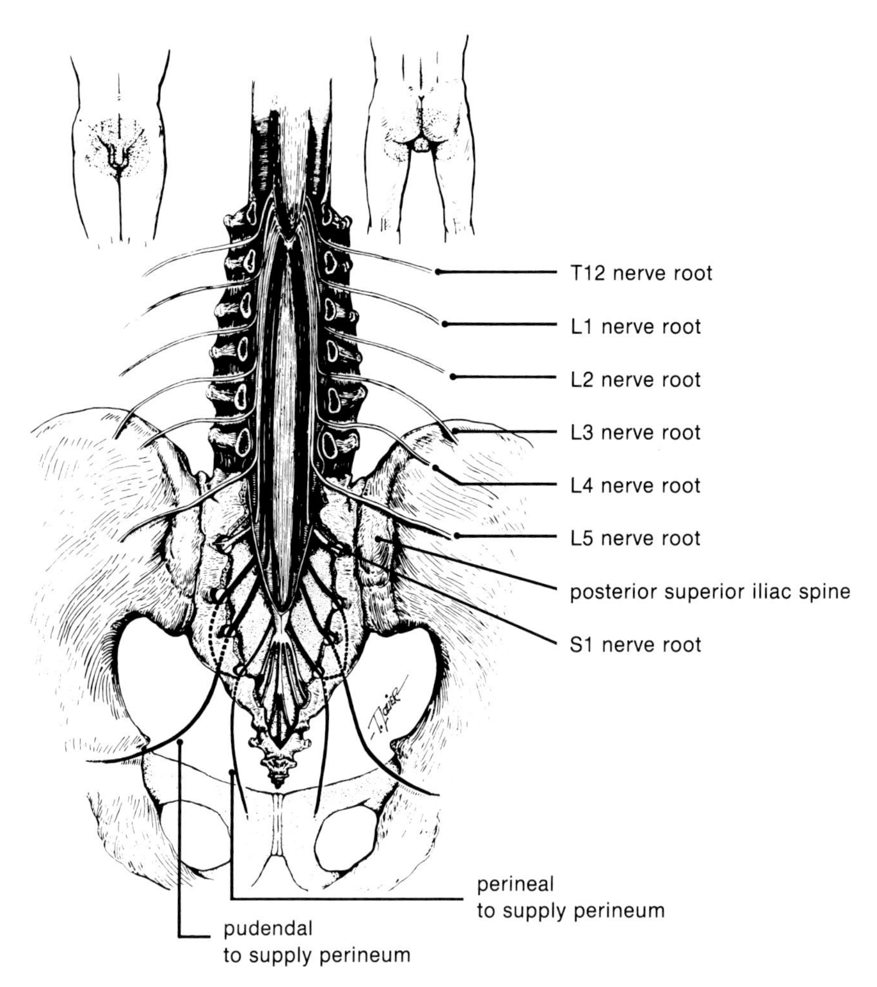

FIGURE 5-18 Relationship of the first sacral nerve root to the posterior superior iliac spine (for first sacral nerve root stimulation study). (Pitkin GP: Conduction Anesthesia, p 788. Southworth JL, Hingson RA [eds]: Philadelphia, JB Lippincott, 1946)

ligament and into the thigh. In the false pelvis it contributes a branch of supply to the iliacus, and in its course downward it lies deep to the iliacus fascia.

Entering the thigh, still in the groove between the iliacus and the psoas, the nerve lies lateral to the femoral artery and within 1 cm to 2 cm begins to divide into a number of cutaneous and muscular branches. The muscular branches are the nerve to the pectineus, several branches to the sartorius, and the various branches to the components of the quadriceps femoris. Small branches from some of the muscular nerves also supply the hip joint and the knee joint. The several cutaneous branches are the anterior femoral cutaneous nerves, which supply the skin overlying the rectus femoris and vastus medialis, and the saphenous nerve, which accompanies the great saphenous vein into the leg and is distributed to the skin of the medial half of the leg down to the level of the foot. The saphenous branch of the femoral nerve accompanies the femoral artery and vein into the troughlike space between the vastus medialis and the adductor muscles, which is covered by a lamina of fascia and thin aponeurosis that is in turn covered by the sartorius muscle. This is Hunter's adductor canal. The saphenous nerve descends through this intermuscular space to its lower end, where the nerve leaves the canal with the descending genicular artery by piercing the fascial covering of the canal (the lamina vastoadductoria) and then passes between the sartorius and gracilis muscles to the subcutaneous level. Just before the saphenous nerve exits the canal, it gives off the infrapatellar branch, which independently leaves the canal by piercing the sartorius muscle and then supplies a small area of skin at the level of the knee joint on the anteromedial side. This small nerve is occasionally damaged in knee joint incisions, resulting in a zone of paresthesia or numbness.

An entrapment syndrome involving the saphenous nerve may occur at the site where the nerve pierces the aponeurotic fascial covering of Hunter's canal. This is at the lower end of that canal, where the posterior border of sartorius comes to overlie the anterior border of gracilis.[112,152] It is a point some 10 cm superior to the adductor tubercle of the medial femoral condyle. Neuropathy of the saphenous nerve by entrapment at this point tends to give pain or paresthesia at the knee level and extending downward over the medial side of the calf, but omitting the more distal portion of the leg. This may be because of particular involvement of the infrapatellar branch and the fibers to the more proximal part of the leg.[78] Walking may precipitate or aggravate the painful sensation and thus give rise to an erroneous suspicion of claudication due to vascular disease. Tinel's sign, elicited by tapping at the lower end of Hunter's canal or along the course of the nerve, aids in the differential diagnosis. Surgical procedures within Hunter's canal may cause scarring that can become a cause of a subsequent neuropathy of the saphenous nerve.

Femoral nerve neuropathy occurring in the main trunk or its roots due to compressive lesions may be found with retroperitoneal tumors, hematomata, trauma, and, of course, radiculopathy from intervertebral disc prolapse. Diabetic neuropathy at the appropriate level of roots, or in the main trunk, may appear as a femoral nerve neuropathy.[182,205] A position of extreme hip flexion or extension, held for some time in a comatose or narcotized patient, may damage the femoral nerve by compression from the inguinal ligament. However, no specific femoral nerve entrapment syndrome has yet been described. Lacerations or surgical manipulations in the femoral trigone below the inguinal ligament may, if high enough, damage the entire nerve. Because of the shortness of the main trunk of the nerve within the femoral trigone, due to the early formation of multiple branches, most injuries here traumatize only a limited number of these branches.

Compressive neuropathies of the main trunk of the femoral nerve are more likely to be in the false pelvis or at the roots of the femoral nerve (L2, L3, and L4) in the retroperitoneal area of the posterior abdominal wall. Here, retroperitoneal hematomata, metastatic neoplasms, and lymphomas may compress the roots of the femoral nerve and simulate a lesion of the main trunk because the findings are paresis and atrophy of the quadriceps femoris and the sartorius plus sensory loss and paresthesia over the total distribution of the cutaneous branches of the femoral nerve. The quadriceps weakness results in loss of power in extension of the leg (or knee) and hence instability and buckling of the knee in walking or climbing stairs. Because the proximal roots of the femoral nerve and the ventral primary rami from which they arise give branches of supply to the psoas major, while lower down the femoral nerve itself sends branches into the iliacus, it is evident that high retroperitoneal compressive lesions can cause paresis of the iliopsoas muscle. This compound muscle is the primary flexor of the thigh (or hip joint), and its weakness is noticed by the patient in climbing stairs, owing to the inability to lift the leg and foot high enough for the next step. This deficit stands in contrast to the weakness of knee extension seen in lesions of the femoral nerve just above and just below the inguinal ligament when the only muscles involved are the quadriceps femoris, the sartorius, and the pectineus. The hip flexor capability of the adductor longus and brevis (supplied by the obturator nerve) and the tensor fasciae latae (supplied by the superior gluteal nerve) is insufficient to compensate for the loss of iliopsoas muscle power. Conversely, if the nerve lesions are scattered foci in the lumbar plexus and ventral primary rami that selectively damage the innervation of the iliopsoas but do not destroy the innervation of the rectus femoris, sartorius, and pectineus, the preserved competence for flexion at the hip joint by these latter muscles will not be sufficient to compensate for the loss of the iliopsoas in routine hip flexion.

An isolated lesion of the L4 nerve root, as for instance from a herniated intervertebral disc, might closely simulate an incomplete femoral nerve lesion. In the former, however, there would

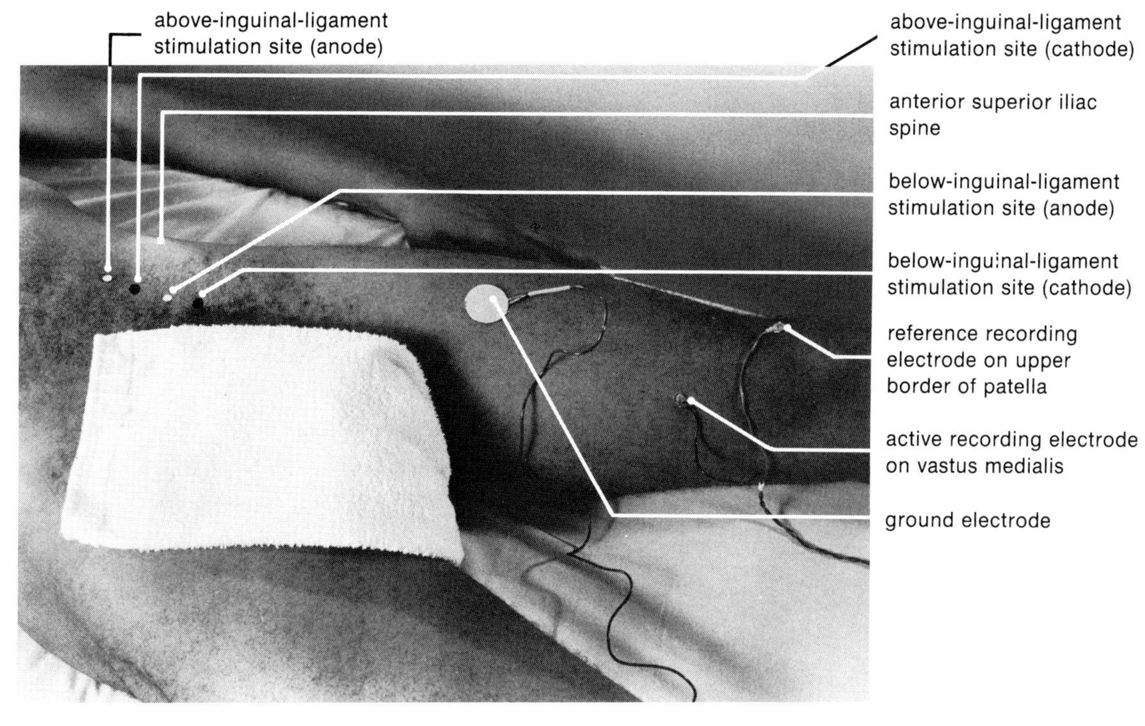

FIGURE 5-19 Femoral nerve motor conduction study.

be no loss of sensory innervation to the anterior aspect of the thigh in the distribution of the femoral nerve, and there would be weakness of dorsiflexion of the foot because of the partial loss of innervation to the tibialis anterior. EMG abnormalities would be expected throughout the L4 myotome, and this would include the erector spinae and other paraspinal muscles. Besides these differentiating physical signs, radiographic studies of the spinal and retroperitoneal areas would aid in the diagnosis.

Because of the common origin of the femoral and obturator nerves from the anterior primary rami of L2, L3, and L4, there is a strong likelihood that retroperitoneal tumors or hematomata that cause a femoral neuropathy at the plexus level will also cause an obturator neuropathy.

Motor Conduction Study (*Fig. 5-19*)

Conduction Time

Amplifier setting:
- Sweep speed: 2 msec/div.
- Sensitivity: 5 mV/div.
- Filter setting: 20 Hz–10 kHz

Recording technique:
- Active electrode: Over the most prominent part of the vastus medialis
- Reference electrode: Over the quadriceps tendon
- Ground electrode: About the middle of the thigh

Stimulation technique:
- Use supramaximal current. Surface or needle stimulation may be used. Stimulation of the femoral nerve can be performed below or above the level of the inguinal ligament.
- Below inguinal ligament: Feel for the groin crease between the pubic crest and the anterior superior iliac spine and stimulate distal to this crease. Keep the stimulation lateral to the pulsation of the femoral artery. (Stimulus duration is usually 0.2–0.5 msec, stimulus strength 200–300 V.)
- Above inguinal ligament: Stimulate approximately 5 cm to 6 cm proximal to the distal stimulation site. (Stimulus duration is usually 0.2–0.5 msec, stimulus strength 200–300 V.)

Normal Values[88]

Latency above inguinal ligament: 7.1 ± 0.7 msec (range: 6.1 – 8.4 msec)
Latency below inguinal ligament: 6.0 ± 0.7 msec (range: 5.5–7.5 msec)
Conduction velocity above inguinal ligament: 66.7 ± 7.4 m/sec (range: 50–96 m/sec)
Conduction velocity below inguinal ligament: 69.4 ± 9.2 m/sec (range: 50–90 m/sec)
Distance across inguinal ligament: 5.5 ± 1.6 cm (range: 4.2–6.6 cm)
Delay across inguinal ligament: 1.2 ± 0.4 msec (range: 0.8–1.8 msec)

Electrodiagnosis in Femoral Nerve Lesions

Anatomy

See Figures 1-45 through 1-47 and Appendix Figure 28.

Nerve Conduction Studies

SENSORY

The sensory potential of the saphenous nerve may be reduced in amplitude or absent. This nerve can be studied by recording between the tibialis anterior tendon and the medial malleolus and stimulating between the medial gastrocnemius and the tibia. One study reports normal values for the conduction velocity to be 41.7 ± 3.4 m/sec and for amplitude to be 9.0 ± 3.4 μV.[235] Since the recording of this nerve may be technically difficult, bilateral studies should be done. The interpretations should be cautious if no response is obtained on either side. In such situations, sensory studies of the sural nerves are best performed to rule out peripheral neuropathy.

MOTOR

The amplitude of the evoked motor response along the femoral nerve may be depressed on stimulation above the inguinal ligament but not on stimulation below the ligament. Entrapments at this level primarily cause conduction block. The conduction velocity of the segment across this level is slowed, and the conduction time (*e.g.*, to the vastus medialis) is prolonged.[88]

EMG

Evidence of denervation is seen in muscles supplied by the femoral nerve, the muscles easily and commonly examined being the rectus femoris, sartorius, vastus lateralis, and medialis. In lesions above the level of the inguinal ligament the iliacus is also involved. It is essential to rule out associated peripheral neuropathy or proximal radiculopathy, and the examination must include muscles supplied by the L3–S2 myotomes.

SCIATIC NERVE

Applied Anatomy (See Appendix Fig. 15)

The sciatic nerve arises from the anterior primary rami of nerves L4 and L5 and S1, S2, and S3. The anterior primary ramus of L4 sends part of its substance into the lumbar plexus and part into the sacral plexus. All of the anterior primary ramus of L5 passes downward into the pelvic cavity to be joined by the contribution from L4 described above. The combined trunk so formed is called the lumbosacral trunk. The union of the lumbosacral trunk (L4, L5) with the anterior primary rami of S1, S2, and S3, which have entered the pelvic cavity through the anterior sacral foramina, forms the broad flattened plate of nerve fibers that is the beginning of the sciatic nerve. Retroperitoneal bleeding either in the lower abdomen or in the pelvis in patients undergoing anticoagulant therapy, as well as bleeding resulting from pelvic or lower abdominal surgery, may be a cause of compressive neuropathy of the roots of origin of the sciatic nerve.[236] The sciatic nerve passes through the foramen infrapiriforme in company with the inferior gluteal nerve, the posterior femoral cutaneous nerve, the pudendal nerve, the nerve to the gemellus superior and obturator internus, and the nerve to the gemellus inferior and quadratus femoris. The inferior gluteal artery and vein and the internal pudendal artery and veins also exit the pelvic cavity to enter the gluteal area through the foramen infrapiriforme. Most of these nerves and vessels, plus those that enter the gluteal area through the foramen suprapiriforme, are fully distributed within the gluteal region. However, the sciatic nerve and the posterior femoral cutaneous nerve merely descend through the gluteal area to pass on into the posterior thigh. In contrast, the pudendal nerve and the internal pudendal vessels with the nerve to the obturator internus descend across the sacrospinous ligament in the most medial position and then enter the perineum or ischiorectal fossa by passing forward below the sacrospinous ligament and through the lesser sciatic foramen.

The sciatic nerve itself is, virtually from the beginning, divisible into two parts because of the union of its ventral rami into the tibial nerve and the union of its dorsal rami into the common peroneal nerve. Each draws its fibers from five anterior primary rami—L4 and L5 and S1, S2, and S3—except that the common peroneal nerve usually has no contribution from S3. The common peroneal nerve, arising from the dorsal divisions of the plexus, accordingly supplies the muscles and skin of the morphologically dorsal or extensor aspect of the lower limb. The tibial nerve, in turn, arising from the ventral divisions of the plexus, supplies the muscles and skin of the morphologically ventral or flexor aspect of the lower limb. In all considerations of the morphological flexor and extensor surfaces of the limbs, it is helpful to think of the posture of the limbs in the human fetus, which allows the palms and soles to be pressed together as if to clap hands and clap feet. In the infant the lower limb gradually rotates medially through 90° for assumption of the upright posture.

Once in the gluteal region, deep to the gluteus maximus, the sciatic nerve becomes more ovoid but is separable into two great nerves bound together in a common sheath of epineurium, so that they appear on casual scrutiny to be one nerve. The tibial nerve is medial and supplies branches to the hamstring muscles. These branches all pass medialward to these muscles, since the latter attach above to the ischium. However, the branch to the short head of the biceps femoris is an exception, since it arises from the common peroneal nerve. In this connection recall that the short head of the biceps femoris arises from the linea aspera of the femur rather than from the ischium, as do the other hamstring muscles. The tibial nerve is still medial as it crosses the popliteal fossa and enters the leg. The common peroneal nerve lies laterally throughout its course down the thigh, and after separating from the tibial nerve at the upper end of the rhomboid popliteal fossa, it hugs the lateral border of the fossa and the biceps femoris tendon to leave the fossa at its lateral angle. In passing across the superficial surfaces of the lateral head of the gastrocnemius and soleus, it winds around the neck of the fibula to gain the lateral and anterior compartments of the leg.

In the gluteal area the sciatic nerve is directly behind the hip joint and may be damaged by the projecting head of the femur in posterior dislocations of the hip, by fractures of the acetabulum, or by hemorrhage associated with these injuries. The upper tip of the greater trochanter is at approximately the same level as the foramen infrapiriforme and is therefore a rough guide to the level of emergence of the sciatic nerve into the gluteal region. To be more accurate, one may bisect an imaginary line drawn from the posterior superior spine of the ilium to the coccyx and from that point draw a line to the upper tip of the greater trochanter with the thigh extended. Halfway along this latter line is the site of emergence of the sciatic nerve into the gluteal region through the foramen infrapiriforme. The sciatic nerve descends below the lower border of the covering gluteus maximus at approximately the level of the lower surface of the posterior end of the ischial tuberosity (a palpable point). Here the nerve is approximately midway between the ischial tuberosity and the level of the epiphyseal line or the base of the greater trochanter (not the upper tip). A less reliable, but useful, guide to the level where the sciatic nerve comes out from under cover of the lower border of the gluteus maximus is to note the level of the gluteal fold as it crosses the midpoint between the tuberosity of the ischium and the base of the greater trochanter (provided that the hip joint is extended).

For a short interval below the gluteus maximus, the sciatic nerve is not fully and securely covered by muscle. Pressure here may separate the muscles and allow the skin to approach the nerve. As the nerve continues its vertical course downward in the posterior thigh, it passes under cover of the long head of the biceps femoris as this muscle runs obliquely downward from the ischial tuberosity to the head of the fibula. In the short interval where the nerve is uncovered between the gluteus maximus and biceps femoris, the nerve may be exposed to external trauma, as by falling in a sitting position on a rock, a curbstone, or the edge of a step. Even prolonged sitting on a narrow edge, as by soldiers or workmen in the back end of a truck, can traumatize the nerve here. Local tenderness of the nerve with pain radiating distally into the thigh may signal damage to the nerve. The upper angle of the popliteal fossa is formed as the semimembranosus (overlaid by the semitendinosus) and the long (ischial) head of the biceps femoris diverge from each other to pass to their respective sides of the knee. At this upper angle of the fossa the sciatic nerve, now separating into its two components, is again out from under cover of any overlying muscle. The level of full separation of the two components of the sciatic nerve varies and may be much higher than usual, although the two components lie side by side even when each is in its own epineurial sheath. Indeed, the tibial and common peroneal nerves may fully separate before they leave the pelvic cavity. The most common arrangement (12% of body sides) when there is such a high separation is for the tibial nerve to take its usual course through the foramen infrapiriforme while the common peroneal pierces the substance of the piriformis and thereafter descends to regain proximity to the tibial nerve. In some 3% of body sides the common peroneal nerve comes into the gluteal region through the foramen suprapiriforme (above the piriformis) while the tibial nerve takes its usual course. Again, in this arrangement, the tibial and common peroneal nerves regain proximity to each other inferior to the piriformis. Least common of all (occurring in fewer than 1%) are cases in which the entire sciatic nerve pierces the piriformis. This leaves approximately 85% of cases as the typically described arrangement. In years past much has been made of a piriformis syndrome believed due either to pinching of the sciatic nerve as it pierces the foramen infrapiriforme or pinching or to traction on the common peroneal as it pierces the piriformis in the variant patterns described above.[173]

For some researchers, if external rotation of the femur against resistance reproduced the symptoms of gluteal pain, this was believed to be confirmation of the syndrome. Certainly the syndrome is rare if not dubious.

In the thigh the tibial nerve component gives off branches to the long head of the biceps, the semitendinosus, the semimembranosus, and the ischiatic portion of the adductor magnus. These branches may spring from a common nerve branch that arises high in the thigh, or they may arise individually at varying levels. The common peroneal component gives only one branch, the twig to the femoral (short) head of the biceps femoris, which usually arises in the upper half of the thigh. Trauma to the sciatic nerve above the origin of these branches may cause weakness and atrophy of the hamstring muscles, so the strength of these muscles should be tested in the initial examination.

Through the mid-thigh level the sciatic nerve lies in a muscular trough between the semimembranosus and the adductor magnus on the medial side and the short (femoral) head of the biceps femoris on the lateral side. The unyielding bone of the linea aspera lies along the deep angle of the trough. The semitendinosus and the long head of the biceps femoris form a roof over the trough on its superficial or posterior aspect. If a person is seated for a prolonged time on a wooden or other unyielding seat or chair with his legs outstretched, the forward edge of the seat compresses the hamstrings and presses the nerve into the unyielding floor of the trough. Thus, depending on the nature of the seat, the duration of the sitting, and the posture of the person's lower limbs, a compressive trauma to the sciatic nerve may occur. The extended posture of the knee, plus flexion at the hip, puts tension on the sciatic nerve (cf., straight leg raising test). This mechanism probably explains many cases of sciatic tenderness and paresthesias occurring in some on long drives or at their desk or workbench. Certainly, if changing posture, particularly increasing flexion at the knees, and preventing posterior thigh compression alleviates or prevents the condition, it would seem likely that this mechanism, rather than a radiculopathy caused by a faulty tilt of the pelvis or exaggerated lumbar lordosis, is the basis of the distress. If the condition is severe enough to produce sensory changes, it should be recalled that sciatic neuropathy produces sensory loss or paresthesias in the sole of the foot (the medial and lateral plantar and calcaneal nerves), while radiculopathy due to root compression does not cause sensory changes in the sole unless the L5

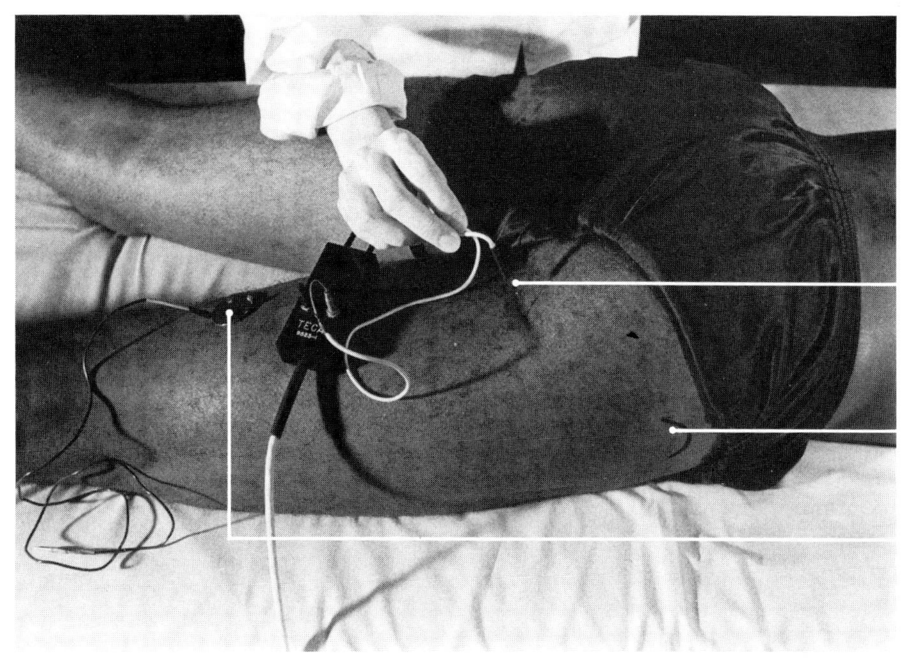

FIGURE 5-20 Sciatic nerve conduction study.

or S1 spinal nerve root is involved (S1 over the lateral half of the sole and the full width of the heel and L5 over the medial portion of the sole but none of the heel). How much the injury to the sciatic nerve, by compression in the thigh, is due to direct nerve injury and how much to ischemia of the nerve, by compression of its arterial supply (arteria comitans nervi ischiadici), is not known. Since the artery has multiple sources of collateral circulation, compression can cause only local ischemia.

Of rare occurrence as causes of entrapment neuropathy of the sciatic nerve are anomalous myofascial bands between the adductor magnus and biceps femoris in the distal portion of the thigh just superior to the popliteal fossa.[3] Morant Baker cysts of the popliteal fossa in patients with rheumatoid arthritis involving the knee joints have been reported as causes of entrapment. In this latter case either the tibial or common peroneal nerves may be affected by the expanding cyst.

Two iatrogenic causes of sciatic neuropathy deserve mention. Surgical trauma associated with total hip replacements plus the leakage of acrylic plastic in the posterior hip area has been reported to cause severe and permanent damage to the sciatic nerve as it descends through the gluteal area.[25,49,238] The repeated intramuscular injection of pentazocine has been reported to cause a severe fibrosis of muscle and connective tissue with entrapment of the sciatic nerve in the fibrotic sites.[190]

Conduction Study (*Fig.* 5-20)

Conduction Velocity

- Amplifier setting:
  - Sweep speed: 2 msec/div.
  - Sensitivity: 5 mV/div.
  - Filter setting: 20 Hz–10 kHz
- Recording technique:
  - Patient position: Prone
  - For tibial portion:
    - Active electrode: On the motor point of the abductor hallucis
    - Reference electrode: On the base of the proximal phalanx of the great toe
  - For peroneal portion:
    - Active electrode: On the extensor digitorum brevis at about the junction of the medial border of this muscle and the tendon of the extensor digitorum longus to the fifth digit

Reference electrode: On the base of the fifth digit
Ground electrode: At mid-thigh
Stimulation technique:
Use supramaximal current. Stimulation is done with a 50-mm monopolar needle with a surface electrode as a reference kept approximately 1 cm from the stimulating electrode.
Proximal: Stimulate 1 cm medial to the middle of an imaginary line joining the ischial tuberosity and the greater trochanter just below the junction of the gluteal crease and the thigh. The needle can be directed medially for stimulation of the tibial components and more laterally for stimulation of the peroneal components.[133]
Distal: Stimulate the tibial nerve 1 cm lateral to the midpoint of the popliteal fossa. Stimulate the peroneal nerve at the bend of the knee, medial to the tendon of the long head of the biceps femoris. The stimulation may be done with a needle at these levels.

Normal Values[133]

Tibial component:
Conduction velocity of between gluteal fold/popliteal fossa: 52.75 ± 4.66 m/sec (range: 46.7–59.6 m/sec)
Peroneal component:
Conduction velocity of between gluteal fold/popliteal fossa: 54.33 ± 4.36 m/sec (range: 48.5–61.5 m/sec)

Electrodiagnosis in Sciatic Nerve Lesions

Anatomy

See Figures 1-41 through 1-43 and 1-48 through 1-50 and Appendix Figure 30.

Nerve Conduction Studies

SENSORY

The sural nerve may show a depressed amplitude. If the sciatic nerve entrapment is severe, sural nerve sensory potential is absent. The H reflex is depressed in amplitude and the conduction time delayed. With more severe lesions the H reflex is absent.

MOTOR

Evoked motor responses on stimulation of the peroneal and tibial nerves may be depressed, and the conduction velocities and F responses of these nerves may be slowed. The conduction velocity along the sciatic nerve from the sciatic notch to the popliteal fossa may be slowed.

EMG

Evidence of denervation may be seen in the semitendinosus, semimembranosus, biceps femoris (long and short heads), and all of the muscles supplied by the superficial and deep peroneal and tibial nerves. Commonly, muscles supplied by the peroneal portion of the nerve are more involved than those supplied by the tibial portion.[216,218,] Abnormal EMG findings in the piriformis may suggest that this muscle is the cause of the sciatic neuropathy.

Comments

The peroneal division is more susceptible to injury in most sciatic nerve lesions, especially in lesions due to trauma. This has been attributed to the fact that the peroneal division is in a more exposed position in the thigh. Its epineurium also contains less adipose tissue than does that of the tibial division. It consists of fewer and bigger funiculi and hence has less connective-tissue packing. The path of the peroneal division is oblique and fixed at both the sciatic notch and the fibular neck,[216,218] and this factor also contributes to making it more susceptible to injury.

PERONEAL AND SURAL NERVES

Applied Anatomy

Common Peroneal Nerve (See Appendix Figs. 30 and 31)

The common peroneal nerve separates from the tibial nerve at the upper angle of the rhomboid popliteal fossa and descends obliquely downward and laterally. Hugging the biceps femoris tendon and crossing superficial to the plantaris and the lateral head of the gastrocnemius, the nerve leaves the fossa, running forward across the upper end of the soleus to wind around the neck of the fibula deep to the upper end of the peroneus longus. With the fibers of origin of the peroneus longus bridging over the nerve, a tunnel-like passage is created for the nerve. Within, or just before entering, this "fibular tunnel" the common peroneal nerve divides into the superficial and deep peroneal nerves. Entrapment in the fibular tunnel may result in compression neuropathy of either the deep or superficial peroneal nerves, or both. Just before entering this tunnel the common peroneal nerve is palpable by pressing it against the posterior and posterolateral surfaces of the neck of the fibula approximately 2 cm below the upper tip of the head of the fibula. In some persons it may be palpated above this level against the tendon of the biceps femoris if the latter is made taut. The common peroneal nerve also gives off the lateral sural cutaneous nerve and a small recurrent branch. The recurrent branch, which may also arise from the deep peroneal nerve, passes deep to the upper end of the extensor digitorum longus and enters and supplies the upper end of the tibialis anterior muscle as well as giving tiny twigs to the knee joint and the adjacent tibiofibular joint.

Superficial Peroneal Nerve

The superficial peroneal nerve, having passed through the fibular tunnel on the lateral side of the neck of the fibula, next turns downward in the connective tissue (the intermuscular septum) between the peroneus longus and brevis of the lateral compartment of the leg and the four muscles of the anterior compartment. It supplies the peroneus longus and then the peroneus brevis as the nerve continues its descent in the intermuscular septum, lying between the two peronei laterally and the extensor digitorum longus medially or anteriorly. At approximately the junction of the middle and lower thirds of the leg the superficial peroneal pierces the deep fascia and divides into medial and lateral branches (respectively, the medial dorsal cutaneous and intermediate dorsal cutaneous nerves of the foot). Recall that the lateral dorsal cutaneous nerve of the foot is the termination of the sural nerve. This latter nerve anastomoses with the intermediate dorsal cutaneous nerve, and the size of the two is reciprocal, one sometimes totally replacing the other.

Deep Peroneal Nerve

After passing around the lateral aspect of the neck of the fibula, deep to the upper end of the peroneus longus (the "fibular tunnel"), the deep peroneal nerve continues medially by piercing or lying deep to the upper end of the extensor digitorum longus. The nerve arrives in the intermuscular cleft between the extensor digitorum longus and the tibialis anterior and then descends in this connective-tissue cleft, lying on the anterior surface of the interosseous membrane accompanied by the anterior tibial artery and veins. Below the upper third of the leg, the extensor hallucis longus is added to the lateral wall of the intermuscular space housing the vasculoneural structures so that this muscle replaces the extensor digitorum longus as the immediate lateral wall of the cleft. As the deep peroneal nerve descends in this interval, it gives off muscular branches in sequence to the extensor digitorum longus, the tibialis anterior, the extensor hallucis longus, and the peroneus tertius. This last muscle is actually a partially separated portion of the extensor digitorum longus that inserts into the base of the fifth metatarsal.

When the deep peroneal nerve passes across the front of the ankle, it lies at first deep to the superior extensor retinaculum (the transverse crural ligament) and then, more distally, deep to the inferior extensor retinaculum (the cruciate ligament). At the level of the inferior retinaculum the tendon of the extensor hallucis longus crosses over the deep peroneal nerve as the tendon heads to the great toe. Thereafter, the nerve proceeds distally on the dorsum of the foot between the tendon of the extensor hallucis longus medially and the separating tendons of the extensor digitorum longus laterally. This nerve ends as a cutaneous branch to the first dorsal interdigital cleft, and it sends an important lateral twig of supply to the extensor digitorum brevis. This latter muscle is not, however, always supplied by the branch from the deep peroneal nerve. Electromyographers have adduced evidence that there is another pathway occasionally taken (in approximately one fourth of cases) by the motor fibers to the extensor digitorum brevis.[68,73,80,126] This is presumed to be a branch of the superficial peroneal nerve that continues downward with the tendons of the peronei and lies just posterior to them as the tendons and this nerve descend behind the lateral malleolus. The nerve then curves forward below the malleolus and reaches the extensor digitorum brevis.

Such a nerve pathway has indeed been demonstrated in human dissections by Bryce (J Anat 31:1897 and 35:1900) and by Winckler (Arch Anat Hist Embryol 18:1934). The muscular branch of the superficial peroneal nerve that supplies the peroneus brevis was occasionally found to be prolonged beyond the muscle belly of the latter muscle and to follow its tendon downward behind and then below the lateral malleolus. This very slender variant branch was found to proceed forward, or distally, on the lateral side of the foot finally to innervate the lateral half of the extensor digitorum brevis. It also gives sensory fibers to the lateral tarsal and metatarsal joints and ligaments. Bryce found this variant nerve to be present in three of 110 extremities in 55 cadavers (2.7% of limbs). It was bilateral in only one body. It was a very slender twig in most cases, and in one nerve that was studied microscopically it had no more than 25 medullated neurons. Winckler found this accessory deep peroneal nerve in four of 19 limbs studied. He also noted that it finally entered the lateral ligaments of the ankle area but had no muscular branch. Thus its occurrence rate in his specimens was 21%. In all instances this accessory deep peroneal branch to the extensor digitorum brevis seemed to be supplementary to the usual supply from the lateral branch in the foot of the deep peroneal nerve. This variant nerve always entered the foot by passing down behind the lateral malleolus and then going forward, and it was always very near to the sural nerve in this location. Cases of the sural nerve replacing both the superficial peroneal nerve and the continuation of the deep peroneal nerve into the foot have been seen in cadavers. Thus the sural nerve carried the fibers that should have traveled in those nerves and became the source of innervation to the extensor digitorum brevis as well as to the skin of the dorsum of the foot (Harmon, J Anat 33:22, 1899).

When the whole of the extensor digitorum brevis is not supplied by the lateral branch in the foot of the deep peroneal nerve, two supplemental sources are possible, as indicated above. The sural nerve and the accessory deep peroneal nerve may carry fibers to the lateral half of the extensor digitorum brevis. Electromyographic evidence indicates that the accessory deep peroneal nerve is by far the more common and important route.[73,80,126] Unless the sural nerve has been ruled out by appropriate higher-level stimulation, however, one cannot be positive that it is the accessory deep peroneal nerve that is responsible in any given case.

Intrinsic entrapment neuropathies of the common peroneal nerve or its two major branches at the neck of the fibula are uncommon and do not occur as often as traumatic compressive neuropathies at that site along with fractures of the fibular neck. Common peroneal nerve palsy or paresis causes some degree of footdrop and a sensory loss over the lateral aspect of the leg and the dorsum of the foot. The precise area of sensory loss varies with the level and degree of nerve damage and the variational pattern of cutaneous innervation. In the physical examination it is found that the evertors of the foot (the peroneus longus, brevis, and tertius) are weakened, although the patient may not have become as aware of this as he is of the weakness of dorsiflexion of the foot. The tibialis anterior is an invertor, but its weakness in that role is masked by the strength of the other invertors supplied by the tibial nerve. Important in differential diagnosis is this prominent loss of evertor power with only minimal loss of invertor strength, since a lesion at the lumbosacral root level tends to weaken both invertors and evertors, as well as dorsiflexors and plantar flexors. The patient in this case, however, is more aware of the dorsiflexor weakness because of the toe-catching tendency in footdrop. Preservation of normal sensibility along the lateral area of the dorsum of the foot indicates that the sural nerve is intact and that the lesion is below the origin of the lateral sural cutaneous nerve with its communicating branch. Preservation of normal sensibility in the region of the first interdigital cleft while the rest of the dorsum of the foot (except the lateral area) shows reduced or altered sensibility indicates a lesion involving the superficial peroneal nerve, but not the deep peroneal nerve. To simplify or schematize the relationship, it can be said that the superficial peroneal nerve supplies a large area of skin and few muscles (the peroneus longus and peroneus brevis), while the deep peroneal nerve supplies a small area of skin and many muscles (the extensor digitorum longus, peroneus tertius, extensor hallucis longus, tibialis anterior, and extensor digitorum brevis).

Mechanisms that may be involved in creating a lesion of the common peroneal nerve or of either of its two major branches at the fibular neck (in the fibular tunnel) are many.[4,7,65,113,127,138] Traumatic compression of the nerve by external violence and fractures of the neck of the fibula are perhaps the most common mechanisms. A variety of constrictive objects have been cited, such as plaster casts, elastic bands, and bandages; compression may also result from leg supports or operating room stirrups or pressure from protruding objects as the patient lies drunken or drugged. Prolonged kneeling or squatting, as in carpet laying, floor painting, gardening, and strawberry picking, have been incriminated as the basis of nerve compression from acute knee flexion.[41,108,206,244] Placing one's own forefinger behind the head of the fibula while adopting such a posture soon reveals the compressive force available.

Synovial cysts or ganglia extruded through clefts in the articular capsule of the proximal tibiofibular joint have been found compressing, and even invading, the substance of the common peroneal nerve or its branches as they pass around the neck of the fibula.[154,155,169,212] Cases have been reported of peroneal nerve lesions occurring at the fibular tunnel in patients who have suffered sprains of the ankle, or at least, forceful inversion and plantar flexion of the foot.[32,143] The mechanism for producing a lesion of the common peroneal or superficial peroneal nerve at the fibular tunnel in these cases appears to be as follows. The plantar flexion and inversion places a downward stretching force on the superficial peroneal nerve. The common peroneal and its branch, the superficial nerve, are well tethered in their rather horizontal position in the fibular tunnel. As the superficial peroneal nerve is drawn tautly downward, with extreme inversion and plantar flexion, its point of separation from the common peroneal and the deep peroneal (which passes onward deep to the upper end of the extensor digitorum longus) is placed under stress, with resultant damage to fibers and intraneural hemorrhage.

As the deep peroneal nerve descends through the anterior compartment of the leg, it may become a victim in the anterior compartment syndrome. The high intracompartmental pressure due to edema of the muscles can impair the microcirculation within the compartment, including that to the nerve, resulting in a deep peroneal nerve palsy. This is manifested over the distal distribution of the deep peroneal nerve beyond the anterior compartment of the leg. When the deep peroneal nerve descends across the anterior aspect of the ankle region, it successively lies deep to the superior extensor retinaculum (the transverse crural ligament) and then the inferior extensor retinaculum (the cruciate ligament). Descending deep to the latter in company with the extensor hallucis longus tendon, the nerve may be traumatized, constricted, or excessively fixed by adhesions and thereby suffer a lesion localized to this distal part of the deep peroneal nerve.[15,119] Physical examination reveals a loss of normal sensibility, and perhaps paresthesia, in the first dorsal interdigital web space plus paralysis and, in time, atrophy of the extensor digitorum brevis muscle. Paralysis of the extensor digitorum brevis cannot be readily detected by any change in extension of the toes in this syndrome because the extensor digitorum longus is normal and performs this function. The palpable inactivity of the muscle belly and its atrophy are the physical signs. This entrapment of the nerve passing deep to the inferior retinaculum has been called by some the "anterior tarsal tunnel syndrome." The nerve is held close to the superior aspect of the talonavicular joint, which provides a firm background against which the nerve can be compressed and damaged, either acutely or by chronic trauma of pressure and friction. The patient's history may or may not reveal trauma to the dorsum of the foot. Prolonged pressure from tight shoelaces or shoe straps may at times play some role in causation.

Sural Nerve

Before the common peroneal nerve passes into the fibular tunnel, it gives off the lateral sural cutaneous nerve, which in turn usually quickly gives off the peroneal communicating branch. This latter nerve descends nearly vertically for a short distance and anastomoses with the medial

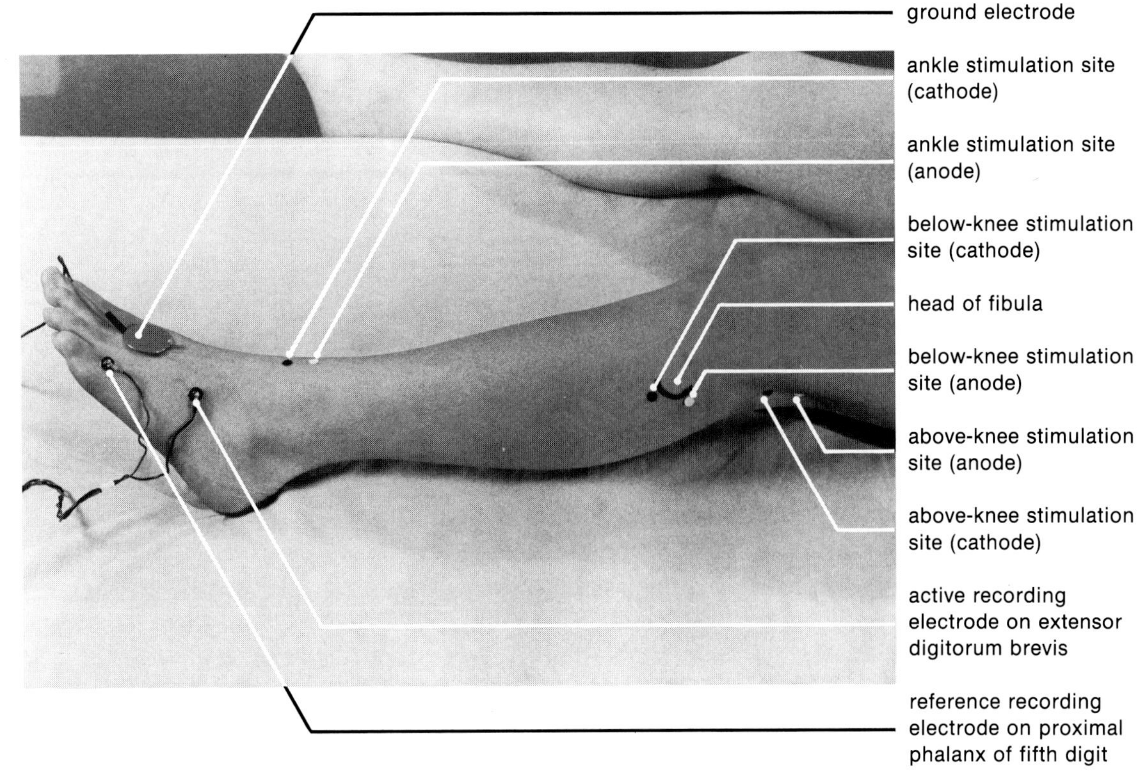

FIGURE 5-21 Peroneal nerve motor conduction study.
Note: The ankle stimulation site is 8 cm proximal to the active recording electrode. The below-knee stimulation site is at the neck of the fibula. The above-knee stimulation site is at the bend of the knee, medial to the tendon of the biceps femoris.

sural cutaneous nerve (called "sural" in many anatomy texts), which is a branch of the tibial nerve that arises within the popliteal fossa. The lateral sural cutaneous nerve distributes its fibers to the posterolateral aspect of the upper half of the leg (the calf level). The union of the medial sural cutaneous nerve and the peroneal communicating nerve from the lateral sural cutaneous nerve allows the continuing trunk (known as the sural nerve) to carry fibers from both the common peroneal nerve and the tibial nerve. The sural nerve continues distally to pass immediately behind the lateral malleolus and then curves forward along the lateral side of the dorsal aspect of the foot as the lateral dorsal cutaneous nerve of the foot. Sometimes the peroneal communicating branch arises directly from the common peroneal nerve rather than from the lateral sural cutaneous nerve. The level of union of the peroneal communicating nerve and the medial sural cutaneous nerve varies greatly up and down the posterior aspect of the leg. Accordingly, the length of the sural nerve beyond that union also varies. Usually the single sural nerve will have been formed and be present in the distal third of the leg, where it lies in close company with the small saphenous vein.

In spite of the superficial course of the sural nerve, compression neuropathies are very uncommon here, and entrapment neuropathies are even more rare. However, compression by boots and casts has been cited. Paresthesias in such cases have been aggravated by dorsiflexion of the foot, presumably due to tensing the sural nerve around the lateral malleolus. Naturally, the nerve is subject to laceration and incision because of its superficial position.

Peroneal Nerve Motor Conduction Study (Fig. 5-21)

Conduction Velocity

Amplifier setting:
Sweep speed: 2 msec/div.

Sensitivity: 5 mV/div.
Filter setting: 20 Hz–10 kHz

Recording technique:

Active electrode: On the extensor digitorum brevis at about the junction of the medial margin of this muscle and the most lateral tendon of the extensor digitorum longus to the fifth digit

Reference electrode: On the dorsum of the proximal phalanx of the fifth digit

Ground electrode: Over the dorsal aspect of the foot

Stimulation technique:

Use supramaximal current.

Ankle: Stimulate 8 cm proximal to the recording electrode. Keep the stimulator on the dorsum of the ankle approximately 1.5 cm lateral to the anterior crest of the tibia. (Stimulus duration is usually 0.1–0.5 msec, stimulus strength 150–300 V.)

Below knee: Feel for the head of the fibula and slide your index finger distally until you feel the neck of the fibula. Place the cathode of the stimulator at this level. (Stimulus duration is usually 0.1–0.2 msec, stimulus strength 200–300 V.)

Above knee: Feel for the tendon of the long head of the biceps femoris and stimulate medial to this tendon approximately 10 cm proximal to the below-knee stimulation site. (Stimulus duration is usually 0.1–0.2 msec, stimulus strength 250–300 V.)

F Wave

Amplifier setting:

Sweep speed: 10 msec/div.
Sensitivity: 200 μV/div.
Filter setting: 20 Hz–10 kHz

Method: Stimulate 10 to 20 times with supramaximal current at the ankle and measure the F wave with the shortest latency. Keep the cathode distal to the anode. (Stimulus duration is usually 0.1–0.5 msec, stimulus strength 150–300 V.) The peroneal nerve F response is difficult to elicit and is frequently absent.

Normal Values

See Table 5-7.

TABLE 5-7
Normal Values for Peroneal Nerve Motor Conduction Studies

Age (Years)	*Data (No.)*	*Amplitude (mV)*	*Distal Latency (msec)*	*Conduction Velocity (m/sec)*	*F Latency Minus Distal Latency (msec)*
20–29	100	6.2 ± 2.2 (3.1–10.6)	4.7 ± 0.7 (3.3–6.1)	49.2 ± 3.8 (41.6–56.8)	42.4 ± 4.6 (33.2–51.6)
30–39	100	6.2 ± 2.3 (3.1–10.8)	4.7 ± 0.6 (3.5–5.9)	49.2 ± 3.3 (42.6–55.8)	42.1 ± 3.9 (34.3–49.9)
40–49	100	5.9 ± 2.2 (3.1–10.3)	4.6 ± 0.6 (3.4–5.8)	48.2 ± 3.8 (40.6–55.8)	44.2 ± 4.4 (35.4–53.0)
50–59	60	5.5 ± 1.6 (3.1–8.7)	4.7 ± 0.7 (3.3–6.1)	46.9 ± 3.2 (40.5–54.1)	43.1 ± 3.5 (36.1–50.1)
Below 60	360	6.0 ± 2.0 (3.1–10.0)	4.7 ± 0.7 (3.3–6.1)	48.4 ± 3.5 (41.4–55.4)	43.0 ± 4.1 (34.8–51.2)
Above 60	45	4.6 ± 1.7 (3.1–8.0)	5.0 ± 0.7 (3.6–6.4)	45.3 ± 3.0 (39.3–51.3)	45.0 ± 4.2 (36.8–53.2)
All ages combined	405	5.6 ± 2.0 (3.1–9.6)	4.7 ± 0.7 (3.3–6.1)	48.8 ± 3.4 (42.0–55.6)	43.4 ± 4.1 (35.2–51.6)

Accessory Deep Peroneal Nerve

The accessory deep peroneal nerve is believed by electromyographers to be an anomalous branch of the superficial peroneal nerve. When present it supplies the lateral portion of the extensor digitorum brevis.[73] The presence of this nerve can be suspected when the amplitude of the proximal evoked response is larger than that of the distal response. The presence of the accessory deep peroneal nerve can be confirmed by obtaining an evoked CMAP from the extensor digitorum brevis on stimulation of this nerve at the posterior border of the lateral malleolus.

Comments

Most laboratories perform F-wave conduction studies by keeping the cathode proximal to the anode to avoid anodal block.[102] F-wave latencies are also noted to increase with increasing height of the subject.

Sural Nerve Conduction Study (Fig. 5-22)

Conduction Velocity

- Amplifier setting:
  - Sweep speed: 2 msec/div.
  - Sensitivity: 20–50 μV/div.
  - Filter setting: 20 Hz–2 kHz
- Recording technique (antidromic):
  - Active electrode: Place the recording electrode at the junction of the lower end of the fibular and lateral malleolus within 1 cm of the posterior border of the lateral malleolus.
  - Reference electrode: Place approximately 4 cm distal to the active recording electrode at the lateral aspect of the foot, at about the level of the junction of the plantar and dorsal skin. *Note*: Recording may be easier if you use a bar electrode, since it can be more firmly applied to the surface of the skin.
  - Ground electrode: Place at the lower third of the leg between the stimulating and recording electrodes.
- Stimulation technique:
  - Use supramaximal current.
  - Stimulate approximately 1 cm lateral to the tendo achillis, 14 cm from the active recording electrode.

Normal Values

See Table 5-8.

Electrodiagnosis in Peroneal Nerve Entrapment at the Knee

Anatomy

See Figures 1-48 through 1-54 and 1-56 and Appendix Figure 31.

Nerve Conduction Studies

SENSORY

The amplitude of the evoked sensory response along the superficial peroneal nerve may be depressed and the conduction velocity slowed. This nerve can be recorded just anterior to the lateral malleolus with the reference electrode placed 4 cm distally. Stimulation is done 14 cm proximally over the belly of the extensor digitorum longus. One study reports a normal latency value of 2.9 ± 0.3 msec, with an amplitude 20.5 ± 6.1 μV and a conduction velocity of 65.7 ± 3.7 m/sec.[82] The sural nerve potential is normal if the lesion is below the level of the lateral sural nerve from the common peroneal nerve, for example, in fibular tunnel lesions. If above this level, the sural nerve potential is depressed in amplitude, and the conduction time may be delayed.

MOTOR

The conduction velocity along the peroneal nerve across the knee level is slower by more than 10 m/sec compared to the velocity distal to the neck of fibula.[204] The CMAP may also drop by more than 25% on stimulation above the fibular head. If no CMAP is obtained from the extensor digitorum brevis, the conduction velocity across the knee can be determined by recording from the tibialis anterior.[37,183,204] Bilateral peroneal and tibial nerve studies help rule out the presence of peripheral neuropathy.

EMG

Evidence of denervation is seen in all muscles supplied by the superficial and deep peroneal

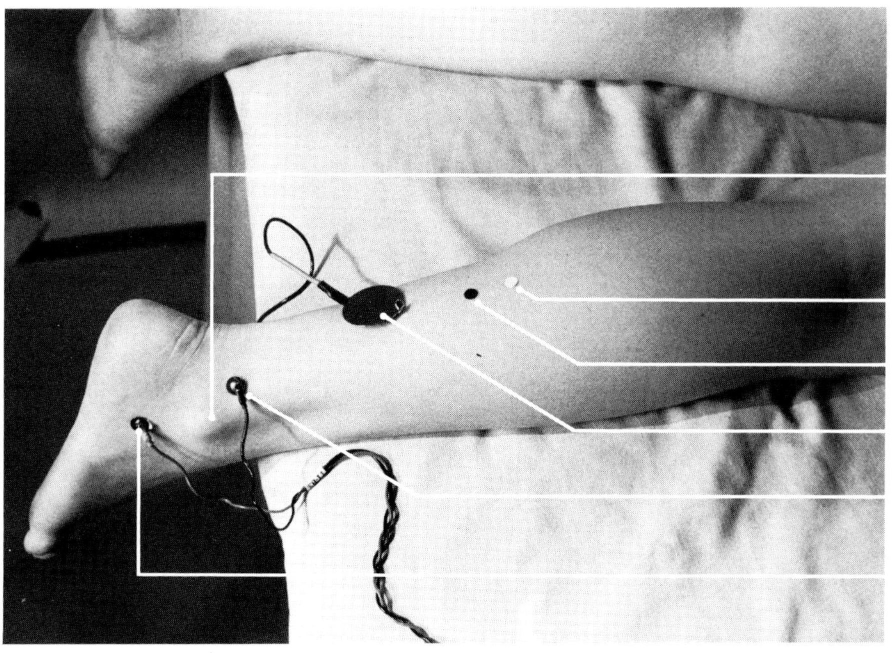

FIGURE 5-22 Sural nerve conduction study.
Note: The stimulation site is 14 cm proximal to the active recording electrode. Stimulate approximately 1 cm lateral to the lateral border of the tendo Achillis.

nerves. When a common peroneal nerve lesion is found, the EMG should also include muscles supplied by the L5 nerve root to rule out the presence of a concurrent L5 radiculopathy.

Electrodiagnosis in Peroneal Nerve Entrapment at the Ankle

Anatomy

See Figures 1-56, 1-57, and 1-66 and Appendix Figure 31.

Nerve Conduction Studies

SENSORY

No sensory abnormalities are seen. The superficial peroneal nerve is not involved, since it passes in front of the extensor retinacula.

MOTOR

The distal latency along the peroneal nerve from the ankle to the extensor digitorum brevis is delayed. The amplitude of the CMAP from this muscle is smaller than normal. In the presence of an accessory deep peroneal nerve the evoked motor response on stimulation of the peroneal nerve at the knee is larger than that obtained at the ankle. The presence of this accessory nerve branch can be confirmed by obtaining a response from the extensor digitorum brevis on stimulation behind the lateral malleolus.[73,126]

EMG

GENERAL

Evidence of denervation can be seen in the extensor digitorum brevis.

REST

The presence of fibrillations and positive sharp waves of higher amplitudes[117] may signify recent denervation. This is a useful criterion, since the extensor digitorum brevis may show some denervation in normal subjects. A comparison between the two sides may be helpful.

MINIMAL CONTRACTION

Recent neurogenic changes can be documented by the presence of complex polyphasic MUPs

TABLE 5-8
Normal Values for Sural Nerve Conduction Studies (Antidromic)

Age (Years)	*Data (No.)*	*Amplitude (μV)*	*Onset Latency (msec)*	*Conduction Velocity (m/sec)*
20–29	100	22.6 ± 8.4 (9.0–39.4)	2.9 ± 0.2 (2.5–3.3)	49.0 ± 4.3 (40.4–57.6)
30–39	100	21.9 ± 7.8 (9.0–37.5)	2.8 ± 0.2 (2.4–3.2)	50.0 ± 3.8 (42.4–57.6)
40–49	100	18.8 ± 8.7 (9.0–36.2)	2.9 ± 0.2 (2.5–3.3)	49.0 ± 4.2 (40.6–57.4)
50–59	100	17.3 ± 6.1 (9.0–29.5)	2.9 ± 0.2 (2.5–3.3)	48.1 ± 4.0 (40.0–56.0)
Below 60	400	20.2 ± 7.8 (9.0–35.8)	2.9 ± 0.2 (2.5–3.3)	49.0 ± 4.1 (40.8–57.2)
Above 60	100	15.2 ± 5.9 (5.0–27.0)	3.0 ± 0.2 (2.6–3.4)	47.1 ± 3.8 (39.5–54.7)
All ages combined	500	19.2 ± 7.5 (5.0–34.2)	2.9 ± 0.2 (2.5–3.3)	48.6 ± 4.0 (40.6–56.6)

with increased jitter and blocking. Chronic neurogenic changes may be observed in trauma from tight shoe straps around the ankle.

MAXIMAL CONTRACTION

The interference pattern is reduced proportional to the degree of neurogenic changes.

TIBIAL NERVE

Applied Anatomy (*See Appendix Fig.* 30)

The tibial nerve arises from the same roots as does the common peroneal nerve except that one more is added; thus its origin is from L4 and L5 and S1, S2, and S3. As has already been pointed out, the tibial nerve is typically alongside of, and bound in the same epineural sheath as, the common peroneal nerve, with the former lying to the medial side of the latter until they reach the apex of the popliteal fossa, where they separate. The tibial nerve descends essentially vertically through the height of the popliteal fossa. The popliteal artery and vein, which appear in the popliteal fossa to the medial side of the nerve by coming through the adductor hiatus, descend at a slightly oblique angle. This allows them to pass to the lateral side of the nerve as all three exit the fossa inferiorly by descending deep to the converging borders of the two heads of the gastrocnemius and plantaris and then under the fibrous arcade between the fibular and tibial heads of origin of the soleus. In the popliteal fossa the nerve is superficial to the vessels and is close to the deep fascia forming the roof of the fossa. Just distal to the popliteal fossa, the descending vessels and nerve all cross the surface of the popliteus so that the tibial nerve lies on the fascia of that muscle.

In the popliteal fossa the tibial nerve usually gives off three articular branches to the knee joint and five muscular branches. These latter nerves pass to the plantaris, the medial and lateral heads of the gastrocnemius, the soleus, and the popliteus. A cutaneous branch is also given off within the fossa. This nerve is the medial sural cutaneous (or sural) nerve.

The medial sural cutaneous nerve (a branch of the tibial nerve) unites with the peroneal communicating branch from the lateral sural cutaneous nerve (which springs from the common peroneal nerve) to form the sural nerve. Confusion is created by the variety of names applied to these nerves and the multiple ways in which the sural nerve may be formed. The typical pattern is a Y-shaped union between the contribution from the tibial nerve (variously called the medial sural cutaneous nerve, the tibial communicating nerve, and the sural nerve) and the contribution from the peroneal nerve that comes via the peroneal communicating branch from the lateral sural cutaneous nerve (this peroneal communicating branch is also called the peroneal anastomotic branch). These two nerves that unite to form the sural nerve usually pierce the deep fascia in the middle third of the leg and lie in the superficial fascia below that level. The level at which the contributions from the tibial and common peroneal nerves unite to form the sural nerve, or the lower segment of the Y-shaped union, varies from high in the leg to near the level of the ankle. Typically, the united trunk called the sural nerve (also called the external saphenous or small saphenous nerve because it runs with the small saphenous vein) exists throughout the lower third of the leg, lying lateral to the tendo Achillis and passing behind and then inferior to the lateral malleolus to run forward as the lateral dorsal cutaneous nerve of the foot. The lateral dorsal cutaneous nerve of the foot supplies the lateral border of the foot and the adjacent dorsum and ends as branches to the fifth toe and at least the lateral half of the fourth toe. It anastomoses with the intermediate dorsal cutaneous nerve from the superficial peroneal nerve. As might be expected, there is variability in the precise position of the cutaneous line of junction of the fibers from the two different sources here on the dorsum of the foot. This is readily understood when one remembers that the size of the contributions into the sural nerve from either the tibial or the common peroneal nerve may vary from large to small, or may even be absent in any given limb.

Below the Popliteal Fossa

After passing downward beneath the fibrous arch between the tibial and fibular origins of the soleus, the nerve comes to lie in the intermuscular septum between the triceps surae and the deep posterior muscles of the leg. These latter deep muscles are, from medial to lateral, the flexor digitorum longus, the tibialis posterior, and the flexor hallucis longus. The tibial nerve, with the posterior tibial artery and veins accompanying, is centered over the tibialis posterior in essentially the midline of the leg, but it gradually moves medially as it descends in the groove between the flexor digitorum longus and flexor hallucis longus. The tibialis posterior is crowded out of its intermediate position, and it gradually passes medially, deep to the flexor digitorum longus, so that between the medial malleolus and the tendo Achillis, the lineup of tendons is as follows: tibialis posterior, flexor digitorum longus, and flexor hallucis longus, in that order, from the malleolus to the tendo Achillis. The tibial nerve and the posterior tibial vessels are escorted downward in the interval between the tendons of the flexor digitorum longus and flexor hallucis longus and still occupy this position when passing behind the medial malleolus. In this position posterior to the malleolus the posterior tibial artery is flanked on both sides by its accompanying venae comitantes, and all three vessels are anterior to the tibial nerve.

As the tibial nerve passes underneath the fibrous or tendinous arch at the upper end of the soleus, it begins to give off a series of four muscular branches. These pass in succession from above downward, to the deep surface of the soleus, the tibialis posterior, the flexor digitorum longus medially, and the flexor hallucis longus laterally. The soleus receives a dual innervation: one branch to its superficial surface and another to its deep surface. Both are from the tibial nerve.

It has already been mentioned that Morant Baker cysts of the popliteal fossa may cause a compressive neuropathy of either of the two great divisions of the sciatic nerve, and that aneurysms of the popliteal artery may compress the tibial nerve as it descends through the fossa superficial to the artery. Pain radiating over the distribution of the tibial nerve may be a result of the compression. Popliteal artery aneurysms are nearly always due to arteriosclerosis, and therefore the condition is seen primarily in the elderly.

Entrapment neuropathy syndromes of the tibial nerve in the leg have not been described, but a compressive neuropathy as a compartment syndrome due to edema of the three muscles of the deep posterior compartment may occur, owing to muscle damage from overuse or compression by external trauma or from fracture with hematoma. The high pressure in the compartment interferes with the blood supply to the nerve, thus adding sensory changes in the foot to the signs due to the muscle damage within the deep posterior compartment.

When the tibial nerve reaches the level of the medial malleolus, it must, along with several other structures, pass deep to the flexor retinaculum (or laciniate ligament). This structure is essentially a dense thickening of the deep fascia that extends ribbonlike between the posterior border of the medial malleolus and the medial process of the tuber calcanei. A deeper layer of the flexor retinaculum blends with the periosteum of the calcaneus, talus, and medial malleolus, as well as with the articular capsules of the talocalcaneal and talocrural joints. Anteriorly and posteriorly, or, more accurately, medially and laterally, the two layers of the retinaculum fuse. However, in the area behind the medial malleolus and talus the two layers are separated except for three septa that convert the space into four compartments or tunnels. The medialmost of these (the anterior) transmits the tendon of the tibialis posterior, the next the tendon of the flexor digitorum longus, followed by a common tunnel for the posterior tibial artery, flanked by its two venae comitantes, and medial to the vessels, and within the same tunnel, the tibial nerve. The fourth and most lateral tunnel (the posterior) transmits the tendon of the flexor hallucis longus. Generations of British doctors have recalled this sequence of structures by the mnemonic "Turner doth vex all very nervous hearts," in recognition of the anxiety produced in students by the great anatomist Sir Edward Turner, who served the University of Edinburgh from 1867 to 1916. American students have often converted this to "Timothy doth vex all very nervous horses." The vertical length of the tunnel through which the tibial nerve and its accompanying vessels descends is approximately 1.5 cm. While the tibial nerve is deep to the flexor retinaculum, it gives off the medial calcaneal branch, which pierces the retinaculum and supplies the skin of the heel. Before the nerve emerges from the lower end of the tunnel, it has divided into the medial and lateral plantar nerves.

There is a great similarity between the medial plantar nerve and the median nerve of the hand, and between the lateral plantar nerve and the ulnar nerve of the hand. This is understandable, since these nerves are serially homologous.

The lateral plantar nerve descends deep to the abductor hallucis and passes obliquely laterally and forward, toward the base of the fifth metatarsal. In this part of its course it lies between the plantar aponeurosis and the flexor digitorum brevis superficially and the flexor digitorum accessorius (quadratus plantae), which lies deep to the nerve. On its way the lateral plantar nerve supplies the flexor digitorum accessorius and the abductor digiti minimi as it lies alongside the latter muscle. At the base of the fifth metatarsal the nerve divides into superficial and deep branches, again reminiscent of the ulnar nerve in the hand. The superficial branch continues distally, adjacent to the tendon of the abductor digiti minimi and the flexor digiti minimi brevis. In this part of its course it supplies the latter muscle. Occasionally, as a variant, it gives twigs of supply to the two most lateral interosseous muscles (the third plantar interosseous and the fourth dorsal interosseous). The other branches of the superficial branch of the lateral plantar nerve are cutaneous and supply the lateral portion of the sole of the foot, the fifth toe, and half of the fourth toe. The deep branch of the lateral plantar nerve plunges into the deep interval between the metatarsals and the interossei on the dorsal side and the adductor hallucis on its plantar side. Passing medially, this deep branch supplies the four dorsal and the three plantar interossei, the adductor hallucis, and the lateral three lumbricals (the medialmost lumbrical is supplied by the medial plantar nerve). Typically, all interossei are supplied by the deep branch of the lateral plantar nerve, but occasionally some fibers destined for the plantar and dorsal interosseous muscles of the fourth interspace fail to turn into the deep branch of the lateral plantar nerve and run onward for a few millimeters into the superficial branch before turning off as small twigs to these lateralmost interossei, hence the variability in their nerve supply, as previously cited.

The medial plantar descends toward the sole of the foot, lying deep to the adductor hallucis, and then curves forward in the axis of the second metatarsal. As the nerve proceeds forward in the foot, it lies deep to the plantar aponeurosis and the flexor digitorum brevis, while the flexor digitorum accessorius (quadratus plantae) and the common tendon of the flexor digitorum longus lie deep or dorsal to the nerve. As the medial plantar nerve passes deep to the abductor hallucis, it gives a branch of supply to that muscle and a lateral branch to supply the flexor digitorum brevis. As the nerve crosses the tendon of the flexor digitorum longus (at about the level of the navicular bone), it gives off a proper digital branch to the medial side of the great toe. On its way to the great toe this branch supplies both heads of the flexor hallucis brevis and gives cutaneous branches to the medial two thirds of the sole of the forefoot. Two or three centimeters further forward, the continuing trunk of the medial plantar nerve divides into three common digital nerves that pass toward the first, second, and third interdigital clefts to then divide into proper digital branches, each supplying its respective side of the toes. The proper digital branch to the medial side of the fourth toe communicates with the proper digital branch from the lateral plantar nerve, which passes to the lateral side of that toe. Again, note the comparability to the pattern of cutaneous innervation in the hand. The common digital nerve passing to the first interdigital space is the source of a branch to the first, or medialmost, lumbrical muscle. The three lateral lumbricals are supplied by the lateral plantar nerve.

One of the more classic entrapment neuropathies is that of the tibial nerve as it passes through its loge deep to the flexor retinaculum in company with the posterior tibial artery and its two flanking venae comitantes.[93,124,125] This is the third of the four compartments deep to the retinaculum, and to its medial (anterior) side is the tunnel for the flexor digitorum longus, while to its lateral (posterior) side is the tunnel for the flexor hallucis longus. The artery, its accompanying veins, and the tibial nerve are all embraced in a web of fatty areolar tissue as they pass through their common osseofibrous tunnel. The talus and calcaneus (covered with periosteum) and the posterior part of the medial or deltoid ligament of the ankle, plus a layer of deep fascia, form the floor of this tunnel, while the dense fibrous band of the flexor retinaculum (laciniate ligament) is the roof. The lineup of the four compartments is as much medial-to-lateral as it is anterior-to-posterior, and all are posterior to the medial malleolus. For the purposes of this chapter, the compartment for the tibial nerve and its accompanying artery and vein will be referred to simply as the "tarsal tunnel," and entrapment of the nerve here will be called the "tarsal tunnel syndrome." To distinguish it from the anterior tarsal tunnel syndrome (the deep peroneal nerve beneath the inferior extensor retinaculum), some clinicians have referred to the one under discussion here as the "posterior tarsal tunnel syndrome," but this additional adjective is not routinely used. Since the floor of the tarsal tunnel is formed by the talus covered by the posterior part of the deltoid or medial ligament (also called the posterior tibiotalar part of the deltoid ligament), it is obvious that ankle sprains or dislocations, with tearing of these special parts of the fibrous capsule of the ankle joint, could cause, after healing, increased thickness or fibrosis of the ligament and consequent encroachment on the space of the tarsal tunnel. Fracture of the talus, or of the calcaneus, in the vicinity of the tarsal tunnel could, on healing with bone proliferation or deformity, result in encroachment on the tarsal tunnel space. The flexor retinaculum itself (the roof of the tunnel) could be torn or injured in severe ankle-area trauma with subsequent fibrous thickening and reduction of the tunnel space. The two venae comitantes within the tunnel offer the possibility that varicosities will compress the nerve or that thrombophlebitis will cause edema and inflammation of the nerve. The fatty areolar tissue within the tunnel may give rise to the development of a lipoma. The presence of the nerve itself gives the possibility of neurinoma formation, while the underlying joint affords the opportunity of inflammation and thickening of the tissues, as in rheumatoid arthritis, and the formation and encroachment of ganglia on the tibial nerve. Inflammation associated with tenosynovitis of the two adjacent synovial sheaths (those of the flexor digitorum longus and flexor hallucis longus) might cause compression of the tibial nerve. Each of the above has been cited in various case studies as a causal factor in tarsal tunnel syndrome.[39,44,69,92,130,137,164] From several collected series of cases, it may be said that roughly one third of cases fall into the category of posttraumatic etiology. Another third are due to a conglomeration of causes, most of which have been cited above. A final third may be said to be unexplained or of unknown etiology. Still another explanation has been offered by Radin, who notes the high frequency of occurrence of inverted or varus heels in combination with pronated and splayed forefeet in patients with tarsal tunnel syndrome.[178] He proposes the varus heel as the fundamental flaw precipitating tarsal tunnel syndrome by angulating the axis of the tarsal tunnel with reference to the axis of the tibial nerve just above the tunnel. This diminishes the space available at the upper end of the tunnel and leads to folding or kinking of the nerve within the tunnel, which would add to the overcrowding in the canal. The pronated and splayed forefoot is not primary, but is compensatory to the varus heel, affording the forefoot weight-bearing contact with the ground. However, Radin suggests that the pronated forefoot may put traction and stretch on the lateral plantar nerve, thus exacerbating the nerve damage. This mechanism, which has been offered to explain the cause of the tarsal tunnel syndrome, may account for some of the heretofore unexplained cases and may also be operative in combination with other causes that have in the past been held to be solely responsible. Kopell and Thompson, however, state that in some cases the symptoms may be increased by forcing the heel into the valgus position, while forcing the heel into a varus position may alleviate the symptoms.[113] The contradiction in these ideas awaits elucidation by further study.

The history usually reveals a unilateral syndrome. If there has been trauma of sprain, dislocation, or fracture, it is likely to have been months or years before the onset of symptoms. The patient reports a burning pain in the sole of the forefoot, but there is no point of local tenderness. This pain may increase with standing or walking, perhaps due to increased venous congestion within the tarsal tunnel. However, some patients emphasize the increase of pain when resting at the end of the day, and nocturnal pain is common. This may, however, be only an increased psychological awareness of the pain. This local pain and radiating tingling is quite regularly present. Tinel's sign is present when percussion is done over the tarsal tunnel. Sensory loss is often difficult to demonstrate and is best tested in the thin skin under the medial longitudinal arch. Weakness of the intrinsic muscles of the foot may be present but is often masked by the strength of the flexor digitorum longus and flexor hallucis longus. Testing the strength of plantar flexion of the second to fifth toes may be helpful. The patient's inability to spread or fan his toes may be evident.

Kopell and Thompson cite another location for medial and lateral plantar nerve entrapment: distal to the tarsal tunnel. As these two nerves descend toward the sole of the foot, lying deep to the abductor hallucis, the medial plantar nerve is anterior to the lateral plantar nerve. Both are deep to the abductor hallucis just anterior to where the muscle arises from its several sites of attachment. Deeper, more tendinous strands of the abductor hallucis may impinge against the medial or lateral plantar nerves and strap them against the medial border of the flexor digitorum accessorius. The medial plantar nerve curves strongly forward while deep to the abductor hallucis and passes underneath the plantar calcaneonavicular ligament (spring ligament) as the nerve runs forward to cross beneath the tendon of the flexor digitorum longus. Deep tendinous fibers of the abductor hallucis may pinch the medial plantar nerve against the inferior aspect of the plantar calcaneonavicular ligament. Excessive pronation of the forefoot, either chronic, or acute from sudden, severe downward force applied to the dorsum of the foot, may stress and compress the medial plantar nerve beneath the spring ligament where the nerve is held *in situ* by deep fibers of the abductor hallucis. Nerve entrapment here may involve one or the other of the plantar nerves, perhaps both. Thus it may simulate the tarsal tunnel syndrome, except that percussion over the tarsal tunnel does not elicit Tinel's sign. Or, the signs being localized to only one nerve (the medial or the lateral), they may at once suggest that the nerve lesion is distal to the tarsal tunnel, since lesions within the tarsal tunnel are far more likely to involve both branches.

As the common digital nerves reach the level of the heads of the metatarsal bones, each divides into two proper digital nerves. Each proper digital nerve then passes forward into its respective toe. The level of division of the common digital nerves is at approximately the anterior or distal border of the deep transverse metatarsal ligaments, in each interspace between the heads of the metatarsals. Here both the nerves and the lumbrical muscles lie on the plantar or inferior side of the deep transverse metatarsal ligaments, while the interosseous muscles run forward dorsal to the ligaments. When the toes are hyperextended at the metatarsophalangeal joint, as they are in the kneeling position, the distal end of each common digital nerve (often called the interdigital nerve) is drawn taut across the anterior border of the unyielding ligament. This trauma of the nerve, if severe enough, of long enough duration, or of frequent enough episodes, can lead to a lesion of the nerve that is essentially a cicatricial "neuroma" of a nerve that is still in continuity, although some fibers may be destroyed.[58,105,106,129] To some degree the trauma to the nerve may also be due to the compression of the nerve between the heads of the metatarsals. This is suggested by the fact that the pain of the condition may be somewhat relieved in certain cases by wearing wider shoes that allow the metatarsal heads to spread apart. But in most instances the trauma of nerve compression against the deep transverse metatarsal ligament is the fundamental cause of the neuroma. This condition, long known as Morton's toe or foot, and metatarsalgia, can occur with any one of the four common digital nerves, but it is much more likely to be an involvement of the nerve to the interspace between the third and fourth toes. Sometimes it occurs on the nerve to the interspace between the second and third toes, and very rarely with the remaining two nerves.

In the push-off phases of walking and when one is wearing high-heeled shoes, the toes are hyperextended, as they are when one is crouching, as in "sitting on one's heels." Thus certain occupations and activities predispose to the development of Morton's neuroma. Metatarsal fractures may precipitate the formation of the neuroma. Running on rocky or uneven terrain may lead to sudden, severe hyperextension of the toes and therefore becomes a causal mechanism.

The history is one of pain in the metatarsal area with a tendency to radiate into the toes receiving the branches of the nerve with the neuroma. Pressure applied to the sole of the foot between the metatarsal heads reveals painfulness, since the neuroma is put under compression by the fingertip. Extending the toes also causes pain. No motor loss is to be expected because the nerves do not innervate muscle beyond the level of the neuroma. Sensory loss may be detectable in both pain and tactile modalities, but the patient is often not aware of this until the time of the examination.

Motor Conduction Study (*Fig.* 5-23)

Conduction Velocity

Amplifier setting:
- Sweep speed: 2 msec/div.
- Sensitivity: 5 mV/div.
- Filter setting: 20 Hz–10 kHz

Recording technique:
- Active electrode: Feel for the navicular bone and place the active electrode 1 cm below and 1 cm posterior to it.
- Reference electrode: At the medial aspect of the base of the proximal phalanx of the great toe
- Ground electrode: Over the dorsal aspect of the foot

Stimulation technique:
- Use supramaximal current.
- Ankle: Stimulate 8 cm proximal to the recording electrode, between the medial malleolus and the tendo Achillis on the medial aspect of the ankle. (Stimulus duration is usually 0.1–0.2 msec, stimulus strength usually 200–300 V.)
- Knee: Feel for the bend of the knee and stimulate approximately 1 cm lateral to the midline of the knee. Stimulation is best done if you approach the patient from the lateral aspect of the knee. If you place the cathode slightly more proximally, it will be over the popliteal fat and will produce submaximal stimulation. The nerve is relatively deep, and usually a stimulus duration of 0.2 msec to 0.5 msec and a stimulus strength of 200 V to 300 V are needed. The cathode must be firmly pressed into the popliteal fossa. If the stimulation is unsatisfactory with the patient supine, the lateral recumbent or the prone positions should be used. Generally, satisfactory recordings can be obtained by stimulating the nerve while the knee is kept bent approximately 45° and the hip is kept in internal rotation.

F Wave

Amplifier setting:
- Sweep speed: 10 msec/div.
- Sensitivity: 200 μV/div.
- Filter setting: 20 Hz–10 kHz

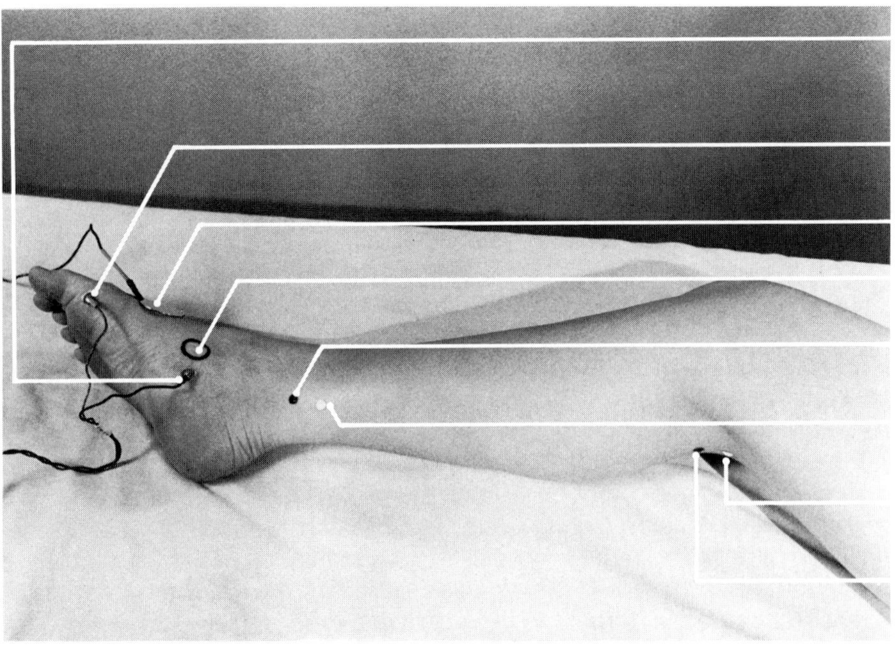

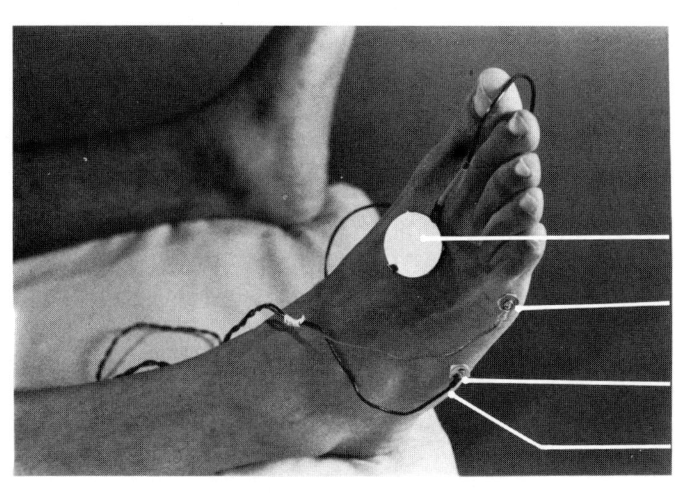

FIGURE 5-23 Tibial nerve motor conduction study.
Note: The ankle stimulation site is 8 cm proximal to the active recording electrode. The knee stimulation site is at the distal knee crease approximately 1 cm lateral to the midline of the popliteal fossa.

Method: Stimulate 10 to 20 times with supramaximal current at the ankle and measure the F wave with the shortest latency. Keep the cathode distal to the anode.

Normal Values

See Table 5-9. The distal latency for the abductor digiti minimi (quinti) is less than 7 msec.

Comments

Most laboratories perform F-wave studies by keeping the cathode distal to the anode to avoid anodal block.[102] F-wave latencies increase with an increase in the subject's height.

One study[193] reports examination of the sensory potential along the medial and lateral plantar nerves by stimulating at the sole of the foot 14 cm from the recording point, which is above

TABLE 5-9
Normal Values for Tibial Nerve Motor Conduction Studies

Age (Years)	*Data (No.)*	*Amplitude (mV)*	*Distal Latency (msec)*	*Conduction Velocity (m/sec)*	*F Latency Minus Distal Latency (msec)*
20–29	100	13.5 ± 4.4 (5.1–17.9)	4.9 ± 0.7 (3.5–6.3)	49.6 ± 3.8 (42.0–57.2)	42.0 ± 4.1 (33.8–50.2)
30–39	100	13.1 ± 4.3 (4.5–21.7)	5.0 ± 0.6 (3.8–6.2)	49.2 ± 3.8 (41.6–56.8)	42.1 ± 4.0 (34.0–50.1)
40–49	100	10.8 ± 4.1 (4.1–19.0)	5.1 ± 0.6 (3.9–6.3)	48.5 ± 3.7 (41.1–55.9)	44.1 ± 4.0 (36.0–52.0)
50–59	60	11.3 ± 4.3 (4.0–19.9)	5.2 ± 0.6 (4.0–6.4)	46.9 ± 3.2 (40.5–53.3)	43.2 ± 3.4 (36.4–50.0)
Below 60	360	12.2 ± 4.3 (3.6–20.8)	5.1 ± 0.6 (3.9–6.3)	48.6 ± 3.6 (41.4–55.8)	42.9 ± 3.9 (35.1 – 50.7)
Above 60	45	7.4 ± 3.8 (4.0–15.0)	5.4 ± 0.6 (4.2–6.6)	46.0 ± 3.6 (38.8–53.2)	44.7 ± 3.9 (36.9–52.5)
All ages combined	405	11.2 ± 4.2 (3.0–19.4)	5.1 ± 0.6 (3.9–6.3)	48.0 ± 3.6 (40.8–55.2)	43.2 ± 3.9 (35.4–51.0)

the flexor retinaculum. The normal latencies obtained with this method for both nerves have been reported to be 3.2 ± 0.3 msec.

Electrodiagnosis in Tarsal Tunnel Syndrome

Anatomy

See Figures 1-59, 1-60, and 1-63 through 1-65 and Appendix Figure 30.

Nerve Conduction Studies

SENSORY

Conduction studies of the medial and lateral plantar nerves may show a delayed or absent response.[164] Saeed and Gatens[193] report an orthodromic method of recording the sensory potentials of the medial and lateral plantar nerves by recording above the flexor retinaculum and stimulating 14 cm along the medial and lateral border of the sole. This can sometimes be performed without an averager and is useful in detecting sensory abnormalities along these two nerves. These sensory responses are frequently abnormal or absent in tarsal tunnel syndrome, while the distal motor latency is still normal.[164]

MOTOR

Conduction times to the abductor hallucis and abductor digiti minimi may be delayed. A difference in motor conduction time of more than 1 msec between one muscle and the same muscle on the contralateral foot may indicate slowing on the symptomatic side.[137]

EMG

Since the medial and lateral plantar nerves may be involved separately, muscles supplied by both nerves must be examined.

REST

A few positive sharp waves may occasionally be seen in the intrinsic foot muscles.[57] The presence of fibrillations is considered the most suggestive evidence of ongoing denervation. The presence of fibrillations and positive sharp waves with larger amplitudes may signify recent denervation.[117]

MINIMAL CONTRACTION

Chronic neurogenic changes due to previous trauma may be seen. Evidence of recent neurogenic involvement is confirmed by the presence of complex polyphasic MUPs with late components showing increased jitter and blocking on contraction.

MAXIMAL CONTRACTION

The interference pattern is reduced relative to the degree of neurogenic involvement.

REFERENCES

*1. Adson AW: Cervical ribs: Symptoms, differential diagnosis for section of the insertion of the scalenus anticus muscle. J Int Coll Surg 16:546, 1951

*2. Adson AW, Coffey JR: Cervical rib. Ann Surg 85:839, 1927

3. Banerjee T, Hall CD: Sciatic entrapment neuropathy. J Neurosurg 45:216, 1976

4. Banerjee T, Koons DD: Superficial peroneal nerve entrapment. J Neurosurg 55:991, 1981

5. Basmajian JV, Griffin WR: Function of the anconeus muscle: An electromyographic study. J Bone Joint Surg 54A:1712–1714, 1972

6. Bendler EM, Greenspun B, Yu J, Erdman WJ: The bilaterality of carpal tunnel syndrome. Arch Phys Med Rehabil 58:362–364, 1977

7. Berry H, Richardson PM: Common peroneal nerve palsy: A clinical and neurophysiological review. J Neurol Neurosurg Psychiatry 39:1162, 1976

*8. Beyer JA, Wright JS: Hyperabduction syndrome. Circulation 4:161, 1951

9. Bhala RP, Goodgold J: Motor conduction in the deep palmar branch of the ulnar nerve. Arch Phys Med Rehabil 49:460–466, 1968

10. Blanquez GM, Delwaide PJ: The thoracic outlet syndrome: An electrophysiological study. Electromyogr Clin Neurophysiol 22:255–263, 1982

11. Blevins CE: Innervation patterns of the human stapedius muscle. Arch Otolaryngol 86:136–142, 1967

12. Blom S, Dahlback LO: Nerve injuries in dislocations of the shoulder joint and fractures of the neck of the humerus: A clinical and electromyographical study. Acta Chir Scand 136:461, 1970

13. Blunt MJ: The blood supply of the facial nerve. J Anat 88:520–526, 1954

14. Bora FW, Osterman AL: Compression neuropathy. Clin Orthop 163:20–32, 1982

15. Borges LF, Hallett M, Selkoe DJ, Welch K: The anterior tarsal tunnel syndrome: Report of two cases. J Neurosurg 54:89, 1981

16. Braddom R, Wolfe C: Musculocutaneous nerve injury after heavy exercise. Arch Phys Med Rehabil 59:290, 1978

* Recommended for further reading

17. Buchthal F, Rosenfalck A: Sensory conduction from digit to palm and from palm to wrist in the carpal tunnel syndrome. J Neurol Neurosurg Psychiatry 34:243, 1971

18. Buchthal F, Rosenfalck A, Trojaborg W: Electrophysiological findings in entrapment of the median nerve at wrist and elbow. J Neurol Neurosurg Psychiatry 37:340, 1974

19. Caldwell W, Crane CR, Krusen EM: Nerve conduction studies: An aid in the diagnosis of the thoracic outlet syndrome. South Med J 64:210, 1971

20. Capener N: The vulnerability of the posterior interosseous nerve of the forearm: A case report and an anatomical study. J Bone Joint Surg 48B:770, 1966

21. Carfi J, Ma DM: Posterior interosseous nerve syndrome revisited. Muscle Nerve 8:499–502, 1985

22. Checkles N, Russakov A, Piero D: Ulnar nerve conduction velocity—effect of elbow position on measurement. Arch Phys Med Rehabil 52:362, 1971

23. Cherington M: Anterior interosseous nerve syndrome: Straight thumb sign. Neurology 27:800, 1977

24. Collins DN, Weber ER: Anterior interosseous nerve avulsion. Clin Orthop 181:175–177, 1983

25. Combs MA, Clark WK: Sciatic nerve injury following intragluteal injection: Pathogenesis and prevention. Am J Dis Child 160:579, 1960

*26. Coni NK: Pall-bearer's palsy. Br Med J 2:808, 1966

27. Corbin KB, Harrison F: The sensory innervation of the spinal accessory and tongue musculature in the rhesus monkey. Brain 62:191, 1939

*28. Cunningham DP, Basmajian JV: Electromyography of genioglossus and geniohyoid muscles during deglutition. Anat Rec 165:401, 1969

*29. Daube JR: Rucksack paralysis. JAMA 208:2447, 1969

30. Daube JR: Nerve conduction studies in the thoracic outlet syndrome. Neurology 25:347, 1975

31. Daube JR: Percutaneous palmar median nerve stimulation for carpal tunnel syndrome. Electroenchephalogr Clin Neurophysiol 43:139, 1977

32. Davies JAK: Peroneal compartment syndrome secondary to rupture of the peroneus longus. J Bone Joint Surg 61A:783, 1979

33. Dawson DM, Hallett M, Millender LH: Entrapment Neuropathies. Boston, Little, Brown & Co, 1983

34. Day MH, Napier JR: The two heads of flexor pollicis brevis. J Anat 95:123–130, 1961

*35. DeLisa JA, Saeed MA: The Tarsal Tunnel Syndrome. Case Report 8. Rochester, MN, American Association of Electromyography and Electrodiagnosis, 1983

*36. Deschuytere J, Rosselle N, De Keyser C: Monosynaptic reflexes in the superficial forearm flexors in man and their clinical significance. J Neurol Neurosurg Psychiatry 39:555, 1976

37. Devi S, Lovelace RE, Duarte N: Proximal peroneal nerve conduction velocity: Recording from anterior tibial and peroneus brevis muscles. Ann Neurol 2:116, 1977

38. DiBenedetto M: Thoracic outlet slowing. Electromyogr Clin Neurophysiol 17:191–204, 1977

39. DiStefano V, Sack J, Whittaker R, Nixon J: Tarsal tunnel syndrome. Clin Orthop 88:76, 1972

40. Drachman DA: Bell's palsy: A neurological point of view. Arch Otolaryngol 89:147, 1969

41. Eaton LM: Paralysis of the peroneal nerve caused by

crossing the legs: Report of case. Mayo Clin Proc 12:206, 1937
42. Ebeling P, Gilliatt RW, Thomas PK: A clinical and electrical study of ulnar nerve lesion in the hand. J Neurol Neurosurg Psychiatry 23:1, 1960
43. Eckman PB, Perlstein G, Altrocchi PH: Ulnar neuropathy in bicycle riders. Arch Neurol 32:130, 1975
44. Edwards WG et al: The tarsal tunnel syndrome: Diagnosis and treatment. JAMA 207:716, 1969
45. Eisen A: Early diagnosis of ulnar nerve palsy: An electrophysiologic study. Neurology (Minneap) 24:256, 1974
*46. Eisen A, Odusote K: Amplitude of the F wave: A potential means of documenting spasticity. Neurology (NY) 29:1306, 1979
*47. Falconer MA, Weddell G: Costoclavicular compression of the subclavian artery and vein: Relation to scalenus anticus syndrome. Lancet 2:539, 1943
48. Feindel W, Stratford J: The role of the cubital tunnel in tardy ulnar palsy. Can J Surg 287:300, 1958
49. Fleming RE: Sciatic paralysis: A complication of bleeding following hip surgery. J Bone Joint Surg 61A:37, 1979
50. Flowers RS: Meralgia paresthetica: A clue to a retroperitoneal malignant tumor. Am J Surg 116:89, 1968
51. Forrest WJ: Motor innervation of human thenar and hypothenar muscles in 25 hands: A study combining EMG and percutaneous nerve stimulation. Can J Surg 10:196–199, 1967
*52. Fullerton PM, Gilliatt RW: Axon reflexes in human motor nerve fibres. J Neurol Neurosurg Psychiatry 28:1, 1965
*53. Garcia-Mullin R, Mayer RF: H reflexes in acute and chronic hemiplegia. Brain 95:559, 1972
*54. Gardner B, Hood RH Jr: Vascular compression at the shoulder girdle: Analysis of normal subjects by means of radial pulse tracings. Ann Surg 153:23, 1961
*55. Gassel MM: A test of nerve conduction to muscles of the shoulder girdle as an aid in the diagnosis of proximal neurogenic and muscular disease. J Neurol Neurosurg Psychiatry 27:200, 1964
56. Gassel MM, Diamantopoulos E: Pattern of conduction times in the distrubution of the radial nerve. Neurology 14:222, 1964
57. Gatens PF, Saeed MA: Electromyographic findings in the intrinsic muscles of normal feet. Arch Phys Med Rehabil 63:317–318, 1982
58. Gauthier G: Thomas Morton's disease: A nerve entrapment syndrome. Clin Orthop 142:90, 1979
59. Ghent WR: Further studies on meralgia paresthetica. Can Med Assoc J 85:871, 1961
60. Gilliatt RW, Thomas PK: Changes in nerve conduction with ulnar lesions at the elbow. J Neurol Neurosurg Psychiatry 23:312, 1960
61. Gilliatt RW et al: Peripheral nerve conduction in patients with a cervical rib and band. Ann Neurol 4:124–129, 1978
*62. Gilroy J, Meyer JS: Compression of the subclavian artery as a cause of ischaemic brachial neuropathy. Brain 86:733, 1963
63. Ginzburg M, Lee M et al: Median and ulnar nerve conduction in Erb's point-axilla segment in normal subjects. J Neurol Neurosurg Psychiatry 41:444–448, 1978
64. Gleason TF, Goldstein WM, Ray RD: The function of the anconeus muscle. Clin Orthop 192:147–148, 1985
65. Gloobe H, Chain D: Fibular fibrous arch: Anatomical considerations in fibular tunnel syndrome. Acta Anat (Basel) 85:84, 1973
66. Goldberg EE, Amelar RD: Causalgia in inguino-genital area. US Armed Forces Med J VII:901, 1956
67. Goldman S et al: Posterior interosseous nerve palsy in the absence of trauma. Arch Neurol 21:435, 1969
68. Goodgold J, Eberstein A: Electrodiagnosis of Neuromuscular Disease, 3rd ed. Baltimore, Williams & Wilkins, 1983
69. Goodgold J, Kopell HP, Spielholz NI: The tarsal-tunnel syndrome: Objective diagnostic criteria, N Engl J Med 273:742, 1965
*70. Goor C, Ongerboer de Visser BW: Jaw and blink reflexes in trigeminal nerve lesions: An electrodiagnostic study. Neurology (Minneap) 26:95, 1976
71. Gross MS, Gelberman RH: The anatomy of the distal ulnar tunnel. Clin Orthop 196:238–247, 1985
72. Guerrier Y: Le nerf facial: Quelques points d'anatomie topographique. Ann Otolaryngol 92:161–171, 1975
73. Gutmann L: Atypical deep peroneal neuropathy in presence of accessory deep peroneal nerve. J Neurol Neurosurg Psychiatry 33:453, 1970
74. Gutmann L: Median–ulnar nerve communications and carpal tunnel syndrome. J Neurol Neurosurg Psychiatry 40:982, 1977
*75. Harness D, Sekeles E: The double anastomotic innervation of the thenar muscles. J Anat 109:461–466, 1971
76. Harness D, Sekeles E, Chaco J: The double motor innervation of the opponens pollicis muscles: An electromyographic study. J Anat 117:329–331, 1974
77. Highet WB: Innervation and function of the thenar muscles. Lancet 1:227, 1943
78. House JH, Ahmed K: Entrapment neuropathy of the infrapatellar branch of the saphenous nerve: A new peripheral nerve entrapment syndrome? Am J Sports Med 5:217, 1977
79. Hunt JR: Occupational neuritis of the deep palmar branch of the ulnar nerve. J Nerve Ment Dis 35:673, 1908
80. Infante E, Kennedy WR: Anomalous branch of the peroneal nerve detected by electromyography. Arch Neurol 22:162, 1970
81. Jabre JF: Ulnar nerve lesions at the wrist: New technique for recording the sensory dorsal branch of the ulnar nerve. Neurology (Minneap) 30:873, 1980
82. Jabre JF: The superficial peroneal sensory nerve revisited. Arch Neurol 38:666, 1981
*83. Jabre JF: Surface recording of the H reflex of the flexor carpi radialis. Muscle Nerve 4:435, 1981
84. Jebsen RH: Motor conduction velocity in proximal and distal segments of the radial nerve. Arch Phys Med Rehabil 47:597, 1966
85. Jefferson D, Eames RA: Subclinical entrapment of the lateral femoral cutaneous nerve. Muscle Nerve 2:145, 1979
86. Johnson EW, Kukla RD, Wongsam PE, Piedmont A: Sensory latencies to the ring finger: Normal values and relation to carpal tunnel syndrome. Arch Phys Med Rehabil 62:206, 1981
87. Johnson EW, Melvin JL: Sensory conduction studies of median and ulnar nerves. Arch Phys Med Rehabil 48:25–30, 1967

88. Johnson EW, Wood PK, Powers JJ: Femoral nerve conduction studies. Arch Phys Med Rehabil 49:528, 1968
*89. Jonsson B: Morphology, innervation and electromyographic study of the erector spinae. Arch Phys Med Rehabil 50:638, 1969
*90. Kaplan P, Sahgal V: Residual latency: New applications of an old technique. Arch Phys Med Rehabil 59:24, 1978
*91. Kaplan PE: Sensory and motor residual latency measurements in healthy patients and patients with neuropathy. Part 1. J Neurol Neurosurg Psychiatry 39:338, 1976
92. Kaplan PE, Kernahan WT: Tarsal tunnel syndrome: An electrodiagnostic and surgical correction. J Bone Joint Surg 63A:96, 1981
93. Keck C: The tarsal-tunnel syndrome. J Bone Joint Surg 44A: 180, 1962
94. Keret D, Porter KM: Synovial cyst and ulnar nerve entrapment: A case report. Clin Orthop Rel Res 188:213–216, 1984
95. Kerr AT: The brachial plexus of nerves in man, the variations in its formation and branches. Am J Anat 23:285, 1918
96. Kiloh LG, Nevin S: Isolated neuritis of the anterior interosseous nerve. Br Med J 1:850, 1952
97. Kim DJ, Kalantri A, Guha S, Wainapel SF: Dorsal cutaneous ulnar nerve conduction: Diagnostic aid in ulnar neuropathy. Arch Neurol 38:321, 1981
98. Kimura J: Alterations of the orbicularis oculi reflex by pontine lesions: Study in multiple sclerosis. Arch Neurol 22:156, 1970
99. Kimura J: The carpal tunnel syndrome: Localization of conduction abnormalities within the distal segment of the median nerve. Brain 102:619, 1979
100. Kimura J: Clinical uses of the electrically elicited blink reflex. In Desmedt JE (ed): Brain and Spinal Mechanisms of Movement Control in Man: New Developments and Clinical Applications. New York, Raven Press, 1982
101. Kimura J: Conduction abnormalities of the facial and trigeminal nerves in polyneuropathy. Muscle Nerve 5:S142, 1982
102. Kimura J: Electrodiagnosis in Diseases of Nerve and Muscle: Principles and Practice. Philadelphia, FA Davis, 1983
103. Kimura J, Lyon LW: Orbicularis oculi reflex in the Wallenberg syndrome: Alteration of the late reflex by lesions of the spinal tract and nucleus of the trigeminal nerve. J Neurol Neurosurg Psychiatry 35:228, 1972
104. Kimura J, Power JM, Van Allen MW: Reflex response of orbicularis oculi muscle to supraorbital nerve stimulation: Study in normal subjects and peripheral facial palsies. Arch Neurol 21:193–199, 1969
105. King LS: Note on the pathology of Morton's metatarsalgia. Am J Clin Pathol 16:124, 1946
106. Kite JH: Morton's toe neuroma. South Med J 59:20, 1966
107. Kleinert HE, Hayes JE: The ulnar tunnel syndrome. Plast Reconstr Surg 47:21, 1971
108. Koller RJ: Strawberry picker's palsy. Arch Neurol 37:320, 1980
*109. Komar J, Varga B: Syndrome of the rectus abdominis muscle. J Neurol 210:121, 1975
110. Kopell H, Goodgold J: Clinical and electrodiagnostic features of the carpal tunnel syndrome. Arch Phys Med Rehabil 49:371–375, 1968
111. Kopell HP, Thompson WAL: Pronator syndrome. N Engl J Med 259:713–715, 1958
112. Kopell HP, Thompson WAL: Knee pain due to saphenous nerve entrapment. N Engl J Med 263:351–353, 1960
113. Kopell HP, Thompson WAL: Peripheral entrapment neuropathies of the lower extremity. N Engl J Med 262:56–60, 1960
114. Kopell HP, Thompson WAL, Postel H: Entrapment neuropathy of the ilioinguinal nerve. N Engl J Med 266:16–19, 1962
*115. Kopell HP, Thompson WAL: Peripheral Entrapment Neuropathies, 2nd ed. New York, Kruger, 1976
116. Kraft GH: Axillary, musculocutaneous and suprascapular nerve latency studies. Arch Phys Med Rehabil 53:384–385, 1972
117. Kraft GH: Decay of fibrillation potential amplitude following nerve injury (abstr). Muscle Nerve 7:565, 1984
118. Kraft GH, Halvorson GA: Median nerve residual latency: Normal value and use in diagnosis of carpal tunnel syndrome. Arch Phys Med Rehabil 64:221–226, 1983
119. Krause KH, Witt T, Ross A: The anterior tarsal tunnel syndrome. J Neurol 217:67, 1977
120. Kudo H, Nori S: Topography of the facial nerve in the human temporal bone. Acta Anat 90:467–480, 1974
121. Laha RK, Dujovny M, DeCastro C: Entrapment of median nerve by supracondylar process of the humerus. J Neurosurg 46:252, 1977
122. Laha RK, Lunsford LD, Dujovny M: Lacertus fibrosus compression of the median nerve: Case report. J Neurosurg 48:838, 1978
123. Lake PA: Anterior interosseous nerve syndrome. J Neurosurg 41:306, 1974
124. Lam SJS: A tarsal tunnel syndrome. Lancet 2:1354, 1962
125. Lam SJS: Tarsal tunnel syndrome. J Bone Joint Surg 49B:87, 1967
126. Lambert EH: The accessory deep peroneal nerve: A common variation in innervation of extensor digitorum brevis. Neurology 19:1169, 1969
127. Large DF, Ludlam CA, Macnicol MF: Common peroneal nerve entrapment in a hemophiliac. Clin Orthop 181:165–166, 1983
128. Lascelles RG, Mohr PD, Neary D, Bloor K: The thoracic outlet syndrome. Brain 100:601, 1977
129. Lassmann G, Lassmann H, Stockinger L: Morton's metatarsalgia: Light and electronmicroscopic observations and their relation to entrapment neuropathies. Virchows Arch [A] 370:307, 1976
130. Linscheid RL, Burton RC, Fredericks EJ: Tarsal tunnel syndrome. South Med J 63:1313, 1970
*131. London GW: Normal ulnar nerve conduction velocity across the thoracic outlet: Comparison of two measuring techniques. J Neurol Neurosurg Psychiatry 38:756–760, 1975
132. Lyon EK: Genitofemoral causalgia. Can Med Assoc J 53:213, 1945
133. Ma DM, Liveson JA: Nerve Conduction Handbook. Philadelphia, FA Davis, 1983
134. MacLean IC: Nerve root stimulation to evaluate conduction across the brachial and lumbosacral plexuses.

Third Annual Continuing Education Course. Rochester, MN, American Association of Electromyography and Electrodiagnosis, 1980
135. Magee RK: Genitofemoral causalgia (new syndrome) Can Med Assoc J 46:325–329, 1942
*136. Magladery JW, McDougal DB Jr: Electrophysiological studies of nerve and reflex activity in normal men. 1. Identification of certain reflexes in the electromyogram and the conduction velocity of peripheral nerve fibres. Bull Johns Hopkins Hosp 86:265, 1950
137. Mann RA: Tarsal tunnel syndrome. Orthop Clin North Am 5:109, 1974
138. Maudsley RH: Fibular tunnel syndrome. J Bone Joint Surg 49B:384, 1967
139. McCormack LJ, Cauldwell EW, Anson BJ: The surgical anatomy of the facial nerve. Surg Gynecol Obstet 80:620, 1945
140. McGregor J, Moncur JA: Meralgia paresthetica: A sports lesion in girl gymnasts. Br J Sports Med 11:16, 1977
141. McLellan DL, Swash M: Longitudinal sliding of the median nerve during movement of the upper limb. J Neurol Neurosurg Psychiatry 39:566, 1976
142. Mead S: Posterior triangle operations and trapezius paralysis. Arch Surg 64:752, 1952
143. Meals RA: Peroneal nerve palsy complicating ankle sprain. J Bone Joint Surg 59A:966, 1977
144. Melvin JL, Harris DH, Johnson EW: Sensory and motor conduction velocities in ulnar and median nerves. Arch Phys Med Rehabil 47:511–519, 1966
145. Melvin JL, Schuchmann JA, Lanese RR: Diagnostic specificity of motor and sensory nerve conduction variables in carpal tunnel syndrome. Arch Phys Med Rehabil 54:69–74. 1973
146. Miller RG: The cubital tunnel syndrome: Diagnosis and precise localization. Ann Neurol 6:56, 1979
147. Mills RHB, Mukherjee K, Bassett IB: Anterior interosseous nerve palsy. Br Med J 2:555, 1969
148. Milton GW: The mechanism of circumflex and other nerve injuries in dislocation of the shoulder, and the possible mechanism of nerve injuries during reduction of dislocation. Aust NZ J Surg 23:25, 1953
149. Moldover J: Tinel's sign: Its characteristics and significance. J Bone Joint Surg 60A:412, 1978
150. Morris HH, Peters BH: Pronator syndrome: Clinical and electrophysiological features in seven cases. J Neurol Neurosurg Psychiatry 39:461, 1976
151. Moscona AR, Sekel R: Posttraumatic meralgia paresthetica: An unusual presentation. J Trauma 18:288, 1978
152. Mozes M, Ouaknine G, Nathan H: Saphenous nerve entrapment simulating vascular disorder. Surgery 77:299, 1975
153. Moyers RE: An electromyographic analysis of certain muscles involved in temporomandibular movement. Am J Orthodontia 36:481, 1950
154. Muckart RD: Compression of the common peroneal nerve by intramuscular ganglion from the superior tibiofibular joint. J Bone Surg 58B:241, 1976
155. Nakano KK: Entrapment neuropathy from Baker's cyst. JAMA 239:135, 1978
156. Nakano KK, Lundergan C, Okihiro MM: Anterior interosseous nerve syndromes: Diagnostic methods and alternative treatments. Arch Neurol 34:477, 1977
157. Nielsen HO: Posterior interosseous nerve paralysis caused by a fibrous band compression of the supinator muscle: A report of four cases. Acta Orthop Scand 47:304, 1976
158. Norden A: Peripheral injuries to the spinal accessory nerve. Acta Chir Scand 94:515, 1946
159. Nunley JA, Bassett FH: Compression of the musculocutaneous nerve at the elbow. J Bone Joint Surg 64A:1050, 1982
160. O'Brien MD: Genitofemoral neuropathy. Br Med J 1:1052, 1979
161. O'Brien MD, Upton ARM: Anterior interosseous nerve syndrome: A case report with neurophysiological investigation. J Neurol Neurosurg Psychiatry 35:531, 1972
162. Ochoa J, Marotte L: Nature of the nerve lesion underlying chronic entrapment. J Neurol Sci 19:491, 1973
163. Ogata K, Manske PR, Lesker PA: The effect of surgical dissection on regional blood flow to the ulnar nerve in the cubital tunnel. Clin Orthop 193:195–198, 1985
164. Oh SJ, Sarala PK et al: Tarsal tunnel syndrome: Electrophysiological study. Ann Neurol 5:327–330, 1979
165. Olarte M, Adams D: Accessory nerve palsy. J Neurol Neurosurg Psychiatry 40:1113, 1977
166. Olsen PZ: Prediction of recovery in Bell's palsy. Acta Neurol Scand 61 (Suppl):1, 1975
167. Ongerboer de Visser BW, Goor C: Electromyographic and reflex study in idiopathic and symptomatic trigeminal neuralgias: Latency of the jaw and blink reflexes. J Neurol Neurosurg Psychiatry 37:1225, 1974
*168. Panayiotopoulos CP: F chronodispersion: A new electrophysiologic method. Muscle Nerve 2:68–72, 1979
169. Pankes A: Intraneural ganglion of the lateral popliteal nerve. J Bone Joint Surg 43B:784, 1961
170. Parkinson CE: The supracondyloid process. Radiology 62:556, 1954
*171. Payan J: Electrophysiological localization of ulnar nerve lesions. J Neurol Neurosurg Psychiatry 32:208, 1969
172. Pearson MG: Meralgia paresthetica with reference to its occurrence in pregnancy. Br J Obstet Gynaecol 64:427, 1957
173. Pezina M: Contribution to the etiological explanation of the piriformis syndrome. Acta Anat (Basel) 105:181, 1979
174. Phalen GS: The carpal tunnel syndrome: Seventeen years' experience in diagnosis and treatment of 654 hands. J Bone Joint Surg 48A:211, 1966
175. Phalen GS: The carpal tunnel syndrome: Clinical evaluation of 598 hands. Clin Orthop 83:29–40, 1972
176. Pleet AB, Massey EW: Palmaris brevis sign in neuropathy of the deep palmar branch of the ulnar nerve. Ann Neurol 3:468, 1978
177. Powers WH: Peripheral facial paralysis and systemic disease. Otolaryngol Clin North Am 7:397, 1974
178. Radin EL: Tarsal tunnel syndrome. Clin Orthop 181:167–170, 1983
179. Rask MR: Anterior interosseous nerve entrapment (Kiloh-Nevin syndrome). Clin Orthop 142:176, 1979
180. Rask MR: Superior gluteal nerve entrapment syndrome. Muscle Nerve 3:304, 1980
181. Ray RD, Johnson RJ, Jameson RM: Rotation of the fore-

arm: An experimental study of pronation and supination. J Bone Joint Surg 33A:993, 1951
182. Razzuk MA, Linton RR, Darling RC: Femoral neuropathy secondary to ruptured abdominal aortic aneurysms with false aneurysms. JAMA 201:817, 1967
183. Redford JB: Nerve conduction in motor fibers to the anterior tibial muscle in peroneal palsy. Arch Phys Med Rehabil 45:500, 1964
184. Rennels GD, Ochoa J: Neuralgic amyotrophy manifesting as anterior interosseous nerve palsy. Muscle Nerve 3:160, 1980
185. Richmond DA: Carpal ganglion with ulnar nerve compression. J Bone Joint Surg 45B:513, 1963
186. Roles NC, Maudsley RH: Radial tunnel syndrome: Resistant tennis elbow as a nerve entrapment. J Bone Joint Surg 54B:499, 1972
*187. Roos DB, Owen JC: Thoracic outlet syndrome. Arch Surg 93:71, 1966
*188. Roth G: Intranervous regeneration: The study of motor axon reflexes. J Neurol Sci 41:139, 1979
*189. Roth G: Intranervous regeneration of lower motor neuron. 1. Study of 1153 motor axon reflexes. Electromyogr Clin Neurophysiol 18:225, 1978
190. Rousseau JJ, Reznick M, LeJeune GN, Franck G: Sciatic nerve entrapment by pentazocine induced muscle fibrosis. Arch Neurol 36:723, 1979
191. Rowntree T: Anomalous innervation of the hand muscles. J Bone Joint Surg 31B:505–510, 1949
*192. Rubin A: Birth injuries: Incidence, mechanisms and end results. Obstet Gynecol 23:218, 1964
193. Saeed MA, Gatens PF: Compound nerve action potentials of the medial and lateral plantar nerves through the tarsal tunnel. Arch Phys Med Rehabil 63:304–307, 1982
194. Salgeback S: Ulnar tunnel syndrome caused by anomalous muscles. Scand J Plast Surg 11:255, 1977
195. Sarala PK, Nisihara T, Oh SJ: Meralgia paresthetica: Electrophysiologic study. Arch Phys Med Rehabil 60:30, 1979
*196. Schiller HH, Stålberg E: F responses studied with single fibre EMG in normal subjects and spastic patients. J Neurol Neurosurg Psychiatry 41:45, 1978
197. Seddon HJ: Carpal ganglion as a cause of paralysis of the deep branch of the ulnar nerve. J Bone Joint Surg 34B:386, 1952
*198. Shahani BT, Potts F, Domingue J: F response studies in peripheral neuropathies. Neurology (NY) 30:409, 1980
199. Shahani BT, Young RR, Potts F, Maccabee P: Terminal latency index (TLI) and late response studies in motor neuron disease (MND), peripheral neuropathies and entrapment syndromes. Acta Neurol Scand (Suppl 73) 60:118, 1979
200. Sharrard WJW: Anterior interosseous neuritis: Report of a case. J Bone Joint Surg 50B:804, 1968
201. Shea J, McClain E: Ulnar-nerve compression syndromes at and below the wrist. J Bone Joint Surg 51A:1095, 1969
202. Simpson JA: Electrical signs in the diagnosis of carpal tunnel and related syndromes. J Neurol Neurosurg Psychiatry 19:275, 1956
203. Singer E: Human brachial plexus united into a single cord. Anat Rec 55:411, 1933
204. Singh N, Behse F, Buchthal F: Electrophysiological study of peroneal nerve palsy. J Neurol Neurosurg Psychiatry 37:1202, 1974
205. Sisto D, Chiu WS, Geelhoed GW, Lewis R: Femoral neuropathy after renal transplantation. South Med J 73:1464, 1980
206. Sorell DA et al: Traumatic common peroneal nerve palsy: A retrospective study. Arch Phys Med Rehabil 57:361, 1976
207. Spindler HA, Felsenthal G: Sensory conduction in the musculocutaneous nerve. Arch Phys Med Rehabil 59:20, 1978
208. Spinner M: The arcade of Frohse and its relationship to posterior interosseous nerve paralysis. J Bone Joint Surg 50B:809–812, 1968
209. Spinner M: The anterior interosseous nerve syndrome with special attention to its variations. J Bone Joint Surg 52A:84, 1970
210. Spinner M: Injuries to the Major Branches of Peripheral Nerves of the Forearm, 2nd ed. Philadelphia, WB Saunders, 1978
211. Spinner M, Schreiber SN: The anterior interosseous nerve paralysis as a complication of supracondylar fractures in children. J Bone Joint Surg 51A:1584, 1969
212. Stack RE, Bianco AJ Jr, MacCarty CS: Compression of the common peroneal nerve by ganglion cysts: Report of nine cases. J Bone Joint Surg 47A:773, 1965
213. Stevens H: Meralgia paresthetica. Arch Neurol Psychiatry 77:557, 1957
*214. Streib E, Daube JR: Electromyography of paraspinal muscles. Neurology (NY) 25:386, 1975
215. Sunderland S: Intraneural topography of the radial, median, and ulnar nerves. Brain 68:243, 1945
216. Sunderland S: The relative susceptibility to injury of the medial and lateral popliteal divisions of the sciatic nerve. Br J Surg 41:300, 1953
217. Sunderland S: Nerve lesion in the carpal tunnel syndrome. J Neurol Neurosurg Psychiatry 39:615, 1976
218. Sunderland S: Nerves and Nerve Injuries, 2nd ed. Edinburgh, Churchill Livingstone, 1978
*219. Takabe K, Vitti M, Basmajian JV: The functions of semispinalis capitis and splenius capitis: An electromyographic study. Anat Rec 179:477, 1974
220. Tanzer RC: The carpal tunnel syndrome: A clinical and anatomical study. J Bone Joint Surg 41A:626, 1959
221. Taylor AR: Ulnar nerve compression at the wrist in rheumatoid arthritis. J Bone Joint Surg 56B:142, 1974
222. Telford ED, Mottershead S: Pressure at the cervicobrachial junction: An operative and anatomical study. J Bone Joint Surg 30B:249, 1948
223. Terry RJ: A study of the supracondyloid process in the living. Am J Phys Anthropol 4:129, 1921
224. Thomander L, Stålberg E: Electroneurography in the prognostication of Bell's palsy. Acta Otolaryngol 92:221–237, 1981
225. Thomas DF: Kiloh-Nevin syndrome. J Bone Joint Surg 44B:962, 1962
*226. Thomas JE, Lambert EH: Ulnar nerve conduction velocity and H reflex in infants and children. J Appl Physiol 15:1, 1960

227. Thomas JE, Lambert EH, Cseuz KA: Electrodiagnostic aspects of the carpal tunnel syndrome. Arch Neurol 16:635, 1967
228. Thompson WHL, Kopell HP: Peripheral entrapment neuropathies of the upper extremity. N Engl J Med 260:1261–1265, 1959
229. Trojaborg W: Rate of recovery in motor and sensory fibres of the radial nerve: Clinical and electrophysiological aspects. J Neurol Neurosurg Psychiatry 33:625, 1970
*230. Trontelj JV: A study of the H reflex by single fibre EMG. J Neurol Neurosurg Psychiatry 36:951, 1973
231. Trontelj MA, Trontelj JV: Reflex arc of the first component of the human blink reflex: A single motoneurone study. J Neurol Neurosurg Psychiatry 41:538, 1978
*232. Tung AS, Tenicela R, Giovannitti: Letter: Rectus abdominis nerve entrapment syndrome. JAMA 240:738, 1978
233. Urschel HC, Razzuk MA et al: The technique of measuring conduction velocity for thoracic outlet syndrome. In Pain in Shoulder and Arm: An Integrated View, pp 165–172. The Hague, Martinus Nijhoff, 1979
*234. Vitti M et al: Electromyographic investigations of the tongue and circumoral muscular sling with fine wire electrodes. J Dent Res 54:844, 1975
235. Wainapel SF, Kim DJ, Ebel A: Conduction studies of the saphenous nerve in healthy subjects. Arch Phys Med Rehabil 59:316, 1978
236. Wallach HW, Oren ME: Sciatic nerve compression during anticoagulation therapy: Computerized tomography aids in diagnosis. Arch Neurol 36:448, 1979
237. Warren JD: Anterior interosseous nerve palsy as a complication of forearm fracture. J Bone Joint Surg 45B:511, 1963
238. Weber ER, Daube JR, Coventry MB: Peripheral neuropathies associated with total hip arthroplasty. J Bone Joint Surg 58A:66, 1976
239. Weber RJ, Piero DL: F wave evaluation of thoracic outlet syndrome: A multiple regression derived F wave latency predicting technique. Arch Phys Med Rehabil 59:464, 1978
240. Weber RJ, Piero D: Entrapment syndromes. In Johnson EW (ed) Practical Electromyography. Baltimore, Williams & Wilkins, 1980
241. Wiederholt WC: Median nerve conduction velocity in sensory fibers through carpal tunnel. Arch Phys Med Rehabil 51:328, 1970
242. Wilbourn AJ: True Neurogenic Thoracic Outlet Syndrome. Case Report 7, Rochester, MN, American Association of Electromyography and Electrodiagnosis, 1982
243. Wilbourn AJ, Lambert E: The forearm median-to-ulnar nerve communication: Electrodiagnostic aspects. Neurology 26:368, 1976
244. Woltman H: Crossing the legs as a factor in the production of peroneal palsy. JAMA 93:670, 1929
245. Woodhall B: Trapezius paralysis following minor surgical procedures in the posterior cervical triangle: Results following cranial nerve suture. Ann Surg 136:375–380, 1952
*246. Wright JS: The neurovascular syndrome produced by hyperabduction of the arms. Am Heart J 29:1, 1945
*247. Wulff CH, Gilliatt RW: F waves in patients with hand wasting from a cervical rib. Muscle Nerve 2:452–457, 1979
*248. Yap C, Hirota T: Sciatic nerve motor conduction velocity study. J Neurol Neurosurg Psychiatry 30:233, 1967
249. Yu J, Bendler EM, Mentari A: Neurological disorders associated with carpal tunnel syndrome. Electromyogr Clin Neurophysiol 19:27–31, 1979

6
H *Reflex and* F *Wave*

Jennifer Chu-Andrews
Francis L. Bruyninckx

H REFLEX

The H reflex, originally described by Hoffmann, is the electrical analogue of the ankle jerk. It is usually recorded from the soleus in the adult but may be recorded from the flexor carpi radialis.[4,9] In infants the H reflex may also be recorded on stimulation of the ulnar nerve.[8,17]

The H reflex is a monosynaptic reflex obtained by using subthreshold current to stimulate the group Ia afferent fibers from the muscle spindle. This reflex thus bypasses stimulation of the spindles themselves. The H reflex is a measure of the conduction along the sensory Ia afferent fibers and the conduction from the spinal cord along the motor axons. It is affected by any lesion along its path. Routinely, subthreshold stimulation is used to record the H reflex. If this stimulation is done repeatedly, it excites the same motor neuron pool each time. Hence, the latency of the H reflex is constant when recorded with surface electrodes. However, with single-fiber electromyographic (SFEMG) studies the H-reflex latency is variable because the time involved for synaptic transmission of single axons is observed.[15,18]

F WAVE

The F wave, originally described by Magladery and McDougal,[11] is obtained by antidromic stimulation of the anterior horn cells by using supramaximal stimulation of a peripheral nerve and recording from the distal muscles supplied by this nerve. The more proximal the stimulation, the shorter the latency. The F response is a measure of conduction along the most proximal segments of the motor nerve. Because it excites primarily the larger motor neurons, conduction along the fastest fibers is measured. Since different motor neurons are activated on successive stimulations, the F-response latency, if recorded with surface electrodes, shows considerable variation. However, with SFEMG recordings, very little variation is seen between the successive F responses because no synapses are involved. This is in contrast to the variability seen in SFEMG recordings of the H reflex.

An increase in F-wave latencies does not signify delayed proximal conduction times in the presence of either distal pathology or an entrapment along the peripheral nerve supplying the muscle from which the recording is obtained. Therefore, F-wave latency minus distal latency is the parameter employed for estimation of conduction of the proximal segments (see Chap. 5 for our normal values). In measuring F-wave latencies, the shortest latency of 10 to 20 discharges is recorded, but the longest latency may also be measured to determine the degree of dispersion of the conduction times along different axons.[12]

Kimura[10] uses the "F ratio" to assess pathology along the proximal nerve segment. This ratio is obtained by using the following formula:

$$\text{Proximal latency} = \frac{F_{prox} - M_{prox} - 1\ \text{msec}}{2}$$

$$\text{F ratio} = \frac{\text{Proximal latency}}{M_{prox}}$$

F_{prox} = F latency obtained by proximal stimulation at the elbow or knee

M_{prox} = motor latency obtained by proximal stimulation.

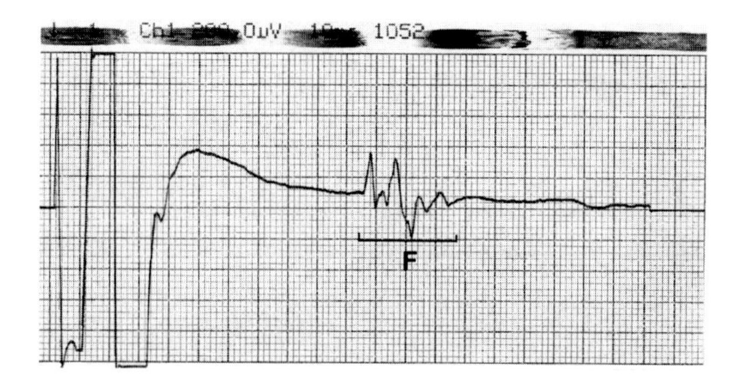

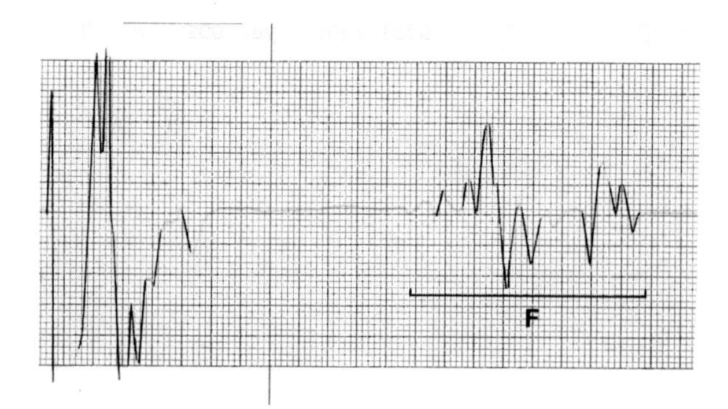

FIGURE 6-1 The F wave. The top trace illustrates an F wave recorded from the abductor hallucis with stimulation of the tibial nerve in a normal subject. The bottom trace is the recording of an F wave from the same muscle in a patient with peripheral neuropathy. Note that in this trace the M response is smaller than normal, and the F wave is large in amplitude and prolonged in duration. Sweep speed 10 msec/div., sensitivity 200 μV/div.

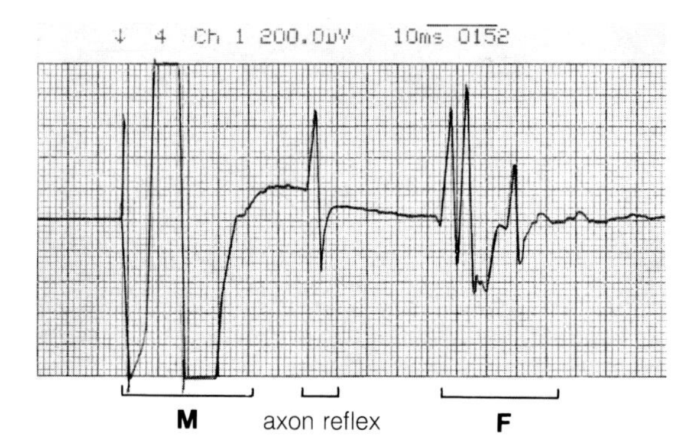

FIGURE 6-2 The axon reflex. The arrow indicates the position of the stimulus artifact. From left to right, the responses are the M wave, the axon reflex, and the F wave. The axon reflex, when present, is usually between the M and F waves. Note also that in this trace the F wave is large in amplitude and prolonged in duration. This trace was obtained from a patient with tarsal tunnel syndrome, and the recording was from the abductor hallucis, with stimulation of the tibial nerve at the ankle. Sweep speed 10 msec/div., sensitivity 200 μV/div.

One millisecond is subtracted because this is the time delay encountered by the stimulus at the level of the anterior horn cell.

F ratios are as follows[10]:

Median nerve stimulation at the elbow crease: 0.98 ± 0.08
Ulnar nerve stimulation 3 cm proximal to the medial epicondyle: 1.05 ± 0.09
Peroneal nerve stimulation immediately above the head of the fibula: 1.05 ± 0.09
Tibial nerve stimulation at the popliteal fossa: 1.11 ± 0.11

An increased F ratio indicates proximal slowing in the presence of either normal or slow peripheral nerve conduction.

F waves may increase in amplitude in the presence of upper motor neuron lesions and spasticity.[5,7] F-wave amplitude also increases in lower motor neuron lesions with chronic extensive reinnervation (Fig. 6-1).[16]

AXON REFLEX

The axon reflex is a reflex response that, when present, ususally occurs between the M response and the F wave (Fig. 6-2).[6] This reflex is seen because of collateral reinnervation and thus is commonly seen with peripheral neuropathies and chronic entrapment syndromes.[13,14] The re-

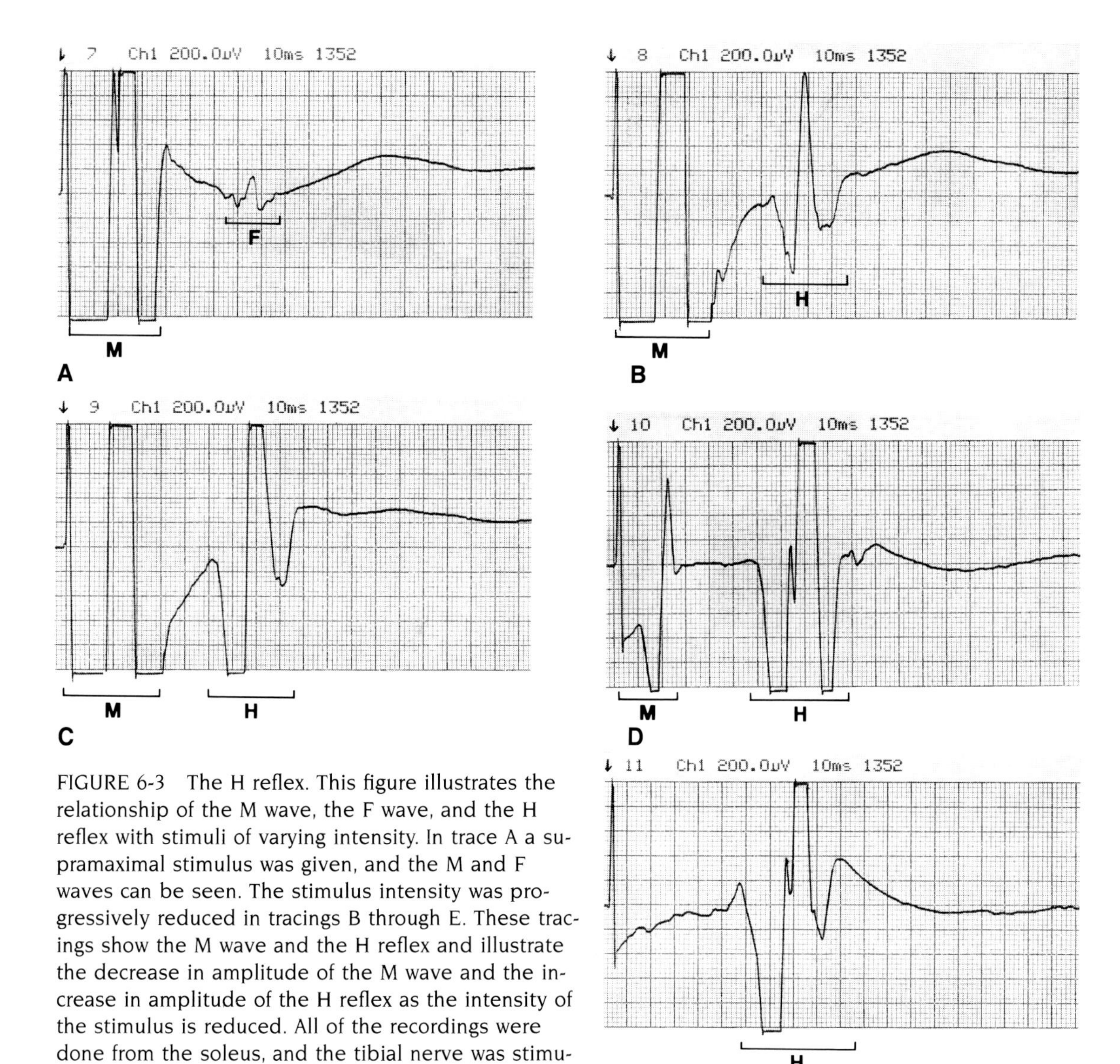

FIGURE 6-3 The H reflex. This figure illustrates the relationship of the M wave, the F wave, and the H reflex with stimuli of varying intensity. In trace A a supramaximal stimulus was given, and the M and F waves can be seen. The stimulus intensity was progressively reduced in tracings B through E. These tracings show the M wave and the H reflex and illustrate the decrease in amplitude of the M wave and the increase in amplitude of the H reflex as the intensity of the stimulus is reduced. All of the recordings were done from the soleus, and the tibial nerve was stimulated at the popliteal fossa. Calibrations: Sweep speed 10 msec/div., sensitivity 200 μV/div.

flex occurs when a distal and submaximal stimulus applied to a nerve with a collateral branch travels antidromically to the branching site and returns along the collateral branch. This reflex is not seen if the stimulus applied is supramaximal, since the collateral branch is stimulated simultaneously. The strong stimulus also generates an antidromic stimulus along the collateral branch, and this collides with the orthodromic impulse coming back down the same collateral from the branching point of the main nerve. Similarly, stimulation of the nerve proximal to the branching point blocks the reflex.

COMPARISON OF THE H REFLEX AND THE F WAVE (Fig. 6-3)

There are several differences between the H reflex and the F wave:

The H reflex is a monosynaptic reflex obtained with low-threshold stimulation and appears before the M response. The F wave is a response obtained by high-intensity antidromic stimulation of the anterior horn cells and therefore is always preceded by an M response.

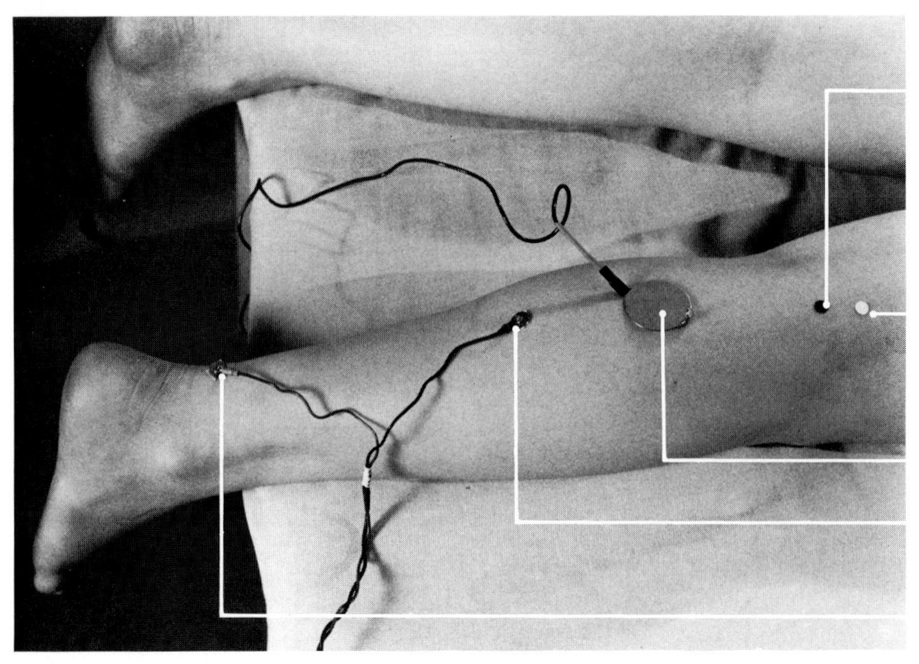

FIGURE 6-4 H reflex and F wave studies.
Note: The active recording electrode is placed at the junction of the lower borders of the lateral and medial gastrocnemii.

The amplitude of the H reflex when it first appears is larger than that of the direct M response. The amplitude decreases as the intensity of the stimulus is increased. The amplitude of the F wave is usually only about 1% that of the M response.[7]

The shape of the H reflex obtained from the soleus is usually triphasic, with an initial and terminal positivity and a central negativity. The F response appears less well summated. Its major deflection is usually negative, although it may be preceeded by a small positive wave.

The H reflex is constant in latency owing to activation of the same motor neuron pool. The F wave has a variable latency and is inconsistent in its appearance. This is due to activation of different groups of motor neurons.

In the adult the H reflex can be obtained readily only from the soleus muscle, whereas the F wave is readily obtainable from the intrinsic hand and foot muscles as well as from other muscles by stimulation of more proximal nerves (*e.g.*, from the facial muscles on stimulation of the facial nerve and from the vastus medialis and lateralis on stimulation of the femoral nerve).

PRACTICAL ASPECTS OF RECORDING THE H REFLEX AND F WAVE

Conduction Time

Amplifier setting:
- Sweep speed: 10 msec/div.
- Sensitivity: 200 μV/div.
- Filter setting: 20 Hz–10 kHz

Recording technique (Fig. 6-4):
- Patient position: Prone, ankle hanging off the edge of the bed
- Active electrode: Over the soleus muscle at about the junction of the lower borders of the medial and lateral gastrocnemius
- Reference electrode: Over the Achilles tendon
- Ground electrode: On the calf, between the

TABLE 6-1
Normal Values for H-Reflex and F-Wave Latencies (Soleus)

Age (Years)	*Data (No.)*	*H-Reflex Latency (msec)*	*F-Wave Latency (msec)*
20–29	100	28.5 ± 2.4 (23.7–33.3)	30.6 ± 2.7 (25.2–36.0)
30–39	100	28.6 ± 2.4 (23.8–33.4)	30.4 ± 2.8 (25.2–36.0)
40–49	100	29.4 ± 1.9 (25.6–33.2)	32.0 ± 1.9 (28.2–35.8)
50–59	100	29.4 ± 1.9 (25.6–33.2)	31.2 ± 2.2 (26.8–35.6)
Below 60	400	29.0 ± 2.2 (24.6–33.4)	31.1 ± 2.4 (26.7–35.9)
Above 60	40	30.1 ± 2.2 (25.7–34.5)	32.7 ± 2.2 (28.3–37.1)
All ages combined	440	29.2 ± 2.2 (24.8–33.6)	31.4 ± 2.4 (26.6–36.2)

stimulating electrode and the active recording electrode

Stimulation technique: Stimulate at the bend of the knee approximately 1 cm lateral to the midline of the popliteal fossa. Stimulation is done with the cathode distal to the anode. Give a submaximal stimulus at a rate of about one stimulus every 2 seconds. Adjust the stimulus so that a maximal amplitude for the H reflex is obtained. The M wave is absent or of minimal amplitude in normal patients. The amplitude of the H reflex is considered to be depressed if the M wave appears before the H reflex with subthreshold stimulation. In such cases an abnormality in conduction along the afferent pathway should be considered. H-reflex latency is measured when amplitude is maximal. The muscles of the anterior compartment of the leg must be relaxed. Otherwise the H reflex may be suppressed or absent.

The F wave is obtained by applying high-intensity stimulation to the tibial nerve. You may find it easier to differentiate the H reflex from the F wave by obtaining the F wave first and then reducing the intensity of the stimulus to obtain the H reflex. This method helps in cases in which the H reflex, though present, has a depressed amplitude. In such cases the H reflex is sometimes mistaken for the F wave, since the amplitude of the H reflex is smaller than that of the M response. By decreasing the stimulus you can more easily observe the change in shape and amplitude occurring as the F wave is replaced by the H reflex. Also helpful in differentiating the two waves is assessment of their respective amplitudes at a low sensitivity (*e.g.*, 1000 μV/div.) so that the relationship between the late responses and the M response can be adequately assessed.

Normal Values* (Table 6-1)

Comments

Most laboratories examine the H reflex and F wave by stimulating with the cathode placed proximal to the anode to avoid anodal block.[2] F ratios are also studied with the cathode proximal to the anode.[10] Refer to our values only when our method, as described in the text, is used. H reflex can also be predicted by using a formula that incorporates the patient's leg length and age.[1]

H-reflex latency may be increased or the reflex may be absent in peripheral neuropathies and S1 radiculopathy.[1,3] In the absence of peripheral neuropathy, a difference of 2 msec in latency

*Values from the authors' laboratory

between the left and right or an asymmetric absence of the H reflex is a useful indicator for the diagnosis of S1 radiculopathy. In our experience, a difference of more than 3 msec between the H reflex and the F response from the soleus may also indicate conduction delay along the S1 motor fibers.

REFERENCES

1. Braddom RL, Johnson EW: Standardization of H reflex and diagnostic use in S1 radiculopathy. Arch Phys Med Rehabil 55:161, 1974
2. Daube JR: F-wave and H-reflex measurements. American Academy of Neurology Course 16: Clinical Electromyography, pp 93–101, 1979
3. Deschuytere J, Roselle N: Diagnostic use of monosynaptic reflexes in L5 and S1 root compression. In Desmedt JE (ed): New Developments in Electromyography and Clinical Neurophysiology, Vol 3, pp 360–366. Basel, S Karger, 1973
4. Deschuytere J, Roselle N, DeKeyser C: Monosynaptic reflexes in the superficial forearm flexors in man and their clinical significance. J Neurol Neurosurg Psychiatry 39:555, 1976
5. Eisen A, Odusote K: Amplitude of the F wave: A potential means of documenting spasticity. Neurology (NY) 29:1306, 1979
6. Fullerton PM, Gilliatt RW: Axon reflexes in human motor nerve fibres. J Neurol Neurosurg Psychiatry 28:1, 1965
7. Garcia-Mullin R, Mayer RF: H reflexes in acute and chronic hemiplegia. Brain 95:559, 1972
8. Hodes R: Effects of age, consciousness, and other factors on human electrically induced reflexes (EIRs). Electroencephalogr Clin Neurophysiol (Suppl) 25:80, 1967
9. Jabre JF: Surface recording of the H reflex of the flexor carpi radialis. Muscle Nerve 4:435, 1981
10. Kimura J: Electrodiagnosis in Diseases of Nerve and Muscle: Principles and Practice. Philadelphia, FA Davis, 1983
11. Magladery JW, McDougal DB Jr: Electrophysiological studies of nerve and reflex activity in normal man. I. Identification of certain reflexes in the electromyogram and the conduction velocity of peripheral nerve fibres. Bull Johns Hopkins Hosp 86:265, 1950
12. Panayiotopoulos CP: F chronodispersion: A new electrophysiologic method. Muscle Nerve 2:68–72, 1979
13. Roth G: Intranervous regeneration of lower motor neuron. I. Study of 1153 motor axon reflexes. Electromyogr Clin Neurophysiol 18:225, 1978
14. Roth G: Intranervous regeneration: The study of motor axon reflexes. J Neurol Sci 41:139, 1979
15. Schiller HH, Stålberg E: F responses studied with single fibre EMG in normal subjects and spastic patients. J Neurol Neurosurg Psychiatry 41:45, 1978
16. Shahani BT, Potts F, Domingue J: F response studies in peripheral neuropathies (abstr.) Neurology (NY) 30:409, 1980
17. Thomas JE, Lambert EH: Ulnar nerve conduction velocity and H-reflex in infants and children. J Appl Physiol 15:1, 1960
18. Trontelj JV: A study of the H reflex by single fibre EMG. J Neurol Neurosurg Psychiatry 36:;951, 1973

7
Newer Techniques in Electrodiagnosis

Jennifer Chu-Andrews

SINGLE-FIBER ELECTROMYOGRAPHY

Single-fiber electromyography (SFEMG) is the most selective method of recording myoelectric signals. This method was developed by Ekstedt and Stålberg.[12] The importance of this method is that it enables the examiner to measure the combined variability in neuromuscular transmission time (jitter) in motor end-plates in pairs of muscle fibers belonging to the same motor unit. SFEMG is also used to determine fiber density, the average number of muscle fibers in one motor unit that can be recorded by the SFEMG needle within its pickup area of 300 μm.[11] The average number of muscle fibers is obtained after recording from 20 different sites within the muscle.

SFEMG is very sensitive in the detection of neurogenic changes, in addition to being the single most important test for detecting diseases of the neuromuscular junction such as myasthenia gravis and myasthenic syndrome. Other uses of SFEMG include the study of reflexes (*e.g.*, the axon reflex, H reflex, and blink reflex)[12] and the firing pattern of motor units.

Characteristics of the SFEMG Needle

The SFEMG needle is a microelectrode 25 μm in diameter encased in a stainless steel outer cannula (see Fig. 7-7). A side port in the cannula serves as the recording area. Because of the small size of the active electrode, the SFEMG needle can record the electrical activity of single muscle fibers.

Amplifier Characteristics and Settings

The amplifier must have a high input impedance, on the order of 100 MΩ. The common mode rejection ratio should be better than 200.[12] These requirements of the amplifier are needed because of the high impedance of the SFEMG needle. The amplifier must also have a trigger circuit and a delay line so that the signal can be displayed in its entirety at fast sweeps. Settings are as follows:

Sweep speed: 0.2 msec–0.5 msec/div.

Sensitivity: 200 μV–5 mV/div. (occasionally 10 mV/div.) Amplitude fluctuates dramatically with slight movements of the needle away from the active muscle fibers. This is due to the small recording surface of the SFEMG needle.[4] Therefore, the recording position is critical.

Filter setting: 500 Hz–10 kHz. The low-frequency (high-pass) filter is set at 500 Hz so that low-frequency contributions from the distant fibers can be attenuated. With this filter the background activity is selectively reduced. The amplitudes of the action potentials of the muscle fibers close to the needle are attenuated by only about 10%.[3,4] The high-frequency (low-pass) filter must be set to at least 10 kHz so that amplitude distortions of the fast components are avoided.[12]

Jitter and Blocking

Jitter is the term used to express normal variability in neuromuscular transmission time. Using

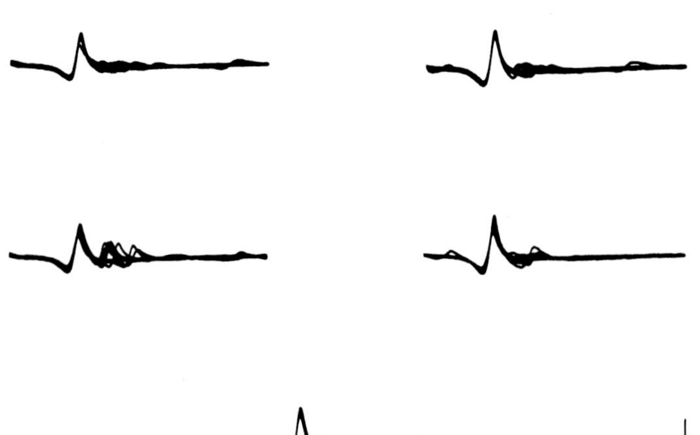

FIGURE 7-1 Superimposed tracings of a pair of single-fiber potentials showing increased jitter and blocking. Calibrations: Sweep speed 0.5 msec/div., sensitivity 500 μV/div.

SFEMG, you can record the interpotential interval (IPI) variation between two or more muscle fibers belonging to the same motor unit. The IPI is the duration between two action potentials, usually approximately 1 msec. IPIs vary at consecutive discharges of the muscle fibers of the same motor unit. This variability is termed the *jitter*. Jitter results from the variation in the time that impulses take to propagate from the common branching point of the axon along the individual nerve branches, motor end-plates, and muscle fibers. Variability in impulse transmission time at the end-plate is believed to be the main contribution to jitter.

Blocking occurs when there is failure of neuromuscular transmission. There will be failure of discharge of one of the muscle fibers of a potential pair (Figs. 7-1 and 7-2). Blocking usually occurs when jitter values exceed 100 μsec.

Blocking is common in early reinnervation, especially during the first 3 months. This is because of the presence of immature nerve terminals and end-plates.[5,12] Occasionally two or more muscle fibers belonging to the same motor unit may block at the same time. This indicates that the blocking has taken place at the branching point of the nerve twig (Fig. 7-3).[12]

Calculation of Jitter

Jitter values can be calculated manually or automatically. Manual measurements consist in calculation of jitter from superimposed tracings of potential pairs recorded on fiberoptic paper (Fig. 7-4). Usually, five groups of ten superimposed discharges of a fiber pair are analyzed. The range is measured between two identical points on the fast positive/negative deflections of the action potentials. The mean IPI or jitter value obtained in this fashion is multiplied by a conversion factor of 0.37, and the resulting value is known as the mean of the consecutive time interval differences (MCD). The MCD is a measure of the short-term variability and is unaffected by slow trends, which can occur because of the differences in the degree of slowing of propagation velocity along the two muscle fibers with continuous contraction. Also, slight displacements of the needle can distort the shape of the action potential, which can affect the ranges measured. In such situations the standard deviation would increase, thus affecting the jitter measurements. Therefore, the jitter values obtained are always converted to and expressed as MCD values. Different conversion factors can be used depending on the number of consecutive discharges superimposed.[1] Calculation of MCD is done on 20 pairs of potentials. Ideal measurements of jitter are made on line with the aid of a computer.[7] Softwear is available to analyze the jitter off line with the aid of a digitizer connected to a computer. A jitter meter is also available to analyze the jitter on line. The jitter meter uses a microprocessor that can be plugged into a computer.

METHOD OF RECORDING

Insert the SFEMG needle into the patient's muscle when the patient is contracting it very slightly. Instruct the patient to contract the muscle very slightly, to listen to the firing rate of the poten-

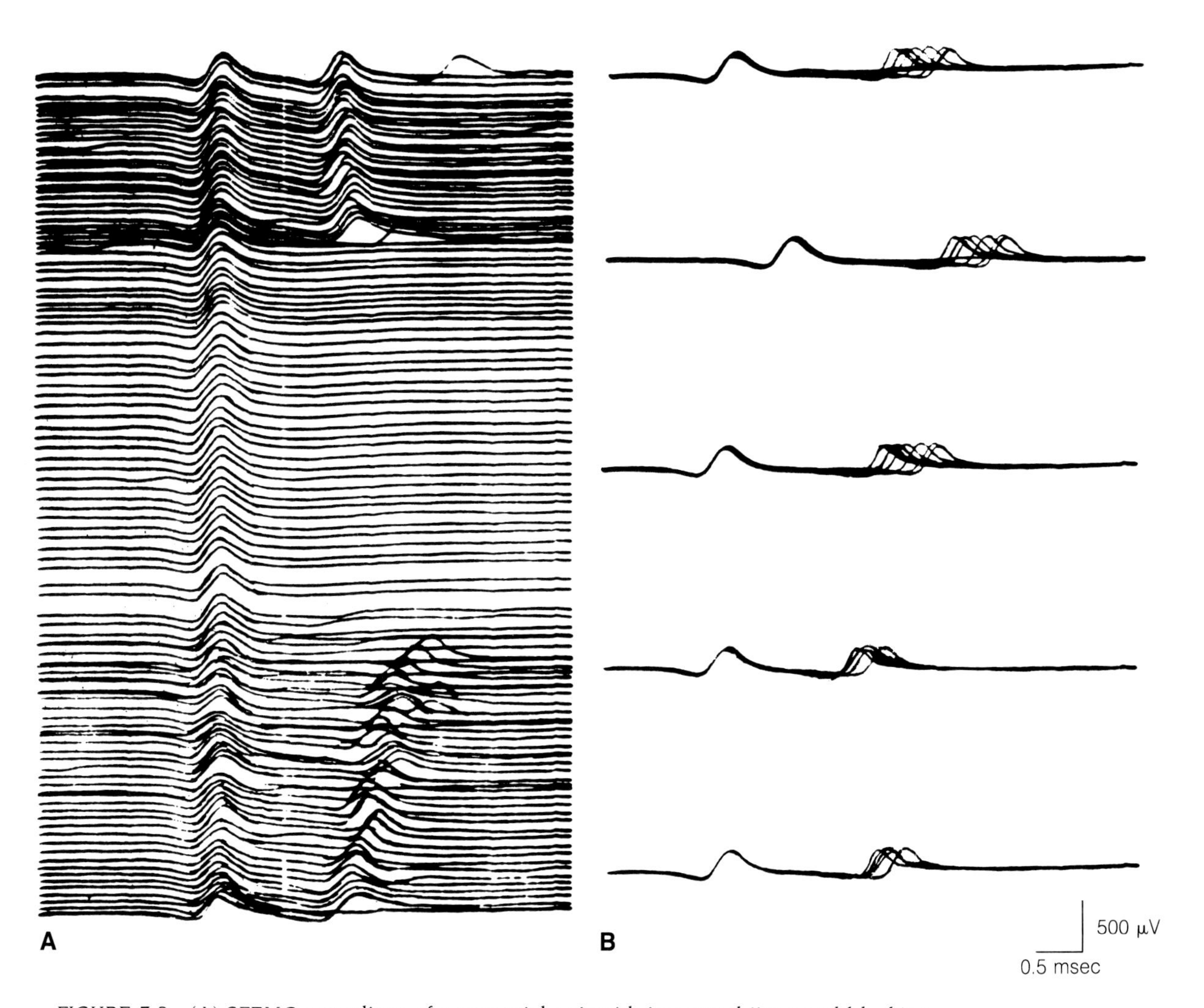

FIGURE 7-2 (A) SFEMG recordings of a potential pair with increased jitter and blocking. The initial tracing is at the bottom of the strip. The second potential in this trace has increased jitter in the lower part and eventually blocks in the middle part. In the upper part the second potential reappears, and the jitter is less than that seen before the blocking took place. The five tracings in B are five groups of ten superimposed discharges of the same pair of single-fiber potentials as seen in A. The superimposed tracings demonstrate the variations in interpotential intervals. The upper two traces also demonstrate blocking of the second potential. Calibrations: Sweep speed 0.5 msec/div., sensitivity 500 μV/div.

tials, and to keep them firing steadily. Position the needle to record two or more muscle fibers firing in a time-locked manner. There should be no variation in the amplitude of the action potentials from discharge to discharge. Record 20 pairs of potentials. The number of pairs of potentials with increased jitter and/or blocking is expressed as a percentage of the total number of pairs recorded. In the measurement of jitter it is essential to have a stable trigger so that erroneous measurements are avoided. The trigger point is most stable when positioned on the negative portion of the rise time of the action potential, close to the baseline.

NORMAL VALUES

Normal values are 5 μsec to 55 μsec. Two or more potential pairs must exceed this normal

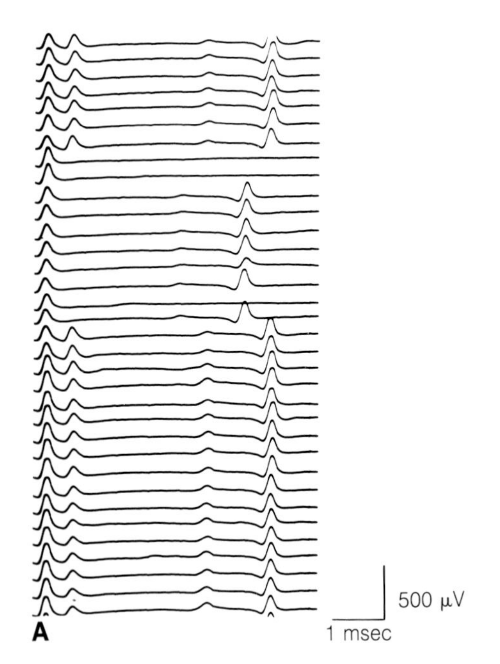

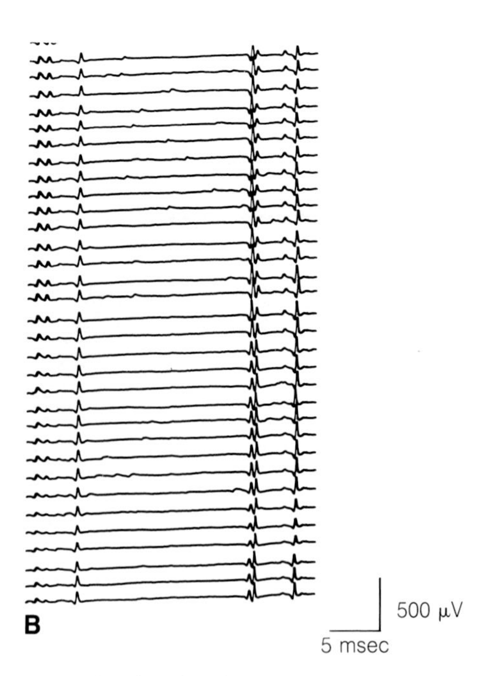

FIGURE 7-3 (A) Axonal blocking in a potential recorded from the rhomboideus major in a patient with C5 radiculopathy. The third and fourth potentials block together and also show increased jitter in relation to the rest of the complex. Axonal jitter and blocking can be identified only when a potential complex consists of at least four muscle fibers. Note also in this trace the increased jitter and blocking of the second potential. This potential shows blocking irrespective of the axonal blocking of the third and fourth potentials. The blocking seen in the second potential is that associated with uncertain neuromuscular transmission, in this case probably due to immature end-plates related to reinnervation. Calibrations: Sweep speed 1 msec/div., sensitivity 500 μV/div. (B) A multispike potential recorded from the same muscle as in A. Frequent blocking is present in the small potentials seen between the more stable parts of the potential complex. The stable parts of the potential complex are at the far left and far right of the trace. Calibrations: Sweep speed 5 msec/div., sensitivity 500 μV/div.

limit before a study is interpreted as abnormal. The study is still regarded as normal when only a single potential pair out of the 20 studied shows increased jitter, even when blocking is present in that pair.[12]

MEANING OF INCREASED VALUES

Increased jitter is seen with disturbances in neuromuscular transmission. Examples of this are diseases of the neuromuscular junction (myasthenia gravis, myasthenic syndrome), ischemia, curare poisoning, and early reinnervation.[10] In reinnervation, jitter may remain increased for up to 6 months.[5,12]

SFEMG is the most sensitive test for documentation of myasthenia gravis.[8] It can detect this disease before its clinical manifestations become apparent.[10] Jitter is increased in this disease, and it increases with exercise. By the time the patient manifests clinical weakness, blocking is usually observed on SFEMG.[2,8,12,13] A combination of the repetitive stimulation study and the SFEMG examination is highly sensitive for detecting myasthenia gravis.[8] If cranial myasthenia is suspected, facial muscles (*e.g.*, frontalis or orbicularis oculi) must be studied. The SFEMG examination can be performed without withholding the patient's anticholinesterase medications. In myasthenia gravis, blocking is inherent in patients with a positive decremental result on slow repetitive stimulation.

Jitter and blocking are observed in myasthenic

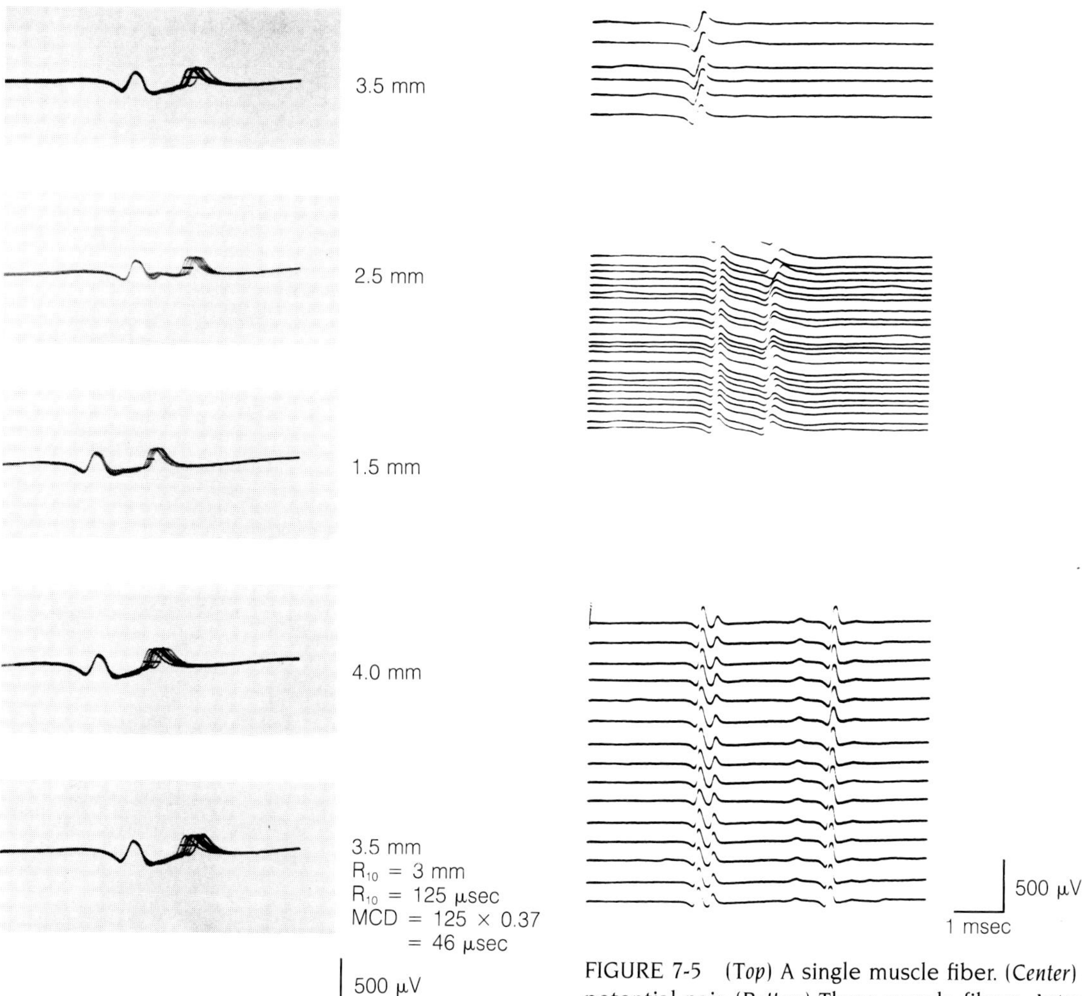

FIGURE 7-4 Superimposed tracings of a pair of single-fiber potentials. Usually, ten discharges are superimposed in each trace, and five different traces of the same potential pair are recorded. The IPI variation in each trace is measured, and the mean is obtained. The mean value is multiplied by a conversion factor of 0.37 to obtain the mean of the consecutive differences. Calibrations: Sweep speed 0.5 msec/div., sensitivity 500 μV/div.

FIGURE 7-5 (*Top*) A single muscle fiber. (*Center*) A potential pair. (*Bottom*) Three muscle fibers. Actually, four muscle fibers are seen by the SFEMG needle, but the third fiber is not counted in fiber density measurements, since it does not have an amplitude of 200 μV. The third muscle fiber is not within the 300-μm uptake area of the SFEMG needle. See also Fig. 7-3 for a complex potential showing multiple muscle fibers. Calibrations: Sweep speed 1.0 msec/div., sensitivity 500 μV/div.

syndrome. In contrast to myasthenia gravis, however, jitter and blocking decrease with exercise.[10]

Increased jitter values are also seen with decreasing intramuscular temperature. Jitter values increase 2 μsec to 3 μsec per degree Celsius fall in intramuscular temperature from 36°C to 32°C. They increase 7.5 μsec per degree Celsius drop in temperature below 32°C.[9]

MEANING OF DECREASED VALUES

Decreased jitter is seen in muscular dystrophies. The jitter values are frequently less than 5 μsec.[12] The second muscle fiber of a given pair is frequently a branch of the first muscle fiber that has resulted from fiber splitting or budding. Con-

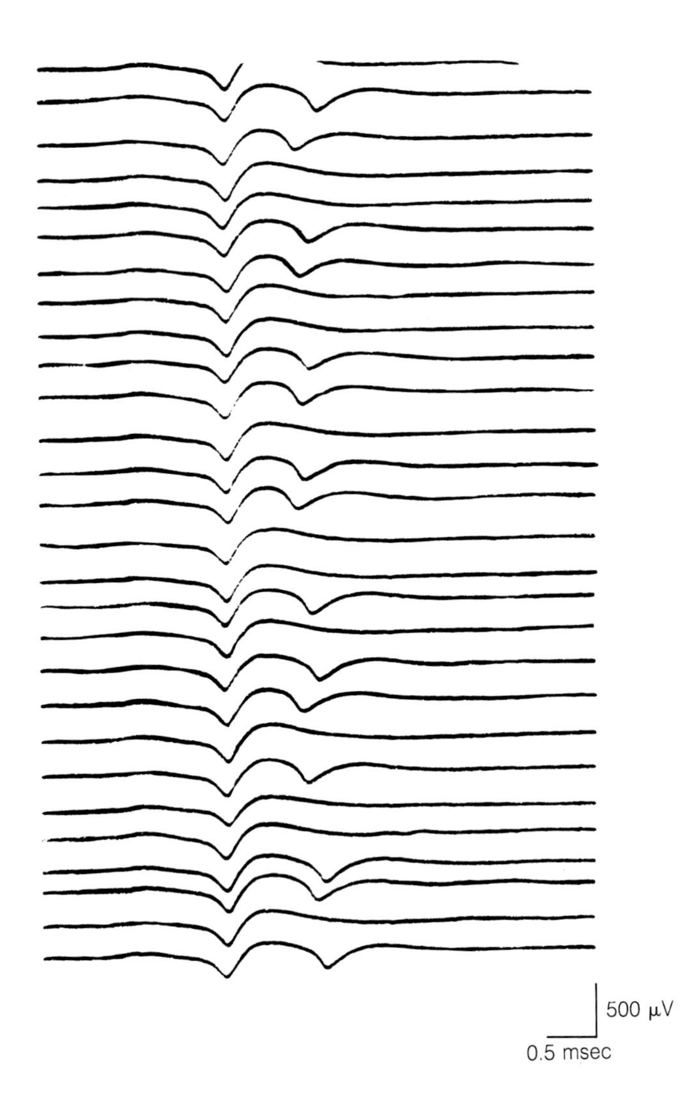

FIGURE 7-6 Serial tracings of a single-fiber potential that has been damaged by the tip of the single-fiber electrode. The second action potential is seen to block occasionally. These types of potentials are not accepted for jitter or fiber density measurements. Calibrations: Sweep spread 0.5 msec/div., sensitivity 500 μV/div.

sequently, no neuromuscular transmission time is involved in the IPI.

Fiber Density

Fiber density is a sensitive measure of the arrangement of muscle fibers within a focal area. It is calculated as the mean number of muscle fibers that can be recorded by the SFEMG needle, which records from a hemisphere area of 300 μm in diameter.[11]

Method of Measurement

Fiber density measurements should be done independently of jitter measurements. Manipulate the needle until the triggering potential has a rise time of 300 μsec and has reached its maximal amplitude. Count each potential with an amplitude of at least 200 μV and a rise time of less than 300 μsec. Include the trigerring potential in this calculation (Fig. 7-5; see also Fig. 7-3). The sweep speed must be slower than that used for measurement of jitter. Typically, a sweep speed of 0.5 msec to 1 msec is needed to accommodate all of the muscle fibers firing in synchrony with the triggering potential. Sweep speeds up to 5 msec are sometimes necessary. Occasionally the tip of the needle may damage some muscle fibers, and the activity from these fibers is seen as positive waves. Do not include these positive waves in the measurement of fiber density or jitter (Fig. 7-6). Perform the recording from 20

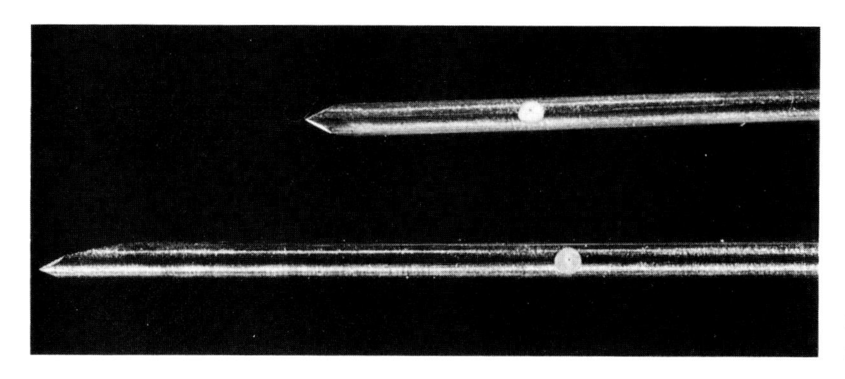

FIGURE 7-7 (*Top*) SFEMG needle. (*Bottom*) Macro EMG needle.

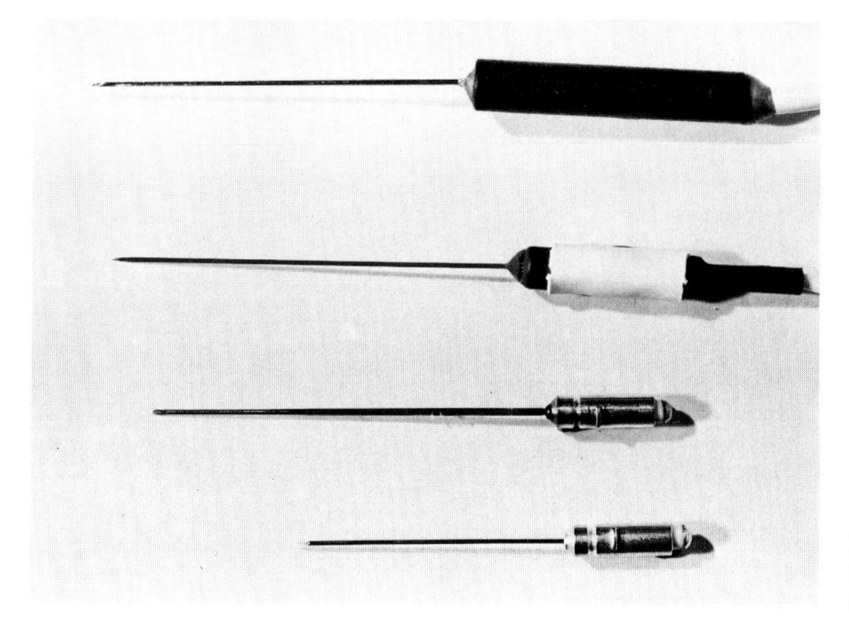

FIGURE 7.8 (*Top to bottom*) Concentric, monopolar, macro, and SFEMG needles.

different recording sites, using at least four skin insertion sites. Then calculate the mean of the number of action potentials from these sites. Normally, only about 30% to 50% of the recording sites reveal a potential pair. The average fiber density is 1.3 to 1.5. This average is different for different muscles: the biceps brachii seems to have the lowest fiber density, and the extensor digitorum brevis seems to have the highest.[12] The fiber density increases with age. Higher fiber densities are seen particularly in the tibialis anterior and extensor digitorum (communis) after age 70 years.[12]

An increase in fiber density (see Fig. 7-3) is seen with collateral reinnervation (*e.g.*, in diseases of the anterior horn cells and peripheral neuropathies) and in muscular dystrophies and polymyositis[6] from fiber splitting and budding.

MACRO EMG

Macro EMG is a newer EMG technique developed by Stålberg.[17,22] This method is used to determine the electrical activity of the total motor unit. Macro EMG, when used in conjunction with conventional EMG and SFEMG, is very useful in helping one to understand the motor unit in the normal patient and in disease.

Characteristics of the Macro EMG *Needle*[17]

The needle consists of a stainless steel cannula coated with Teflon up to 15 mm proximal to the tip. A side port is placed at the center of the exposed cannula shaft so that an SFEMG needle is exposed (Figs. 7-7 and 7-8).

Method of Recording[17]

Two-channel recordings are done. In the first channel, filter settings are adjusted to 500 Hz–10 kHz, and the SFEMG signals are recorded via the SFEMG needle referenced to the cannula. In the second channel, filter settings are adjusted to 8 Hz–8 kHz, and signals from the cannula are referenced to a concentric or monopolar needle placed subcutaneously in an area remote from the muscle where the recording is being performed (*e.g.*, on the tendon of the biceps femoris for recording of the quadriceps). Recording of macro EMG potentials is done with a sweep speed of 5 msec to 7 msec/div. Averaging of the cannula signals that are time locked to the triggering SFEMG signal gives the macro EMG potential. The macro MUP is usually delayed before it is averaged and displayed. This MUP represents the temporal and spatial summation of the electrical activity of the majority of the muscle fibers of the motor unit to which the triggered SFEMG potential belongs (Fig. 7-9). Fiber density recordings are done on the SFEMG channel.

Twenty macro MUPs are collected from at least four skin insertions. If two macro MUPs have exactly the same shape, the second potential is discarded. Usually only the SFEMG channel is monitored while one is searching for new macro MUPs to avoid bias in the selection of the macro MUPs.

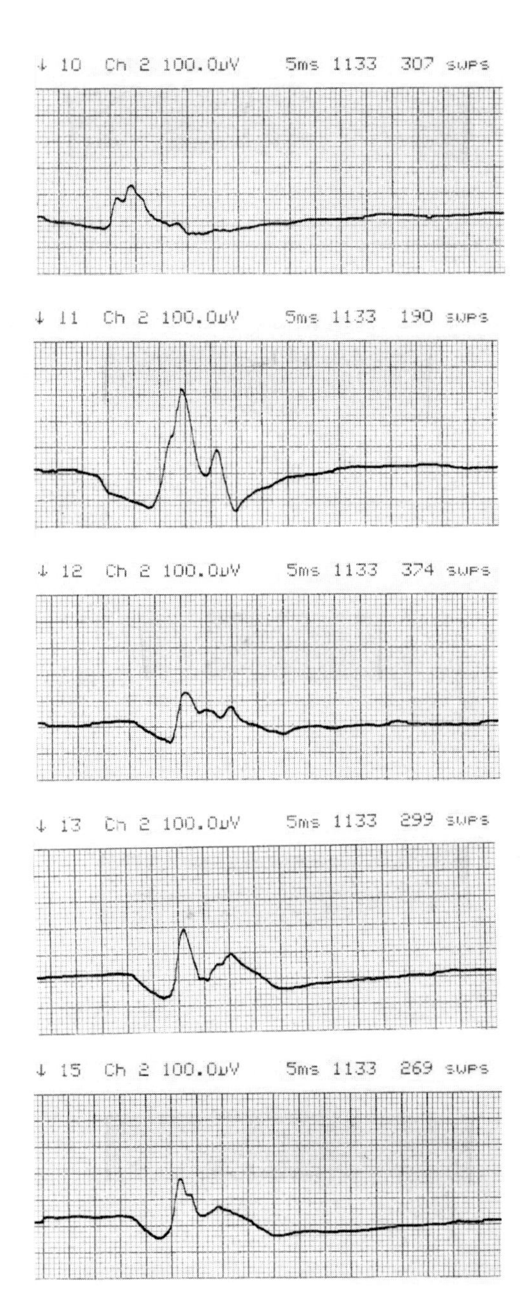

FIGURE 7-9 Macro MUPs recorded from the biceps brachii.

Characteristics

The shape of the macro MUP depends on the number and size of muscle fibers in the motor unit, the arrangement of the end-plates, and the distance of the needle from the end-plate region. The shape of a macro MUP differs from muscle to muscle.[17]

Normally, there is great variation in the amplitudes of the macro MUPs. This variation has been attributed to (1) the different sizes (number of muscle fibers) of different units, (2) the recording position within the motor unit (*i.e.*, the amplitudes of MUPs recorded close to the center of the motor unit are twice as big as those recorded in the periphery of the motor unit), (3) the difference in the size of the motor units at different depths (the smaller motor units are recorded more deeply),[2] and (4) the difference in the recruitment threshold of motor units (the larger-threshold motor units are recruited later).[14,16]

In disease the changes of macro MUPs are similar to those seen with conventional EMG. In myopathies in general, the macro MUPs are of smaller amplitude. Even though the mean values of the amplitudes may not change, an increased number of MUPs with small amplitudes is seen.[15]

In reinnervation an increase in the number of MUPs with larger amplitudes is observed. If there is uneven reinnervation, discrepancies can be seen. For example, in amyotrophic lateral sclerosis the macro MUPs may be normal, enlarged, or small. A mixture of these findings reflects the different stages of the disease process and its progression, as well as the duration of the disease.[18] The findings are best interpreted together with the fiber density and jitter studies of SFEMG (see Anterior Horn Cell Diseases in Chap. 4).

In Guillain-Barré syndrome the amplitudes of the macro MUPs have been seen to be increased within the first week of the symptoms. This is found in association with normal fiber density on SFEMG. The underlying mechanism is believed to be the earlier recruitment of larger, higher-threshold MUPs.[19–21]

REFERENCES

Single-Fiber Electromyography

1. Ekstedt J, Nilsson G, Stålberg E: Calculation of the electromyographic jitter. J Neurol Neurosurg Psychiatry 37:526–539, 1974
2. Ekstedt J, Stålberg E: Myasthenia gravis: Diagnostic aspects by a new electrophysiological method. Opuscula Medica 12:73–76, 1967
3. Gath I, Stålberg E: On the volume conduction in human skeletal muscle: In situ measurements. Electroencephalogr Clin Neurophysiol 43:106, 1977
4. Gath I, Stålberg E: The calculated radial decline of the extracellular action potential compared with in situ measurements in the human brachial biceps. Electroencephalogr Clin Neurophysiol 44:547, 1978
5. Hakelius L, Stålberg E: Electromyographical studies of free autogenous muscle transplants in man. Scand J Plast Reconstr Surg 8:211, 1974
6. Henriksson KG, Stålberg E: The terminal innervation pattern in polymyositis: A histochemical and SFEMG study. Muscle Nerve 1:3 1978
7. Mihelin M, Trontelj JV: Automatic measurement of random interpotential intervals in single fibre electromyography. Int J Biomed Comput 6:181, 1975
8. Sanders DB, Howard JF, Johns TR: Single fiber electromyography in myasthenia gravis. Neurology (Minneap) 29:68–76, 1979
9. Stålberg E, Ekstedt J, Broman A: The electromyographic jitter in normal human muscles. Electroencephalogr Clin Neurophysiol 31:429, 1971
10. Stålberg E, Sanders DB: Electrophysiological tests of neuromuscular transmission. In Stålberg E, Young RR (eds): Clinical Neurophysiology, pp 89–116. Cornwall, England, Butterworth & Co, 1981
11. Stålberg E, Thiele B: Motor unit fibre density in the extensor digitorum communis muscle: Single fibre electromyographic study in normal subjects at different ages. J Neurol Neurosurg Psychiatry 38:874, 1975
12. Stålberg E, Trontelj J: Single Fibre Electromyography. Old Woking, Surrey, Mirvalle Press, 1979
13. Stålberg E, Trontelj J, Schwartz MS: Single muscle fibre recording of the jitter phenomenon in patients with myastenia gravis and in members of their families. Ann NY Acad Sci 274:189–262, 1976

Macro EMG

14. Clamann HP: Activity of single motor units during isometric tension. Neurology (Minneap) 20:254–260, 1970
15. Hilton-Brown P, Stålberg E: Motor unit size in muscular dystrophy, a macro EMG and scanning EMG study. J Neurol Neurosurg Psychiatry 46:996–1005, 1983
16. Milner Brown HS, Stein RB, Yemm R: The orderly recruitment of human motor units during voluntary isometric contractions. J Physiol (Lond) 230:359–370, 1973
17. Stålberg E: Macro EMG, a new recording technique. J Neurol Neurosurg Psychiatry 43:475–482, 1980
18. Stålberg E: Electrophysiological studies of re-innervation in ALS. In Rowland L (ed): Human Motor Neurone Diseases, pp 49–61. New York, Raven Press, 1982
19. Stålberg E: Macro electromyography in reinnervation. Muscle Nerve 5:S135–138, 1982
20. Stålberg E: Macro EMG. Minimonograph 20. Rochester, MN, American Association of Electromyography and Electrodiagnosis, 1983
21. Stålberg E, Antoni L: Computer-aided EMG analysis. In Desmedt JE (ed): Progress in Clinical Neurophysiology, Vol 10, pp 186–234. Basel, S Karger, 1983
22. Stålberg E, Fawcett PRW: Macro EMG in healthy subjects of different ages. J Neurol Neurosurg Psychiatry 45:870–878, 1982

APPENDIX

Diagrams of the Attachments of the Muscles

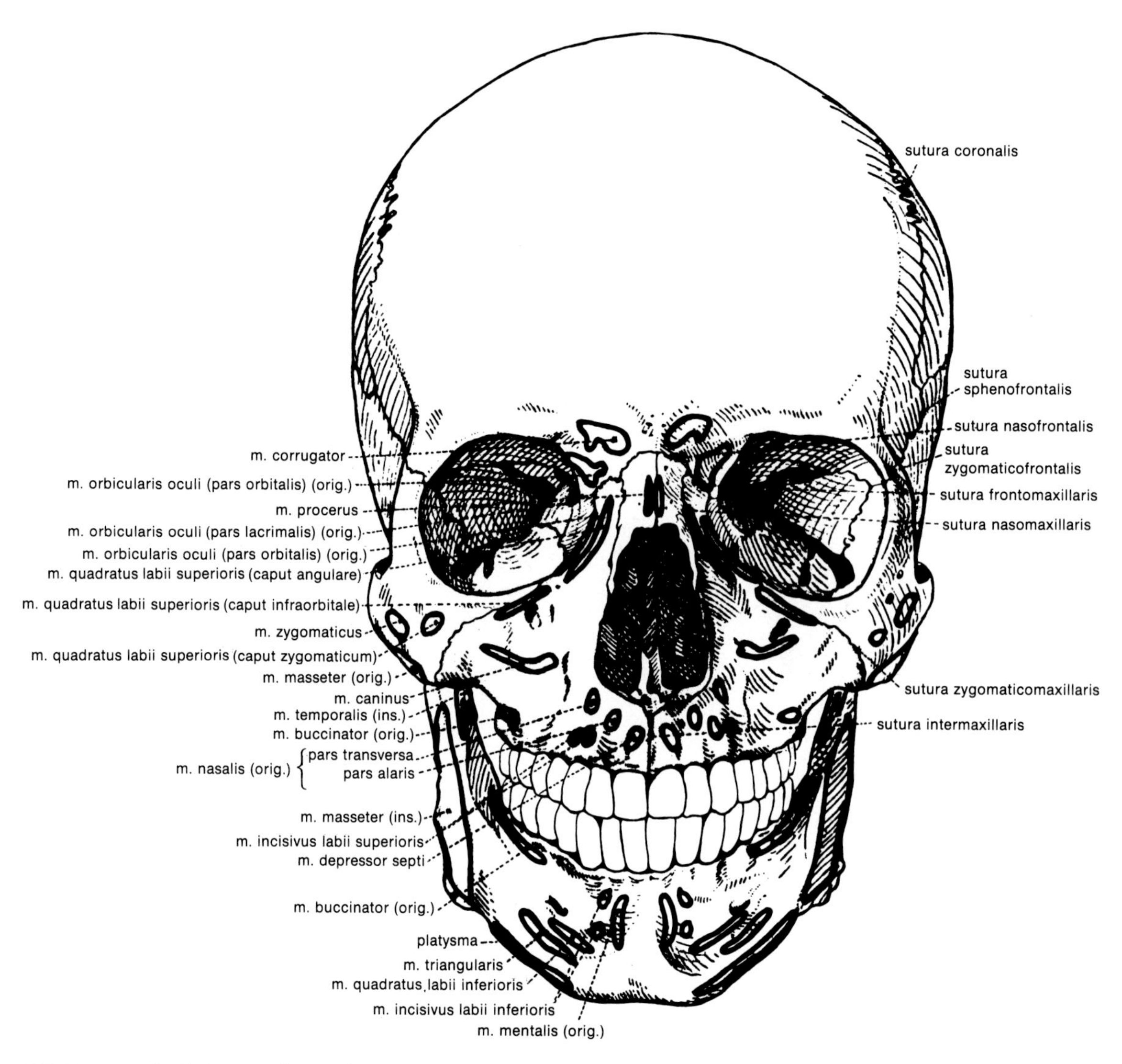

FIGURE 1 Skull, from in front, showing muscular attachments.
Note: Since 1955, certain facial muscles have different names, according to *Nomina Anatomica* (3rd ed. Amsterdam, Excerpta Medica, 1966).

Old Terminology	*New Terminology*
m. quadratus labii superioris, (caput angulare)	m. levator labii superioris alaeque nasi
m. quadratus labii superioris (caput infraorbitale)	m. levator labii superioris
m. quadratus labii superioris (caput zygomaticum)	m. zygomaticus minor
m. zygomaticus	m. zygomaticus major
m. caninus	m. levator anguli oris
m. nasalis (pars transversa)	m. compressor naris
m. nasalis (pars alaris)	m. depressor nasi
m. triangularis	m. depressor anguli oris

ins., insertion; *orig.*, origin
(Spalteholz W: Hand-Atlas of Human Anatomy, 7th ed., Vol 1. Philadelphia, JB Lippincott, 1937)

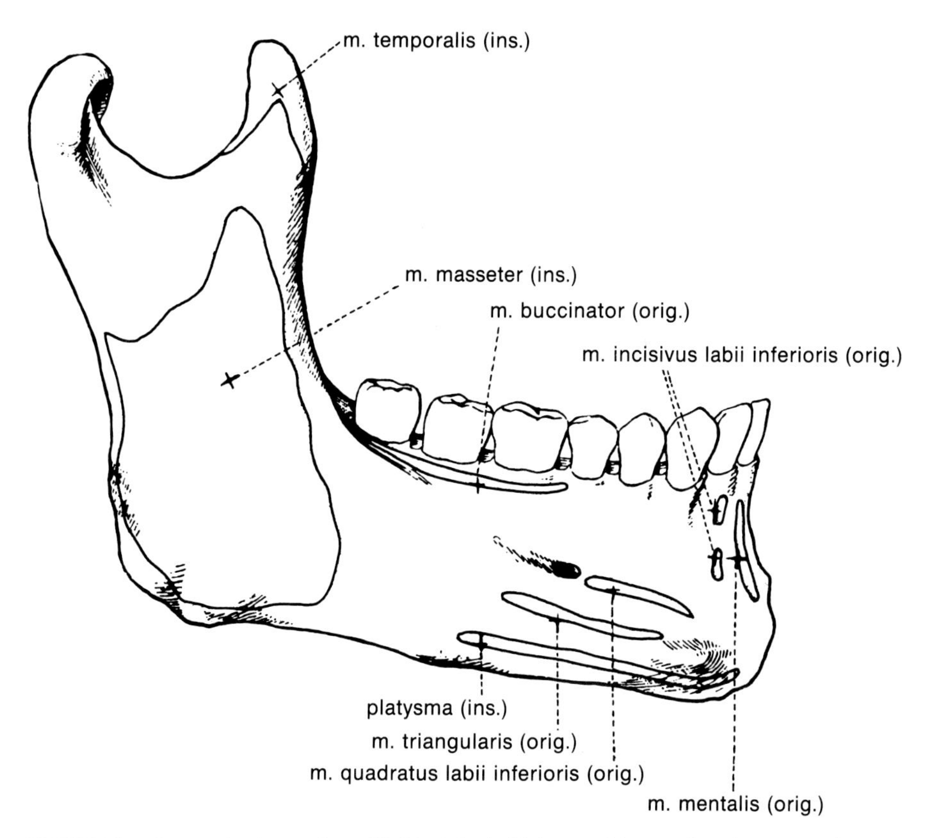

FIGURE 2 Lower jawbone (*mandibula*) right half, from without, showing muscular attachments.
ins., insertion; *orig.*, origin
(Spalteholz W: Hand-Atlas of Human Anatomy, 7th ed., Vol 1. Philadelphia, JB Lippincott, 1937)

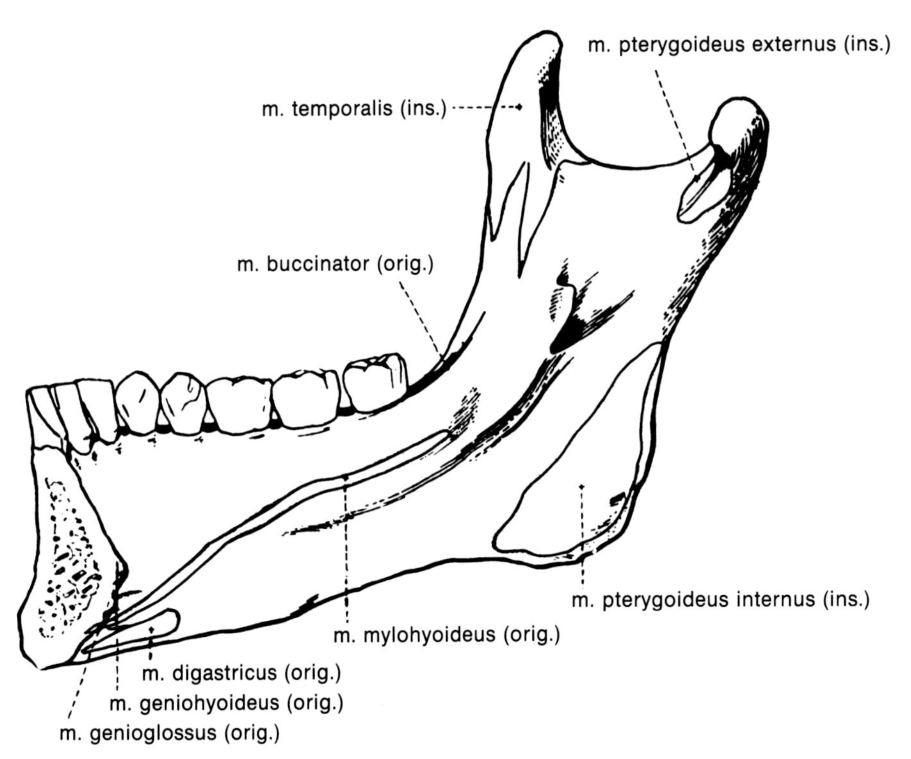

FIGURE 3 Lower jawbone (*mandibula*), right half, from within, showing muscular attachments.
ins., insertion; *orig.*, origin
(Spalteholz W: Hand-Atlas of Human Anatomy, 7th ed., Vol 1. Philadelphia, JB Lippincott, 1937)

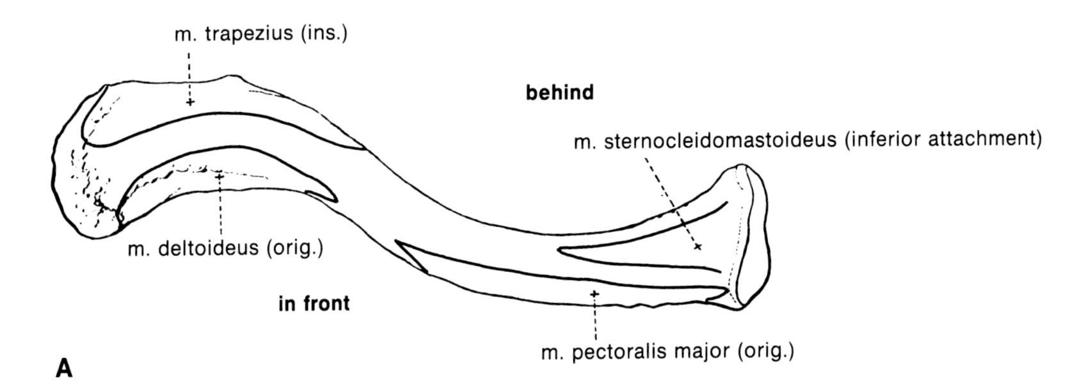

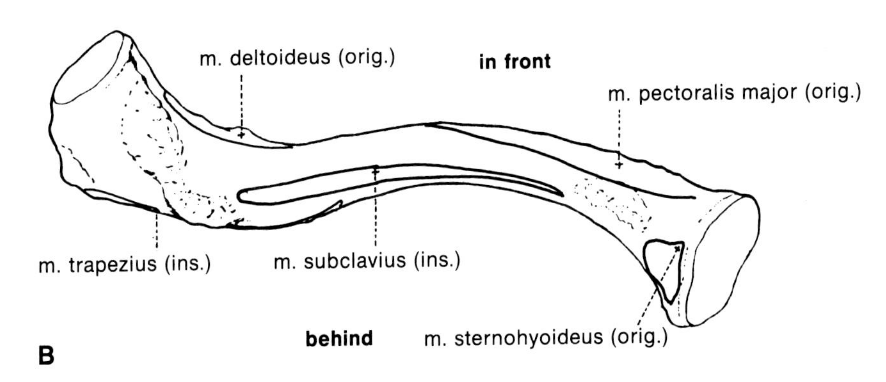

FIGURE 4 (A) Right collarbone, or clavicle (*clavicula*), from above, showing muscular attachments. (B) Right collarbone from below, showing muscular attachments.
ins., insertion; *orig.*, origin
(Spalteholz W: Hand-Atlas of Human Anatomy, 7th ed., Vol 1. Philadelphia, JB Lippincott, 1937)

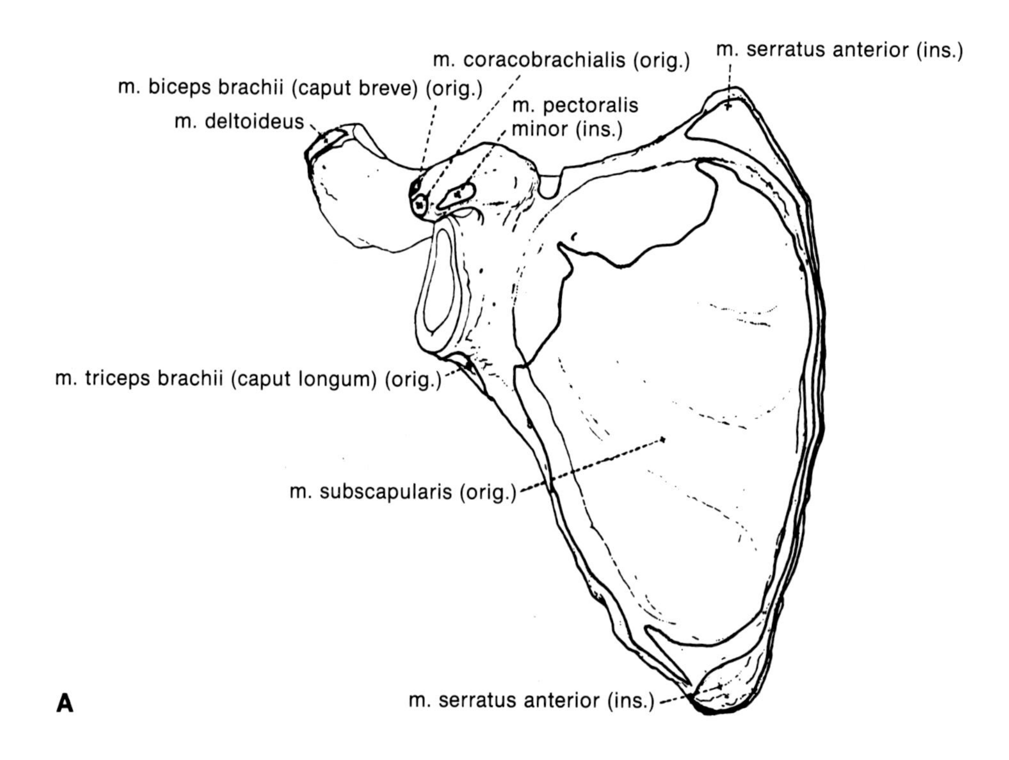

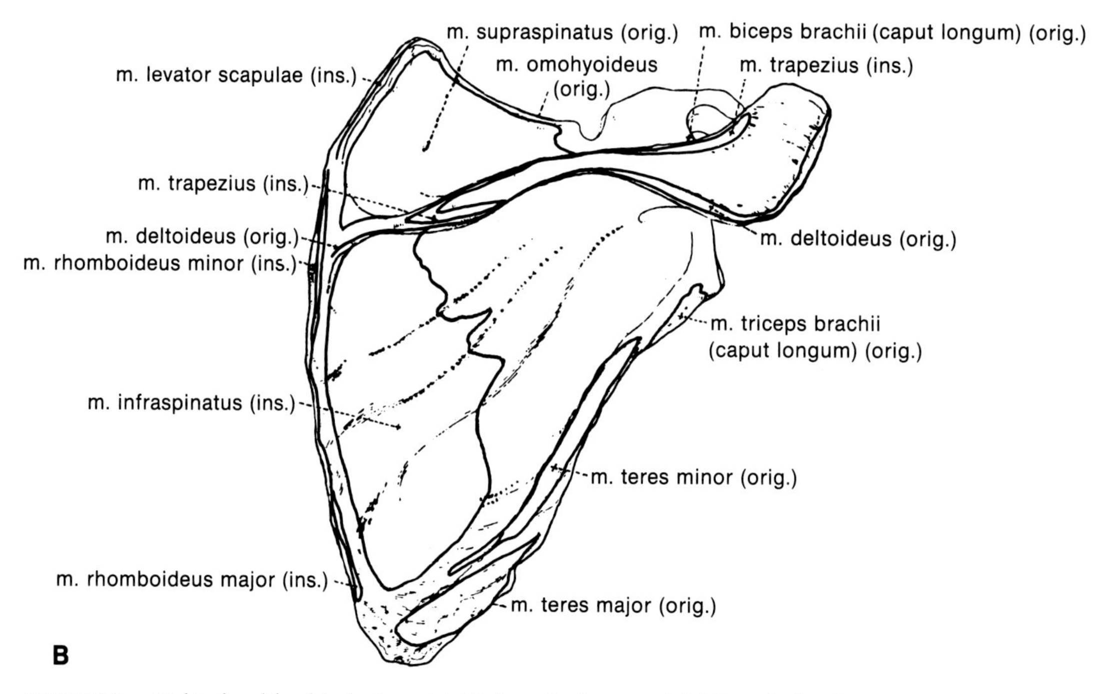

FIGURE 5 Right shoulder blade (*scapula*) (A) from in front and (B) from behind, showing muscular attachments.
ins., insertion; *orig.*, origin
(Spalteholz W: Hand-Atlas of Human Anatomy, 7th ed., Vol 1. Philadelphia, JB Lippincott, 1937)

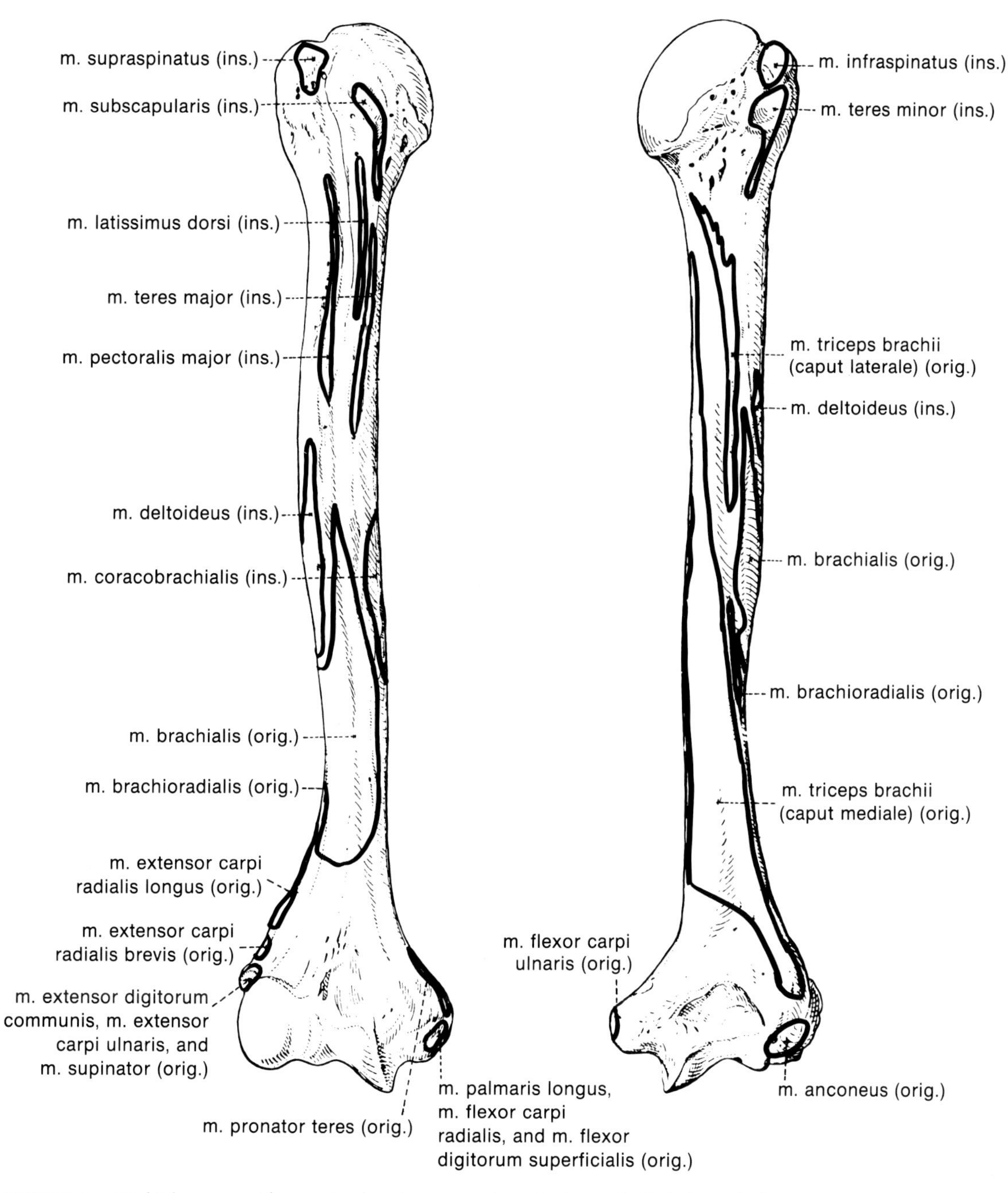

FIGURE 6 Right humerus (*humerus*), showing muscular attachments. *Left*, from in front. *Right*, from behind.
ins., insertion; *orig.*, origin
(Spalteholz W: Hand-Atlas of Human Anatomy, 7th ed., Vol 1. Philadelphia, JB Lippincott, 1937)

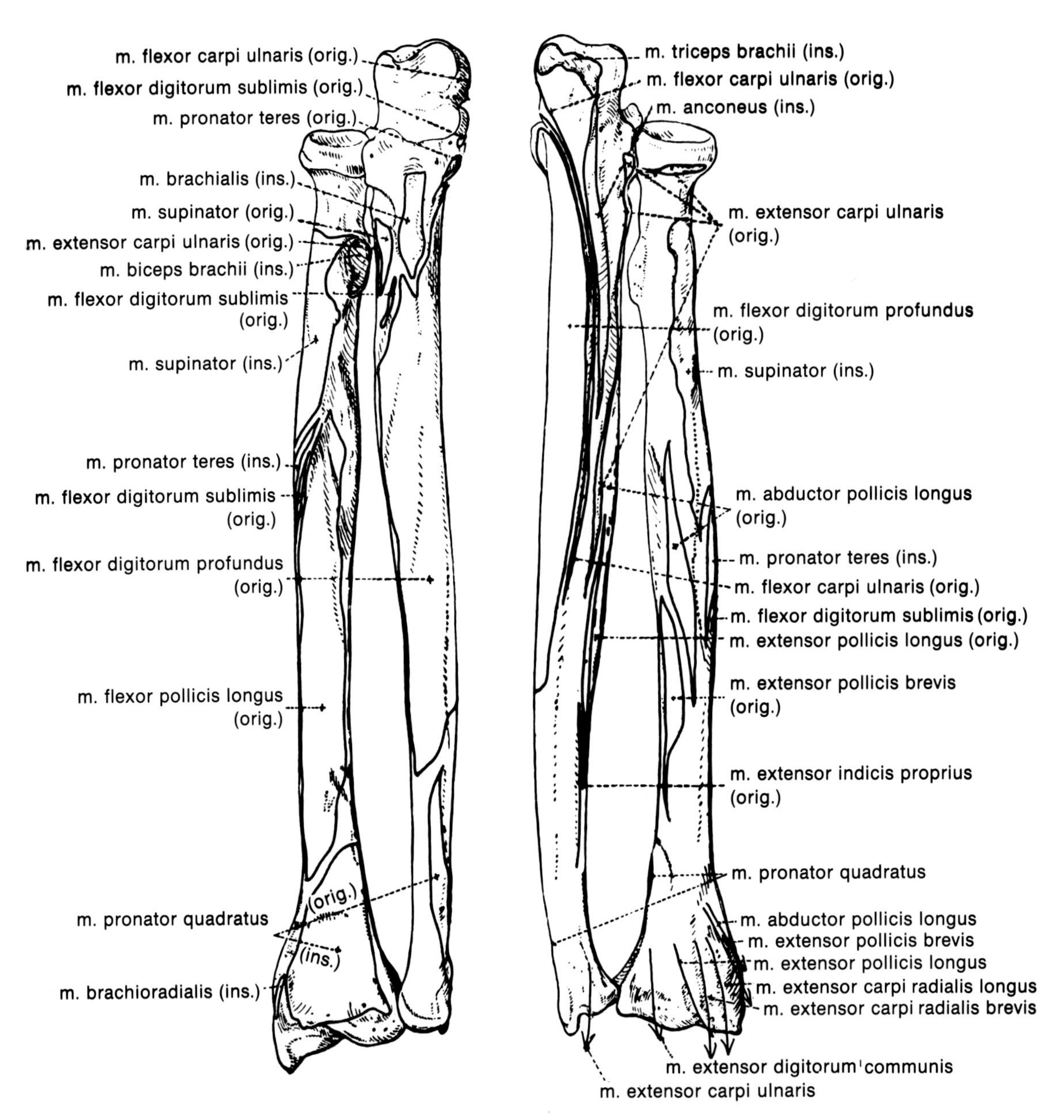

FIGURE 7 Bones of the right forearm, in supination, showing muscular attachments. *Left*, from the surface corresponding to the hollow of the hand. *Right*, from the side corresponding to the back of the hand.
Note: Old terminology, m. flexor digitorum sublimis; new terminology, m. flexor digitorum superficialis
ins., insertion; *orig.*, origin
(Spalteholz W: Hand-Atlas of Human Anatomy, 7th ed., Vol 1. Philadelphia, JB Lippincott, 1937)

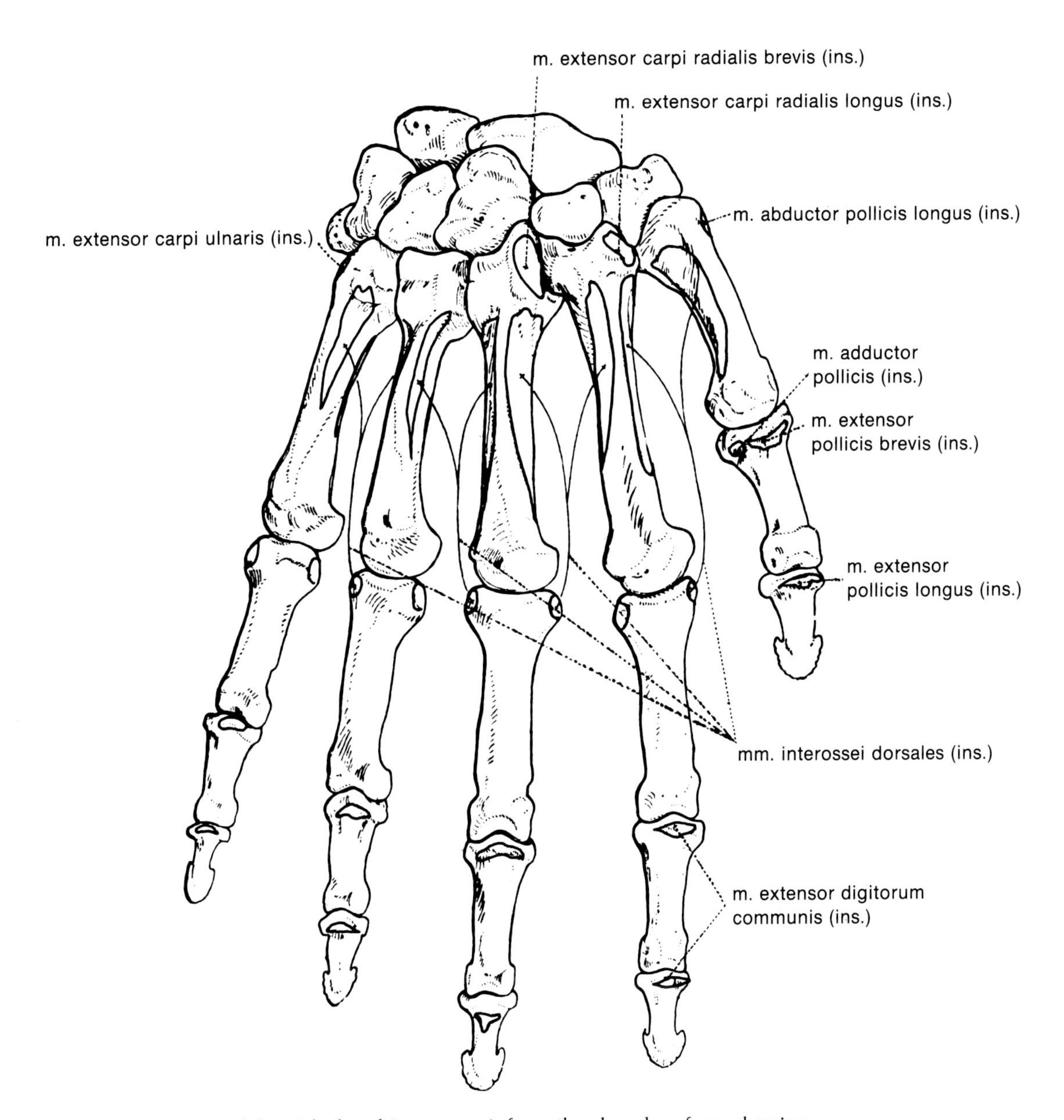

FIGURE 8 Bones of the right hand (*ossa manus*), from the dorsal surface, showing muscular attachments.
ins., insertion
(Spalteholz W: Hand-Atlas of Human Anatomy, 7th ed., Vol 1. Philadelphia, JB Lippincott, 1937)

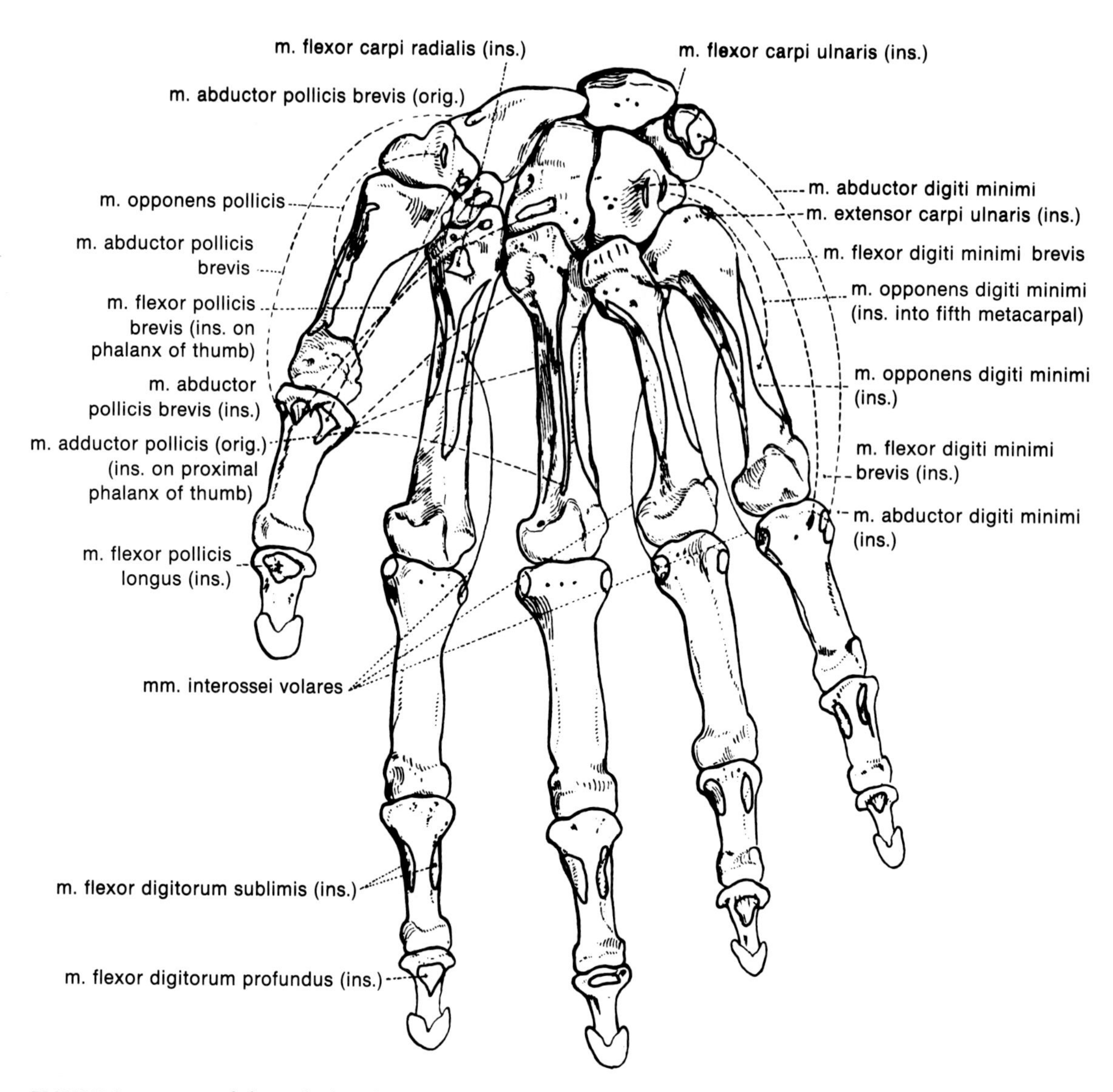

FIGURE 9 Bones of the right hand (*ossa manus*), from the volar surface, showing muscular attachments.

Note:

Old Terminology	*New Terminology*
mm. interossei volares	mm. interossei palmares
m. flexor digitorum sublimis	m. flexor digitorum superficialis
m. abductor digiti v	m. abductor digiti minimi
m. flexor digiti v brevis	m. flexor digiti minimi brevis
m. opponens digiti v	m. opponens digiti minimi

ins., insertion; *orig.*, origin

(Spalteholz W: Hand-Atlas of Human Anatomy, 7th ed, Vol. 1. Philadelphia, JB Lippincott, 1937)

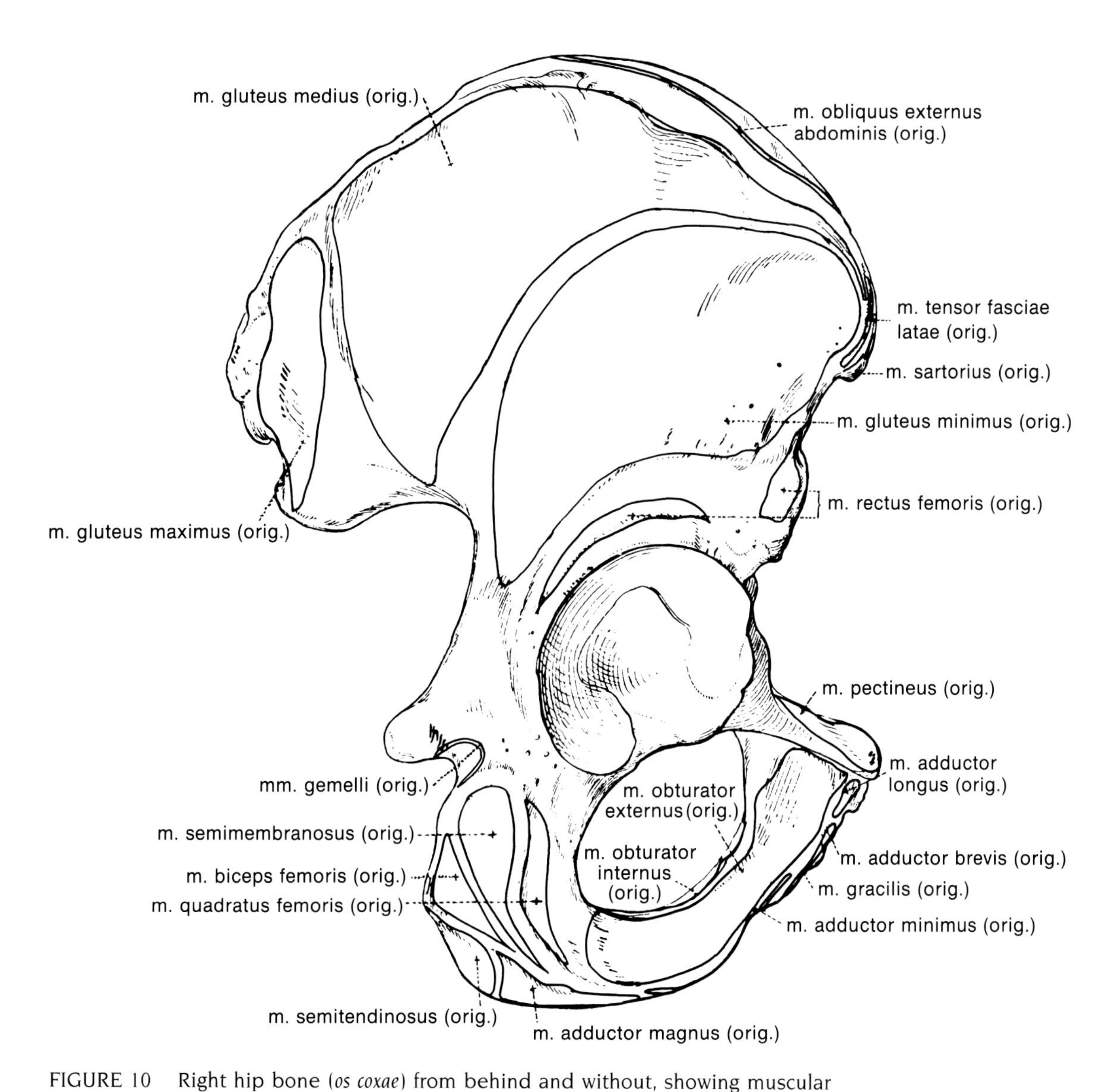

FIGURE 10 Right hip bone (*os coxae*) from behind and without, showing muscular attachments.
orig., origin
(Spalteholz W: Hand-Atlas of Human Anatomy, 7th ed., Vol 1. Philadelphia, JB Lippincott, 1937)

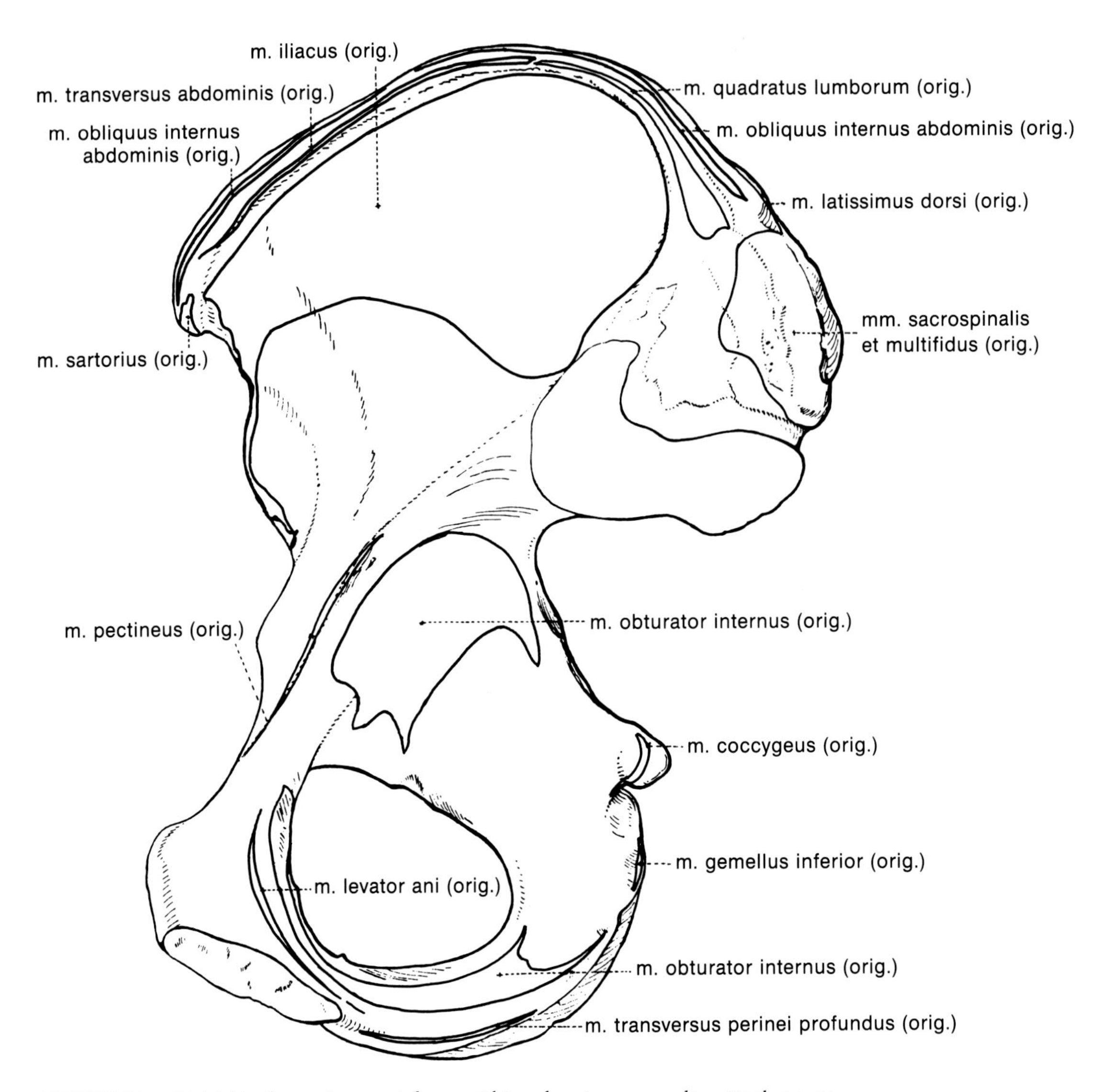

FIGURE 11 Right hip bone (*os coxae*) from within, showing muscular attachments.
orig., origin
(Spalteholz W: Hand-Atlas of Human Anatomy, 7th ed., Vol 1. Philadelphia, JB Lippincott, 1937)

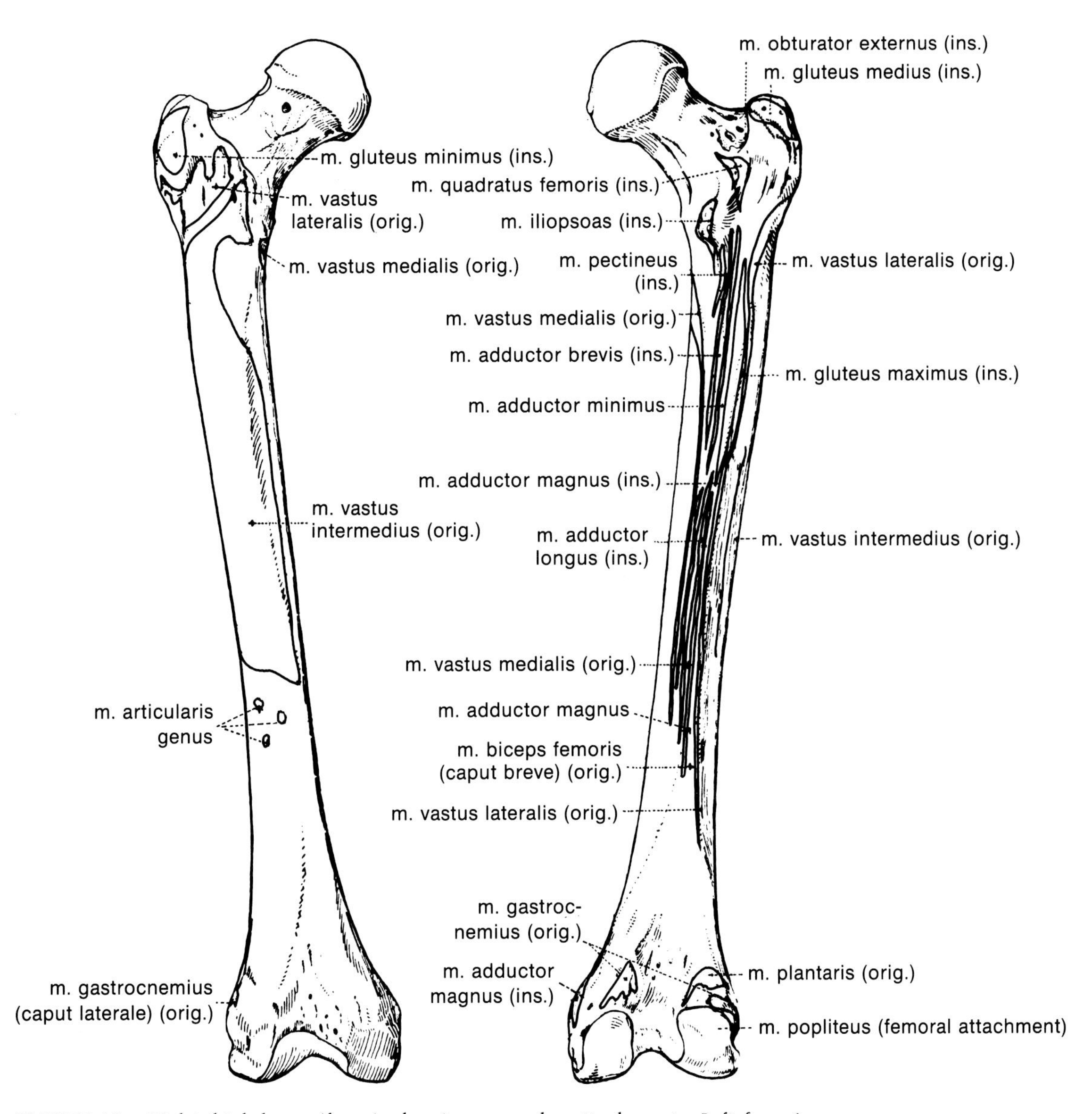

FIGURE 12 Right thigh bone (*femur*), showing muscular attachments. *Left*, from in front. *Right*, from behind.
ins., insertion; *orig.*, origin
(Spalteholz W: Hand-Atlas of Human Anatomy, 7th ed., Vol 1. Philadelphia, JB Lippincott, 1937)

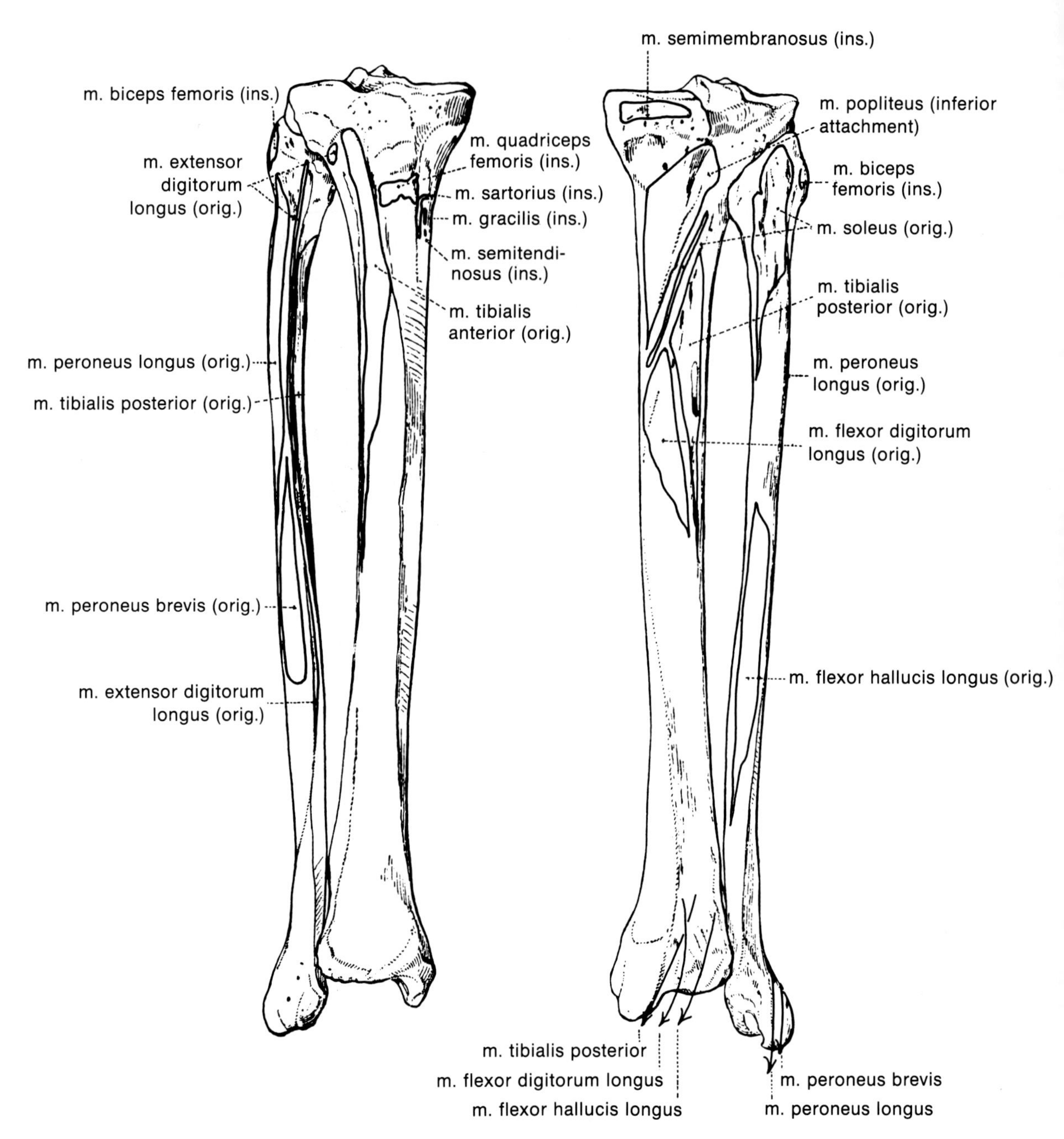

FIGURE 13 Right tibia and fibula (*tibia et fibula*), showing muscular attachments. *Left*, from in front. *Right*, from behind.
ins., insertion; *orig.*, origin
(Spalteholz W: Hand-Atlas of Human Anatomy, 7th ed., Vol 1. Philadelphia, JB Lippincott, 1937)

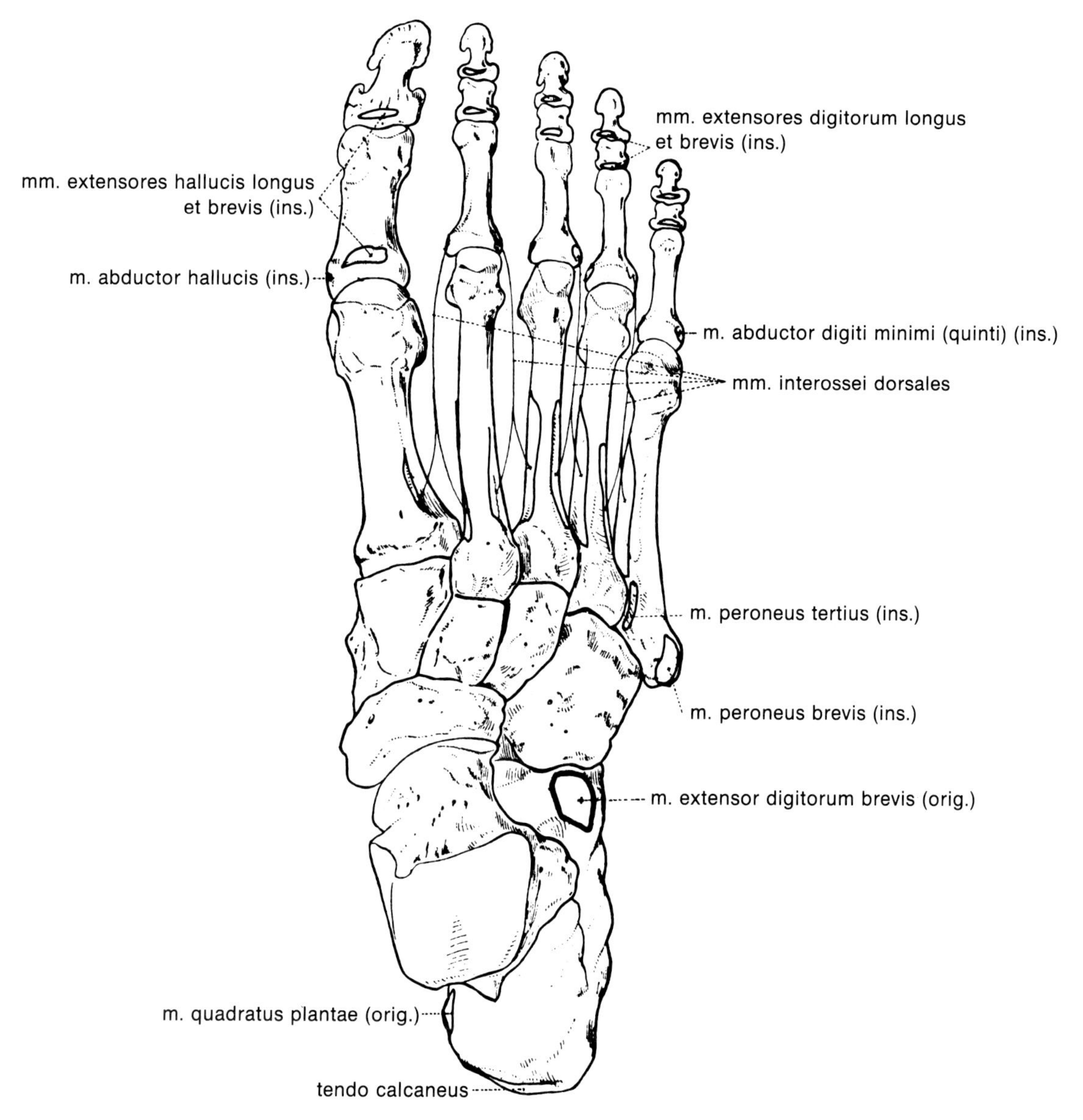

FIGURE 14 Bones of the right foot (*ossa pedis*), viewed from the back of the foot, showing muscular attachments. The position of the phalanges, especially in the second toe through the fifth toe, does not correspond exactly to reality.
Note: Old terminology, m. abductor digiti v; new terminology, m. abductor digiti minimi (quinti)
ins., insertion; *orig.*, origin
(Spalteholz W: Hand-Atlas of Human Anatomy, 7th ed., Vol 1. Philadelphia, JB Lippincott, 1937)

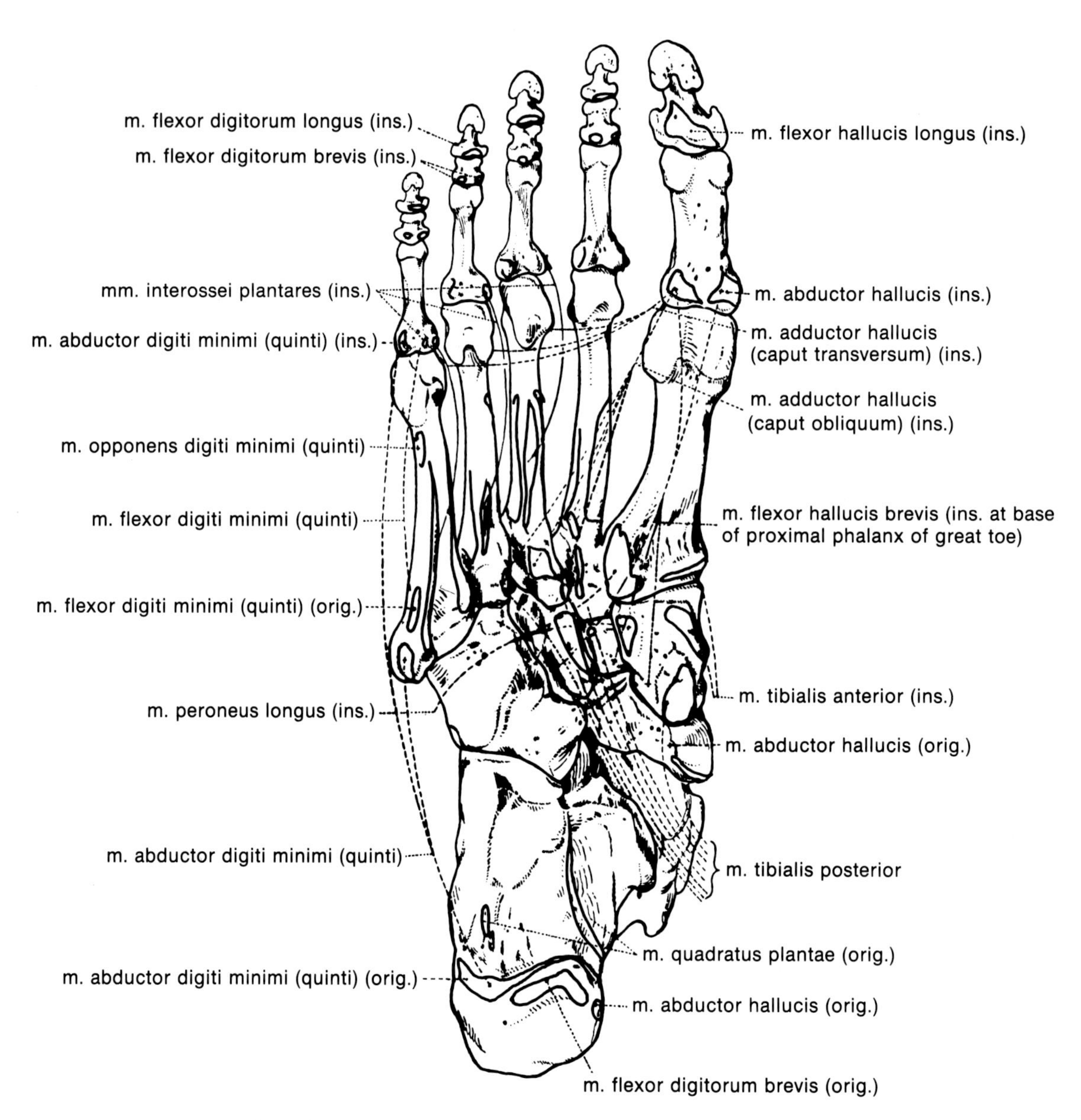

FIGURE 15 Bones of the right foot (*ossa pedis*), viewed from the sole of the foot, showing muscular attachments. The position of the phalanges, especially in the second through the fifth toe, does not correspond exactly to reality.

Note:

Old Terminology	*New Terminology*
m. abductor digiti v	m. abductor digiti minimi (quinti)
m. flexor digiti v brevis	m. flexor digiti minimi (quinti)
m. opponens digiti v	m. opponens digiti minimi (quinti)

ins., insertion; *orig.*, origin
(Spalteholz W: Hand-Atlas of Human Anatomy, 7th ed., Vol 1. Philadelphia, JB Lippincott, 1937)

Diagrams of the Dermatomes and Peripheral Nerves

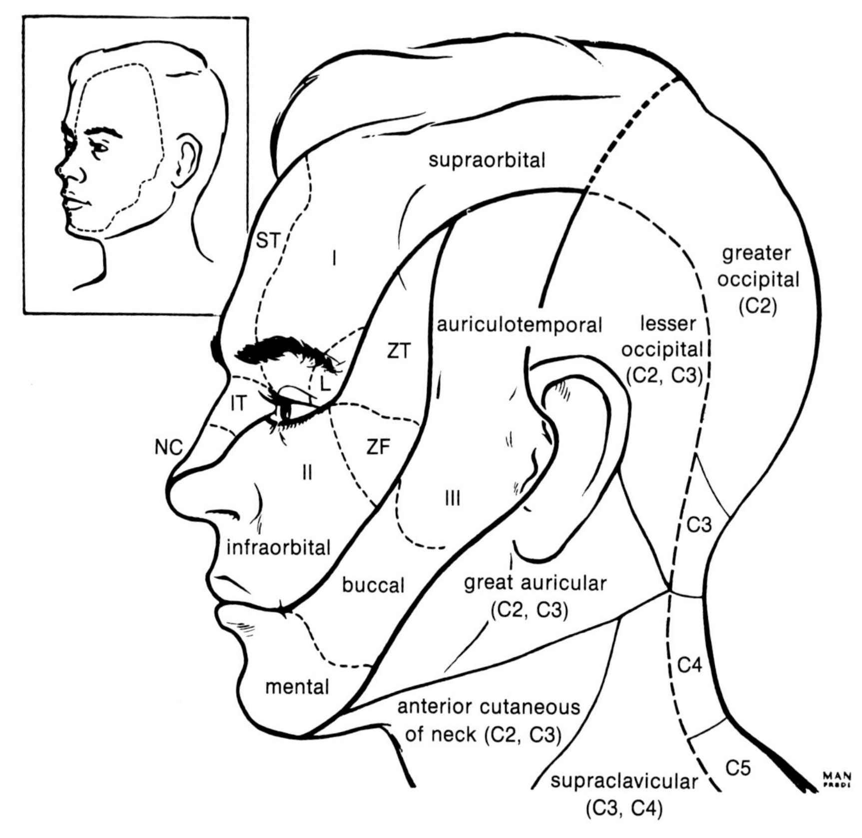

FIGURE 16 Cutaneous fields of the head and the upper part of the neck. The fields supplied by the three divisions of the trigeminal nerve (I, ophthalmic; II, maxillary; III, mandibular) are indicated by heavy lines, and their subdivisions by light broken lines. The conjunctivae are innervated by the ophthalmic division. The lateral and superior boundaries of the posterior primary rami are indicated by broken lines. The caudal boundary of the manidbular division is taken from a publication by Foerster (1933), as is the area of sensory loss in the face following resection of the trigeminal nerve (*inset*). IT, infratrochlear nerve; L, lacrimal nerve; NC, external nasal branch of the nasociliary nerve; ST, supratrochlear nerve; ZF, zygomaticofacial nerve; ZT: zygomaticotemporal nerve. (Haymaker W, Woodhall B: Peripheral Nerve Injuries: Principles of Diagnosis. Philadelphia, WB Saunders, 1945)

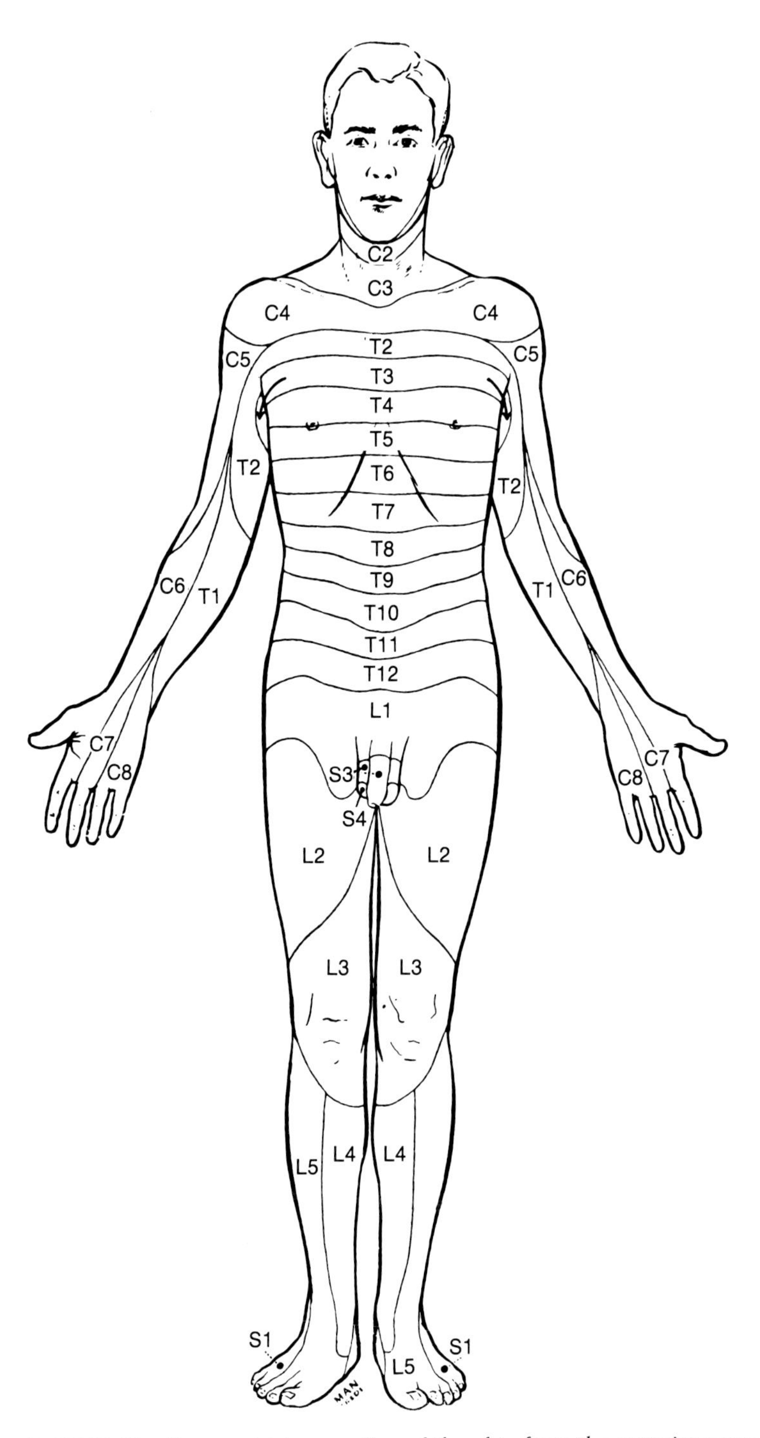

FIGURE 17 Segmental innervation of the skin from the anterior aspect. The uppermost dermatome adjoins the cutaneous field of the mandibular division of the trigeminal nerve. The arrows indicate the lateral extensions of dermatome T3. (Haymaker W, Woodhall B: Peripheral Nerve Injuries: Principles of Diagnosis: Philadelphia, WB Saunders, 1945, after Foerster, 1933)

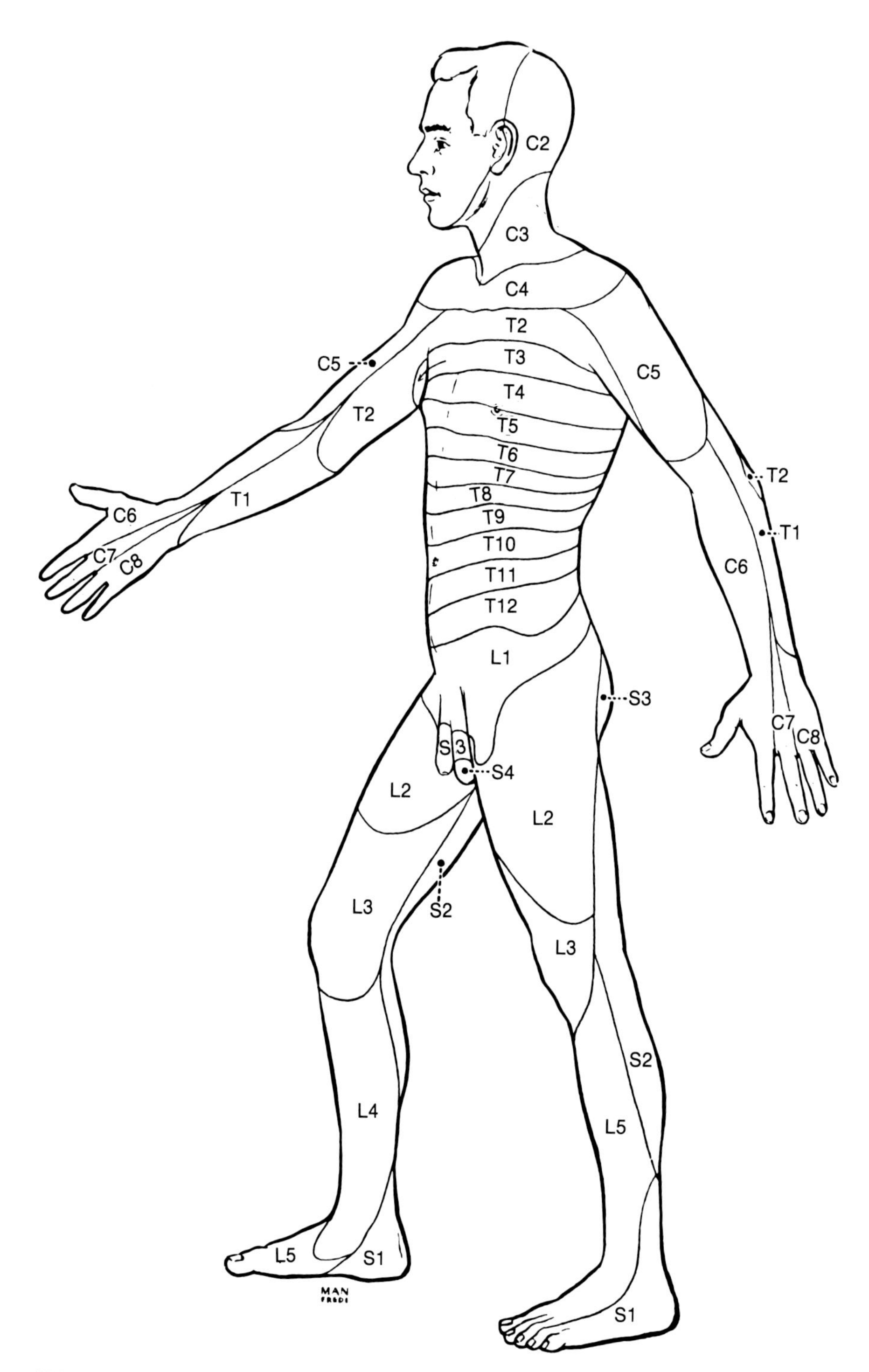

FIGURE 18 Side view of the dermatomes. (Haymaker W, Woodhall B: Peripheral Nerve Injuries: Principles of Diagnosis. Philadelphia, WB Saunders, 1945, after Foerster, 1933)

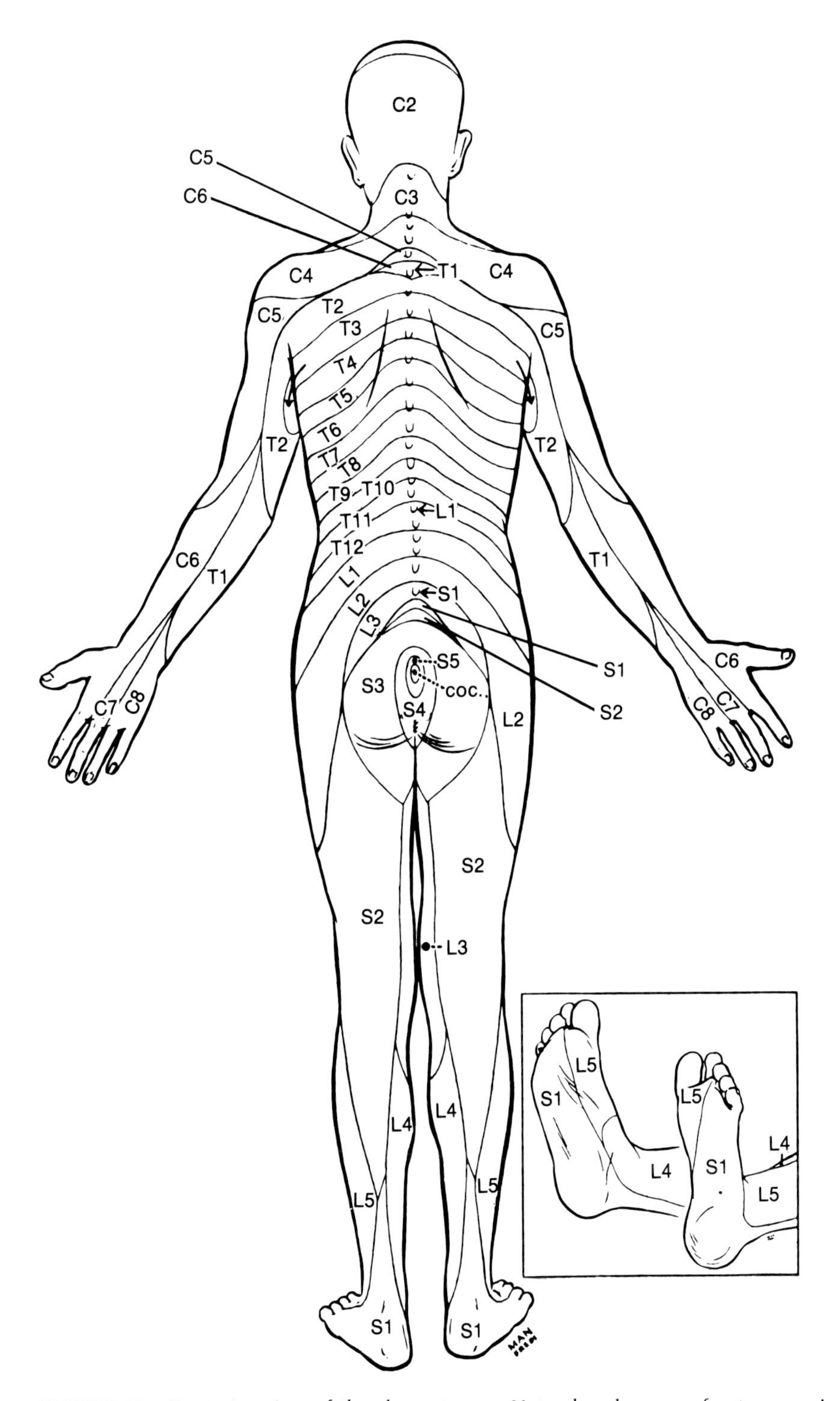

FIGURE 19 Posterior view of the dermatomes. Note the absence of cutaneous innervation by the first cervical segment. The arrows in the axillary regions indicate the lateral extent of dermatome T3; those in the region of the vertebral column point to the first thoracic, the first lumbar, and the first sacral spinous processes. (Haymaker W, Woodhall B: Peripheral Nerve Injuries: Principles of Diagnosis. Philadelphia, WB Saunders, 1945, after Foerster, 1933)

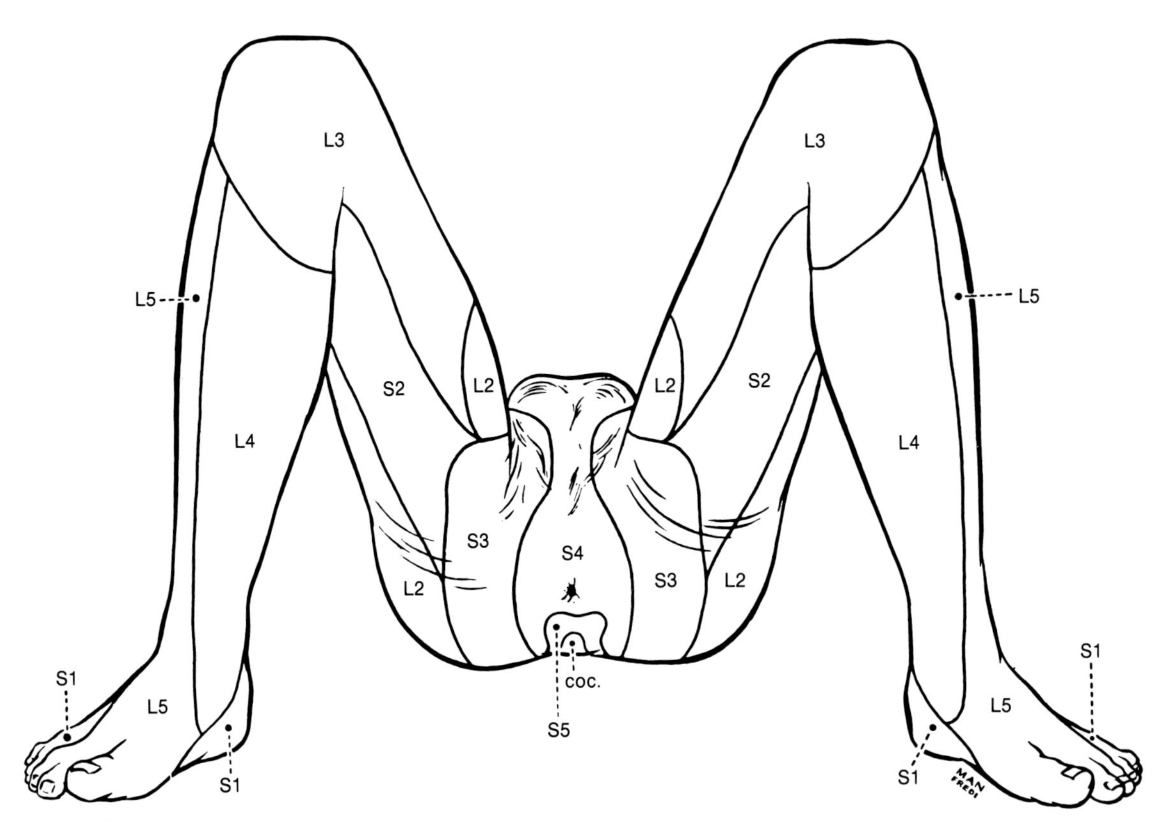

FIGURE 20 Dermatomes of the perineum and limbs. (Haymaker W, Woodhall B: Peripheral Nerve Injuries: Principles of Diagnosis. Philadelphia, WB Saunders, 1945)

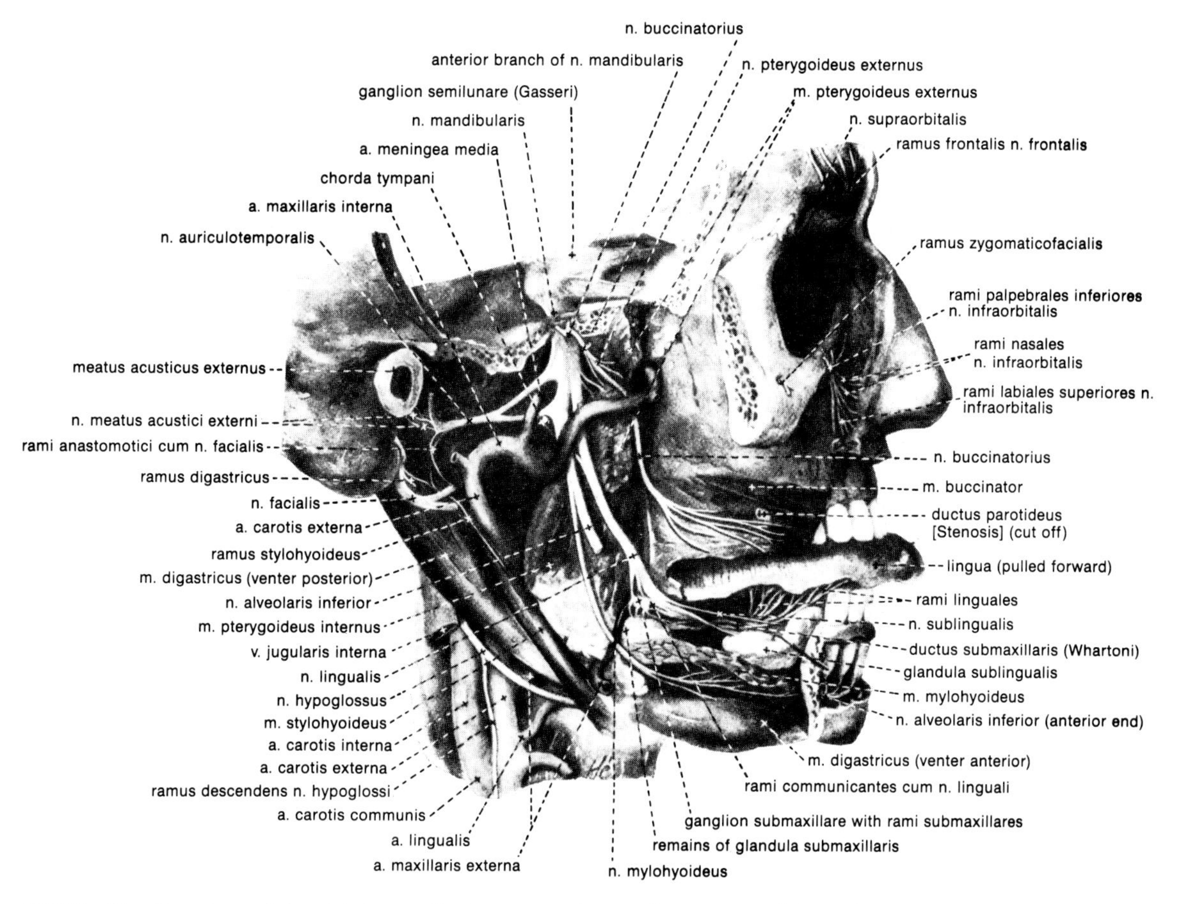

FIGURE 21 Branches of the right mandibular nerve, deeper layer, viewed from the right. (The lower jaw and masticatory muscles have been almost completely removed; all but a small part of the glandula submaxillaris has been removed.) (Spalteholz W: Hand-Atlas of Human Anatomy, 7th ed., Vol 3. Philadelphia, JB Lippincott, 1937)

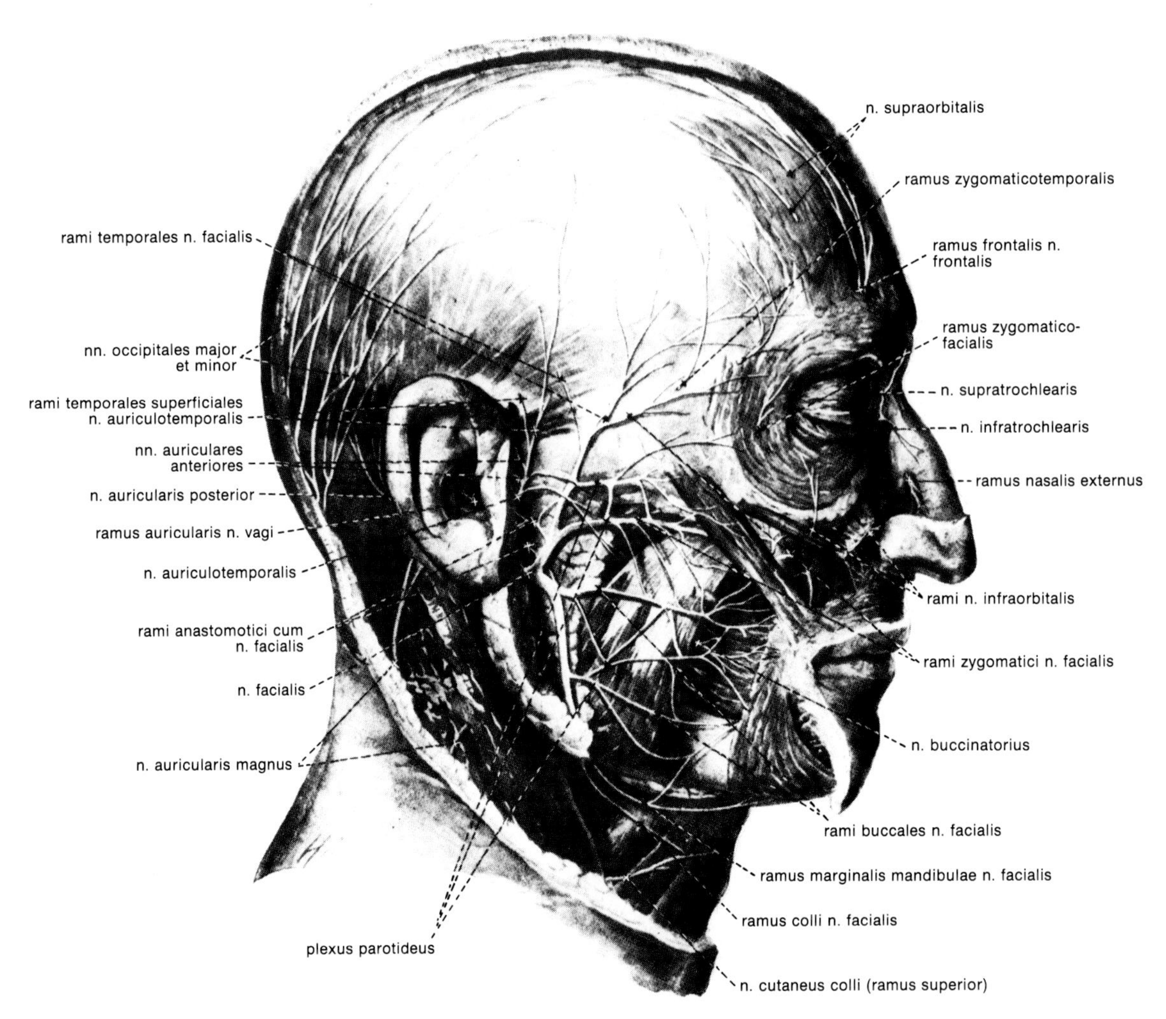

FIGURE 22 Nerves of the face, viewed from the right. (The platysma has been removed; a piece has been cut out of the glandula parotis.) (Spalteholz W: Hand-Atlas of Human Anatomy, 7th ed, Vol 3. Philadelphia, JB Lippincott, 1937)

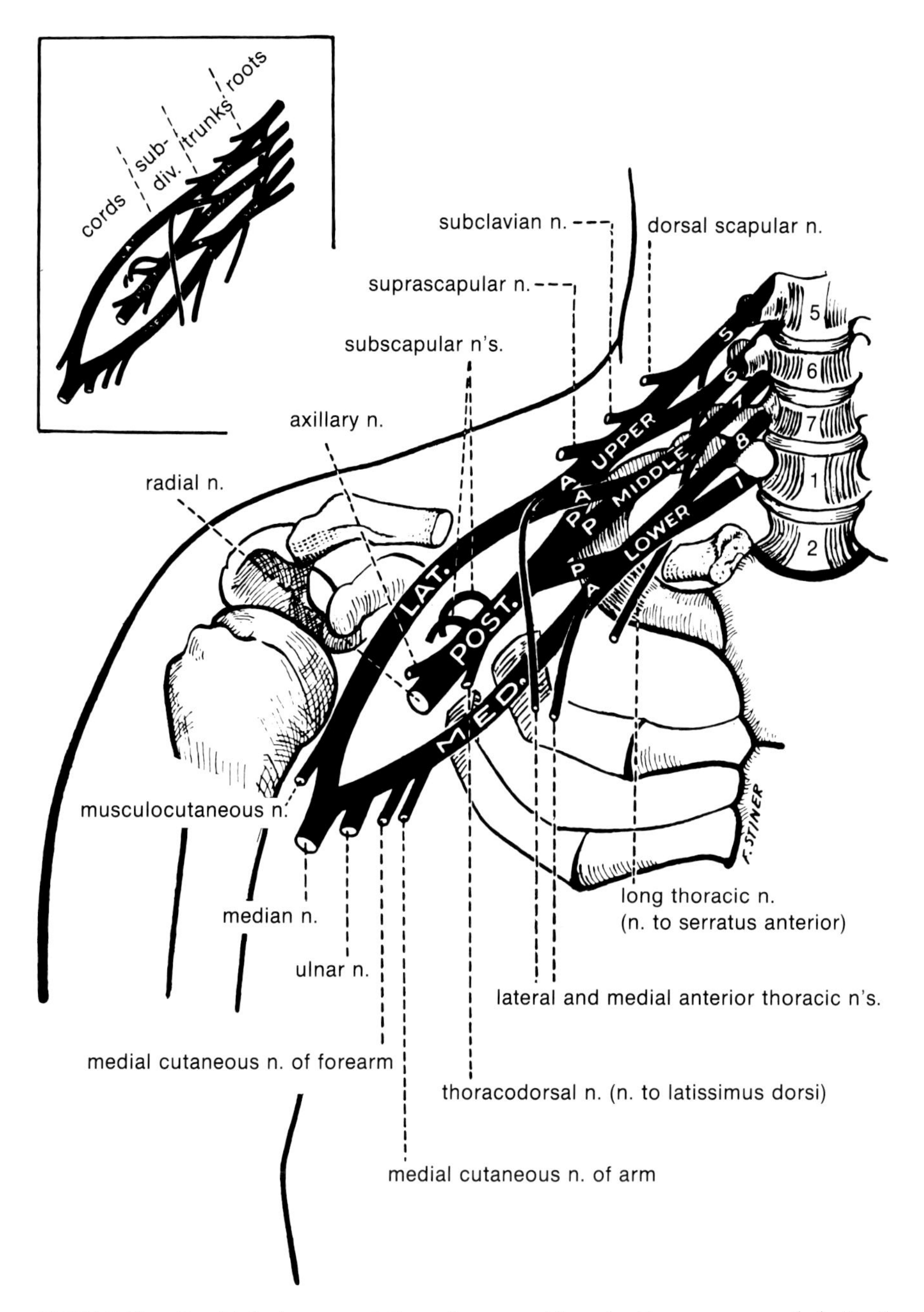

FIGURE 23 Brachial plexus and its various constituents. For purposes of clarity the components of the plexus have been separated and drawn out of scale. Peripheral nerves arise from various components of the plexus: undivided anterior primary rami ([C] 5, 6, 7, and 8 and [T]1), trunks (upper, middle, and lower), divisions (anterior and posterior), and cords (lateral, posterior, and medial). The median nerve arises from the heads of the lateral and medial cords. Not infrequently, an anterior division of the middle trunk connects with the medial cord. (Haymaker W, Woodhall B: Peripheral Nerve Injuries: Principles of Diagnosis. Philadelphia, WB Saunders, 1945)

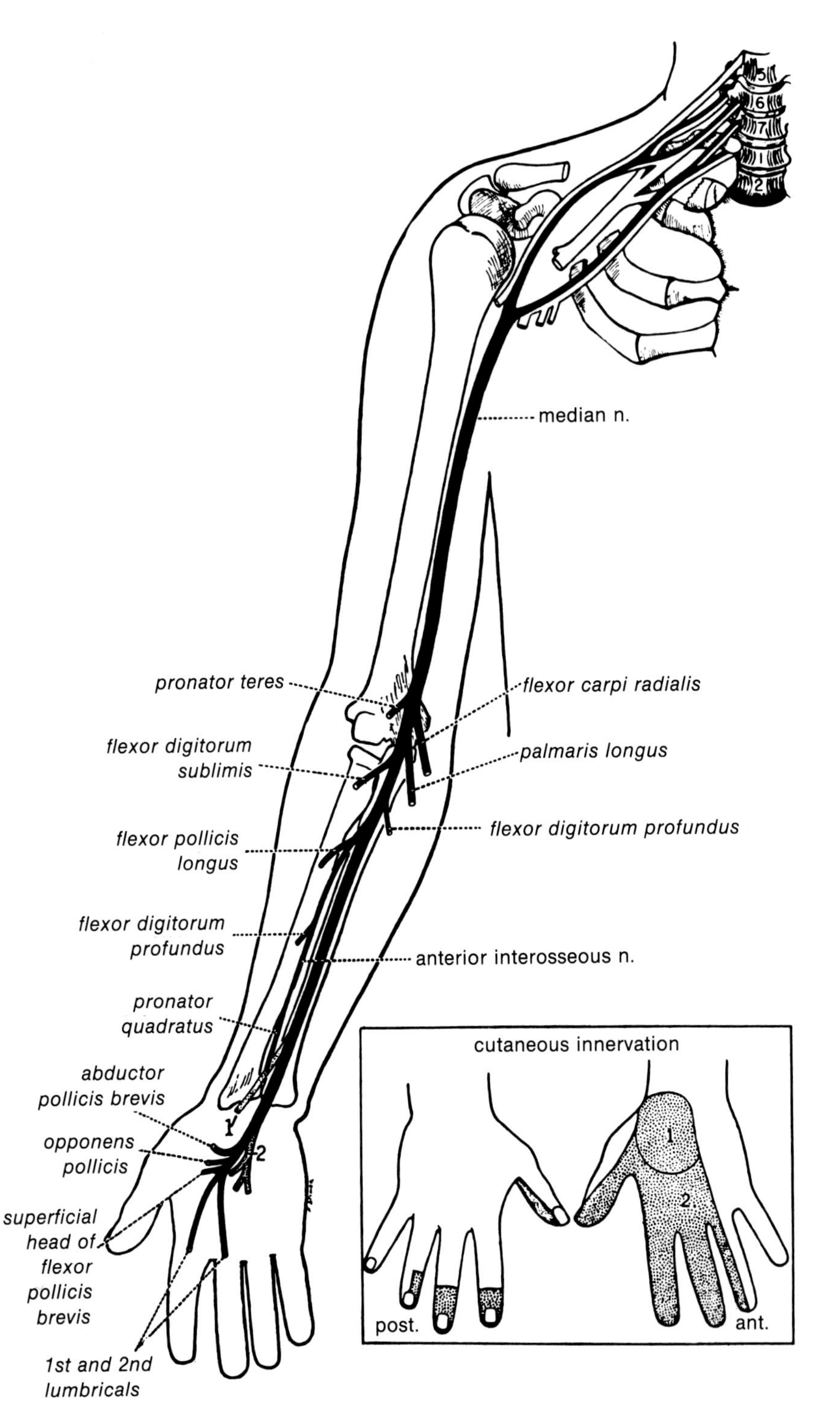

FIGURE 24 Course and distribution of the median nerve. The muscles supplied are indicated in *italics*. In the hand the cutaneous branches are marked by stippling, as is the field of cutaneous innervation (*inset*). The nerve indicated by 1 is the palmar cutaneous branch of the median nerve. Those marked 2 are the palmar digital nerves. The corresponding areas of cutaneous innervation are indicated in the inset. In some people the region of innervation of the dorsal aspect of the fingers is somewhat more proximal than is indicated in this drawing.) (Haymaker W, Woodhall B: Peripheral Nerve Injuries: Principles of Diagnosis, 2nd ed. Philadelphia, WB Saunders, 1953)

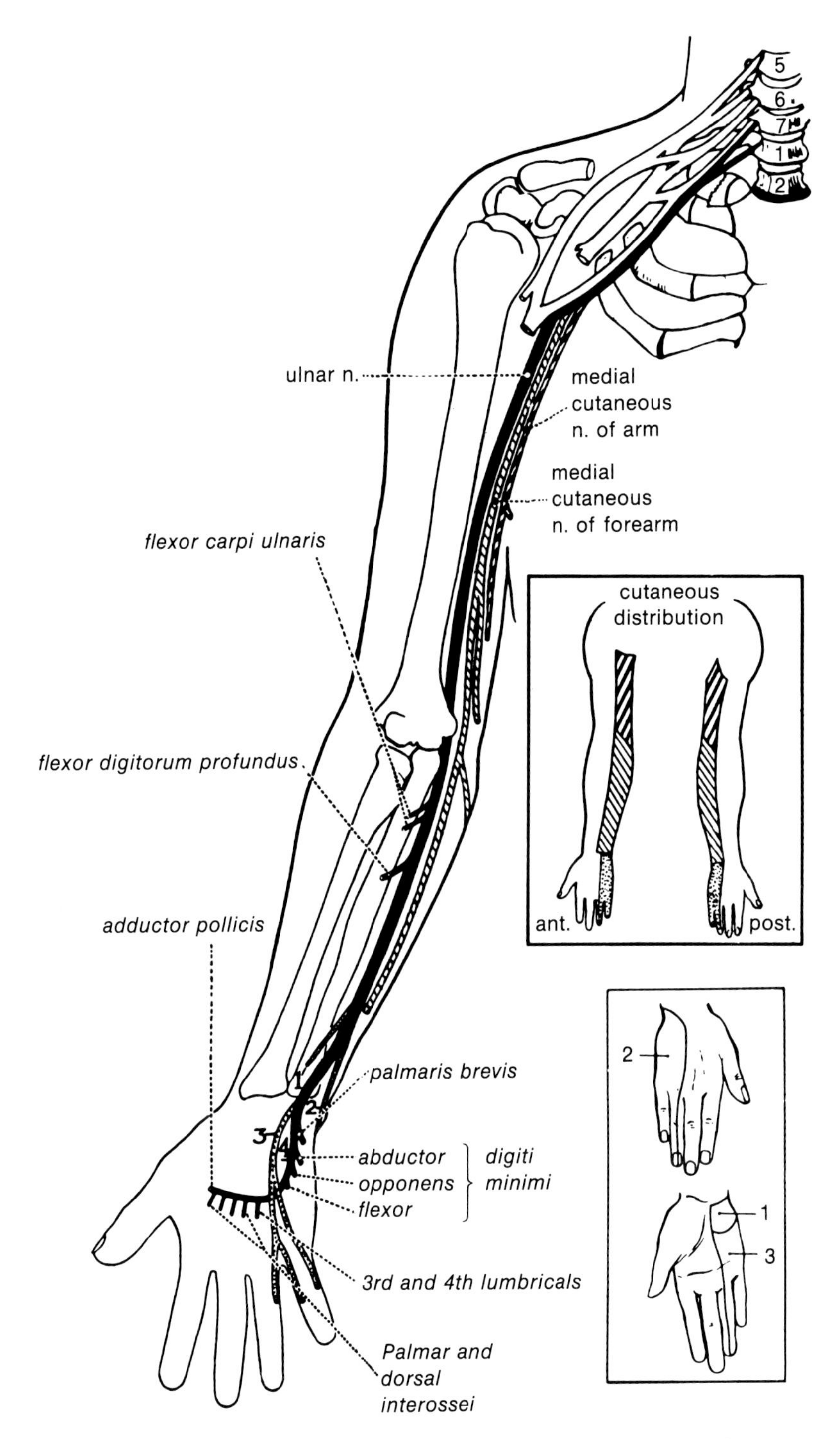

FIGURE 25 Origin and distribution of the ulnar nerve, the medial cutaneous nerve of the forearm, and the medial cutaneous nerve of the arm. The muscles supplied are indicated in *italics*. The patterns of the different nerves are duplicated in the upper inset. The numbered nerves are as follows: 1, palmar branch; 2, dorsal branch; 3, superficial terminal branch; 4, deep terminal branch. The fields of innervation of cutaneous branches, 1, 2, and 3 are illustrated in the lower inset. (Haymaker W, Woodhall B: Peripheral Nerve Injuries: Principles of Diagnosis, 2nd ed. Philadelphia, WB Saunders, 1953)

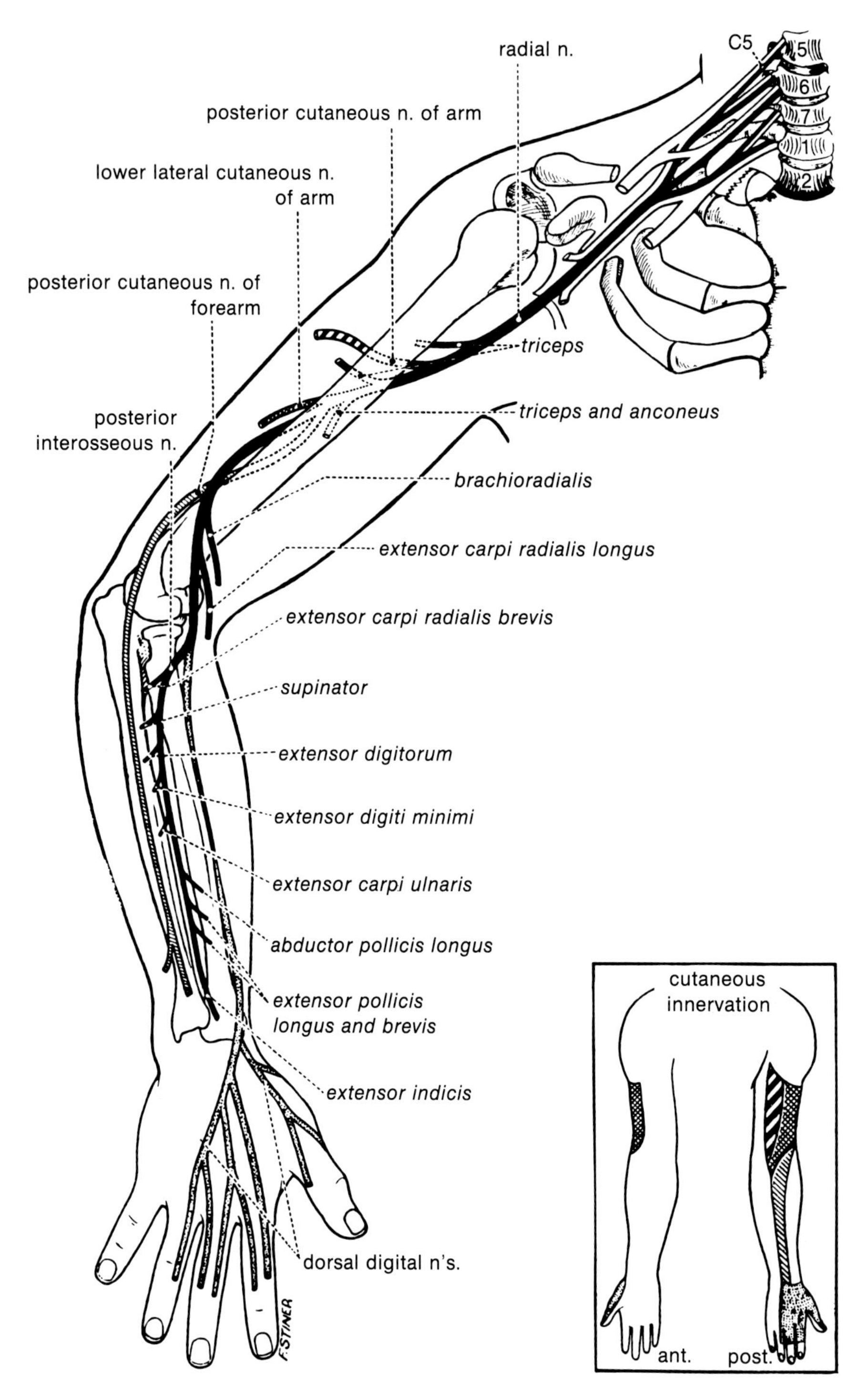

FIGURE 26 Course and distribution of the radial nerve. The patterns of the cutaneous nerves are duplicated in the inset. The names of the various muscles supplied by the radial nerve are in *italics*. (Haymaker W, Woodhall B: Peripheral Nerve Injuries: Principles of Diagnosis, 2nd ed. Philadelphia, WB Saunders, 1953)

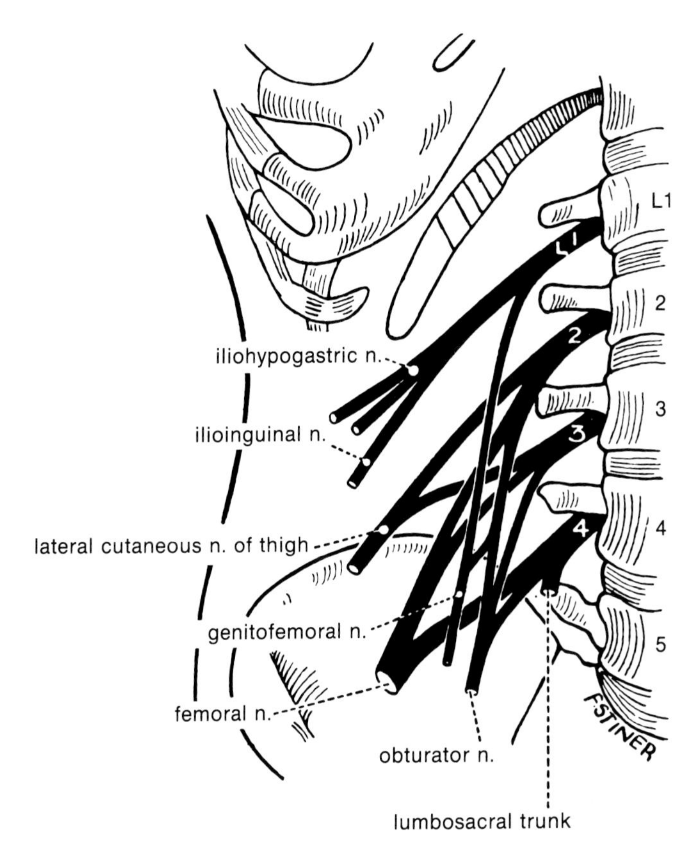

FIGURE 27 Constituents of the lumbar plexus. The lumbosacral trunk is the liaison between the lumbar and sacral plexuses. (Haymaker W, Woodhall B: Peripheral Nerve Injuries: Principles of Diagnosis. Philadelphia, WB Saunders, 1945)

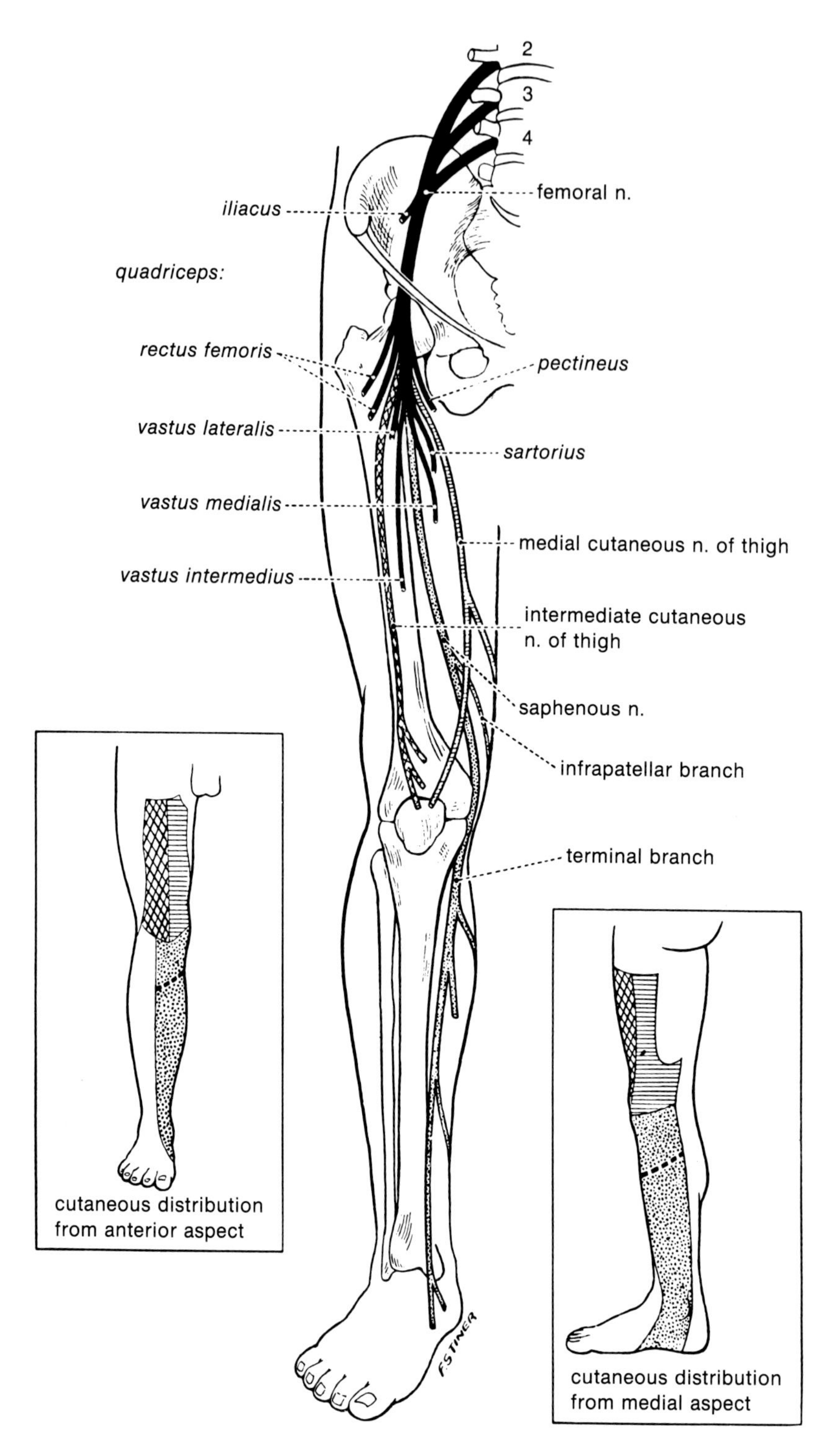

FIGURE 28 Course and distribution of the femoral nerve. The names of the muscles supplied by this nerve are in *italics*. The patterns of the cutaneous nerves are duplicated in the insets. In the field of the saphenous nerve the broken line represents the boundary between the fields of the infrapatellar and terminal branches. (Haymaker W, Woodhall B: Peripheral Nerve Injuries: Principles of Diagnosis, 2nd ed. Philadelphia, WB Saunders, 1953)

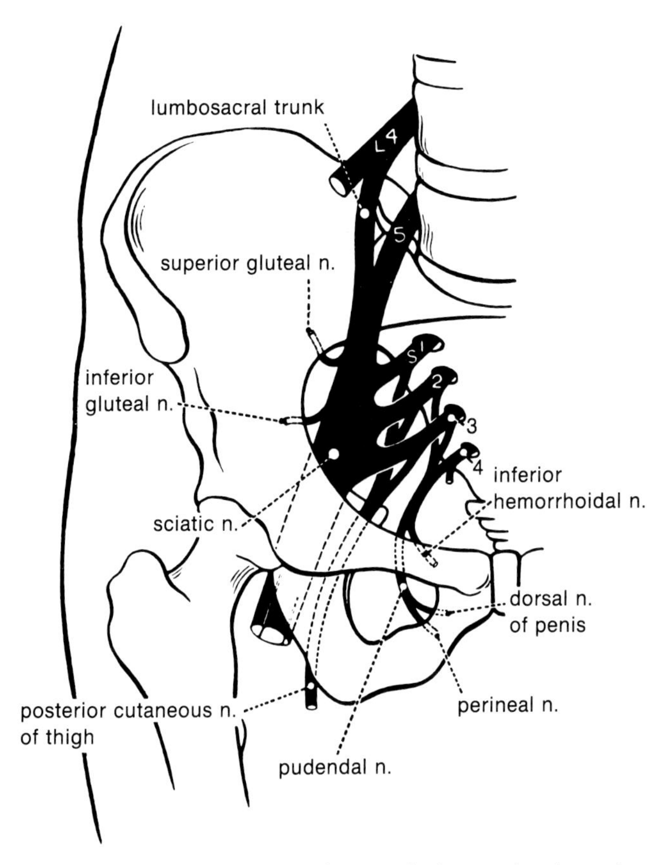

FIGURE 29 Constituents of the sacral plexus. The three divisions of the sciatic nerve are indicated. Not illustrated is the inferior medial clunical nerve, which arises from anterior primary rami S2 and S3 and courses downward between the posterior cutaneous nerve of the thigh and the pudendal nerve. (Haymaker W, Woodhall B: Peripheral Nerve Injuries: Principles of Diagnosis. Philadelphia, WB Saunders, 1945)

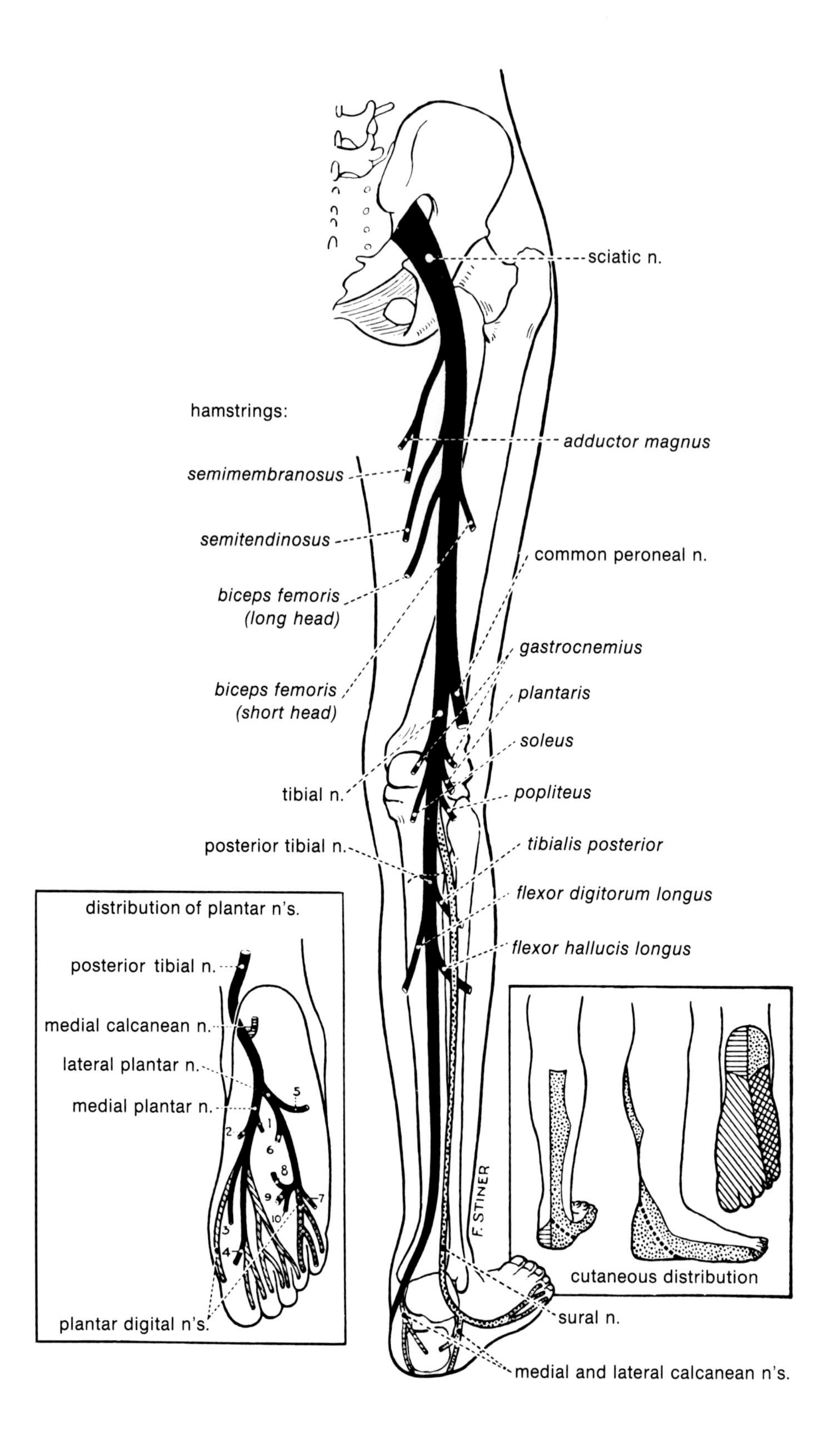
sciatic n.
hamstrings:
adductor magnus
semimembranosus
semitendinosus
common peroneal n.
biceps femoris
(long head)
gastrocnemius
biceps femoris
(short head)
plantaris
soleus
tibial n.
popliteus
posterior tibial n.
tibialis posterior
flexor digitorum longus
flexor hallucis longus
distribution of plantar n's.
posterior tibial n.
medial calcanean n.
lateral plantar n.
medial plantar n.
plantar digital n's.
F. STINER
cutaneous distribution
sural n.
medial and lateral calcanean n's.

◀ FIGURE 30 Course and distribution of the sciatic, tibial, posterior tibial, and plantar nerves. A dotted line marks the transition between the tibial and posterior tibial nerves. The cutaneous fields of the medial calcanean and medial plantar nerves are indicated in the inset by lines, the field of the sural nerve and its lateral calcanean branch by dots, and that of the lateral plantar nerve by crosshatching. The names of the muscles supplied are in *italics*. The numbered branches of the plantar nerves are as follows: 1, flexor digitorum brevis; 2, abductor hallucis; 3, flexor hallucis brevis; 4, first lumbrical; 5, abductor digiti minimi (quinti); 6, flexor digitorum accessorius; 7, flexor digiti minimi (quinti); 8, adductor hallucis; 9, interossei; 10, second, third, and fourth lumbricals. To simplify, the sural nerve is indicated as arising solely from the tibial nerve; actually, it usually receives an anastomotic branch from the common peroneal nerve. (Haymaker W, Woodhall B: Peripheral Nerve Injuries: Principles of Diagnosis, 2nd ed. Philadelphia, WB Saunders, 1953)

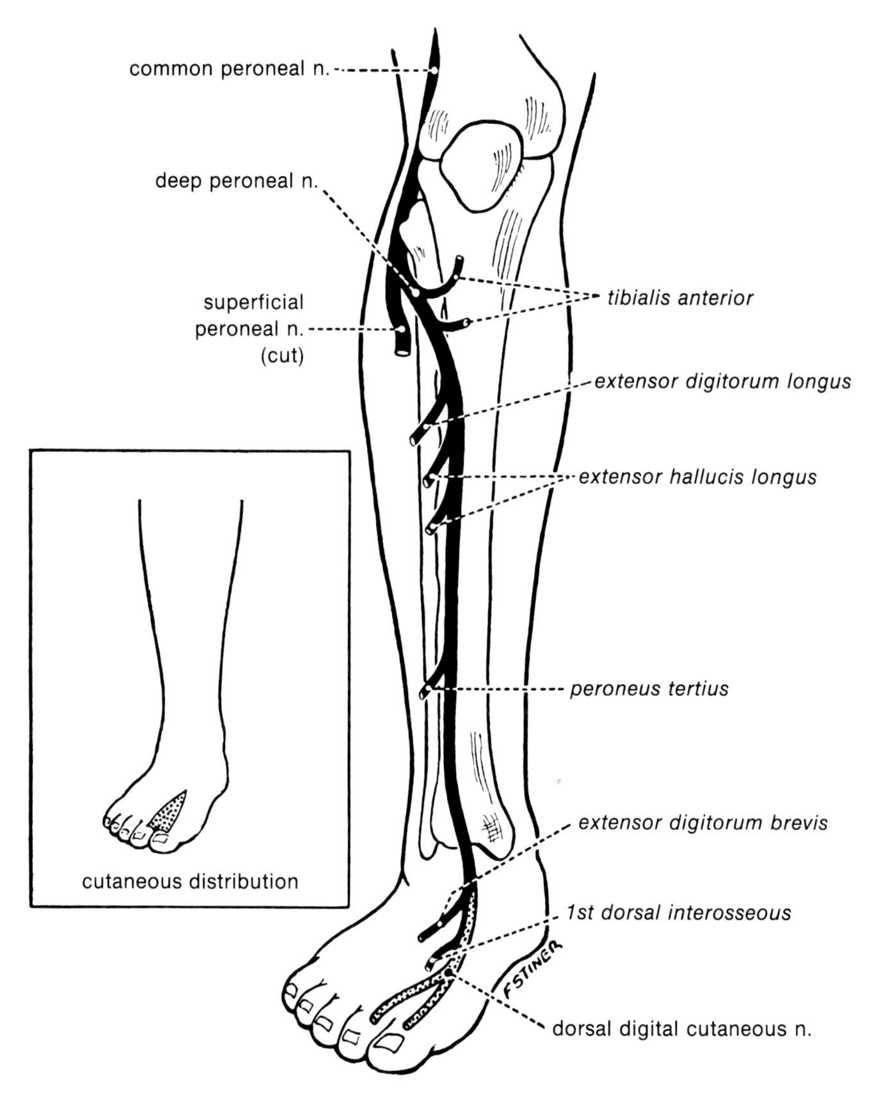

FIGURE 31 Course and distribution of the deep peroneal nerve. The muscles supplied are indicated in *italics*. The cutaneous distribution of the nerve is shown in the inset. (Haymaker W, Woodhall B: Peripheral Nerve Injuries: Principles of Diagnosis, 2nd ed. Philadelphia, WB Saunders, 1953)

BIBLIOGRAPHY

Haymaker W, Woodhall B: Peripheral Nerve Injuries: Principles of Diagnosis, 2nd ed. Philadelphia, WB Saunders, 1953

International Anatomical Nomenclature Committee: Nomina Anatomica, 3rd ed. Amsterdam, Excerpta Medica, 1966

Spalteholz W: Hand-Atlas of Human Anatomy, 7th ed, Vol 1. Philadelphia, JB Lippincott, 1937

Spalteholz W: Hand-Atlas of Human Anatomy, 7th ed, Vol 3. Philadelphia, JB Lippincott, 1937

A Glossary of Terms Used in Clinical Electromyography*

Absolute Refractory Period See *Refractory Period*.

Accommodation The reduced efficacy of a prolonged constant current or a gradually increasing current in generating action potentials from nervous tissue

Accommodation Curve A curve obtained by plotting the strength of current (in multiples of *Rheobase*) required to produce a response from an excitable tissue against the time required by a slowly rising current pulse to reach that value

Action Current The electrical current associated with an *Action Potential*

Action Potential (abbr. AP). Strictly defined, the all-or-none, self-propagating, nondecrementing voltage change recorded from an excitable cell. The scource of the action potential should be specified, *e.g.*, nerve (fiber) action potential or muscle (fiber) action potential. Commonly, the term refers to the nearly synchronous summated action potentials of a group of cells, *e.g.*, *Motor Unit Potential*. To avoid ambiguity in reference to the recording of nearly synchronous summated action potentials of nerve and muscle as done in nerve conduction studies, it is recommended that the terms *Compound Nerve Action Potential* and *Compound Muscle Action Potential*, respectively, or the specific named responses (*e.g.*, *M Wave*, *F Wave*, *H Wave*, *R1 and R2 Waves*) be used.

* Reprinted from *A Glossary of Terms Used in Clinical Electromyography*, 1980, with permission of the American Association of Electromyography and Electrodiagnosis, Copyright © 1980. Compiled by the Nomenclature Committee: The American Association of Electromyography and Electrodiagnosis: George H. Kraft, Chairman; Jasper R. Daube; Joel A. DeLisa; Joseph Goodgold; Charles K. Jablecki; Edward H. Lambert; J. A. Simpson; Albrecht Struppler; and David O. Wiechers

Active Electrode Synonymous with *Exploring Electrode*. See *Recording Electrode*

Adaptation A transient state at the initiation of an abrupt depolarization in which the impulse frequency first increases and then diminishes before the cell reaches a steady firing frequency

After Discharge Repetitive electrical firing that persists after initiation by some other process, usually muscle contraction. It may have variable form and be regular or irregular at long or short intervals.

Afterpotential Membrane potential following the spike component of an *Action Potential* and not yet returned to a steady resting value. It first has a positive phase (positive afterpotential), followed by a negative phase (negative afterpotential).

Amplitude With reference to an *Action Potential*, the maximum voltage difference between two points, usually baseline to peak or peak to peak. By convention, the amplitude of the *Compound Muscle Action Potential* is measured from the baseline to the most negative peak. In contrast, the amplitude of a *Compound Sensory Nerve Action Potential*, *Motor Unit Potential*, *Fibrillation Potential*, *Positive Sharp Wave*, *Fasciculation Potential*, and most other *Action Potentials* is measured from the most positive to the most negative peak.

Anodal Block A local block of nerve conduction caused by hyperpolarization of the nerve cell membrane by an electrical stimulus. See *Stimulating Electrode*.

Anode The positive terminal of a source of electrical current

Antidromic Said of an action potential or of the stimulation causing the action potential that propagates in the direction opposite the normal (dromic or *Orthodromic*) one for that fiber—*i.e.*, conduction along motor fibers toward the spinal cord and conduction along sensory fibers away from the spinal cord. Contrast with *Orthodromic*.

Artifact A voltage change generated by a biologic or nonbiologic source other than the ones of interest. The *Stimulus Artifact* is the potential recorded at the time that the stimulus is applied and includes the *Electrical* or *Shock Artifact*, which is a potential due to the volume-conducted electrical stimulus. The stimulus and shock artifacts usually precede the activity of interest. A *Movement Artifact* is a change in the recorded activity due to movement of the recording electrodes.

Auditory Evoked Potential An electrical waveform of biologic origin elicited by a sound stimulus. See *Evoked Potential*.

Backfiring Recurrent discharge of an antidromically activated motor neuron

BAER Abbreviation for brain stem auditory evoked response. Synonym: *Brain Stem Auditory Evoked Potential*.

Baseline The potential difference recorded from the biologic system of interest while the system is at rest

Benign Fasciculation Use of term discouraged. See *Fasciculation Potential*.

BER Abbreviation for brain stem evoked response. See *Brain Stem Auditory Evoked Potential*.

Bifilar Needle Electrode See *Bipolar Needle Electrode*.

Biphasic Action Potential An action potential with two phases

Biphasic Spike Potential See *End-Plate Activity, Biphasic*.

Bipolar Needle Electrode A recording electrode with two insulated wires side by side in a metal cannula the bare tips of which act as the active and reference electrodes. The metal cannula may be grounded.

Bizarre High-Frequency Discharge See *Complex Repetitive Discharge*.

Bizarre Repetitive Potential See *Complex Repetitive Discharge*.

Blink Reflex See *Blink Responses*.

Blink Response Strictly defined, one of the *Blink Responses*. See *Blink Responses*.

Blink Responses *Compound Muscle Action Potentials* evoked from the obicularis oculi muscles as a result of brief electrical or mechanical stimuli to the cutaneous area innervated by the supraorbital (or less commonly the infraorbital) branch of the trigeminal nerve. Typically, there is an early compound muscle action potential (R1 *Wave*) ipsilateral to the stimulation site with a latency of about 10 msec and a bilateral late compound muscle action potential (R2 *Wave*) with a latency of approximately 30 msec. Generally, only the R2 *Wave* is associated with a visible twitch of the orbicularis oculi. The configuration, amplitude, duration, and latency of the two components, along with the sites of recording and the sites of stimulation, should be specified. Both R1 and R2 *Waves* are probably due to a polysynaptic brain stem reflex, the *Blink Reflex*, with the afferent arc provided by the sensory branches of the trigeminal nerve and the efferent arc provided by the facial nerve motor fibers.

Brain Stem Auditory Evoked Potential (abbr. BAEP). Early (latency less than 10 msec) electrical waveforms of biologic origin elicited in response to sound stimuli. See *Evoked Potential*.

Brain Stem Auditory Evoked Response (abbr. BAER, BER). Synonymous with *Brain Stem Auditory Evoked Potential*

Breakthrough Voluntary Activity A burst of voluntary activity occurring within the S–X *Interval*

BSAP Abbreviation for brief, small, abundant potentials. Use of term discouraged. It is used to describe a recruitment pattern of brief-duration, small-amplitude, overly abundant motor unit action potentials. Quantitative measurements of motor unit potential duration, amplitude, numbers of phases, and recruitment frequency are to be preferred to qualitative descriptions such as this. See *Motor Unit Potential*.

BSAPP Abbreviation for brief, small, abundant, polyphasic potentials. Use of term discouraged. It is used to describe a recruitment pattern of brief-duration, small-amplitude, overly abundant, polyphasic motor unit action potentials. Quantitative measurements of motor unit potential duration, amplitude, numbers of phases, and recruitment frequency are to be preferred to qualitative descriptions such as this. See *Motor Unit Potential*.

Cathode The negative terminal of a source of electrical current

Cerebral Evoked Potential Electrical waveforms of biologic origin recorded over the head and elicited by sensory stimuli. See specific evoked potentials, *e.g., Somatosensory Evoked Potential, Visual Evoked Potential, Auditory Evoked Potential*.

Chronaxie The time required for an electrical current stimulus at a voltage twice the *Rheobase* to elicit the first muscle twitch. See *Strength–Duration Curve*.

Clinical Electromyography Loosely used to refer to all electrodiagnostic studies of peripheral nerves and muscle. See *Electrodiagnosis*.

Coaxial Needle Electrode See synonym, *Concentric Needle Electrode*.

Collision When used with reference to nerve conduction studies, the interaction of two action potentials propagated toward each other from opposite directions on the same nerve fiber so that the refractory periods of the two potentials prevent propagation past each other

Complex Action Potential See preferred term, *Serrated Action Potential.*

Complex Motor Unit Potential See preferred term, *Serrated Action Potential.*

Complex Repetitive Discharge Polyphasic or serrated action potentials that may begin spontaneously or after a needle movement. They have uniform frequency, shape, and amplitude, with abrupt onset, cessation, or change in configuration. Amplitude ranges from 100 μV to 1 mV and frequency of discharge from 5 Hz to 100 Hz.

Compound Action Potential See *Compound Mixed Nerve Action Potential. Compound Motor Nerve Action Potential, Compound Nerve Action Potential. Compound Sensory Nerve Action Potential,* and *Compound Muscle Action Potential.*

Compound Mixed Nerve Action Potential A compound nerve action potential is considered to have been evoked from afferent and efferent fibers if the recording electrodes detect activity on a mixed nerve with the electrical stimulus applied to a segment of the nerve that contains both afferent and efferent fibers.

Compound Motor Nerve Action Potential A compound nerve action potential is considered to have been evoked from efferent fibers to a muscle if the recording electrodes detect activity only in a motor nerve or a motor branch of a mixed nerve, or if the electrical stimulus is applied only to such a nerve or a ventral root. The amplitude, latency, duration, and phases should be noted. See *Compound Nerve Action Potential.*

Compound Muscle Action Potential The summation of nearly synchronous muscle fiber action potentials recorded from a muscle, commonly produced by stimulation of the nerve supplying the muscle either directly or indirectly. Baseline-to-peak amplitude, duration, and latency of the negative phase should be noted, along with details of the method of stimulation and recording. Use of specific named potentials is recommended, *e.g.*, *M Wave, F Wave, H Wave,* and *R1 Wave* or *R2 Wave* (*Blink Responses*).

Compound Nerve Action Potential The summation of nearly synchronous nerve fiber action potentials recorded from a nerve trunk, commonly produced by stimulation of the nerve directly or indirectly. Details of the method of stimulation and recording should be specified, together with the fiber type (sensory, motor, or mixed).

Compound Sensory Nerve Action Potential A compound nerve action potential is considered to have been evoked from afferent fibers if the recording electrodes detect activity only in a sensory nerve or in a sensory branch of a mixed nerve, if the electrical stimulus is applied to such a nerve or a dorsal nerve root; or if an adequate stimulus is applied synchronously to sensory receptors. The amplitude, latency, duration, and configuration should be noted. Generally, the amplitude is measured as the maximum peak-to-peak voltage, the latency as either the *Latency* to the initial deflection or the *Peak Latency* to the negative peak, and the duration as the interval from the first deflection of the waveform from the baseline to its final return to the baseline. The compound sensory nerve action potential has been referred to as the *Sensory Response* or *Sensory Potential.*

Concentric Needle Electrode The recording electrode that measures the potential difference between the bare tip of a central insulated wire in the bare shaft of a metal cannula. The bare tip of the central wire (active electrode) is flush with the bevel of the cannula (reference electrode).

Conditioning Stimulus A stimulus, preceding a *Test Stimulus*, used to modify the response elicited by the test stimulus alone. See *Stimulus.*

Conduction Block Failure of an action potential to be conducted past a particular point in the nervous system. In practice, a conduction block is documented by demonstration of a reduction in amplitude of an evoked potential greater than that normally seen with electrical stimulation at two different points on a nerve trunk; anatomical nerve variations and technical factors related to nerve stimulation must be excluded as the source of the reduction in amplitude.

Conduction Distance See *Conduction Velocity.*

Conduction Time See *Conduction Velocity.*

Conduction Velocity Speed of propagation of an *Action Potential* along a nerve or muscle fiber. The nerve fiber studied (motor, sensory, autonomic, or mixed) should be specified. For a nerve trunk, the maximum conduction velocity is calculated from the *Latency* of the evoked potential (muscle or nerve) at maximal or supramaximal intensity of stimulation at two different points. The distance between the two points (*Conduction Distance*) is divided by the difference between the corresponding latencies (*Conduction Time*). The calculated velocity represents the conduction velocity of the fastest fibers and is expressed in meters per second (m/sec). As commonly used, the term *Conduction Velocity* refers to the *Maximum Conduction Velocity*. By specialized techniques the conduction velocity of other fibers can be determined as well and should be specified. *e.g.*, minimum conduction velocity.

Contraction A voluntary or involuntary reversible muscle-shortening that may or may not be accompanied by *Action Potentials* from the muscle. This term is to be contrasted with the term *Contracture*, which refers to a condition of fixed muscle shortening.

Contracture An electrically silent, involuntary state of maintained muscle contraction, as seen in phosphorylase deficiency. The term is also used to refer to immobility of a joint due to other local processes.

Cortical Evoked Potential See *Cerebral Evoked Potential*.

Coupled Discharge See preferred term, *Late Component*.

Cramp Discharge Repetitive firing of action potentials with the configuration of *Motor Unit Potentials* at a high frequency in a large area of muscle, associated with an involuntary, painful muscle contraction (cramp).

Cycles Per Second A unit of frequency (abbr. *C/sec* or CPS). The preferred equivalent is *Hertz* (abbr. Hz).

Decrementing Response A progressive decline in the amplitude associated with a decrease in the area of the negative phase of the M *Wave* of successive responses to a series of supramaximal stimuli. The rate of stimulation and the number of stimuli should be specified. Contrast with *Incrementing Response*.

Delay The interval between the onset of oscilloscope sweep and the onset of a stimulus. Was used in the past to designate the interval from the stimulus to the response. Compare with *Latency*.

Denervation Potential Use of term discouraged. See *Fibrillation Potential*.

Depolarization A decrease in the electrical potential difference across a membrane from any cause, to any degree, relative to the normal resting potential. See *Polarization*.

Depolarization Block Failure of an excitable cell to respond to a simulus because of *Depolarization* of the cell membrane

Discharge Synonymous with *Action Potential*

Discharge Frequency the rate of repetition of an *Action Potential*. When potentials occur in groups, the rate of recurrence of the group and the rate of repetition of the individual components in the groups should be specified. See *Firing Rate*.

Discrete Activity The pattern of electrical activity at full voluntary contraction of the muscle is reduced to the extent that each individual *Motor Unit Potential* can be identified. The firing frequency of each of these potentials should be specified together with the force of contraction.

Distal Latency See *Motor Latency* and *Sensory Latency*.

"Dive-Bomber" Potential Use of term discouraged. See preferred term, *Myotonic Discharge*.

Double Discharge Two action potentials of the same form and nearly the same amplitude, occurring consistently in the same relationship to each other at intervals of 2 msec. to 20 msec. Contrast with *Paired Discharge*.

Doublet Synonymous with *Double Discharge*

Duration The time during which something exists or acts. (1) The duration of individual potential *Waveforms* is defined as the interval from the first deflection from the baseline to its final return to the baseline, unless otherwise specified. One common exception is the duration of the M *Wave*, which is usually defined as the interval from the deflection of the first negative phase from the baseline to its return to the baseline. (2) The duration of a single electrical stimulus is the interval of the applied current or voltage. (3) The duration of recurring stimuli or action potentials is the interval from the beginning to the end of the series.

Earthing Electode Synonymous with *Ground Electrode*

Electrical Artifact See *Artifact*.

Electrical Silence the absence of measurable electrial activity due to biologic or nonbiologic sources. The sensitivity, or signal-to-noise level, of the recording system should be specified.

Electrode A device capable of conducting electricity. The material (metal, fabric), size, configuration (disc, ring, needle), and location (surface, intramuscular, intracranial) should be specified. Electrodes may be used to record an electrical potential difference (*Recording Electrodes*) or to apply an electrical current (*Stimulating Electrodes*). In both cases two electrodes are always required. Depending on the relative size and location of the electrodes, however, the stimulating or recording condition may be referred to as *Monopolar*. See *Ground Electrode*, *Recording Electrode*, and *Stimulating Electrode*. Also see specific needle electrode configurations: *Monopolar*, *Concentric*, *Bipolar*, and *Multilead Needle Electrodes*.

Electrodiagnosis (abbr. EDX). General term used to refer to the recording of responses of nerves and muscle to electrical stimulation and the recording of insertional, spontaneous, and voluntary action potentials from muscle. It was originally used to refer to *Strength–Duration Curve* determinations and other early techniques.

Electromyelography the recording and study of electrical activity from the spinal cord. The term is also used to refer to studies of electrical activity from the cauda equina.

Electromyogram The record obtained by *Electromyography*

Electromyograph An instrument for detecting and displaying *Action Potentials* from muscle and nerve

Electromyography (abbr. EMG). Strictly defined, the recording and study of insertional, spontaneous, and voluntary electrical activity of muscle. The term is commonly used to refer to nerve conduction studies as well. Compare with *Clinical Electromyography* and the more general term, *Electrodiagnosis*.

Electroneurography The recording and study of the action potentials of peripheral nerves. See the preferred term, *Nerve Conduction Studies*, and more general term, *Electrodiagnosis*.

Electroneuromyography A newly fabricated word referring to the combined studies of *Electromyography* and *Electroneurography*. See preferred terms, *Clinical Electromyography* and *Electrodiagnosis*.

Electrospinogram The record obtained by *Electromyelography*

End-Plate Activity Spontaneous electrical activity recorded with a needle electrode close to muscle end-plates. May be either of two forms:

Monophasic. Low-amplitude (10–20 μV), short-duration (0.5–1 msec), monophasic (negative) potentials that occur in a dense, steady pattern and are restricted to a localized area of the muscle. Because of the multitude of different potentials occurring, the exact frequency, although appearing to be high, cannot be defined. These potentials are miniature end-plate potentials recorded extracellularly. This form of end-plate activity has been referred to as *End-Plate Noise* and is associated with a sound not unlike that of a seashell, which has been called a *Sea Shell Noise* or *Roar*.

Biphasic. Moderate-amplitude (100–300 μV), short-duration (2–4 msec), biphasic (negative–positive) spike potentials that occur irregularly in short bursts with a high frequency (50–100 Hz), restricted to a localized area within the muscle. These potentials are generated by muscle fibers excited by activity in nerve terminals. These potentials have been referred to as *Biphasic Spike Potentials*, *End-Plate Spikes*, and, incorrectly, "*Nerve*" *Potentials*.

End-Plate Noise See *End-Plate Activity, Monophasic*.

End-Plate Potential Graded, nonpropagated potential recorded by microelectrodes from muscle fibers in the region of the neuromuscular junction

End-Plate Spike See *End-Plate Activity, Biphasic*.

End-Plate Zone The site of the neuromuscular junction, a localized area of the muscle fiber in which activity identified as end-plate activity may be recorded

Evoked Action Potential Action potential elicited by a stimulus

Evoked Compound Muscle Action Potential The electrical activity of a muscle produced by stimulation of the nerves supplying the muscle. Baseline-to-peak amplitude of the negative phase, duration of the negative phase, and *Latency* should be measured, and details of the method of stimulation should be recorded. See specific named potentials: *M Wave*, *F Wave*, *H Wave*, R1 and R2 *Waves*, and *Blink Responses*.

Evoked Potential An electrical waveform elicited by and temporally related to a stimulus, most commonly an electrical stimulus delivered to a sensory receptor or nerve, or applied directly to a discrete area of the brain, spinal cord, or muscle. See *Auditory Evoked Potential, Brain Stem Auditory Evoked Potential, Spinal Evoked Potential, Somatosensory Evoked Potential, Visual Evoked Potential, Cerebral Evoked Potential, Compound Muscle Action Potential*, and *Compound Sensory Nerve Action Potential*.

Evoked Response Tautology. Use of term discouraged. The suggested term is *Evoked Potential*.

Excitability Capacity to be activated by or react to a stimulus

Excitatory Postsynaptic Potential (abbr. EPSP). A local, graded depolarization of a neuron in response to activation by a nerve terminal at a synapse. Contrast with *Inhibitory Postsynaptic Potential*.

Exploring Electrode Synonymous with *Active Electrode*. See *Recording Electrode*.

Facilitation of Neuromuscular Transmission An increase in the amplitude of an end-plate potential of a muscle fiber with stimulation of the axon in a variety of physiological and pharmacologic settings. Use of the term is not recommended for description of the phenomenon recorded in repetitive stimulation studies.

Fasciculation The random, spontaneous twitching of a group of muscle fibers that may be visible through the skin. The electrical activity associated with the spontaneous contraction is called the *Fasciculation Potential*. Compare with *Myokymia*.

Fasciculation Potential The electrical potential associated with *Fasciculation*, which has dimensions of a motor unit potential that occurs spontaneously as a single discharge. Most commonly these potentials occur sporadically and are termed *single fasciculation potentials*. Occasionally the potentials occur as a grouped discharge and are termed *grouped fasciculation potentials*. The occurrence of large numbers of either single or grouped fasciculations may produce a writhing, vermicular movement of the skin called *Myokymia*. Use of the terms *Benign Fasciculation* and *Malignant Fasciculation* is discouraged. Instead, the configuration of the potentials, peak-to-peak amplitude, duration, number of phases, and stability of configuration, in addition to frequency of occurrence, should be specified.

Fatigue Reduction in the force of contraction of muscle fibers as a result of repeated use or electrical stimulation. More generally, it is a state of depressed responsiveness resulting from protracted activity and requiring appreciable recovery time.

Fiber Density (1) Anatomically, a measure of the number of muscle or nerve fibers per unit area. (2) In single-fiber EMG, the mean number of muscle fiber potentials under voluntary control encountered during a systematic search. See *Single-Fiber Electromyography*.

Fibrillation The spontaneous contractions of individual muscle fibers that are ordinarily not visible through the skin. This term has been used loosely in electromyography for the preferred term, *Fibrillation Potential*.

Fibrillation Potential The electrical activity associated with fibrillating muscle fibers, reflecting the action potential of a single muscle fiber. The action potentials may occur spontaneously or after movement of the needle electrode. The potentials usually occur repetitively and regularly. Classically, the potentials are biphasic spikes of short duration (usually less than 5 msec) with an initial positive phase and a peak-to-peak amplitude of less than 1 mV. The firing rate has a wide range (1–50 Hz) and often decreases just before cessation of an individual discharge. A high-pitched regular sound is associated with the discharge of fibrillation potentials and has been described in the old literature as "rain on a tin roof." In addition to this classic form of fibrillation potentials, *Positive Sharp Waves* may also be recorded from fibrillating muscle fibers; the difference in the configuration of the potentials is due to the position of the recording electrode.

Firing Pattern Qualitative and quantitative description of the sequence of discharge of potential waveforms recorded from muscle or nerve

Firing Rate Frequency of repetition of a potential. The relationship of the frequency to the occurrence of other potentials and the force of muscle contraction may be described. See *Discharge Frequency*.

Fractionation of Motor Unit Potentials Use of term discouraged. This term has been used to describe polyphasic, short-duration, low-amplitude motor unit potentials, a configuration thought to imply failure to activate all of the muscle fibers in a motor unit.

F Reflex Use of term discouraged. No reflex is considered to be involved. See F *Wave*.

Frequency Number of complete cycles of a repetitive waveform in 1 second. Measured in *Hertz* (Hz), a unit preferred to its equivalent, *Cycles Per Second* (C/sec).

Frequency Analysis Determination of the range of frequencies composing a potential waveform, with a measurement of the absolute or relative amplitude of each component frequency. It is similar to the mathematical technique of Fourier analysis.

F Response Synonymous with F *Wave*. See F *Wave*.

Full Interference Pattern See *Interference Pattern*.

F Wave A late compound action potential evoked intermittently from a muscle by a supramaximal electrical stimulus to the nerve. Compared with the maximal amplitude M wave of the same muscle, the F wave has a reduced amplitude, variable configuration, and a longer and more variable latency. It can be found in many muscles of the upper and lower extremities, and the latency is longer with more distal sites of stimulation. The F *Wave* is due to antidromic activation of motor neurons. It was named by Magladery and McDougal in 1950. Contrast with H *Wave*.

G1, G2 Synonymous with Grid 1, Grid 2. See *Recording Electrodes*.

"Giant" Motor Unit Action Potential Use of term discouraged. It refers to a motor unit potential with a peak-to-peak amplitude and duration much greater than the range recorded in corresponding muscles in normal subjects of similar age. Quantitative measurements of amplitude and duration are preferable.

Ground Electrode An electrode connected to a large conducting body (such as the earth) used as a common return for an electrical circuit and as an arbitary zero potential reference point

Grouped Discharge Intermittent repetition of a group of *Action Potentials* with the same or nearly the same waveform and a relatively short interpotential interval within the group compared to the time interval between each group. It may occur spontaneously or with voluntary activity and may be regular or irregular in its firing pattern.

Habituation Decrease in amplitude and/or duration of a response with repeated stimuli. Response may be eliminated.

Hertz (abbr. Hz). Unit of frequency representing cycles per second

Hoffmann Reflex see H *Wave.*

H Reflex Abbreviation for Hoffmann reflex. See H *Wave.*

H Response Synonymous with H *Wave*

H Wave A late compound muscle action potential having a consistent latency evoked regularly, when present, from a muscle by an electrical stimulus to the nerve. It is regularly found only in a limited group of physiologic extensors, particularly the calf muscles. The reflex is most easily obtained with the cathode positioned proximal to the anode. Compared with the maximal amplitude M *Wave* of the same muscle, the H wave has a reduced amplitude, a longer latency, and a lower optimal stimulus intensity; its configuration is constant. The latency is longer with more distal sites of stimulation. A stimulus intensity sufficient to elicit a maximal-amplitude M wave reduces or abolishes the H wave. The H wave is thought to be due to a spinal reflex, the Hoffmann reflex, with electrical stimulation of afferent fibers in the mixed nerve to the muscle and activation of motor neurons to the muscle through a monosynaptic connection in the spinal cord. The reflex and wave are named in honor of Hoffmann's description (1918). Compare with F *Wave.*

Hyperpolarization See *Polarization.*

Increased Insertional Activity See *Insertional Activity.*

Incremental Response See synonym, *Incrementing Response.*

Incrementing Response A progressive increase in amplitude associated with an increase in the area of the negative phase of the M *Wave* of successive responses to a series of supramaximal stimuli. The rate of stimulation and the number of stimuli should be specified. Contrast with *Decrementing Response.*

Indifferent Electrode Synonymous with *Reference Electrode.* See *Recording Electrode.*

Inhibitory Postsynaptic Potential (abbr. IPSP). A local graded hyperpolarization of a neuron in response to activation at a synapse by a nerve terminal. Contrast with *Excitatory Postsynaptic Potential.*

Injury Potential The potential difference between a normal region of the surface of a nerve or muscle and a region that has been injured; also called a demarcation potential. This potential was studied before intracellular recording was introduced. The injury potential approximates the potential across the membrane because the injured surface is almost at the potential of the inside of the cell. This term has been loosely used to describe *Insertional Activity* encountered in *Clinical Electromyography.*

Insertional Activity Electrical activity caused by insertion or movement of a needle electrode. The amount of the activity may be described qualitatively as *Normal, Reduced, Increased,* or *Prolonged.*

Interdischarge Interval The time between consecutive discharges of the same potential. Measurements should be made between the corresponding points on each waveform.

Interference Unwanted electrical activity arising outside the system being studied

Interference Pattern Electrical activity recorded from a muscle with a needle electrode during maximal voluntary effort, in which identification of each of the contributing action potentials is not possible because of the overlap or interference of one potential with another. When no individual potentials can be identified, this is known as a *Full Interference Pattern.* A *Reduced Interference Pattern* is one in which some of the individual potentials may be identified while other individual potentials cannot because of overlapping. The term *Discrete Activity* is used to describe the electrical activity recorded when each of the motor unit potentials can be identified. It is important that the force of contraction associated with the interference pattern be specified.

Interpotential Interval The time between two different potentials. Measurement should be made between the corresponding parts on each waveform.

Intramuscular Electrode An electrode ususally used for recording and usually shaped like a needle to facilitate placement within a muscle belly

Involuntary Activity Action potentials that are not under voluntary control. The condition under which they occur (*e.g.*, spontaneous), or, if elicited by a stimulus, the nature of the stimulus, should be described. Compare with *Spontaneous Activity.*

Isoelectric Discharge A recording obtained from a pair of equipotential electrodes

Iterative Discharge See preferred term, *Repetitive Discharge.*

Jitter Synonymous with "single-fiber electromyographic jitter." Jitter is the variability of the *Interpotential Interval* between two muscle fiber action potentials belonging to the same motor unit. It is usually expressed quantitatively as the mean value of the difference between the interpotential intervals of consecutive discharges (the mean consecutive difference, abbr. MCD). Under certain conditions jitter is expressed as the mean value of the difference between the interpotential intervals arranged in order of decreasing interpotential intervals (the mean sorted difference, abbr. MSD).

Jolly Test A technique, described in 1895 by Jolly, of applying a Faradic current to a motor nerve while recording the muscle contraction. This test has been refined and replaced by the technique of *Repetitive Stimulation* of motor nerves and the recording of successive M waves to detect a defect of neuromuscular transmission; use of the term is discouraged for modern testing techniques.

Late Component of a Motor Unit Potential A potential separated from a *Motor Unit Potential* by a segment of baseline recording, but firing in a time-locked relationship to the motor unit potential

Late Response A general term used to describe an evoked potential having a longer latency than the M *Wave*. See H *Wave*, F *Wave*.

Latency The interval between the onset of a stimulus and the onset of a response unless otherwise specified. Latency always refers to the onset unless specified, as in *Peak Latency*.

Latency of Activation The time required for an electrical stimulus to depolarize a nerve. In the past this was estimated to be 0.1 msec.

Latent Period See synonym, *Latency*.

Malignant Fasciculation Use of term discouraged. See *Fasciculation Potential*.

Maximal Stimulus See *Stimulus*.

Maximum Nerve Conduction Velocity See *Conduction Velocity*.

Membrane Instability The tendency of a cell membrane to depolarize spontaneously or after mechanical irritation or voluntary activation

Microneurography The technique of recording peripheral nerve action potentials in man by means of intraneural microelectrodes

Miniature End-Plate Potential When recorded with microelectrodes, monophasic negative discharges with amplitudes less than 100 μV and durations of 4 msec or less, occurring irregularly and recorded in an area of muscle corresponding to the myoneural junction. They are thought to be due to small quantities (quanta) of acetylcholine released spontaneously. Compare with *End-Plate Activty*.

Mixed Nerve Action Potential See *Compound Nerve Action Potential*.

Monophasic Action Potential An action potential with one phase

Monophasic End-Plate Activity See *End-Plate Activity*.

Monopolar Needle Electrode A solid wire, usually of stainless steel, coated, except at its tip, with an insulating material. Variations in voltage between the tip of the needle (active or exploring electrode) positioned in a muscle and a conductive plate on the skin surface or a bare needle in subcutaneous tissue (reference electrode) are measured. By convention this recording condition is referred to as a monopolar needle electrode recording; it should be emphasized, however, that potential differences are always recorded between two electrodes.

Motor Latency The interval between the onset of a stimulus and the onset of the resultant *Compound Muscle Action Potential*. The term may be qualified as *Proximal Motor Latency* or *Distal Motor Latency*, depending on the relative position of the stimulus.

Motor Nerve Action Potential See *Compound Motor Nerve Action Potential*.

Motor Nerve Conduction Velocity (abbr. MNCV). See *Conduction Velocity*.

Motor Point The point over a muscle where a muscle contraction may be elicited by a minimal-intensity, short-duration electrical stimulus

Motor Response Either (1) the compound muscle action potential recorded over a muscle with stimulation of the nerve to the muscle or (2) the muscle twitch or contraction elicited by stimulation of the nerve to a muscle. As commonly used, *motor response* refers only to the evoked potential, the M *Wave*.

Motor Unit The anatomical unit of an anterior horn cell, its axon, the neuromuscular junctions, and all of the muscle fibers innervated by the axon

Motor Unit Action Potential (abbr. MUAP). See synonym, *Motor Unit Potential*.

Motor Unit Potential (abbr. MUP) An action potential reflecting the electrical activity of that part of a single anatomical motor unit that is within the recording range of an electrode. The action potential is characterized by its consistent appearance with and relationship to the force of a voluntary contraction of a muscle. The following parameters should be specified, quantitatively if possible, after the recording electrode is placed so as to minimize the *Rise Time* (which by convention should be less than 0.5 msec), generally also maximizing the amplitude:

- I. Configuration
  - A. *Amplitude*, peak-to-peak (μV or mV)
  - B. *Duration*, total (msec)
  - C. Number of *Phases* (*Monophasic*, *Biphasic*, *Triphasic*, *Tetraphasic*, *Polyphasic*)
  - D. Direction of each *Phase* (negative, positive)

E. Number of *Turns of Serrated Potential*
F. Variation of shape with consective discharges
G. Presence of *Late Components*

II. *Recruitment* characteristics
A. Threshold of activation (first-recruited, low-threshold, high-threshold)
B. *Onset Frequency* (Hz)
C. *Recruitment Frequency* (Hz) or *Recruitment Interval* (msec) of individual potentials

Descriptive terms implying diagnostic significance (*e.g.*, *Myopathic*, *Neuropathic*, *Regeneration*, *Nascent*, *Giant*, BSAP, and BSAPP) are not recommended.

Motor Unit Subunit An abandoned concept of muscle physiology. Fibers of a motor unit were considered to be arranged in groups of subunits containing an average of ten fibers that fired synchronously. This theory is no longer accepted.

Motor Unit Territory (1) The area in which *Motor Unit Potentials* from a single motor unit may be recorded with a *Rise Time* of less than 0.5 msec. (2) The area in a muscle over which the muscle fibers of an individual motor unit are distributed anatomically

Movement Artifact See *Artifact*.

M Response See synonym, *M Wave*.

MUAP Abbreviation for motor unit action potential. See synonym, *Motor Unit Potential*.

Multielectrode See *Multilead Electrode*.

Multilead Electrode Three or more insulated wires inserted through a common metal cannula with their bared tips at an aperture in the cannula and flush with the outer circumference of the cannula. The arrangement of the bare tips relative to the axis of the cannula and the distance between each tip should be specified.

Multiple Discharge Four or more motor unit action potentials of the same form and nearly the same amplitude occurring consistently in the same relationship to one another. See *Double Discharge* and *Triple Discharge*.

Multiplet See *Multiple Discharge*.

MUP Abbreviation for *Motor Unit Potential*

Muscle Action Potential Strictly defined, the action potential recorded from a single muscle fiber. However, the term is commonly used to refer to a compound muscle action potential. See *Compound Muscle Action Potential*.

Muscle Fiber Conduction Velocity The speed of propagation of a single muscle fiber action potential, usually expressed as meters per second. The muscle fiber conduction velocity is usually less than most nerve conduction velocities, varies with the rate of discharge of the muscle fiber, and requires special techniques for measurement.

Muscle Unit An anatomical term referring to the group of muscle fibers innervated by a single motor neuron. See *Motor Unit*.

M Wave A *Compound Action Potential* evoked from a muscle by a single electrical stimulus to its motor nerve. By convention, the M wave elicited by supramaximal stimulation is used for motor nerve conduction studies. The recording electrodes should be placed so that the initial deflection of the evoked potential is negative. The *Latency*, commonly called *Motor Latency*, is the latency (milliseconds) to the onset of the first negative phase. The amplitude (millivolts) is the baseline-to-peak amplitude of the first negative phase, unless otherwise specified. The term *Duration* (milliseconds) refers to the duration of the first negative phase, unless otherwise specified. Normally, the configuration of the M wave (usually biphasic) is quite stable with repeated stimuli at low rates (1–5 Hz). See *Repetitive Stimulation*.

Myokymia Involuntary, continuous quivering of muscle fibers, which may be visible through the skin as a vermiform movement. It is associated with spontaneous, rhythmic discharge of *Motor Unit Potentials*. See *Myokymic Discharges*, *Fasciculation*, and *Fasciculation Potential*.

Myokymic Discharges Action potentials with the configuration of *Motor Unit Potentials* that occur spontaneously, recur regularly, and may be associated with clinical myokymia. Two distinct firing patterns are recognized. Commonly, the discharges are grouped with a short period of firing (up to a few seconds) at a uniform rate (2–20 Hz), followed by a short period (up to a few seconds) of silence, with repetition of the same sequence for a particular potential. Less commonly, the potential recurs continuously at a fairly uniform firing rate (1–5 Hz). Myokymic discharges are a subclass of *Grouped Discharges* and *Repetitive Discharges*.

Myopathic Motor Unit Potential Use of term discouraged. It is used to refer to low-amplitude, short-duration, polyphasic motor unit action potentials. The term incorrectly implies specific diagnostic significance of a motor unit potential configuration. See *Motor Unit Potential*.

Myopathic Recruitment Use of term discouraged. It is used to describe an increase in the number and firing rate of motor unit potentials compared with normal for the strength of muscle contraction.

Myotonic Discharge Repetitive discharge of 20 Hz to 80 Hz of bipasic (positive–negative) spike potentials less than 5 msec in duration or monophasic positive waves of 5 msec to 20 msec recorded after needle insertion, or less commonly after voluntary muscle contraction or muscle percussion. The amplitude and frequency of the potentials must both wax and wane to be identified as myotonic discharges. This change produces a characteristic musical sound in the audio display of the electromyograph, to the corresponding change in pitch, which has been likened to the sound of a dive-bomber. Contrast with *Waning Discharge*.

Myotonic Potential See prefered term, *Myotonic Discharge*.

Myotonic Response Delayed relaxation of muscle after voluntary contraction or percussion and associated with a myotonic discharge. See *Myotonic Discharge*.

Nascent Motor Unit Potential From the Latin *nascens*, to be born. Use of the term is discouraged because it incorrectly implies diagnostic significance of a motor unit potential configuration. The term has been used to refer to very low amplitude, long-duration, highly polyphasic motor unit potentials observed during early stages of reinnervation of muscle. See *Motor Unit Potential*.

Nascent Unit Use of term discouraged. See *Nascent Motor Unit Potential*.

Needle Electrode An electrode for recording or stimulating, shaped like a needle. See specific electrodes: *Bipolar Needle Electrode, Concentric Needle electrode, Monopolar Needle Electrode, Multilead Electrode*.

Nerve Action Potential Strictly defined, an action potential recorded from a single nerve fiber. The term is commonly used to refer to the compound nerve action potential. See *Compound Nerve Action Potential*.

Nerve Conduction Studies Refers to all aspects of electrodiagnostic studies of peripheral nerves. However, the term is generally used to refer to the recording and measurement of *Compound Nerve* and *Compound Muscle Action Potentials* elicited in response to a single supramaximal electrical *Stimulus* under standardized conditions that permit establishment of normal ranges of amplitude, duration, and latency of *Evoked Potentials* and the calculation of the *Maximum Conduction Velocity* of individual nerves. See *Compound Nerve Action Potential, Compound Muscle Action Potential, Conduction Velocity*, and *Repetitive Stimulation*.

Nerve Conduction Velocity (abbr. NCV). Loosely used to refer to the maximum nerve conduction velocity. See *Conduction Velocity*.

Nerve Potential Equivalent to *Nerve Action Potential*. Also commonly, but inaccurately, used to refer to the biphasic form of *End-Plate Activity*. The latter use is incorrect because muscle fibers, not nerve fibers, are the source of these potentials.

Nerve Trunk Action Potential See preferred term, *Compound Nerve Action Potential*.

Neuromyotonia Clinical syndrome of continuous muscle fiber activity manifested as continuous muscle rippling and stiffness. It may be associated with a variety of electrical discharges.

Neuromyotonic Discharges Bursts of *Motor Unit Potentials* firing at more than 150 Hz for 0.5 sec to 2 sec. The amplitude of the response typically wanes. Discharges may occur spontaneously or be initiated by needle movement.

Neuropathic Motor Unit Potential Use of term discouraged. It is used to refer to abnormally high amplitude, long duration, polyphasic *Motor Unit Potentials*. The term incorrectly implies a specific diagnostic significance of a motor unit potential configuration. See *Motor Unit Potential*.

Neuropathic Recruitment Use of term discouraged. It has been used to describe a recruitment pattern with a decreased number of *Motor Unit Potentials* firing at a rapid rate. See preferred terms, *Discrete Activity, Reduced Interference Pattern*.

Noise Strictly defined, an *Artifact* consisting of low-amplitude, random potentials produced by a amplifier and unrelated to the input signal. It is most apparent when high gains are used. The term is loosely used to refer to end-plate noise. Compare with *End-Plate Activity*.

Onset Frequency The lowest stable frequency of firing for a single *Motor Unit Potential* that can be voluntarily maintained by a subject

Onset Latency Tautology. See *Latency*.

Order of Activation The sequence of appearance of different *Motor Unit Potentials* with increasing strength of voluntary contraction. See *Recruitment*.

Orthodromic Said of *Action Potentials* or stimuli eliciting action potentials propagated in the same direction as physiologic conduction, *e.g.*, motor nerve conduction away from the spinal cord and sensory nerve conduction toward the spinal cord. Contrast with *Antidromic*.

Paired Discharge Two action potentials of the same form and nearly the same amplitude occurring consistently in the same relationship to each other at intervals of 20 msec to 80 msec. Contrast with *Double Discharge*.

Paired Response Loosely used to refer to either the *Paired Discharge* or the *Late Component*.

Paired Stimuli Two temporally linked stimuli. The time interval between the two stimuli and the intensity of each stimulus should be specified. The first is called the *Conditioning Stimulus* and the second the *Test Stimulus*.

Parasite Potential See preferred term, *Late Component of a Motor Unit Potential*.

Peak Latency The interval between the onset of a

stimulus and a specified peak of the evoked potential (usually the negative peak)

Phase That portion of a *Wave* between the departure from and the return to the *Baseline*

Polarization As used in neurophysiology, the presence of an electrical *Potential* difference across an excitable cell membrane. The potential across the membrane of a cell when it is not excited by input or spontaneously active is termed the *Resting Potential*; it is at a steady state with regard to the electrical potential difference across the membrane. *Depolarization* is a decrease in polarization to any degree, relative to the normal resting potential. *Hyperpolarization* is an increase in polarization relative to the resting potential. *Repolarization* is an increase in polarization from the depolarized state toward, but not above, the normal or resting potential.

Polyphasic Action Potential An *Action Potential* having five or more phases. See *Phase*. Contrast with *Serrated Action Potential*.

Positive Sharp Wave Strictly defined, one form of electrical activity associated with fibrillating muscle fibers. It is recorded as a biphasic, positive-negative *Action Potential* initiated by needle movement and recurring in a uniform, regular pattern at a rate of 2 Hz to 50 Hz, which may decrease just before cessation of the discharge. The amplitude and duration vary considerably, but the initial positive deflection is usually less than 5 msec in duration and up to 1 mV in amplitude. The negative phase is of low amplitude, with a duration of 10 msec to 100 msec. A sequence of positive sharp waves is commonly referred to as a *Train of Positive Sharp Waves*. Positive sharp waves are recorded from the damaged area of fibrillating muscle fibers. Loosely defined, a positive sharp wave is any action potential recorded with the waveform of a positive wave, without reference to the firing pattern or method of generation.

Positive Wave Strictly defined, the positive phase of a waveform. Loosely defined, the term refers to a positive sharp wave. See *Positive Sharp Wave*.

Postactivation Depression The reduction in amplitude of an *Evoked Potential* in response to a single *Stimulus* that occurs after *Repetitive Stimulation* or after voluntary contraction

Postactivation Exhaustion The reduction in amplitude associated with a decrease in the area of the negative phase of the initial M *Wave* and/or the exaggeration of the *Decrementing Response* seen 2 to 4 minutes after either a brief (10–30-sec), strong voluntary contraction or a period of nerve stimulation causing tetanic muscle contraction. Compare with *Postactivation Facilitation*.

Postactivation Facilitation The increase in amplitude associated with an increase in the area of the negative phase of the initial M *Wave* and/or the diminution of the *Decrementing Response* seen a few seconds after either a brief (10–30-sec), strong voluntary contraction or a period of nerve stimulation causing tetanic muscle contraction. Compare with *Postactivation Exhaustion*.

Postactivation Potentiation Synonymous with preferred term, *Postactivation Facilitation*

Posttetanic Potentiation Enhancement of excitability following a long period of high-frequency stimulation. This phenomenon is known mainly in the mammalian spinal cord, where it lasts minutes or even hours. Use of the term is not recommended to describe the phenomenon of *Postactivation Facilitation*.

Potential Strictly, *Voltage*; loosely, synonymous with *Action Potential*. See *Polarization*.

Prolonged Insertional Activity See *Insertional Activity*.

Propagation Velocity of a Muscle Fiber The speed of transmission of a muscle fiber action potential

Proximal Latency See *Motor Latency* and *Sensory Latency*.

Pseudofacilitation (of Neuromuscular Transmission) Use of term discouraged. It refers to an increase in amplitude with a corresponding reduction in duration of the negative phase of the M *Wave*, resulting in no change in the area of the negative phase of the M wave. This probably reflects a reduction in the temporal dispersion of a constant number of summated muscle fiber action potentials and must be differentiated from *Postactivation Facilitation*. See *Postactivation Facilitation*.

Pseudomyotonic Discharge Use of term discouraged. It has been used to refer to various phenomena, including (1) *Myotonic Discharges* occurring in the presence of a neurogenic disease, (2) *Complex Repetitive Discharges*, and (3) *Repetitive Discharges* that wax or wane in either frequency or amplitude but not in both. See *Waning Discharge*.

Pseudopolyphasic Action Potential Use of term discouraged. See preferred term, *Serrated Action Potential*.

R1, R2 Waves See *Blink Responses*.

Recording Electrode Device used to monitor electrical current or potential. All electrical recordings require two *Electrodes*. The electrode close to the source of the activity to be recorded is called the *Active* or *Exploring Electrode*, and the other is called the *Reference Electrode*. The term *active electrode* is synonymous with the older terminology G1 or *Grid* 1, and the reference electrode with G2 or *Grid* 2. By current convention, a potential difference that is negative at the active electrode relative to the reference electrode causes an upward deflection on the oscilloscope screen. The term *monopolar recording* is not recommended because all recording requires two electrodes; however, it is commonly used to describe the use of an intramuscular needle exploring electrode in combination with a surface disc or subcutaneous needle reference electrode.

Recruitment The orderly activation of the same and new motor units with increasing strength of voluntary muscle contraction. See *Motor Unit Potential*.

Recruitment Frequency Firing rate of a *Motor Unit Potential* when an additional motor unit potential first appears during gradually increasing voluntary muscle contraction.

Recruitment Interval The *Interdischarge Interval* between two consecutive discharges of a *Motor Unit Potential* when an additional motor unit potential first appears during gradually increasing voluntary muscle contraction. The reciprocal of the recruitment interval is the *Recruitment Frequency*.

Recruitment Pattern A qualitative and/or quantitative description of the sequence of appearance of *Motor Unit Potentials* with increasing voluntary muscle contraction. The *Recruitment Frequency* and *Recruitment Interval* are two quantitative measures commonly used. See *Interference Pattern* for commonly used qualitative terms.

Reduced Insertional Activity See *Insertional Activity*.

Reduced Interference Pattern See *Interference Pattern*.

Reference Electrode See *Recording Electrode*.

Reflex A stereotyped *Motor Response* elicited by a *Stimulus*

Refractory Period Time after an *Action Potential* during which the response to an additional stimulus is altered. The *Absolute Refractory Period* is that segment of the refractory period during which no stimulus, however strong, evokes an additional action potential. The *Relative Refractory Period* is that segment of the refractory period during which a stimulus must be greater than a normal threshold stimulus to evoke a second action potential.

Relative Refractory Period See *Refractory Period*.

Repetitive Discharges General term for the recurrence of an *Action Potential* with the same or nearly the same form. The term may refer to recurring potentials recorded in muscle at rest, during voluntary contraction, or in response to single nerve stimulus. The discharge may be named for the number of times a potential recurs in a group (*e.g.*, *Double Discharge*, *Triple Discharge*, *Multiple Discharge*, *Coupled Discharge*) or other characteristics (*e.g.*, *Complex Repetitive Discharge*, *Myokymic Discharge*).

Repetitive Stimulation The technique of using repeated supramaximal stimulation of a nerve while quantitatively recording M *Waves* from muscles innervated by the nerve. It should be described in terms of the frequency of stimuli and number of stimuli (or duration of the total group). For descriptions of specific patterns of responses, see *Incrementing Response*, *Decrementing Response*, *Postactivation Facilitation*, and *Postactivation Exhaustion*.

Repolarization See *Polarization*.

Residual Latency The calculated time difference between the measured distal latency of a motor nerve and the expected distal latency, calculated by dividing the distance between the stimulus cathode and the active recording electrode by the maximum conduction velocity measured in a more proximal segment of a nerve

Response An activity elicited by a *Stimulus*

Resting Membrane Potential Voltage across the membrane of an excitable cell at rest. See *Polarization*.

Rheobase The intensity of an electrical current of infinitely long duration necessary to produce a minimal visible twitch of a muscle when the cathode is applied to the motor point of the muscle. In practice a duration of at lease 300 msec is used to determine the *Rheobase*.

Rise Time By convention, the shortest interval from the nadir of a positive phase to the peak of a negative phase of a *Wave*

Satellite Potential Synonymous with preferred term, *Late Component*

Sea Shell Noise (Sea Shell Roar) Use of term discouraged. See *End-Plate Activity*, *Monophasic*.

Sensory Delay See preferred terms, *Sensory Latency* and *Sensory Peak Latency*.

Sensory Latency The interval between the onset of a stimulus and the onset of the *Compound Sensory Nerve Action Potential*. This term has been loosely used to refer to the *Sensory Peak Latency*. The term may be qualified as *Proximal Sensory Latency* or *Distal Sensory Latency*, depending on the relative position of the stimulus.

Sensory Nerve Action Potential See *Compound Sensory Nerve Action Potential*.

Sensory Nerve Conduction Velocity See *Conduction Velocity*.

Sensory Peak Latency The interval between the onset of a *Stimulus* and the peak of the negative phase of the *Compound Sensory Nerve Action Potential*. Note that the term *Latency* refers to the interval between the onset of a stimulus and the onset of a response.

Sensory Potential Used to refer to the compound sensory nerve action potential. See *Compound Sensory Nerve Action Potential*.

Sensory Response Used to refer to a sensory evoked potential, *e.g.*, *Compound Sensory Nerve Action Potential*

Serrated Action Potential An action potential waveform with several changes in direction (turns) that do not cross the baseline. This term is preferred to the terms *Complex Action Potential* and *Pseudopolyphasic Action Potential*. See *Turns*.

Shock Artifact See *Artifact*.

Silent Period Time during which there is no electrical activity in a muscle following rapid unloading of a muscle

Single-Fiber Electromyography (abbr. SFEMG). General term referring to the technique and conditions that permit recording of a single muscle fiber *Action Potential*. See *Single-Fiber Needle Electrode*.

Single-Fiber Needle Electrode A needle *Electrode* with a small recording surface (usually 25 μm in diameter), permitting the recording of single muscle fiber action potentials. See *Single-Fiber Electromyography*.

Somatosensory Evoked Potential (abbr. SSEP). Electrical *Waves* recorded from the head or trunk in response to electrical or physiological stimulation of peripheral sensory fibers. Recordings over the spine may be referred to as *Spinal Evoked Potentials*.

Spike A transient *Wave* with a pointed peak and short duration (a few milliseconds or less). See *End-Plate Spike* and *Fibrillation Potentials*.

Spinal Evoked Potential An electrical *Wave* recorded over the spine in response to electrical stimulation of peripheral sensory fibers. See *Somatosensory Evoked Potential*.

Spontaneous Activity Action potentials recorded from muscle or nerve at rest after insertional activity has subsided and when there is no voluntary contraction or external stimulus. Compare with *Involuntary Activity*.

Staircase Phenomenon The progressive increase in the force of a muscle contraction observed with repeated nerve stimulation at low rates

Stigmatic Electrode Synonymous with active or exploring electrode. See *Recording Electrode*.

Stimulating Electrode Device used to apply electrical current. All electrical stimulation requires two electrodes; the negative terminal is termed the *Cathode*, the positive terminal the *Anode*. By convention, the stimulating electrodes are called *Bipolar* if they are roughly equal in size and separated by less than 5 cm. The stimulating electrodes are called *Monopolar* if the cathode is smaller than the anode and is separated from it by more than 5 cm. Electrical stimulation for *Nerve Conduction Studies* generally requires application of the cathode to produce depolarization of the nerve trunk fibers. If the anode is inadvertently placed between the cathode and the recording electrodes, a focal block of nerve conduction (*Anodal Block*) may occur and cause a technically unsatisfactory study.

Stimulus Any external agent, state, or change that is capable of influencing the activity of a cell, tissue, or organism. In clinical *Nerve Conduction Studies* an electrical stimulus is generally applied to a nerve or muscle. The electrical stimulus may be described in absolute terms or with respect to the evoked potential of the nerve or muscle. In absolute terms the electrical stimulus has a strength or intensity measured in voltage (volts) or current (milliamperes) and a duration (milliseconds). With respect to the evoked potential, the stimulus may be graded as subthreshold, threshold, submaximal, maximal, or supramaximal. A *Threshold Stimulus* is that electrical stimulus just sufficient to produce a detectable response. Stimuli less than the threshold stimulus are termed *Subthreshold*. The *Maximal Stimulus* is the stimulus intensity after which a further increase in the stimulus intensity causes no increase in the amplitude of the evoked potential. Stimuli of intensity below this and above threshold are *Submaximal*. Stimuli of intensity greater than the maximal stimulus are *Supramaximal*. Ordinarily, supramaximal stimuli are used for nerve conduction studies. By convention, an electrical stimulus of approximately 20% greater voltage than required for the maximal stimulus may be used for supramaximal stimulation. The frequency, number, and duration of a series of stimuli should be specified.

Stimulus Artifact See *Artifact*.

Strength–Duration Curve A graphic representation of the relationship between the intensity (Y axis) and various durations (X axis) of the threshold electrical stimulus for a muscle with the stimulating cathode positioned over the motor point

Submaximal Stimulus See *Stimulus*.

Subthreshold Stimulus See *Stimulus*.

Supramaximal Stimulus See *Stimulus*.

Surface Electrode A conducting device for stimulating or recording placed on a skin surface. The material (metal, fabric), configuration (disc, ring), size, and separation should be specified. See *Electrode (Ground, Recording, Stimulating)*.

S–X Interval The total duration of the *Silent Period* produced by electrical stimulation of the mixed nerve to a voluntarily contracting muscle, measured from the stimulus artifact to resumption of uninterrupted voluntary activity

Temporal Dispersion A waveform of longer duration than normal. Commonly used to refer to an increase in the duration of an evoked potential with more proximal sites of stimulation of a greater degree than that normally seen.

Terminal Latency Synonymous with preferred term, *Distal Latency*. See *Motor Latency* and *Sensory Latency*.

Test Stimulus The stimulus producing the event being measured. Contrast with *Conditioning Stimulus.*

Tetanic Contraction The state of a muscle in sustained contraction resulting from stimulation at a frequency high enough for individual twitches to summate to a smooth tension and with associated electrical activity of muscle action potentials. It may be attained in normal muscle voluntarily or in response to repetitive nerve stimulation. Contrast with *Cramp Discharge.*

Tetanus Loosely used to refer to *Tetanic Contraction.* The term is also used to refer to the acute infectious disease. See *Tetanic Contraction* and *Tetany.*

Tetany A clinical syndrome manifested by muscle twitching, cramps, and sustained muscle contraction (*Tetanus*). These clinical signs are manifestations of peripheral and central nervous system nerve irritability from several causes. In these conditions *Repetitive Discharges* (double discharge, triple discharge, multiple discharge) occur frequently with voluntary activation of motor unit potentials or may appear as spontaneous activity with systemic alkalosis or local ischemia.

Tetraphasic Action Potential An *Action Potential* with four phases

Threshold the level at which a clear and abrupt transition occurs from one state to another. The term is generally used to refer to the voltage level at which an *Action Potential* is initiated in a single axon or a group of axons. It is also operationally defined as the intensity that produced a response in about approximately 50% of equivalent trials.

Threshold Stimulus See *Stimulus.*

Time Constant of Accommodation (lambda, λ). The time constant of the rate at which, after accommodation, the threshold of an excitable tissue reverts to its initial level. It is the reciprocal of the slope of the *Accommodation Curve.*

Train of Positive Sharp Waves See *Positive Sharp Waves.*

Train of Stimuli A group of stimuli. The duration of the group and the frequency of the individual components should be specified.

Triphasic Action Potential An *Action Potential* with three phases

Triple Discharge Three action potentials of the same form and nearly the same amplitude, occurring consistently in the same relationship to one another. The interval between the second and the third action potentials often exceeds that between the first two, and both are usually in the range of 2 msec to 20 msec.

Triplet See *Triple Discharge.*

Turns Changes in the direction of a waveform that do not necessarily pass through the baseline. The minimal excursion required to constitute a turn should be specified.

Unipolar Needle Electrode See synonym, *Monopolar Needle Electrode.*

Visual Evoked Potential Electrical waveforms of biologic origin recorded over the cerebrum and elicited by light stimuli

Visual Evoked Response (abbr. VER). See *Visual Evoked Potential.*

Voltage The potential difference between two points

Volume Conduction The spread of current from a potential source through a conducting medium, such as the body tissues

Voluntary Activity In electromyography, the electrical activity recorded from a muscle with consciously controlled muscle contraction. The effort made to contract the muscle (*e.g.*, minimal, moderate, or maximal) and the strength of contraction in absolute terms or relative to a maximal voluntary contraction of a normal corresponding muscle should be specified.

Waning Discharge General term referring to a repetitive discharge that decreases in frequency or amplitude. Compare with *Myotonic Discharge.*

Wave An undulating line constituting a graphic representation of a change, *e.g.*, a changing potential difference

Waveform The shape of a *Wave.* The term is often used synonymously with *Wave.*

Wedensky-like Neuromuscular Failure Use of term discouraged. The term has been used to describe a decrease in the strength of the sustained muscle contraction during repeated nerve stimulation at frequencies within the physiologic range (less than 50 Hz). See preferred term, *Decrementing Response.*

Wedensky Phenomenon A decrease in strength of a sustained muscle contraction during sustained nerve stimulation at frequencies above the physiologic range, (greater than 50 Hz). This phenomenon is seen in normal muscle.

Suggestions for Compiling an Electrodiagnostic Report

Mark down findings of abnormal muscles while performing the examination. The report should indicate and describe findings in different muscles at rest, minimal contraction, and maximal contraction. We find that listing muscles with similar EMG findings together and giving a narrative description of findings under the listed muscles is best.

Summarize findings of nerve studies and EMG findings in an anatomical or physiological diagnosis when reporting the conclusion: for example, "Partial chronic denervation and reinnervation seen in muscles supplied by the lt. L5 nerve root, no evidence of new-onset denervation seen at the present time."

Keep clinical impressions separate from the description of the electrophysiological findings and from the anatomical and physiological interpretations of these findings. At times, a separate letter to the referring physician about your clinical impressions may be helpful.

Relay reports promptly, within 24 to 48 hours. If the results are urgent, contact the referring physician and convey the results by phone.

In describing your findings, include the activity of the disease process and its changes from previous investigations. Comment on a reasonable prognosis if possible. Include approximate intervals at which you might like to reexamine the patient for followup studies.

The following is a sample electrodiagnostic report.

ELECTRODIAGNOSTIC REPORT, HOSPITAL OF THE UNIVERSITY OF PENNSYLVANIA DEPARTMENT OF PHYSICAL MEDICINE AND REHABILITATION

Patient History

39-yr.-old female who noticed that for 6 months she had been unable to bend the tip of the rt. thumb. Rt. index finger seems strong. No history of trauma, pain, or loss of sensation. Patient has a 20-month-old baby whom she cradles on the rt. forearm while feeding, and the baby sometimes falls asleep for about 1 to 2 hours on the rt. forearm. Past history includes an auto accident 5 years ago and treatment for neck pain at that time.

Findings on Nerve Studies

1. Normal conduction studies along the rt. and lt. median, rt. ulnar, and rt. and lt. radial sensory nerves.

2. No evoked motor response from the rt. flexor pollicis longus on stimulation of the rt. anterior interosseous nerve. Normal latency from the lt. flexor pollicis longus on stimulation of the lt. anterior interosseous nerve.

Date: 850523	ID: 460408	Name: Jane Doe
Sex: F	Operator:	Code: Jennifer Chu, M.D.
Age: 39	Height: 163	

Nerve		*dlat (msec)*	*ampl (mV)*	*plat (msec)*	*dist (mm)*	*cv (m/sec)*	*sd*	*f-dlat (msec)*	*sd*	*dlsd*	*% amp*	*% area*
med	dx:	2.6	14.5	7.0	235	53.4	**	22.6	***		−8	−2
	sin:	2.3	15.8	6.6	230	54.2	**	23.7	***	−2.4	−6	1
uln	dx:	2.3	8.3	6.3	215	53.8	**	22.9	***	−2.2	−16	−4
	sin:											
uln	dx:	6.3	6.9	8.2	100	52.1	**	(across elbow)			3	1
	sin:											

Nerve		*lat (msec)*	*dur (msec)*	*ampl (μV)*	*dist (mm)*	*(m/sec)*	*sd*
rad	dx:	2.1		40	140	67.3	2.2
	sin:	2.2		29	140	62.5	****

ant. inteross dx: Recording from flex. poll. longus—no response
sin: Recording from flex. poll. longus—2.60 msec

Nerve		Palm *lat*	Palm *amp*	I *lat*	I *amp*	II *lat*	II *amp*	III *lat*	III *amp*	IV *lat*	IV *amp*	V *lat*	V *amp*
Med	dx:	1.5	125					2.5	104	2.6	66		
	sin:	1.4	125					2.3	117	2.3	63		
uln	dx:											2.2	104
	sin:											2.2	78

Findings on EMG Studies (*Monopolar* Recordings)

Rt. flex. poll. longus: 10 out of 10 sites with fibrillations and positive sharp waves at rest, no MUPs on minimal or maximal contraction

Rt. pron. quad.: 10 out of 10 sites with fibrillations and positive sharp waves at rest. Few MUPs were seen on minimal contraction with discrete interference on maximal contraction.

Rt. flex. dig. prof. (slips to the index and middle fingers): Increased insertional activity at rest, normal MUPs, and increased incidence of normal-duration polyphasic MUPs (30%). Some of the polyphasic MUPs were complex and were seen on minimal contraction. Interference on maximal contraction was reduced (poor).

Impression: Evidence of severe recent denervation and complete absence of MUPs seen in the rt. flex. poll. longus supplied by the rt. ant. interosseous nerve. Few MUPs were seen in the rt. pron. quad., but there is no evidence of ongoing reinnervation in this muscle. The rt. flex. dig. prof. (slips to the index and middle fingers) shows the least evidence of denervation, and there is evidence of beginning reinnervation in the residual MUPs.

Rt. and lt. rhomboids (C5), rt. and lt. paraspinals (C5), rt. and lt. post. deltoid (C6), rt. and lt. biceps (short head—C6), rt. and lt. teres major (C6), rt. and lt. brachialis (C6), rt. and lt. paraspinals (C6): Silence at rest, normal MUPs, and long-duration triphasic MUPs (20%) were seen on minimal contraction. Interference on maximal contraction was reduced (rich).

Impression: Evidence of mild chronic reinnervation seen in muscles supplied by the rt. and lt. C5 and C6 roots

Rt. and lt. triceps (C7), rt. and lt. ext. dig. comm. (C7), rt. and lt. flex. carp. rad. (C7), rt. and lt. paraspinals (C7), rt. and lt. flex. dig superficialis (C8), rt. and lt. flex. carp. uln. (C8), rt. and lt. 1st dorsal interosseous (C8, T1), rt. and lt. abd. poll. brev. (C8): Silence at rest, normal MUPs on minimal contraction, and full interference on maximal contraction

Impression: Normal EMG findings in muscles supplied by the rt. and lt. C7 and C8 roots

Lt. flex. poll. longus, lt. flex. dig. prof. (slips to the index and middle fingers), lt. pron. quadratus: Silence at rest, normal MUPs on minimal contraction, and full interference on maximal contraction

Impression: Normal EMG findings in muscles supplied by the lt. anterior interosseous nerve

Conclusions

1. Severe recent involvement of the rt. anterior interosseous nerve in the forearm.

   The rt. flex. poll. longus is totally denervated at present. The rt. pron. quadratus shows a few functioning MUPs, but there is no evidence of ongoing reinnervation in these MUPs. The slips of the rt. flex. dig. prof. to the rt. index and middle fingers are the least involved. There is also evidence of beginning reinnervation in this muscle.

   The prognosis for further reinnervation in the rt. flex. dig. prof. to the index and middle fingers should be good. The prognosis for recovery for the rt. pron. quadratus should be fair, since there are functioning MUPs in these muscles. The potential for recovery for the rt. flex. poll. longus is uncertain.
2. Mild chronic reinnervation seen in muscles supplied by the rt. and lt. C5 and C6 nerve roots.

Comments

1. Patient gives a history of letting her 20-month-old baby sleep on her forearm, especially the rt. forearm, for 1 to 2 hours at a stretch. This may be a possible cause of pressure on the rt. anterior interosseous nerve. Entrapment syndromes of the anterior interrosseous nerve should be ruled out. The lt. anterior interosseous nerve distribution shows no evidence of lower motor neuron changes. The involvement of the rt. anterior interosseous nerve in this patient is not part of a diffuse shoulder girdle–type neuropathy. Follow-up studies at about 8 weeks are suggested.
2. The mild chronic changes seen in the distribution of the rt. and lt. C5 and C6 nerve roots are probably related to the neck injury she sustained 5 years ago in an auto accident. There is no active or new-onset denervation along these nerve roots.

INDEX

Index

The letter *f* after a page number indicates a figure; *t* following a page number indicates tabular material. The anatomical structures are listed under the noun that describes them, rather than the descriptive adjective. For example, the trapezius muscle is listed under "muscle(s), trapezius." Other categories are aponeurosis, artery, bone(s), fascia, ligament(s), nerve(s), retinaculum, tendon(s), vein(s).